LEGAL MUSCLE
Anabolics in America

LEGAL MUSCLE
Anabolics in America

Rick Collins, J.D.

Legal Muscle Publishing, Inc.
2083 Hempstead Turnpike
PMB #420
East Meadow, New York 11554

Legal Muscle Publishing, Inc.
2083 Hempstead Tpke.
PMB #420
East Meadow, NY 11554
1-800-525-6758 · Fax (516) 294-0477
Website: www.legalmusclebooks.com
E-mail: sales@legalmusclebooks.com

ISBN 0-9726384-07
Printed in the United States of America
10 9 8 7 6 5 4 3

Table of Contents

Acknowledgments

It's with my deepest gratitude that I acknowledge the many individuals without whose expertise, time or support this project could never have been realized. In the area of anabolic chemistry, Patrick Arnold, Bill Llewellyn and Dave Palumbo were all great assets. Will Brink, Dr. Jack Darkes, Nick Evans, M.D., Alan Mintz, M.D., Michael Mooney, Dr. Mark Myhal, and Eric Serrano, M.D., were terrific sources regarding steroid health risks and other medical and scientific issues. My colleagues in the legal profession who provided their assistance were too numerous to name; over a hundred lawyers, including some prosecutors, from all across America offered their practical comments on the material. Of particular help were Terri R.Z. Jacobs, Esq., Lawrence Kessler, Esq., John McEntee, Esq., Barbara Raney, Esq., Peter Tomao, Esq., and John Williams, Esq.. Pat McCloskey, Esq., was especially giving of his time and valuable advice. Dr. Simon Davis was a wonderful aid on the topic of drug testing, and Brent Allen, Bob Cuccinello and Nelson Montana were terrific sounding boards on various issues. Many of my past and present clients, including Jeff, Keith, Mike and Todd, made valuable contributions that were greatly appreciated. I also want to thank the many research assistants who aided me over a two-year course, including Doug Spencer, June Reiter, Antonetta Stancu, Robert Scalera and Jen Imundo. *Legal Muscle* became, especially toward its completion, a team effort. Fred Harper's awesome art, Allen Dittrich's terrific cover design, Donna DiBiase's meticulous proofing, and the wonderful Julie Fleck's superb layout skills all contributed toward a first-rate publication. Steve Rogers should also be noted, for his design of www.teamlegalmuscle.com and, nearly five years ago, my original and still popular site, www.steroidlaw.com. I also want to especially thank John Romano and *Muscular Development* magazine for all their support; I want my monthly column to continue for as long as they'll have me. My thanks also go out to my law partners, Marc Gann, Esq., and Bob McDonald, Esq., for their encouragement and support over our many years of practice, to Allyson Levine and the rest of the staff at Collins, McDonald & Gann for putting up with me during this unexpectedly lengthy project, and to the heart of Team Legal Muscle, Mike DiMaggio and Rob Conti, Esq., whose tremendous and tireless efforts were unparalleled. Most of all, I thank my family, Kathy, Lauren and Caitlin, without whose great patience and sacrifice over these last two years this book could not have been written.

Foreword

By John Romano

I've been in the iron game a long time. I started lifting religiously when I was 15, and other than requisite layoffs due to various injuries, I've been throwing down hard with as much gumption and sheer will as any seasoned musclehead for the last 28 years. For the last 15 of those 28 years, I've made my living in bodybuilding, first as a freelance writer for various publications and now in the seat of Senior Editor for the internationally distributed *Muscular Development* magazine. I'm also a seasoned juice head.

During this tenure in muscledom, to say I've seen it all is a severe understatement, especially considering I spent 20 years of it training at the "Mecca of bodybuilding," Gold's Gym in Venice, California. I witnessed firsthand the evolution of the legalities surrounding androgens and related gear, and how this evolution ravaged the lives of some really good people.

Back in the day, even before my time, anabolics were regarded as nothing more than "super vitamins." They were not criminalized, characterized, nor demonized. They were just a tool that muscleheads used in order to do their thing. No one really cared. Well, unless you live in Mexico, Thailand, India or China, those days are long gone. Today, if you're a bodybuilder in America who chooses to exercise your sovereignty over your own body and stick gear into your hide, you are effectively a felon. In the last 15 years, juice has gone from being an innocuous prescription item to being listed on Schedule III of the DEA's list of controlled substances, carrying with it potentially major prison time for its sale, possession with intent to sell, distribution, importation or trafficking – *if* you get caught and convicted.

Has that stopped anyone from using them? Even the most conservative estimates say, absolutely not! As you will find later in this book, the laws haphazardly forced through Congress, as unfounded and grievously biased as they are, were specifically intended to curtail the use of performance-enhancing drugs in sports. Unfortunately, the vast majority of those affected by these laws are *not* Olympic and professional athletes. They are otherwise law-abiding, tax-paying citizens; and every year more and more of them put their liberty in jeopardy because they have opted to break the law and gear up. These otherwise normal people – your co-workers or next-door neighbors – have had their lives turned upside down. They have in many cases lost their homes, jobs, money, professional licenses, relationships, and most importantly, their freedom. But that hasn't stopped anyone from using steroids. In fact, the numbers keep rising.

Digesting these facts, and the fact that the medical community has successfully treated many sick people with these drugs with little ill effect for the last 60 years, I eventually began to realize the greatest risk to a steroid user was not to his health, but to his freedom. I figured that the average juice desperado would have no idea that his door could get kicked in and a SWAT team of federal agents could point MP-5s at his head, tackle him, cuff him, and start ransacking his house with his wife and kids watching in horror, confined to the couch. I realized that he would have no idea that his subsequent interrogation (without his lawyer present) would cause him to spill his guts, give up his sources, be labeled as a dealer (while his stash was only for personal use), and end up doing time as a convicted felon.

I thought it would be a great idea to get that point across in my magazine, and searched for a lawyer who could provide the dirty details of a real case and describe just how nasty things can get when a cop – disguised as the mailman and supported by a hidden back-up team – delivers a package of D-bol from Thailand. I didn't have to look far. Rick Collins is the only true steroid lawyer in America. Who better to defend a musclehead than a fellow musclehead with an extensive knowledge of the gear listed in your indictment? Oddly, few if any criminal defense lawyers know squat about juice and the mentality of the guy using it – I know because I searched around. Rick, on the other hand, has a completely unique "dual" perspective.

First, he is a former competitive bodybuilder. He's eaten as many chicken breasts and cans of tuna as any of you; he's done the contest thing, and has more than a few physique trophies collecting dust on a mantelpiece at home to prove it. While he once completed the stiff and standard ACE personal trainer certification program, with all the requisite courses in anatomy, exercise performance, nutrition and kinesiology, his ideas about diet and training to build healthy muscularity have always been two steps ahead of the pack. He co-founded and developed a personal training business, Innovation Fitness, in the 1990s. When it comes to muscle, he knows what he's talking about. To put it bluntly, the guy fills out his Italian suits in a way only custom tailoring can accommodate.

Second, Rick knows the criminal laws and courts like the back of his hand. A veteran criminal defense lawyer and a former prosecutor, he has defended more anabolic steroid cases in more places than anyone who ever picked up a briefcase. Not a day goes by that someone desperately seeking his help on a juice-connected legal problem doesn't contact him. He's personally defended against steroid prosecutions from coast to coast, and at the borders of Canada and Mexico. Muscleheads from all walks of life, professional athletes, physicians, pharmacists, military servicemen, police officers, and even the internal affairs unit of a major metropolitan police force have sought his help on steroid issues, and criminal lawyers frequently consult him for advice and assistance. Rick was retained last year by a coalition of nutritional supplement companies to spearhead a presentation of scientific evidence to the DEA on the relationship between prohormones and anabolic steroids. He is frequently asked to provide legal counsel to physicians seeking to develop anti-aging practices using androgen replacement therapies. He's been consulted as an expert witness on steroid legalities, has been interviewed and quoted as an authority on anabolics by numerous journalists in a variety of media, and has written many articles for print and online magazines. His article "Drugs and the Body Beautiful: A Guide to Defending Anabolic Steroid Prosecutions" was the featured cover story for a recent issue of *The Champion*, the journal of the National Association of Criminal Defense Lawyers. After working with Rick on the eye-popping, original article for *Muscular Development* (which is reprinted here, in Chapter 23), I believed his knowledge to be so necessary for our cause that I implored my publisher to hire Rick as a monthly contributor. Rick has ever since penned the monthly column, *Busted! Legal Q & A.*

What Rick has to say about juice and the law could fill an encyclopedia, and this book will be the authoritative word on the subject for years to come. His comprehensive knowledge spans both sides of the fence and can help make better sense of a topic that has for years been mired in controversy, misinformation, lies, half-truths and negative propaganda. This awesome book explains the realities of non-medical juice use, its true health risks, the various ways that states and the feds deal with it all, and the shocking untold story of how it became criminalized (reading what Congress did made me furious!). The pages are filled with case history after case history of actual clients, detailing exactly what the government did to them and how they responded to it, for better or worse. I think the most valuable thing you muscleheads will learn from Rick is how to *exercise* your rights and preserve your liberties if your door gets kicked in by a SWAT team, or if your car is stopped or you're in a thousand other confrontation scenarios. Absorbing every page of *Legal Muscle* now can help you later if you should ever wind up in court; lending it to your lawyer can make him better able to defend you (Rick can't defend everyone); and reading it may even help you not get busted to begin with. However, I say that cautiously – this is *not* a book about how to get away with breaking the law. Hopefully, it will *discourage* breaking the law, but *encourage CHANGING* the law. In the meantime, if exercising your Constitutional rights in a police confrontation protects you from arrest or conviction, then that's as it should be. If being informed and making the right strategic defense decisions with your lawyer in criminal court results in a dismissal or other favorable outcome, there's nothing wrong with that.

Having been busted myself and having done time under the care of the federal government, I can't emphatically enough tell you that getting busted is about the worst thing that could ever happen to you, and I can't emphatically enough dissuade you from doing anything illegal. But, history and human nature prove I'm at a disadvantage. That being the irrefutable case, you muscleheads better damn well read this book cover to cover *BEFORE* you hit the streets.

If you're *not* a member of the muscle world, you're in for quite an education. That goes for lawyers, judges, prosecutors and law enforcers, as well as for journalists, physicians, pharmacists, personal trainers, college and high school coaches, parents of teens, and anyone else interested in how influential special interest groups can get oppressive laws passed, how the public can be manipulated and misled, and how your tax dollars can be squandered. *Legal Muscle* is practically an encyclopedia of everything connecting gear to the law. If you've got a question, you should find your answer, whoever you are.

Face it: this isn't your typical book about steroids. It serves up the unvarnished, *unbiased truth* – a revolutionary approach to the subject. Hold on tight. What you're about to read will probably shock *everybody*.

John Romano
Senior Editor, *Muscular Development* magazine

Preface

On Truth and Freedom

How do we know that what we believe to be true ... is really true? What if some truths we've come to firmly believe are distortions, like reflections in a fun-house mirror – mere illusions, created and maintained by those who benefit from our misplaced trust? Could such a thing happen in America? Would we let it happen?

It *has* happened. On one subject – anabolic steroids – what passes for common knowledge has little connection to reality. But we've been manipulated to believe it, and it's in the interests of certain influential forces to keep the illusion going. They're quite happy with it, even though many effects of the illusion have been catastrophic, both at the individual and societal levels.

How could it have happened? Easily enough, I'm afraid. Too many of us are sheep in the meadow, content to be herded. We blindly trust what we read in the daily papers or see on the evening news, and save our critical thinking only for those issues that appear to have a direct and immediate personal impact on us. Why question authority? It's easier to let others decide what's best for us. If a sports medicine physician proclaims that anabolics are deadly and dangerous drugs, we believe it without reservation. If a politician or government spokesman says our steroid laws are working, who are we to challenge them? Negative and alarming reports are all we've heard from the mainstream media; the flow of information to the public has been carefully controlled to ensure that. Inextricably binding steroids to cheating athletes has well served the agenda of some powerful special interests. Demonizing steroids has been great for the media. While alternative views exist, they have gone unheralded. Suppression and punishment seem totally natural public responses to the non-medical use of these substances. *Freedom* is never mentioned as having anything to do with it.

Freedom has *everything* to do with it. The more we submit to additional layers of governmental protection from ourselves, the more freedom we sacrifice. Where will it end? Prepare for further losses of freedom. The same players who brought us the Anabolic Steroid Control Act are at it again: this time to dupe us into believing that broadly depriving *everyone* of various over-the-counter health food supplements is in our best interests. Yet another freedom will be lost. Who knows what it will be next time?

British author George Orwell wrote, "Freedom is the freedom to say that two plus two make four" – even though you're being told otherwise. It's the freedom to give voice to the *real* truth, untainted by disinformation and propaganda. Is that freedom of value to you? You have a choice. You can continue to believe what you've been told, or you can open your eyes to examine the facts and discover the truth for yourself. My aim is to help you to do that.

This book is limited to one topic: anabolic steroids. Together, we'll explore all the legal and ethical territory associated with their use. You'll probably be shocked and perhaps appalled by what you will read. You may feel a sense of outrage. If, at the end of our journey, you conclude that you had previously been manipulated and deceived about this subject, you may find yourself asking what other "truths" may be illusory. How accurate and objective is the other information being fed to us on issues of health and science policy? Or even, frighteningly, on issues of the economy, history, or national and world affairs? Take courage. There are many uncharted roads ahead, much to be explored, and a flock in the meadow in need of brave shepherds.

Rick Collins
October, 2002

Chapter 1

OUTLAWING ANABOLICS: A FAIR PITCH?

"To retain respect for sausages and laws, one must not watch them in the making."
– *Otto von Bismarck (1815-1898)*

Picture if you will a smoky, paneled conference room, filled with pale old men in business suits gathered around a long table. Overweight and out of shape, they're preaching to each other about the deadly evils of anabolic steroids, occasionally gesturing with one of their cheese fries left over from lunch. On and on they piously rant about health dangers, pausing only for sips of Scotch-and-soda and wheezy drags on their cigars. They warble away about the importance of role models to our youth, even as they subject innocent bystanders to their second-hand smoke and kill their own brain cells with excess alcohol. It's all in a day's work, as long as a flowery press release gets out to the voters confirming the legislators' attention to the problem.

That's a congressional subcommittee at work, in the eyes of the many members of the muscle world who think that outlawing non-medical steroid use was the height of hypocrisy. It's unfortunate that our elected legislators in Washington are viewed this way by anybody. Most are hard-working public servants whose primary aim is to protect *us*, not their own re-election prospects. We have to believe that our members of Congress mean well. So what if they don't wear Otomix and muscle shirts? They're all right anyway. They draft laws that they determine are necessary and proper, after careful consideration, to ensure our health and safety. Protecting the citizenry from dangerous drugs is precisely the kind of thing they ought to be doing, right? Surely, the action they took toward anabolic steroids was intended to protect us from a deadly scourge. It wasn't just to kowtow to special interest groups, was it? After all, didn't Congress hold lots of hearings before they added anabolic steroids to the list of controlled substances, thereby criminalizing their non-medical use? Certainly, our legislators must have heard powerful evidence from the top experts in the field about the dire consequences that result from these terrible drugs. Our Congress would only have acted with the full and enthusiastic support of these experts, including the physicians of the American Medical Association and the top brass of the Drug Enforcement Administration (DEA). Congress acted primarily to save us from an anabolic steroid health crisis, right? After all, what else would justify subjecting personal users of a substance to arrest and prosecution?

Congress acted primarily to save us from an anabolic steroid health crisis, right?

The Ceremonial First Pitch

Once upon a time, long ago, a physician named John Ziegler dispensed some pills to a group of weight lifters. The year was 1958 and the pills were Dianabol – an anabolic steroid preparation manufactured by a pharmaceutical company named Ciba. Combined with rigorous training and proper nutrition, the pills were reported to help build muscle. They did. Overnight, the genie was out of the bottle. Athletes had discovered a way to get an advantage over their competitors that undermined the basic values of fair sportsmanship. It was wrong because it was cheating. It had to be stopped to keep a level playing field for *all* athletes.

The organized sports establishment decided that they would solve the whole problem by educating the athletes. They would present *facts* to discourage competitive athletes from using steroids. The establishment devised a strategy: to convince competitive athletes that anabolic steroids don't build muscle. But they needed a credible source through which to sell the message. It was decided that the American College of Sports Medicine would be the entity to spread the news, a bit like the "Ministry of Truth" had the job of spreading false propaganda to the masses in George Orwell's classic book about a totalitarian future, entitled *1984*. In 1977, the sports community's Ministry of Truth came out with an emphatic position statement that steroids had *absolutely no effect* on lean muscle or strength, and that any increased size was as a result of "fluid retention" or the placebo effect. It sounded good, but they needed some proof. So, "studies" were conducted to back it up. Obviously not very good studies, but the intended outcome was far more important than accuracy. [For an examination of how results were engineered through the use of intentionally flawed designs, *see* W.N. Taylor, *Anabolic Steroids and the Athlete* (Jefferson, NC; McFarland & Co., 1982)] Then, with absolutely straight faces, the Ministry of Truth publicly pronounced the party line position despite ridiculously overwhelming anecdotal evidence to the contrary. As those in the sport of professional bodybuilding grew to larger and larger proportions, excuses were cooked up to explain away the obvious.

Of course, the truth could be obscured for only so long. Eventually, an alternate plan was required if athletic use was to be deterred. By the time the Ministry of Truth was forced to confess in, of all years, *1984* (an eerie coincidence for Orwell fans), that steroids were effective – actually, *too* effective – a much more convincing argument was brewing: anabolic steroids can *kill*. It seemed like a brilliant and compelling approach: what would be a better disincentive to a health-conscious person than risking the loss of his or her life? Moreover, unlike their earlier argument, this one had a legitimate foundation in the medical literature, which linked anabolic steroids with lots of adverse effects. Also, as increasing numbers of bodybuilders began using and *abusing* anabolics, evidence of side effects began to mount. Reports of the dangers of anabolic steroid abuse appeared in medical journals. A "laundry list" of dangers was compiled and disseminated to the media. The media loved it. An alliance was born that would last to this day.

The Media Take the Field

News is a business. Scare stories sell, which brings us to two fundamental tenets that pervade most of what we see and read in the news: keep it simple and keep it negative. Keeping the story easy to understand reaches the broadest possible audience of viewers, readers, and advertisers, right on down to children, the poorly educated, and the mentally unhinged. My eight-year-old daughter, accidentally catching a minute of the movie "Gladiator" on cable television, asked of the central character, "Is he a good guy or a bad guy?" That's all she needs to know. She doesn't want to hear about moral ambiguities or see shades of gray. She wants it simple. Good or bad,

> Frightening the living daylights out of the great unwashed masses glues their eyes to their television sets and keeps them buying newspapers.

yes or no. Of course, beyond childhood, life is rarely so simple. But that hasn't deterred modern mainstream journalism. To them, by and large, you're an idiot.

Keeping the story negative is even more important. Nobody is rushing home from work to catch a television news report that's balanced and bland. Objective reporting puts people to sleep. Frightening the living daylights out of the great unwashed masses glues their eyes to their television sets and keeps them buying newspapers. Isn't that the prime directive? "*Something in your refrigerator may be poisoning you. What? Watch the News at 11,*" will reel them in like nobody's business. In fact, during slow news periods, our friends in the press aren't above *creating* news to foment a little hysteria. Want an example? A recent John Stossel segment on ABC's *20/20* examined 2001's "Summer of the Shark" phenomenon. Stossel reported:

> "You may have believed that shark attacks were on the rise. That's what some television stations reported. But it wasn't true. Last year, shark attacks off American beaches were hardly different from previous years. Most of the reports mentioned that, but that important truth got lost amid the blare and blur of frightening headlines and images. While the media were busy scaring us out of the water, scientists said there was no increase in the number of sharks off our beaches and stressed that sharks were so unlikely to kill you that you're about 25 times more likely to be killed by lightning."

Quite an effective tool at spreading hysteria, huh? Well, the agenda of the sports establishment suited the media just fine. During the mid-1980s, anti-steroid spokespeople became media darlings. They spoon-fed alarmist statements to the media, which eagerly wolfed them down and regurgitated them to the public. One California physician associated with the NFL made the completely unsupported assertion that "young athletes who take heavy doses of anabolic steroids for 60 to 90 days should expect to die in their 30s or 40s." As time went on, a new angle on steroid use was presented in the press: teen and adolescent usage. Focusing on youthful abuse, despite the fact that the majority of steroid users were and are *not* teens, they attempted to usher in an even higher level of hysteria.

Legally, at that time, anabolics were classified as prescription medicines. They could be prescribed and dispensed only by licensed physicians. They were regulated by the Food and Drug Administration under the Food, Drug and Cosmetic Act [21 U.S.C.A. §§ 351, 352, 353, and 355 (1981 & Supp. 1990)]. The International Olympic Committee had banned them since 1975. Concerns within the National Football League (NFL) had prompted then-Commissioner Pete Rozelle, in November of 1983, to issue a letter to every player warning about the dangers of steroid use and threatening disciplinary action for players caught using them without a legitimate medical basis. Still, rumors of rising use persisted, and other sports were slow to address the issue. The sports bodies weren't doing nearly enough to police themselves. The media kept fanning the flames wherever possible. They began reporting even more widespread use, and even more dangerous effects. For example, among the articles referenced in appendices of the various Congressional subcommittee hearings on steroids was a *Sports Illustrated* story called "The Nightmare of Steroids" by South Carolina lineman Tommy Chaikin and Rick Telander, detailing Chaikin's medical and psychiatric travails after abusing steroids. An article in the June 8, 1987 edition of the *Baltimore Sun* pointed out, "Steroid abuse, once limited to body-building fanatics and some big-time athletes, has trickled down to high school boys and weekend amateurs seeking heroic physiques through chemistry." Pressure was building for some sort of governmental inquiry.

Capitol Hill Steps to the Plate

Congress began exploring the ways that it might curtail anabolic steroid usage. Members of subcommittees in both the House and Senate drafted bills and scheduled hearings to tackle the issue. After examination of the issue within the Subcommittee on Health of the House Committee on Energy and Commerce, Rep. Richard Baker, on July 14, 1987, introduced a bill, H.R. 2928, making it a felony to distribute steroids without a valid prescription. The bill proposed raising the prison penalties for selling anabolics. Senator Joseph Biden introduced a similar Senate bill. On November 18, 1988, President Reagan signed the resulting legislation as part of the Anti-Drug Abuse Act of 1988 [Pub. L. No. 100-690, Sec 2401, 102 Stat. 4181 (1988)]. The new law, 21 U.S.C. 333(e)(1), punished traffickers of anabolic steroids for non-medical reasons with up to three years in prison (up to six years if sold to minors under 18), enabling enforcement against those illegally dispensing steroids, such as shady doctors, and against black market dealers. It also provided for application of federal forfeiture laws. Importantly, it permitted the prosecution of dealers and distributors *without* authorizing the arrest or prosecution of personal *users* of anabolics, and it did *not* classify steroids as controlled substances.

Over 175 steroid trafficking convictions were obtained *without* classification of steroids as controlled substances ...

The new law worked well. A joint task force to prosecute dealers was created with the U.S. Department of Justice, the Food and Drug Administration, and the Federal Bureau of Investigation. By the spring of 1990, there had been 125 legal actions on various steroid-related charges in 27 different federal districts [J.E. Wright and V.S. Cowart, *Anabolic Steroids: Altered States* (Carmel, IN; Benchmark Press, 1990)]. Over 175 steroid trafficking convictions were obtained *without* classification of steroids as controlled substances [Rorie Sherman, "The Big Push," *Nat'l L.J.*, Feb. 10, 1992].

But although trafficking was criminalized and prosecutions were increasing, steroids were still a hot topic. Legislators seemed hungry to jump at any new angle to attack anabolics. When a crotchety 78-year-old man from California received a mail catalog from Mexico offering a price list of steroids for sale, a volcano of activity erupted on Capitol Hill. A new bill, H.R. 995, proposed to create an "Anabolic Steroid Restriction Act of 1989" to criminalize using the mail to transport or sell steroids. Olympic Gold Medallist Carl Lewis testified in favor of the bill, as did a representative of the Criminal Investigations division of the U.S. Postal Inspection Service. While the bill wasn't destined to go far, it focused attention on what would later become the paramount steroid target in criminal justice: steroids by mail.

Since the new bills and laws imposed no federal controls on the *manufacture* of anabolics, they didn't prevent steroid products from being diverted to the black market. There was no way to tell if drug companies were *overproducing* steroids to secretly "slip them out the back door." One way of placing a "control" on this diversion problem would be to schedule steroids federally as a controlled substance. For this reason, a few doctors began suggesting controlled substance status for anabolic steroids. [*See* W.N. Taylor, M.D., "Synthetic Anabolic-Androgenic Steroids: A Plea for Controlled Substance Status," *The Physician and Sportsmedicine* (Vol. 15, Number 5, May 1987).] Not to start dragging personal steroid users screaming off to jail, but just to keep Big Pharmacy honest.

Regulatory Agencies Check their Swing

Under 21 U.S.C. § 812(a), there are five classes, known as *schedules*, of controlled substances. In order to put a drug into Schedule III, the government has to find that it meets the requirements of 21 U.S.C. § 812(b)(3):

A. The drug or other substance has a potential for abuse less than the drugs or other substances in schedules I and II.
B. The drug or other substance has a currently accepted medical use in treatment in the United States.
C. Abuse of the drug or other substance may lead to moderate or low physical dependence or high psychological dependence.

How does the government decide if a drug meets the requirements to become a controlled substance? The process is set forth under 21 U.S.C. § 811. The authority to add new substances to the schedules is given to the Attorney General. To start the inquiry, he's supposed to request an evaluation and recommendations from the Secretary of Health and Human Services (HHS) regarding the drug's potential for abuse and the need for scheduling. That's what Attorney General Edwin Meese did, right by the book. He wrote to both DEA and HHS asking for their views on the possible scheduling of anabolics as controlled substances. The procedures under § 811(c) list the factors to consider as to the drug in question:

(1) Its actual or relative potential for abuse.
(2) Scientific evidence of its pharmacological effect, if known.
(3) The state of current scientific knowledge regarding the drug or other substance.
(4) Its history and current pattern of abuse.
(5) The scope, duration and significance of abuse.
(6) What, if any, risk there is to the public health.
(7) Its psychic or physiological dependence liability.
(8) Whether the substance is an immediate precursor of a substance already controlled under this subchapter.

DEA and HHS evaluated steroids in light of the eight factors. When they were finished, on October 1, 1987, John Lawn, Administrator of DEA, concluded that anabolic steroids should *not* be made controlled substances. On March 15, 1988, HHS Secretary Otis Bowen agreed. *Neither DEA nor HHS viewed anabolic steroids as meeting the criteria for a controlled substance.* At this point, a new law had criminalized steroid trafficking and the appropriate agencies had concluded that scheduling anabolics was inappropriate. Time to take your ball and glove and go home. The issue would seem to have been resolved. But certain members of Congress, it would be seen, had other ideas.

Of course, these legislators were aware of the established administrative process by which a drug was to be made into a controlled substance. They were also aware, however, that Congress had the authority to conduct its own investigative hearings. They simply ignored the decisions of the regulatory agencies that were specifically charged and arguably best qualified to make such decisions. Instead, these politicians lumbered forward with their own investigations.

Capitol Hill Puts Men on Base

In July of 1988, the members of the Subcommittee on Crime of the House Committee on the Judiciary convened to consider a bill introduced by Rep. Dan Lungren, H.R. 3216, which proposed to amend the Controlled Substances Act to add methandrostenolone as a Schedule I controlled substance. Why methandrostenolone alone was chosen, out of all the anabolic steroids, is unclear. Apparently, little if any real thought went into the bill. In fact, the manufacturer had discontinued Dianabol in 1983, and all methandrostenolone had been removed from the legitimate market in 1986. Most likely, Dianabol was the only anabolic steroid that these politicians had heard of.

The subcommittee held a hearing to find out what the experts thought about the actual health dangers and the idea of scheduling steroids. Charles Yesalis, Sc.D., professor of health and human development at Penn State University and probably the world's foremost expert on steroids at that time, began his testimony by repeatedly stressing to the subcommittee that the medical side effects were mostly temporary, and presented a balanced and objective assessment:

> "Steroids do have a medical use. From an epidemiologic point of view of the health dangers, I am much more concerned about heroin; I am much more concerned about cocaine; I am much more concerned about cigarettes than anabolic steroids. This is not to say steroids are not potentially dangerous; rather, from what we know currently, I am more concerned about the other drugs – and you could likely add the abuse of alcohol to that list than anabolic steroids."

Regarding the issue of steroids' addictive potential, Dr. David Bever, an associate professor of health education at George Mason University who had recently conducted a study about steroid usage among bodybuilders and powerlifters in the D.C. area, said: "We did not find that it was as habituating from the standpoint of when the supplies ran out as it was also a financial situation. 'Geez, that was all the money I had for this cycle. Now I'm going to go a number of months without.' They did, with no problem. Now, there were changes in a certain amount of body mass and size of people, and they were disappointed, but was not something that they, again – like psychologically addictive, no. The guys – when they went off, they went off with few or no problems."

Clearly, the experts from the scientific community were lending little support for scheduling. But what would DEA have to say? Would they back down from their earlier position? Gene Haislip, Deputy Assistant Administrator of DEA's Office of Diversion Control, was called to testify. But rather than supporting the bill, Mr. Haislip flat-out *opposed* it on behalf of DEA. He pointed out the inappropriateness of steroid hormones in the Controlled Substances Act, stating, "The Controlled Substances Act is built entirely and exclusively around drugs which are principally psychoactive and are abused almost exclusively by virtue and because of that property. All of these drugs can be described either as narcotics, stimulants, depressants or hallucinogens." He went on to say that he had "doubts as to whether this would be appropriate" and that "when Congress enacted the Controlled Substances Act, I don't think it had in mind this kind of drug or this kind of drug abuse." He noted, "It appears that the motivation is somewhat different from that which is involved in most kinds of drug abuse. It is to develop muscles, to increase physical performance and perhaps simply to look good and appear to be more attractive to members of the opposite sex." The DEA position, he made clear, was to continue its *opposition* to scheduling steroids, stating that DEA was not "the appropriate body to enforce any measures of this kind."

In April 1989, the Senate conducted its own investigation. The Senate's Committee on the Judiciary addressed "The Steroid Abuse Problem in America, Focusing on the Use of Steroids in College and Professional Football Today." Chaired by Senator Biden of Delaware, it was held in a public-friendly forum at the University of Delaware to maximize the potential for the country to see what these politicians were doing about this issue. As the designated voice of the American Medical Association (AMA), Dr. Edward Langston had come to the hearing to acknowledge that steroid abuse is a significant problem but to *oppose* scheduling. The AMA opposed the renegade take-the-ball-and-run approach of these legislators, especially when the regulatory agencies that were officially supposed to make the decision – the Attorney General, DEA and HHS – had already decided *not* to schedule steroids. Further, the AMA opposed scheduling because "abuse of steroids does not lead to the physical or psychological dependence as is required for scheduling ..." Dr. Langston also pointed out that other effective and appropriate approaches to the problem existed, including the recently enacted Anti-Drug Abuse Act of 1988, which permitted aggressive prosecution of traffickers.

Further, the AMA opposed scheduling because "... abuse of steroids does not lead to the physical or psychological dependence as is required for scheduling ..."

Dr. Yesalis was called as an authority before the Senate subcommittee. He again gave an objective review, and explicitly recommended *against* scare tactics, saying, "The other potential loss of credibility is we are telling people they are going to be dropping over dead and the athletes are looking at the longtime user and not seeing people dropping like flies. Now, increased death, probability of death, or morbidity could be taking place, but people apparently are not dropping like flies. And I think we have to be careful not to lose further credibility." He also dismissed the quaint notion, perpetuated by other witnesses, that the effects of steroids could be achieved simply by hard work. He stated, with respect to major strength sports, "... it is almost incomprehensible to think that you could even compete at the high level without these drugs."

The Foul Balls Start Flying

On both occasions, the testimony of Dr. Yesalis was straightforward. Especially in light of more recent statements he has made, it was truly his finest hour. But his comments were a little too honest for the subcommittees. Clearly surprised and disappointed not to be hearing a more unequivocal and "politically correct" condemnation, Rep. Lungren, who had introduced the bill to schedule methandrostenolone, accused Dr. Yesalis of "playing down the side effects." Undeterred, Dr. Yesalis continued to present the facts, including that: "If you stay away from the oral versions of these drugs, the issue of liver toxicity is really not a great one at all." Rep. Lungren countered that a "constituent" of his who supposedly took steroids got a liver tumor and "lost his house trying to pay for all the medical bills" (it later comes out that the patient had been exposed to Agent Orange in Vietnam). When presented with the objective facts about steroids and liver function, Rep. Lungren jumped to the topic of liver tumors. When presented with objective facts on liver tumors that were apparently not to his liking, he switched to "'roid rage." Again Dr. Yesalis addressed the point head-on, condemning the questionable methodological designs of a study by two psychiatrists, Drs. Harrison Pope and David Katz.

In light of all he knew, Dr. Yesalis *opposed* H.R. 3216. He did, however, ultimately concede that placing anabolics into Schedule V, the lowest scheduled status, "would likely apply pressure to manufacturers of these drugs to stem the apparently high level of diversion of their products to 'black markets.'" This, after all, was the original reason that a few physicians had called for scheduling steroids. He emphasized that while he did recommend controlled substance status, it was only as a Schedule V substance. And, most significantly, he cautioned that it was "not to interfere with the physician/patient relationship, but simply to make the drug companies and the wholesalers keep records." Let's stop and think about that. The diversion problem was real. Undeniably, it required a solution. By recommending Schedule V, Dr. Yesalis was attempting to make manufacturers and distributors account for the products to prevent diversion to the black market, while leaving doctors and their patients *alone*. The idea made some sense (although Congress certainly could have legislated such controls *without* formal scheduling). But was it what these determined politicians wanted to hear?

It wasn't what Rep. Lungren wanted to hear. After sparring with Dr. Yesalis, the politician went after Dr. Bever. When Dr. Bever attempted to give a balanced presentation by describing a study correlating high testosterone levels with *positive* social characteristics, Rep. Lungren simply mocked, "I don't know what I am supposed to get out of that except maybe I should avoid bald people with beards." The manner in which politicians who knew next to nothing about the subject matter were attacking qualified experts was becoming ... suspicious.

What Drs. Yesalis and Bever got was nothing compared to what was given to Dr. Langston of the AMA. The physician had barely finished his presentation when the onslaught began. Dr. Katz, the psychiatrist whose flawed work had been criticized by Dr. Yesalis, took the first swing by declaring the AMA statement, as voiced by Dr. Langston, "shocking" and "ridiculous." Those were compliments compared to what Senator Biden had to say. Rude, condescending, and belittling, Senator Biden boxed Dr. Langston around the hearing room. Ultimately, he was mostly dragging him around. It was painful to read, and must have been even worse to watch as the doctor was forced to defend himself against a skilled inquisitor. Was the AMA position weak? Probably. Still, something was going on. Was it coincidence that only the witnesses whose testimony presented speed bumps in the path of scheduling were castigated and ridiculed? It was evident that Senator Biden, along with the subcommittees of both the House and the Senate, had a certain game plan in mind.

The Umpires Are Blind

The legislators were able to call witnesses at the various hearings whose stories would help support the criminalization idea. Former Olympic track and field athlete Diane Williams testified about the masculinization she suffered due to steroid use, breaking down and unable to continue after confessing to sprouting facial hair and the growth of her clitoris to "embarrassing proportions." A nasty business, to be sure. Dr. David Katz, the Harvard psychiatrist whose work had been questioned by Dr. Yesalis, was quick to add, without much if any basis, that, "Thousands more could probably tell similar, if not more saddening stories." Steve Courson, former player for the Pittsburgh Steelers and Tampa Bay Buccaneers, offered articulate but questionable testimony by suggesting – without any basis in fact – that his heart problems were linked to his past steroid use. Pat Croce, conditioning coach for the Philadelphia 76ers and Philadelphia Flyers, insisted "steroids must be considered a controlled substance, no different than cocaine. Steroids, cocaine; the same connotation." In contrast to Dr. Yesalis, Mr. Croce went on to vigorously tout scare tactics, in addition to criminal prosecutions, as the best approach: "I tell them to drop their pants and show me how manly they really are. They want to get bigger and manly, but then their testes shrink. And as [Diane Williams] has told us with regard to the clitoris of the female, it enlarges. You have to scare them. You have to scare them. That is the only way..." *Is* that the only way? I think not, and, with all due respect, let's pull our pants back *up*.

The show wasn't over. Dr Katz, in his testimony, found it "fascinating and very worrisome" that "a large number of phone calls" had come from criminal defense attorneys who read about his "hypotheses" of steroid-induced psychosis. He self-importantly chose to see this as an epidemic that validated his theories, rather than demonstrating how resourceful criminal defense lawyers typically seek novel excuses for their clients' violent crimes. Dr. Katz made a point of telling the committee that there were "fewer and fewer accepted uses for anabolic steroids." Of course, if in fact it was true at that time, his comment seems ridiculous today. Anabolic steroids are now more widely used than ever before. They have proven to be one of the most powerful weapons ever discovered in the fight against the wasting associated with the HIV virus, providing dramatic, life-changing improvements for many sufferers. Further, anabolic steroids are used by many progressive physicians in the battle against age-related hormonal declines in middle-aged men.

It was Kenneth Kashin, MD, Assistant Professor of Psychiatry at Yale University School of Medicine, who spoke the language that the politicians were looking to hear, opining his speculations that "steroid use can cause an addiction with similarities to alcohol, opiate and cocaine addiction." He talked about "dangerous criminal-like behavior while intoxicated on anabolic steroids" and individuals who have "lost control of their behavior." He even resurrected the "placebo effect" theory of steroid gains. Among his more preposterous statements was this one: "Disturbingly, many experts now believe that the profound psychological effects of anabolic steroids may be the single factor that differentiates them from the intensive training with diet alone." He suggested that athletes were taking the drugs primarily for their psychoactive effects of increasing self-confidence and aggressiveness. The doctor recommended the inclusion of "severe penalties" for those afflicted by these disturbances. Quite a compassionate bedside manner, huh? While his opinions would be ridiculed by many authorities, he was clearly speaking the language that the politicians wanted. They even incorporated into the record his co-authored article from the *Journal of the American Medical Association* entitled "Hooked on Hormones? An anabolic steroid addiction hypothesis." All in all, an objective review of the hearings suggests they were as reminiscent of a 17th century witch-hunt as a modern fact-finding proceeding. "The one thing I fear the most," said Senator Biden as he concluded one hearing, "... is sending misinformation to people." Pretty funny.

"The one thing I fear the most," said Senator Biden as he concluded one hearing, "... is sending misinformation to people."

The Final Innings

When the Subcommittee on Crime of the House Committee on the Judiciary held their final steroid hearing in May of 1990, they were armed with a bill: H.R. 4658, the proposed "Anabolic Steroid Control Act of 1990." Only one witness was called: Congressman Mel Levine of California, whose pitch was that it was "time to take strong measures against anabolic steroid use. Steroid abuse may be the quiet side of the drug war, but it is an extremely serious side of it." The bill added steroids to the Controlled Substances Act by inserting them into 21 U.S.C. § 802, effectively making simple possession punishable by up to one year in prison; distribution and possession with intent to distribute punishable by up to five years in prison; and distribution and possession with intent to distribute to an individual under 21 years of age punishable by up to ten years in prison for a first offense and up to 30 years for a second. It also proposed to amend 21 U.S.C. § 844 with a subsection (b), which would have criminalized coaches, managers, trainers or other advisers who endeavor "to persuade or induce" individuals to possess or use steroids. (For all the attention to cheating athletes, this section somehow never made it into the final law.) Finally, the bill added growth hormone into 21 U.S.C. § 333, the so-called Steroid Trafficking Act, replacing anabolic steroids. Effectively, this made it illegal to distribute, but not to possess, growth hormone.

When all was done, despite the position of the AMA, DEA, and the recommendations of the most knowledgeable experts, Congress scheduled steroids as Schedule III controlled substances under Title 21 of the United States Code, which regulates food and drugs. The question is, what really happened?

What Went On in the Clubhouse

What agenda motivated Congress to ignore the advice of the experts and forge ahead with scheduling? The answer is suggested by reading the over five hundred pages of transcripts. While a smattering of testimony about health risks dresses up a few pages, the overwhelming majority of the hearings had nothing to do with that. Page after page focuses on two issues and two issues only.

The primary issue: the unfair advantage that steroid-enhanced professional and top-level athletes have over those who don't use steroids. Words like "unequal playing field," "cheating" and "unfair advantage" were repeatedly used throughout the proceedings by witnesses and legislators alike. And things heated up to boiling after September 1988, when the steroids hit the proverbial fan. Amid an international media circus, Canadian sprinter Ben Johnson was stripped of his Olympic gold medal for testing positive for steroids, much to the humiliation of the International Olympic Committee. Everything changed overnight. Suddenly, elite athletics seemed less about discipline, training, innate gifts and sportsmanship, and more about who's got the better drugs. "Fairness" on the athletic field became front-page news, and the "purity" and ethics of athletic competition became a joke on late night television. Somebody quipped that Dianabol had truly become the "breakfast of champions," referring back to a 1969 story in *Track and Field News*. "Permitting steroid users to compete with drug-free athletes reflects on the fairness of athletic competition at every level. Allowing those with an unfair advantage to compete can pressure drug-free athletes to use anabolic steroids to remain competitive." [Abuse of steroids in Amateur and Professional Athletics: Hearings Before the Subcomm. on Crime of the House Comm. on the Judiciary, 101st Cong., 2d Sess. 92 (Mar. 22, 1990) (statement of Frank D. Uryasz, Director of Sports Sciences, National Collegiate Athletic Association)]

The popularity of Olympic competition appeared to be in jeopardy, and both the politicians and the athletic bodies feared that the spillover could ruin all of sports. On the shakiest ground would be football, where the advantages of steroid-produced size and strength would be most "unfair." Professional sports are big business, good for the economy and good for America.

Imagine the economic disaster that could result if the integrity of sports was to be compromised and the public was to become disenchanted? Understandably, the sports establishments – and Congress – panicked over the potential fallout. At one point, Senator Biden gave voice to what Congress seemed to be really afraid of: "... I think you are going to see, over the next several years, some real backlash from the public about sports in America, from Olympians straight through to college sports, to pro sports. There is a feeling of resentment that is growing, and I do not know how it will manifest itself." Empty seats? Lost profits? International embarrassment? The sports world just couldn't afford another Ben Johnson, and certain members of Congress were determined to find a way, with much flag-waving and politically correct grandstanding, to prevent it.

That's why the great majority of witnesses at the hearings weren't the physicians, pharmacologists or addiction specialists that you'd expect. Instead, they were athletes, coaches, trainers, and sports officials, mostly from professional and college football. That's why seemingly endless time was devoted to examining the minutest details of the NFL drug testing procedures and technology. It was all about fairness in sports. And some of the legislators had rather personal reasons to ensure an equal playing field. Rep. Richard H. Baker from Louisiana, who testified as a witness, expressed concern that the NFL's approach to solving the problem wasn't forceful enough, and mentioned that his own son was "an Olympic hopeful ... committed to winning the right way." Remember Rep. Dan Lungren, who introduced the poorly conceived methandrostenolone bill and attacked the experts who were too honest with him? According to his colleague Rep. George Gekas of Pennsylvania, Rep. Lungren became "insistent" on tackling the subject for his own personal reasons. Rep. Lungren's son, an entrant to the Notre Dame football program, had "implored his dad" to pass legislation on steroids because he didn't want his refusal to use steroids to be a "disadvantage." Is it a coincidence that Sen. Biden opened his hearings, amid much fanfare, by declaring that steroid use "undermines, quite frankly, our value system, the so-called American way"?

It was all about fairness in sports. And some of the legislators had rather personal reasons to ensure an equal playing field.

The secondary consideration of Congress was the message that steroid use in high-level sports sends to our youth. This consideration surfaces repeatedly, expressed by numerous witnesses and legislators alike throughout the hearings. The focus of Sen. Biden in his opening remarks was on the "stars on the athletic field as the role models in our schools, in our colleges, and in our lives." Sen. Herbert Kohl, owner of the Milwaukee Bucks basketball team, also emphasized, "But worst of all, steroid users set an intolerable example for our nation's youth. Every time a sports hero betrays us through drug use, he or she also harms our children." While some concern was expressed about teen use of steroids, much more talk was directed to the demoralizing effect that steroid use by sports stars would have on teens.

Should concerns about the failure of public figures to be worthy role models justify laws that have *ordinary* people arrested? Isn't there some irony to the Congressional chest-thumping about athletes failing to set the "right example for our nation's youth," when many of our elected officials in Washington have demonstrated unparalleled bad behavior, including but not limited to internationally publicized lies, alcohol abuse, and adultery? Our current President won't deny rumors he formerly abused cocaine; our immediate past president had used marijuana (not to mention his scandalous behavior in office). Whatever your views on the hypocrisy of it all, one thing was certain: Congress was very serious about making a major public statement against anabolic steroids in sports.

Given the obvious predisposition of Congress, one has to wonder just how objectively the legislators listened to the health risks information. It's difficult to imagine that they could have been impartial, given their agenda and motivations. A 1990 Senate press release quoted Sen. Biden as decrying from his soapbox, "like crack and other hard drugs, steroids can cause serious medical damage. *Worse yet,* using steroids to increase athletic performance undermines the basic values that we learn in sports: namely, hard work, discipline and fair play" (emphasis added). The Senator's statement that undermining "fair play" in sports was worse than "serious medical damage" speaks volumes about his priorities and agenda. The hyperbolic testimony about health risks on which he and his colleagues chose to rely seems like icing to disguise the true dish they were serving to America. As for the addiction "hypothesis," the politicians knew that the only way to get a substance scheduled was to establish its potential for abuse and dependency. However flimsy and unsubstantiated, the theory was the "missing ingredient" they needed to sell to the rest of Congress to justify scheduling.

With all due respect to the sports establishment's Ministry of Truth, does keeping their games clean justify forbidding physicians from prescribing anabolics to *anybody* who just wants to *look* better? Does it justify arresting and imprisoning informed adults for choosing to use these medications for cosmetic reasons? Let's keep an open mind. Maybe the answers to those questions can be found by better understanding how and why people take anabolic steroids nonmedically, and what the potential health risks really are. We'll take a long, hard, *unbiased* look at that controversial subject in the following two chapters.

Chapter 2

AAS Use for the Uninitiated

"Provided a man is not mad, he can be cured of every folly but vanity."
–Jean Jacques Rousseau (1712–1778)

A long time ago when the earth was young and the curiosity of primitive man began to dawn, an idle cave dweller must have pondered his testicles. They were suspended there for a reason, no doubt. But what was it? It was obvious what the penis was for. More inscrutable were the testicles, which seemed to take little interest in everyday activities. Oddly, they were exclusive to males. What exactly were they doing down there?

Over time, ancient cultures came to understand that the testicles were somehow connected to brute strength and manliness. But how? It wasn't until modern times that scientists conducted experiments to get some solid answers, much to the consternation of some of our feathered barnyard friends. In 1771, a Scotsman transplanted the testes from a rooster to a surprised hen and confirmed his hypothesis that the hen would thereafter act more like a rooster. A German scientist feathered – I mean, furthered the research in 1849 by examining the effects of castration on the secondary sex characteristics of roosters. He proved the existence of a mysterious masculinizing substance produced in the testes and released through the bloodstream. Interest in this unknown chemical grew until, in 1935, scientists working in Amsterdam succeeded in collecting ten milligrams of it from a hundred kilograms of bull testes and identified this chemical as "testosterone." The prospect of what effects this "he hormone" might have on augmenting strength and muscular development was intriguing. By the late 1940's, Russian weightlifters had reportedly discovered testosterone and were using it for building strength. [For further information, *see* C.D. Kochakian, "Anabolic-Androgenic Steroids: A Historical Perspective and Definition," in C.E. Yesalis (Ed.), *Anabolic Steroids in Sport and Exercise* (Champaign, IL; Human Kinetics, 1993)]

The prospect of what effects this "he hormone" might have on augmenting strength and muscular development was intriguing.

What is Testosterone?

Testosterone is the primary male sex hormone, synthesized from cholesterol, and produced mostly by the Leydig cells of the testes. The average man produces about 4 to 7mg (milligrams) of testosterone every day. The normal range for *total* testosterone levels in adult males is 278 to 1,000 ng/dl (nanograms per deciliter of blood) and the average for *free* testosterone levels is 13 to 40 pg/ml (picograms per milliliter) for men aged 18 - 59 and 9 to 26 pg/ml for men aged 60 - 75. A nanogram is one billionth of a gram and a picogram is one trillionth of a gram. So we're not talking about huge amounts, as you can see. Free testosterone levels are important because they represent the "unbound" testosterone molecules that are free and available for interaction with the cells of the body. Women also have testosterone, produced in the ovaries and adrenal glands, but in a greatly reduced amount (10 to 15 times less). The normal range for *total* testosterone in women is usually 14 to 76 ng/dl and the average for *free* testosterone is 1 to 4 pg/ml. The levels for both men and women can vary depending on the time of day. Testosterone is a steroid, it is anabolic, and it is androgenic. Let's look at each of those three characteristics in turn.

Testosterone is called a *steroid* because of its chemical structure. All steroids share the same basic four-ring carbon structure, but differ in the number and arrangement in which hydrogen (H), oxygen (O), and hydroxyl (OH) groups are attached to the carbon atoms. There are various types of steroids. Your dear Aunt Edna's estrogen tablets are steroids. So are birth control pills. In fact, estrogens and birth control pills are pretty similar to androgens from a chemist's point of view. Perhaps the most commonly used steroids are the corticosteroids, such as prednisone and cortisone, which are used to reduce inflammation. These compounds are catabolic; that is, they break tissue down. When your mom tells you that they've put poor Uncle Cosmo on "steroids" at the hospital, it almost always means the use of corticosteroids. Don't worry, Uncle Cosmo won't come home with boulder-sized deltoids or fly into a psychotic 'roid rage.

Testosterone is an *anabolic* steroid. Anabolic steroids are medications that build tissue up, making muscles bigger and stronger. Did I say *medications*? Yes, indeed. While reports in the popular press almost invariably call them *drugs*, anabolic steroids were readily available as prescription medications for many years before they were scheduled as controlled substances. They are *not* drugs in the sense of cocaine or heroin, which have no generally accepted medical uses. Anabolic steroids are very effective medications with a variety of applications. Their ability to increase protein synthesis and nitrogen retention can have extremely positive effects on human physiology. They can stimulate the healing process in burn victims. They can effectively treat certain forms of anemia. One of the big secrets within the medical community is the beneficial effect that anabolic steroids have on the immune response. The crucial role that anabolic steroids can play in the war against AIDS has recently begun garnering support from the clinical community. The quality of life benefits that anabolics can offer those suffering from the muscle wasting associated with the HIV virus are nothing short of miraculous. For more information on the highly positive effects that AAS therapy is having upon HIV+ and AIDS patients, and about the relative safety of anabolic steroids in general, see www.medibolics.com, the web site of researcher Michael Mooney, an internationally recognized expert in the field of AIDS survival strategies and the co-author of *Built to Survive: A Comprehensive Guide to the Medical Use of Anabolic Steroids, Nutrition and Exercise for HIV(+) Men and Women* (PoWeR, 1999).

One of the big secrets within the medical community is the beneficial effect that anabolic steroids have on the immune response.

Now, testosterone is also *androgenic*. As the primary male sex hormone, you'd expect it to have masculinizing properties, right? These masculinizing or androgenic effects include the development of secondary male sex characteristics, such as the growth of your noisy neighbor's back hair and handlebar moustache, or the deepening tone of a man's voice. If a young boy's body doesn't produce its own testosterone, he'll require the administration of testosterone medications in order to fully develop. If an older man completely stops producing testosterone *endogenously* (by his own body), or if his testosterone level becomes abnormally low, he'll need the administration of *exogenous* testosterone to replace it. The problem of insufficient testosterone is called *hypogonadism*, and the age-related decline in testosterone levels experienced by most men is sometimes called *andropause* (see Chapter 12 for the applications of testosterone to age management). As you might guess, testosterone is the hormone that's administered if a woman decides to change her gender and become a man. Oh, there's some surgery to be sure, but there's also lots of testosterone for the rest of that person's life.

So, testosterone is both an anabolic and an androgenic steroid. As we've discussed, the androgenic effects are important in some medical situations but the anabolic effects are more desirable in others. The androgenic effects are much less desirable in fully developed adults – especially women. After all, not everyone likes cuddling with a woman with a full goatee, no matter how well she keeps it trimmed. So, somewhere around 1950, scientists began working hard to isolate testosterone's muscle-building properties from its androgenic effects. They discovered that by making certain modifications to the testosterone molecule, the resulting compound had higher anabolic effects with reduced androgenic effects. Bingo! Although the anabolic and androgenic qualities of these substances could never be completely separated, numerous compounds were synthesized that had more favorable anabolic-to-androgenic ratios than testosterone itself. These synthetically produced variations (*analogs*) of natural testosterone are today's anabolic steroids, also interchangeably referred to as anabolics, steroids, or androgens, or, in a major mouthful, as "anabolic-androgenic steroids" (often thankfully abbreviated as "AAS"). While synthetically produced, they are made from natural ingredients usually derived from wild yams, which are rich in the natural steroid diosgenin. These aren't your ordinary yams – they are not only inedible but they weigh an average of *fifty pounds*! Some steroids are also derived from soy phytosterols. Anabolic steroids can then be made into tablets to take orally, into creams or gels for transdermal application (such as Androgel®, a topical androgen), or into liquid form for *parenteral* injection, commonly into the buttocks or other large muscles.

Oral Anabolic Steroids

Let's talk about oral steroids first. Plain testosterone is ineffective if taken orally. That's because it must proceed through the gastrointestinal tract to the liver. The liver quickly breaks its structure down on its *first pass*, before it has time to enter the blood to be distributed to the muscles. So in order to withstand this rapid breakdown, oral anabolic steroids were purposely modified at the molecular level. One type of modification is a process called "alkylation" – the addition of a carbon atom or atoms at the alpha position of the number 17 carbon atom. Steroids altered in this way are called *C-17 alpha alkylated steroids*. They are more difficult for the liver to break down. They make the liver work really, really hard, especially if administered for a prolonged period of time. That's where the connection of steroids to liver (*hepatic*) problems comes from. Don't blame steroids – blame C-17 alkylation! It's this chemical modification of only certain oral steroids, not the intrinsic nature of all AAS variations, which accounts for the stress placed on the liver. Unfortunately, most oral steroids are modified in this way. Once consumed, oral steroids tend to stay in body for a short time. An oral steroid's *half-life* (the time required for a dose of an administered substance to decrease by half) is generally on the order of several hours. Oral steroids are generally pressed into tablets containing from 2 milligrams of active product on up to 50 milligrams.

Steroids altered in this way are called *C-17 alpha alkylated steroids*. They are more difficult for the liver to break down.

Injectable Anabolic Steroids

Injectable steroids go into the muscle and are then absorbed directly into the blood stream, avoiding a first pass through the liver. The liver thus experiences a much lower concentration than with oral anabolics. For this reason, most injectable steroids have little effect upon liver function. (However, a few C-17 alkylated steroids that are usually used orally in humans are available as injectable veterinary compounds [examples are stanozolol and methandrostenolone], and these have similar hepatic profiles to their oral counterparts.) Most injectable steroids undergo a process called *esterification* to slow their release into circulation. Esterification is the addition of carboxylic acids to the 17-beta hydroxyl group of the testosterone molecule. An ester of testosterone will release more slowly and gradually into the bloodstream from the site of injection than unesterfied testosterone will. Most of the common injectable androgens are esters dissolved in a mixture of plant oil and alcohol. A few injectable steroids are not oil-based, but are shorter-lasting, water-based suspensions (examples are the testosterone and stanozolol suspensions). Injectables tend to have longer half-lives than orals. Injectables are typically packaged in multiple-use vials of a variety of sizes. The standard is a 10cc vial, although some veterinary products come in 50cc vials. The potency of the product is measured in milligrams (mg) per cc. For example, a testosterone ester might have 200mg in each cc. Some injectables come in single use ampoules or in preloaded syringes. All injectable steroids are designed for intramuscular injection – they go into the muscle. The image of someone administering anabolics like a heroin junkie, by intravenous injection, is a flight of pure fancy.

How Do Anabolic Steroids Work?

Are you with me so far? Okay, let's talk about how anabolic steroids actually work to increase muscular size and strength in a way that everyone can understand. Whether taken orally or by injection, all anabolic steroids eventually wind up as molecules in the blood stream, carried along with thousands of other types of molecules. At various points along the way, the cells within the body's tissues have areas called *receptor sites*. These areas are receptive to some free-floating molecules within the blood, but they're very specific. There are receptor sites with an affinity for anabolic steroid molecules in our skeletal muscle cells, for example, and in our scalp and prostate. These sites are sometimes collectively referred to as the *androgen receptor*. Think of the blood stream like a busy Los Angeles freeway. The molecules are like countless vehicles of all sizes and shapes traveling rapidly in the same direction. The steroid molecule is like a delivery van – the "andro-van" – racing along with all the others. The receptor sites are like road stops designed only for the andro-van. They're just waiting for the andro-van to stop by with a delivery.

> There are receptor sites with an affinity for anabolic steroid molecules in our skeletal muscle cells, for example, and in our scalp and prostate.

An anabolic steroid molecule that's being carried along in the blood enters the muscle cell by diffusion and binds to one of these receptor sites, like the andro-van might pull into and park in its specially marked road stop. The connection that is formed permits the steroid molecule to deliver a cellular message, like the andro-van might make a delivery at the road stop. The steroid molecule commands the receptor site to effect certain metabolic changes within the cell, such as increasing the synthesis of proteins and the retaining of nitrogen. Increased protein synthesis and nitrogen retention cause increased size and strength of the skeletal muscle cell. The connection of a steroid molecule and receptor site is fleeting: once the andro-van delivers its cellular command, it moves on to other road stops, delivering its message over and over. Eventually the andro-van breaks down and is scrapped. What happens to it then? Well, a worn-out steroid molecule can be excreted in the urine, or it can be converted into something else, like estrogen or DHT. This capacity of androgens to be converted into other substances by chemical reactions and enzymes within certain tissues of the body will be extremely significant later when we discuss potential side effects.

Anabolics also enhance size and strength through a different mechanism. The intense resistance training typical of bodybuilding causes the body to produce increased levels of *cortisol*. Cortisol is a catabolic substance that causes muscle tissue breakdown, like those damned corticosteroids they were giving to your Uncle Cosmo. Cortisol works to limit the body's ability to make muscular gains, breaking down muscle tissue. Anabolics have an anti-catabolic effect; that is, they work to antagonize cortisol's catabolic effect by suppressing the catabolic cellular mechanisms stimulated by cortisol. Consequently, recovery processes are sped up, and injuries, including the microscopic muscle damage incurred from heavy training, heal faster. Some authorities believe that the anti-catabolic properties of steroids may be of equal or even greater significance than the anabolic properties, but no studies back it up at this time.

Who's Using Anabolics Non-Medically?

All right, now we have a basic working knowledge of how anabolics work, focusing on the medical uses. Let's talk about who's taking them *non-medically*. The most obvious population with an interest in taking them non-medically is the athletic community. While anabolics may not improve eye-hand coordination, reaction time, stamina or judgment, sheer size and strength can provide some major advantages on the playing field. They certainly didn't hurt Olympic Gold Medalist Ben Johnson's running times. Clearly, competitive athletes have an interest in taking anabolics. And the media have let America know about it. Almost without exception, when we hear or read about adults who take steroids we're presented with college, Olympic or professional athletes who use them to enhance performance. In fact, anabolic steroids are commonly referred to as *sports performance-enhancing drugs*. If you're a coach or trainer, it's this application of AAS use that most concerns you.

Well, here's a shocker (unless you're part of the muscle world). The vast majority of people who take steroids for non-medical reasons are *not* doing it for performance enhancement. In fact, they're not even *playing* sports. Most people who take steroids are doing it primarily to improve the way they *look*. Yes, you read that correctly. They're taking steroids for *cosmetic* purposes, not athletic purposes. You haven't heard much about that, have you? Well, that's because most newsworthy items about steroids involve sports scandals – athletes who take them to cheat other athletes. The cosmetic steroid takers, *millions* of them, aren't a press target. A small percentage are top-rated bodybuilders, but most are ordinary people who are taking steroids cosmetically to build their bodies and perhaps boost their self-esteem. Many of them are men in their late twenties to early forties seeking to increase their lean muscle mass and decrease their body fat. Some

Most people who take steroids are doing it primarily to improve the way they *look*.

bring themselves up to a level of size and conditioning to compete in bodybuilding contests, but most never set foot on a competition platform. Some AAS users are teens – which is quite clearly a bad thing – but most of them are *not* teens (see Chapter 11 for a full discussion of why anabolics are totally unsuited for teens). Some of them are women who compete in bodybuilding or fitness competitions, but some women use very low dosages of anabolics in an effort to get more of a "hard body" look. Under today's laws, all of them are risking arrest and prosecution.

How Anabolics are Used for Appearance

As you will see, legal restrictions as well as current medical ethics prevent physicians from prescribing steroids for cosmetic purposes. So, mature healthy adults who want to take them for building their bodies or boosting their self-esteem can't go to a doctor and get a prescription. They have to get them unlawfully, usually from black market sources. To maximize the anabolic effects and minimize the potential adverse effects, most cosmetic AAS users will *cycle* their self-administration of anabolics – often called *juice* or *gear* – by alternating periods of use with periods of steroid-free training. Cycling is *safer* than staying on steroids all the time. Cycle lengths vary considerably. The cycles of most novice to intermediate cosmetic steroid takers last from 4 to 12 weeks, followed by a steroid-free period of the same duration [Perry, P.J., Andersen, K.H., and Yates, W.R., "Illicit Anabolic Steroid Use in Athletes," 18 *Amer. J. of Sports Med.,* 4 (1990)]. Cycles lasting from 12 to 16 weeks are also quite common. Obviously, the goals of hardcore steroid veterans and elite level bodybuilding competitors are different from the more casual users. They often remain on a continuous cycle of steroids for most of the year, sometimes employing reduced dosages and ancillary medications to bridge from one cycle to the next.

Injectable anabolics are generally favored over oral anabolics because of the reduced stress on the liver. Testosterone esters, such as enanthate, propionate and cypionate, are extremely popular, as they are reported to produce gains in size and strength with little or no liver toxicity. All of these esters of testosterone, however, are highly androgenic, meaning there is the potential for unwanted effects at the dosages required to promote muscle growth. For this reason, people will often combine testosterone esters with less androgenic, more anabolic compounds like nandrolone decanoate, popularly referred to by the brand name Deca-durabolin® or simply "Deca." This *stacking* technique is intended to provide for the substantial overall dosages required for growth in a way that minimizes side effects. While Deca is an extremely popular product, its formulation is not sufficiently similar to testosterone to fully duplicate it. When it is used alone, it suppresses natural testosterone production without fully supporting testosterone's more androgenic effects. This characteristic of nandrolone, which metabolizes into a weak metabolite called DHN, is reported to explain the sexual functioning problems of those who use nandrolone without a testosterone "base." By combining both drugs, favorable results may be obtained with minimal side effects. Most users stack more than one compound.

This *stacking* technique is intended to provide for the substantial overall dosages required for growth in a way that minimizes side effects.

Polypharmacy – the combination of various medications – is practiced by over 80% of those who use anabolics. It's common practice to self-administer ancillary medications to avoid or control unwanted side effects like acne, hair loss, water retention or reduced libido. The list of non-controlled substances used in conjunction with steroid cycles may include oral and injectable diuretics, thyroid preparations, finasteride (Proscar® and Propecia®) and human chorionic gonadotropin (HCG). Since excessive androgens can be aromatized by the body's enzymes into estrogens, users often take aromatase-blockers (anastrozole) and/or anti-estrogens (tamoxifen citrate, clomiphene citrate or cyclofenil) to avert or reduce side effects such as chest feminization (gynecomastia). Further, not everyone achieves the same muscle gains with the same dosages and cycles. Individual genetics play a significant part in the equation. Some people will grow on very conservative dosages and cycles, while others will make few gains even at high dosages and extended cycles. Long-term users frequently need to raise dosages to continue growing. Clearly, at some point cosmetic use can become *abuse*. But the issue of whether *any* cosmetic use automatically constitutes abuse is far from settled, and an issue we'll revisit later.

An Example of Cosmetic AAS Use in Practice

Okay, how about getting a sense of cosmetic juice use in practice? Understanding how physique enthusiasts take steroids is essential to our later discussions. Let's invent a typical scenario, *not* to instruct or condone, but to get a feel for why and how an otherwise responsible mature adult might self-administer anabolics. Let's take Lou, 31, a computer programmer who doesn't play any sports but loves working out. He's a solid 190 pounds and looks better than most guys on the beach. But he's been training for over ten years and hasn't made any gains in the last three. He's convinced that he's reached his genetic potential for muscle size and strength, but he's not satisfied with his physique. He knows it's vanity, but he wants to add some muscle to his frame, particularly his chest and calves, and lose some fat. Over-the-counter fad supplements, strict dieting and hard training of every variation haven't helped Lou achieve the goals he set for himself when he first started training. Lou puts in quite a bit of time researching anabolics. Whatever your own feelings about the wisdom of his choice, Lou ultimately makes the informed decision to try steroids.

He speaks to his doctor, but the doctor is afraid of anything to do with steroids. Lou sees a cosmetic surgeon, but the surgeon suggests a combination of prosthetic chest implants, calf implants and liposuction. Lou summarily rejects such radical, invasive and potentially dangerous procedures. Instead, Lou, a guy who's never had anything but some parking tickets, buys some gear on the black market. Most black market anabolics consumed today are of foreign origin. Some of these products surely have substandard quality control, and some are counterfeit products that contain little or no active ingredient or are otherwise contaminated. Lou knows it's illegal, and that he's undertaking significant health risks. Of course, Lou is taking much bigger chances than he realizes, as many of the chapters of this book will show.

Most black market anabolics consumed today are of foreign origin. Some of these products surely have substandard quality control ...

Anyway, Lou isn't interested in staying on anabolics forever. He knows his body has a feedback system, and that taking anabolics will send a message to his body that it can temporarily stop making its own androgens. He wants to cycle on and off them, so that his body's own production won't be too suppressed for too long. He wants a very simple, conservative cycle that, when combined with proper training and diet, will induce muscle growth while minimizing the potential for side effects. He chooses to use exclusively injectable steroids to avoid the stress that orals might place on his liver and kidneys. His cycle will last ten weeks, at which time he will curtail all AAS use and allow his body to recover its natural testosterone production. He's willing to work out hard four days a week, and to consume plenty of calories and protein. He's planning a protein intake of at least one gram per pound of his body weight.

Lou knows that a typical physiological replacement dose might be about 100mg a week. That's what a doctor would give him if he was hypogonadal (had abnormally low testosterone levels). But Lou knows he'll need to take a *supraphysiologic* dose of androgens in order to achieve results. He reasons that simply replacing his body's own levels won't enable him to meet his goals. Lou decides to use 600mg per week. He chooses to use a testosterone enanthate product from Mexico that's available to him from a guy at the gym. It's a long-acting oil-based injectable.

Lou knows that testosterone is highly androgenic and at high doses can lead to unwanted side effects. So rather than taking 600mg of testosterone enanthate, he chooses to stack a dose of only 400mg per week with 200mg of a complimentary steroid. He chooses nandrolone decanoate, as it is primarily anabolic in nature with very little androgenic activity. But because nandrolone has an affinity for the progesterone receptor, high doses of nandrolone can cause side effects not unlike those caused by an excess of estrogen. Combining the two steroids together allows Lou to maximize the benefits of a conservative total dosage while minimizing side effects. Lou has also decided to take tamoxifen citrate (Nolvadex®) throughout his cycle to limit the potential for estrogen related side effects.

From his research, Lou has learned that at the end of his ten-week cycle, his own natural testosterone production will be suppressed. Nandrolone stays active for several weeks after administration. Though blood concentrations will be steadily declining, there's enough activity to continue suppression of natural testosterone production. Lou determines that a combination of human chorionic gonadotropin (HCG) in conjunction with clomiphene citrate is reported to be the optimum approach for recovering natural testosterone production expeditiously. The last week of his injection, Lou will begin administration of HCG in doses of 3000iu's every fifth day for the first two weeks and then 1500iu's every fifth day for the third week. during which time he will continue to take tamoxifen citrate. Three weeks after his last injection, he will curtail his use of HCG and tamoxifen and begin "Clomid therapy," using a daily dose of 150mg per day for the first two weeks, reducing the dosage to 50mg daily for the following two weeks. Clomid therapy is the last step in the process of recovery. (The traditional approach to this stage of recovery has been to use clomiphene citrate while the more progressive approach favors the use of tamoxifen citrate.)

If Lou is lucky, he'll gain from five to fifteen pounds of muscle from this cycle. However, it's unlikely that he'll keep it all after completing his cycle. Most people keep a substantial portion of their gains from a cycle. However, poor training, diet and recovery strategies can make some people lose most or even all of their gains. Most likely, Lou will not have told his physician about his AAS use. Because of the clandestine nature of cosmetic anabolic use, few folks get check-ups during or after their cycles. Of course, the lack of medical supervision greatly escalates the potential risks (see Chapter 3). That's Lou's story. It's based on a real person. It's the first of many true-life tales you'll read here.

Forging Ahead

This chapter was intended to provide a very rudimentary understanding of anabolics and their non-medical use by mature adults. It's sufficient for the understanding of all that is to follow in this book. The book's glossary provides more specific information about some of the medications and over-the-counter products (such as creatine monohydrate and androstenedione) used by the muscle world, as well as descriptions of the various AAS formulations on the market and their unique characteristics. However, any adults interested in a more intensive knowledge of the individual AAS products and their non-medical effects are referred to the book entitled *Anabolics 2002* by Bill Llewellyn (Patchogue, NY: Molecular Nutrition, 2002), which is available at www.molecularnutrition.com.

Now that we have an idea of how people use anabolics non-medically, let's look at what anabolics do to people's health. Honestly, how dangerous are these substances for healthy adults? There are more surprises in store, folks.

Chapter 3

THE REAL DANGERS REVEALED

"Medicine sometimes snatches away health, sometimes gives it."
– *Ovid (43 BC – 18 AD)*

While anabolics were originally outlawed to help purify the Olympics and other competitive sports, they've been the subject of countless horrific health warnings by the athletic establishments and the government. Today, they've been so thoroughly demonized that the public believes that steroids will kill you, plain and simple. That's common knowledge, isn't it? Liver cancer, heart disease, and 'roid rage *always* result from anabolic usage, regardless of dosages, duration of use, or preexisting conditions, right? Won't all your hair fall out? Won't your testicles vanish? Won't your prostate automatically blow up to the size of a cantaloupe? Isn't taking *any* amount of steroids without medical necessity *abuse*, regardless of the circumstances? Wouldn't it be heresy to say otherwise? Isn't it better to arrest and prosecute the poor souls than allow them to destroy themselves?

Isn't taking *any* amount of steroids without medical necessity *abuse*, regardless of the circumstances?

Steroid users themselves, however, haven't bought into any of it. They stopped listening to the mainstream experts back when they were chanting the "steroids don't work" mantra. Like Chicken Little who cried that the sky was falling in countless false alarms, the anti-AAS establishment lost all credibility in the muscle world decades ago. Too many of them have all-too-obvious biases and agendas, like anti-steroid physicians who happen to be sports anti-doping officials. They're now seen as fit only to be ignored or ridiculed. Hardcore physique enthusiasts have amassed their own body of underground anecdotal evidence, derived from their observations of themselves and their peers, or from underground treatises on the self-administration of steroids. Even those in the medical community concede that the real steroid experts are not doctors, but those in the lay community who use them. [Perry et al., 1990]

Let's begin by agreeing that there are health risks involved in the administration of *any* prescription medicine, including hormones like anabolic steroids. Naturally, the risks go up when a drug is *self-administered* in the absence of a physician's advice as to dosages and duration of use. Without an initial screening examination, contraindications or preexisting problems might go undetected. Without regular monitoring by a doctor, some side effects might go unnoticed or untreated until they have serious consequences. Make no mistake, folks, anabolic steroids can have adverse effects on the body, particularly in women and teenagers. [See Chapter 11, Teens and Testosterone.]

But just how dangerous are anabolics for mature healthy adults? We're talking only about fully developed adults – they're the ones who are mostly using them anyway. Let's put aside everything we've been told about anabolic steroids. Let's suspend our preconceived ideas and moral judgments. We'll trust ourselves to the cold, hard facts, and see where they lead us. You're in for a surprise.

Anabolic Steroids and the Liver

Ask most people what steroid use will do to you, and they'll talk about the liver. Of all the reported physical consequences of AAS use, the effects on the liver have been the most alarming to the public. We've been told that not only do AAS's unduly stress the liver, causing damage, but that they can also cause serious liver problems like hepatocellular carcinoma (liver cancer) and peliosis hepatitis (blood-filled sacs within the liver that can rupture, causing the patient to bleed to death). Pretty scary stuff to be sure.

Well, let's examine how oral medications affect the liver. When you take a medicine by mouth, it doesn't go directly into the bloodstream. It gets processed on its first pass through the liver, and its chemical structure may provide a general indication of liver burden (hepatotoxicity). It's interesting to know that many prescription drugs are hepatotoxic. It's more surprising to know that even *over-the-counter pain relievers* are hepatotoxic. Acetaminophen (Tylenol®) has been reported to cause liver damage – even fatal hepatic necrosis – when repeatedly used, particularly among alcoholics. Even more surprising, this damage resulted not at massive dosages, but at *therapeutic* dosages. [Prescott, 1986; Eriksson et al., 1992; Patel, 1992] Just recently, an FDA advisory panel recommended stronger and clearer warnings to highlight the liver risk. Some FDA panelists cautioned against making the warning too strong. "We don't want to make Tylenol look like a dangerous product," said panel member Dr. Nathaniel Katz. A curious position, given that an FDA analysis estimated that there are about *100 deaths* and more than *13,000 emergency room visits* each year in the U.S. from unintentional acetaminophen overdoses.

As discussed in the last chapter, C-17 alkylated oral steroids are stressful for the liver to process. Like Tylenol®, they are hepatotoxic. Even brief administration of alkylated oral steroids can elevate liver enzyme levels in the blood (a sign that liver cells are being damaged). But while liver function test readings go up during a cycle, they don't stay elevated *after* a moderate, short-term anabolic cycle. They simply return to normal.

Further, not all liver stress exhibited by bodybuilders is due to anabolics. Scientists are just beginning to learn that the damage caused by intense resistance training elevates liver counts, with or *without* steroids. A study conducted at the University of North Texas Health Science Center compared the blood chemistries of steroid-using bodybuilders and natural bodybuilders. The focus of the blood chemistry profiles was on aspartate aminotransferase (AST), alanine aminotransferase (ALT), gamma-glutamyltranspeptidase (GGT), and creatine kinase (CK) levels, which are all indicators of liver function. It was found that in *both* groups of bodybuilders, CK, AST, and ALT were elevated, whereas GGT remained in the normal range. The conclusion: "Prior reports of anabolic steroid-induced hepatotoxicity based on elevated aminotransferase levels may have been overstated, because no exercising subjects, including steroid users, demonstrated hepatic dysfunction based on GGT levels. Such reports may have misled the medical community to emphasize steroid-induced hepatotoxicity when interpreting elevated aminotransferase levels and disregard muscle damage." [Dickerman et al., 1999] Got that? Past researchers may have been mistaken when they blamed steroids for elevated liver counts.

As for the more serious liver problems, most cases in the medical literature didn't involve bodybuilders who cycle on and off anabolics. To the contrary, they involved extremely *sick* and *elderly* patients who had been continuously treated with C-17 alkylated steroids for years; and many of whom had a particular type of anemia linked to liver tumors even *without* anabolic steroid therapy. What about the minority of cases with younger patients? Let's take a look at them. In one case, a 20-year-old Japanese girl with aplastic anemia developed hepatic adenomas (HA) following *six years* of continuous treatment with an extremely powerful, C-17 alkylated steroid (oxymetholone) at 30mg per day. Six years? What was that doctor thinking? And yet, when the patient was brought in, her lab tests revealed *normal* liver function. It took ultrasono-graphy and computed tomography to detect the lesions in her liver, which were benign. A MEDLINE search reported only 17 cases of androgen-induced HA published between 1975 and 1998 in the English language literature. [Nakao, 2000] In another case, a 35-year-old woman with aplastic anemia was diagnosed with hepatocellular carcinoma, the most common form of liver cancer. She too had been treated with oxymetholone, but at a dose of 60mg daily for three years. [Kosaka, 1996] Even the most *hard-core* AAS user would acknowledge the danger of using oxymetholone for that duration.

But all those patients were quite sick to begin with. What about serious effects in healthy bodybuilders? Take a study by none other than Dr. Harrison ("Skip") Pope, a staunch anti-anabolics crusader. This one surely didn't help his case. In a study of strength athletes, of the 53 current or past steroid users who underwent laboratory testing only *one* subject displayed an abnormal liver test. [Pope & Katz, 1994] Incidentally, on physical examination, not one user displayed evidence of any major abnormalities possibly attributable to steroids, such as high blood pressure, edema, acne, or hair loss. Not one. Well, let's search the medical literature. Of the untold millions of people who've taken steroids (the last estimate of three million is over a decade old and completely out of date), how many have gotten liver tumors? A 1990 computer search of the medical literature looking for steroid-associated liver tumors could find only *three* in athletes. [Friedl, 1990] Not three thousand. Three. You'd expect a higher number in the general population. Of the three, one was using massive amounts of C-17 alkylated steroids (700mg of oxymetholone a week, which is the dosage equivalent of 20 Dianabol tablets a day) for *five straight years*, and one had a tumor more indicative of classic liver cancer than of steroid-associated tumors.

Virtually all of the reported liver problems seemed to occur with the C-17 oral steroids. But even with respect to them, the case is hardly overwhelming. One study tested oxymetholone for 30 straight weeks on HIV+ men and women in a dosage of over 1,000mg per week (more than that used by most bodybuilders, and for a much longer duration of uninterrupted use). [Hengge et al., 1996] You'd expect the result to be major liver damage, especially since these people already had HIV, were probably taking all sorts of other meds, and would be in far worse physical condition than a healthy athlete, right? Wrong. There were *no* significant problems with liver function (nor with water retention or virilization side effects). On the other hand, there was a significant gain in lean muscle mass – even without any weight lifting.

But enough about the oral steroids. Most bodybuilders rely mainly on injectable anabolics like the testosterone and nandrolone esters. What do they do to the liver? The shocking answer is: *virtually nothing*. There have been *no* cysts or liver tumors reported in athletes using the 17 beta-esterified injectable steroids. [Wright & Cowart, 1990] Contrary to what most folks have been led to believe, injectable oil-based steroids generally have *little if any effect upon liver function*. [Haupt, 1993; Myhal, 2000]

Contrary to what most folks have been led to believe, injectable oil-based steroids generally have *little if any effect upon liver function*.

What can we conclude, but that the dangers of most anabolics to healthy mature adults' livers appear to have been wildly exaggerated? Over-the-counter Tylenol® is statistically a *tremendously* bigger public health hazard, and let's not even talk about the thousands of cases of liver damage and liver failure from alcohol use. When it comes to the liver, the C-17 anabolics are the ones to watch out for. An apparently healthy subject with a previously existing but undiscovered liver problem could cause damage by self-administering C-17 anabolics. It's risky for anyone to take C-17 steroids without having a physician regularly conduct lab tests to monitor liver function. In fact, chronic users, especially those consuming large dosages of oral steroids, "should undergo a periodic liver ultrasound examination because routine blood chemistries may not detect potentially life-threatening hepatic lesions in early stages." [Myhal, 2000] Even in countries where cosmetic steroid use is not outlawed, it would seem foolish for any bodybuilder to use significant amounts of C-17 oral steroids when much safer injectable esters are available.

Anabolic Steroids and the Heart

Conventional wisdom dictates that steroid use is bad for the heart, right? But exactly how cardiac risk might be increased by the use of steroids is a subject of speculation and controversy. A recent examination of two young Italian bodybuilders who died of heart attacks tried to establish a link between steroid use and sudden cardiac death. The study was unable to find "any evidence of a cause-effect relationship." [Fineschi et al., 2001] When cardiac problems do occur in bodybuilders, they may be related to specific types of steroids or to other substances besides androgens. For example, since estrogen has multiple cardiovascular protective effects, the chronic use of estrogen blockers, aromatase inhibitors, or non-aromatizing steroids may play a part in a potential for cardiac disease by decreasing the circulating estrogen concentrations.

In examining cardiovascular risks, often cited is a case report [McNutt et al., 1988] concerning a 22-year-old steroid-using weight lifter who experienced a sudden heart attack. While frequently held out by anti-anabolics proponents as the "smoking gun" connecting steroid use to heart attacks, a reading of the actual report reveals that the subject weighed 330 pounds and had a total serum cholesterol of a whopping 596mg/dl! The fact that so few similar case studies exist may well indicate that the condition of this individual was hardly representative of the majority of healthy men who use steroids. [For a more detailed critique of the "doubtful nature" of this case report, *see* Myhal, 2000] Nonetheless, all strength athletes, including steroid users, should regularly monitor serum cholesterol. Obviously, this poor fellow didn't get his weight to 330 and his cholesterol to 596 overnight, and it's not reported when he last visited a physician prior to his heart attack. Some might speculate that our nation's criminalization approach to steroids, discouraging steroid-users from seeing doctors, contributed to this result.

Researchers have speculated that anabolics cause changes in cardiac structure after observing thickening of the heart's left ventricular wall in steroid users. A University of North Texas study conducted on elite power lifters, however, found "in contrast to previous reports" that left ventricular wall thickening occurs with or *without* anabolic steroid use. [Dickerman et al., 1998] Another recent study from Australia examined arterial and cardiac structure and function in ten bodybuilders using anabolics, compared to ten non-steroid-using bodybuilder controls. The authors concluded that although high-level bodybuilding is associated with impaired vascular reactivity and increased thickening of the arteries, the use of anabolics per se is *not* associated with significant abnormalities of arterial structure or function. [Sader et al., 2001]

Okay, what about cholesterol? Just like with liver problems, the C-17 alkylated steroids seem to be the bad guys. They can affect blood lipids, causing a reduction in HDL (high-density lipoproteins, the "good" cholesterol) in some steroid users, as well as an increase in LDL (low-density lipoproteins, the "bad" cholesterol). [*See*, for example, Welder et al., 1995] Increased LDL levels have been shown to increase platelet sensitivity, which could theoretically increase the chances of blood clots. Increased potential for blood clotting has led some reviewers to speculate that C-17 alkylated steroids could increase the chances of stroke, although no direct evidence exists that androgens cause blood clots in humans. [Street et al., 1996] Further, changes in the blood lipid levels now appear to begin to recover within about a month after discontinued use, and, in fact, most studies do not report an increase in total cholesterol. [Yesalis & Cowart, 1998] Moreover, the great majority of studies suggest that injectable non-C-17 steroids (which are more commonly used anyway) "exert minimal adverse effects on blood lipids." [Myhal, 2000] When C-17 orals are consumed, dosages may play a crucial factor. José Antonio, PhD., a nationally recognized authority on anabolic substances and supplements, cites a study examining serious cardiovascular side effects in four weight lifters using "massive amounts" of steroids. [Antonio, 1998] While there is little doubt that the health problems of these men were caused by their anabolic steroid abuse, these were clearly mega-dose abusers. "[H]igh dose equals high risk," notes Dr. Antonio, but "low-dose androgens (e.g., 200-600mg per week for 10 weeks) pose little threat to health."

Further studies conducted over the last few years continue to refute conventional wisdom connecting anabolic steroid use and cardiac risk. Researchers who recruited competitive bodybuilders for an evaluation of the cardiovascular effects of steroid use concluded steroids do not appear to raise the risk. [Dickerman et al., 1997] Researchers in Poland found that testosterone replacement therapy may actually *lower* the risk of heart disease. [Zgliczynski et al., 1996] In fact, *decreases* in testosterone levels over time are associated with unfavorable heart disease risk. [Zmuda et al., 1997] Some researchers are currently looking into the possibility of using androgens as a therapy for cardiovascular disease! [Shapiro et al., 1999]

Well, what about high blood pressure? As weight gain and water retention can result from anabolic steroid use, hypertension can also result. But while hypertension is often cited as a confirmed consequence of anabolic steroid usage, reports indicate that high blood pressure is perhaps "one of the most exaggerated claims" of steroid-related health risks, and remains difficult to confirm despite numerous studies. [Friedl, 1993] Certainly, those using steroids, particularly highly androgenic steroids, should carefully monitor salt intake and have regular blood pressure tests.

While the question of whether short-term, reversible alterations of these cardiac risk factors are detrimental to long-term cardiac health is "unanswered" at this time [Haupt,1993], it has been suggested that some characteristics of steroid-users — intense exercising, low body fat, and avoidance of smoking — tend to put them in a *low-risk* group for heart disease [Friedl, 1993]. It should be noted that long-term treatment of female-to-male transsexuals with high doses of testosterone results in adverse blood lipid changes, but does not increase the incidence of coronary artery disease in comparison to normal women. [Myhal, 2000] While exactly what role certain anabolic steroids may play in the development of cardiovascular disease is quite unclear, the incidence of "life-threatening circulatory events" linked to steroids over decades represents a very small percentage. If only the same could be said of smoking or carrying too many extra pounds. Still, the high importance of regular physician monitoring should be considered when using these substances for non-medical purposes.

[T]he incidence of "life-threatening circulatory events" linked to steroids over decades represents a very small percentage.

Anabolic Steroids and the Kidneys

Kidney damage is an uncommon side effect of steroid use. It's not even mentioned much. But logic suggests there's a legitimate risk, so let's discuss it. The kidneys play an integral role in filtration and removal of byproducts from the human body. So, you'd expect that anabolic steroids might be stressful on the kidneys. A search of the medical literature reveals that when anabolic steroids are implicated as the cause of a kidney-related disorder, guess which types of steroids are the culprit? You got it: C-17 alkylated steroids, in high dosages and for long periods of continuous use. That's not surprising. Case in point: a 28-year-old bodybuilder was diagnosed with severe cholestasis and acute renal failure after being admitted to the hospital with signs of jaundice. Up until three weeks prior to his admission to the hospital, the patient had been using a daily dose of 10 to 50mg of methandrostenolone in conjunction with 50mg of stanozolol every other day for 80 days. That's right, eleven and a half weeks using high doses of two different C-17 alkylated steroids. [Habscheid , 1999]

What *is* surprising is that androgens like oxymetholone are now being used experimentally to *treat* the malnutrition and catabolism associated with *renal (kidney) failure*, although additional clinical studies must be conducted before this treatment will become a common practice. [Johnson, 2000; Chen et al., 2001] Patients on *kidney dialysis* who were given the anabolic steroid nandrolone decanoate for six months reaped terrific benefits – they gained more lean body mass, had less fatigue, and performed better on physical performance tests than the placebo group. [Johansen, 1999]. This may be because nandrolone and other anabolic steroids can stimulate kidney tissue repair.

Adverse Effects of Excess Androgens

The average adult male production of testosterone is only 4 to 7mg per day. Supplemental androgens can raise blood androgen levels to many times the amount that could be naturally produced. All these extra androgens will affect the body's hormonal balance, including the reproductive system. Anabolics mimic your own naturally-produced testosterone in the negative feedback loop of the hypothalamic-pituitary-testicular axis (HPTA). In other words, your body perceives that it has plenty of circulating testosterone, so it alters its own production. The testicles say, why not close down the shop if there's no work to be done? Exactly how long it takes for the body to shut down the shop is uncertain, although some have estimated it at about three weeks. After that, the testicles go completely off duty. One result is decreased sperm production, which also takes place in the testes. This effect has been the focus of studies testing the use of anabolics as an exciting new form of birth control – male contraception. [W.H.O., 1990] It's also been used as a basis for claiming "sterility" as a side effect of anabolic use. That's kind of like saying that women's birth control pills cause sterility. Anyway, the effect is reversible with discontinuance of the medication [Haupt & Rovere, 1984] and no case of permanent sterility as a result of prolonged high-dose steroid consumption has ever been reliably documented. [Yesalis & Cowart, 1998]

... no case of permanent sterility as a result of prolonged high-dose steroid consumption has ever been reliably documented.

What effects can all this have on a man's reproductive organs? I've heard some folks claim that steroids will cause the penis to shrink. Some people have actually argued the point. Let's get it straight, once and for all. Anabolics will *not* shrink a man's member. That rumor was probably started by somebody seeking a scapegoat for his natural shortcomings. It's *totally* unfounded. In fact, anabolic steroids are effective at *increasing* the size of the penis in young boys who are not developing properly. [Charmandari et al., 2001] Before you get any bright ideas, there is absolutely *no* evidence that they accomplish this feat in mature adults. Men seeking an excuse in this area would be much better served by the "shrinkage" argument presented by George Costanza on "Seinfeld." He blamed it all on swimming in the cold pool.

While the penis is safe from shrinkage, the testicles are not. The shutdown of endogenous production can cause the testicles to decrease in size. Like your muscles, they can get smaller and softer if you don't use them. This effect has been a favorite of anti-steroid propagandists and has been widely reported in the media. Like impaired fertility, testicular shrinkage is generally fully reversible upon discontinuation of use. While decreased testicular size has been a significant problem in the past, today fewer anabolic users suffer from this problem because it is usually easily treated by the administration of an ancillary medication, a gonadotropin-stimulating drug called human chorionic gonadotropin (HCG). It's been shown that the use of HCG during steroid cycles can maintain both testicular size and normal sperm production during high-dose testosterone treatment. [Matsumoto, 1983]

Effects of AAS on Women

What about the effects of excess male hormones on women's reproductive systems? The effect of anabolic steroid use on fertility in women is unknown. Mark Myhal, Ph.D. and David R. Lamb, Ph.D. reviewed the relevant literature, finding that a number of hormonal and physiological changes occur in women who use high doses of androgens. These changes include decreases in circulating Follicle Stimulating Hormone (FSH) and Sex Hormone Binding Globule (SHBG) concentrations. Menstruation may decrease or stop during prolonged steroid use, although women may continue to ovulate. High circulating concentrations of testosterone can effect changes in the tissues of the female genital tract, including symptoms consistent with the diagnosis of polycystic ovaries. In addition, recent data from female-to-male transsexuals suggest an increased risk of ovarian cancer in women exposed to high doses of androgens for prolonged periods of time. [Hage et al., 2000] Further research is warranted before a determination can be made as to the effects of these changes on fertility both during and after steroid use. [Myhal & Lamb, 2000]

Since large exogenous doses of androgens are more foreign to a woman's body than to a man's, their effect on the hormonal balance of a woman is expectedly more profound.

With the exception of oxandrolone and perhaps methenolone (Primobolan), if anabolic steroids are used intermittently and in relatively low doses, most women will experience some form of permanent virilization. Of course the degree depends on the androgenicity of the drug as well as the dosage, duration, and individual response. Since large exogenous doses of androgens are more foreign to a woman's body than to a man's, their effect on the hormonal balance of a woman is expectedly more profound. Excessive growth of body hair (hirsutism), coarsening of the skin, male pattern baldness, and deepening of the voice may occur (especially at massive dosages) in both men and women, and are generally not reversible upon discontinuance of steroids. Other possible effects particular to women include heavy facial masculinization, breast tissue reduction, and clitoral enlargement, besides the less objectionable effects of increased muscularity and decreased body fat. Moreover, and perhaps most importantly, any woman who considers the use of AAS should make absolutely sure she does not become pregnant during or immediately following a cycle, as this could permanently disfigure a developing female fetus. It is also important to mention that the absence of a menstrual cycle does not mean that ovulation is not occurring. Many female AAS users think that because their menstrual cycles have ceased, there is a reduced risk of pregnancy. Nothing could be further from the truth.

It appears at least anecdotally from the discussions on many female fitness message boards and chat rooms that the use of AAS by women for cosmetic purposes, particularly in figure and fitness shows as well as bodybuilding, is the fastest-growing AAS phenomenon in the U.S. Because of this, it is critically important that women are well informed of the short- and long-term, irreversible nature of some cosmetic side effects and the differences between various AAS. While the increase in muscle mass and strength, energy, and feelings of well-being combined with the loss of that stubborn female fat from the hips and buttocks is particularly appealing to many women in the physique culture, a 5cm clitoris and voice that makes James Earl Jones sound like a tenor is not. However, many women are blinded to these developing permanent side effects until it is too late. Furthermore, because of the mislabeling of black-market drugs, many women end up ingesting potent androgens (instead of more anabolic agents) that result in immediate and significant masculinizing side effects.

Steroid use can also affect the libido in both men and women. In fact, physicians may lawfully prescribe steroids medically for this purpose if circumstances warrant. For cosmetic users who cycle, however, it's common for the sex drive to heighten during a cycle but decrease toward the end and after. After the supplemental androgens are discontinued, the androgen blood levels drop before the testes can be "reawakened" and put back to work. The result is a post-cycle crash that can be quite traumatic. However, this effect can be minimized or avoided altogether with the administration of HCG and Nolvadex® or Clomid® to "jump-start" the body's natural production of testosterone. [Llewellyn, 2002; Di Pasquale, 1990]

Mechanisms of Adverse Effects

How else do excessive androgens adversely affect the body? Well, in the last chapter we talked about the steroid molecule as an "andro-van" that raced from one receptor road stop to the next until it broke down. What happens when it breaks down? It can be excreted in the urine, or it can be converted into other hormones or metabolites. This conversion takes place by an enzymatic process. Testosterone can be converted into a strong androgenic metabolite called dihydrotestosterone (DHT) that is primarily responsible for some of the more unpleasant androgenic effects of steroid use like male pattern baldness, acne, and prostate enlargement. Remember that muscle cells aren't the only place to find androgen receptor sites. There are also receptor sites in the scalp, skin, and prostate. While increasing protein synthesis in muscle, the same androgen messenger also binds to a receptor site in the hair follicles that may lead to male pattern baldness, in a sebaceous gland that may cause acne, and in the prostate gland that may cause it to enlarge or become inflamed (prostatitis). The occurrence and extent of these adverse effects depend upon the genetically predetermined concentration of androgen receptor sites in that particular area. Each individual is different. For example, while steroids won't always cause baldness, male pattern baldness can be worsened in those who already have a predisposition to it. Steroids with a high conversion rate to DHT, steroids that are derivatives of DHT, or highly androgenic steroids seem to be particularly responsible for this adverse effect, and reportedly should be avoided, although the effect can be partially controlled by the use of finasteride (Proscar® or Propecia®), a prescription drug which helps to block the conversion of testosterone to DHT. Note that not all anabolic steroids convert to DHT. For example, the popular steroid nandrolone decanoate converts to a metabolite called dihydronandrolone (DHN). Since DHN is a metabolite with a weaker binding affinity for the androgen receptor, it's been speculated that suppressing testosterone levels by taking nandrolone judiciously could theoretically have a *beneficial* effect on hair loss.

Regarding men, recent research suggests that the side effects of even highly androgenic compounds have been overstated. There were no significant side effects of 10 weeks of testosterone enanthate therapy at a dosage of 600mg per week (six times the replacement dose of this highly androgenic steroid and a dose typical of what many bodybuilders might use). [Bhasin et al., 1996] In a discouraging kick in the pants to natural athletes everywhere, study participants receiving the testosterone injections without any exercise at all enjoyed significantly greater increases in fat-free mass, arm size, and leg size than those who worked out hard but without the steroids. Other studies have also reported minimal significant androgenic side effects [Pope & Katz, 1994] including one involving the highly androgenic oral steroid oxymetholone. [Hengge et al., 1996] Despite what sometimes appear to be intentional efforts by researchers to obscure the bottom line, the conclusion on this topic is pretty much common sense. Analogize it to alcohol. By and large, 151-proof rum in massive quantities seems more prone to cause problems than light beers. By and large, highly androgenic oral steroids such as oxymetholone or Halotestin, especially in massive quantities, seem much more prone to cause problems than less androgenic steroids like methenolone or nandrolone. 'Nuff said.

There were no significant side effects of 10 weeks of testosterone enanthate therapy at a dosage of 600mg per week (six times the replacement dose of this highly androgenic steroid ... a dose typical of what many bodybuilders might use).

Adverse Effects of Excess Estrogens

There's also a whole 'nother problem associated with excess androgens. Remember those enzymes that can convert testosterone into DHT? Well, there are additional enzymes that can convert testosterone into *estrogen*. In other words, some of the men's hormones jump the net and play on the women's team. The process that converts testosterone to estrogen is called *aromatization*. Those anabolics that are easily aromatized into estrogen can cause a formation of breast tissue known as *gynecomastia*, sometimes called "bitch tits." While this problem is usually related to high doses, a genetic predisposition among some individuals for this condition can cause it to occur even at moderate dosages. Media reports suggest the growth of pontoon-like appendages that would make porn stars jealous, and the movie "Fight Club" threw fuel on the fire by portraying a character who formerly used steroids with breasts twice the size of Jenna Jameson's. What a joke! Actually, gynecomastia generally looks like swelling or puffiness on and around the nipple area, with accompanying sensitivity. It can happen naturally to teenagers or old folks even without the use of androgens. It's not unusual for only one side to be affected. The problem is often temporary, disappearing after cessation of a steroid cycle. It can often be treated or prevented entirely by the use of anti-estrogenic compounds, such as anastrozole (Arimidex®) at ¼ to 1mg daily, or tamoxifen citrate (Nolvadex®). Many bodybuilders use anti-estrogens throughout their anabolic cycle as a prophylactic measure and never have the problem. Once a serious cosmetic problem exists, however, minor surgery is usually required to correct it. Numerous professional bodybuilders, who are long-term, high-dose steroid users, have had this surgery [Phillips, 1991] and others obviously need it, as can be seen by a close inspection of many of today's contest lineups, including the 2002 Night of the Champions and 2002 Mr. Olympia contest.

Anabolic Steroids and the Prostate

Let's get back to that cantaloupe-sized prostate we were worrying about. Okay, I'm exaggerating, but the concern about androgens having an adverse effect on the prostate is legitimate. What does the medical literature say about it? While there is one case report of prostate cancer in a 40-year-old bodybuilder who reported using numerous androgens as well as somatotropin for about 20 years [Roberts & Essenhigh, 1986], *no* studies have shown an increased risk or incidence of prostatic cancer or hypertrophy with androgen use or indicated that androgens per se predispose to these conditions. [Swerdloff & Wang, 1993] Androgens are not the only or even the main causative factor in prostate cancer, as evinced by a case study in which a chronically testosterone-deficient man developed prostate cancer. [(Boccon et al., 1991] World Health Organization male contraceptive studies using up to 200mg per week for over a year show no evidence of prostate stimulation. [W.H.O., 1990] In one study, researchers examined the prostate effects of the administration for 15 weeks of up to 500mg of androgens per week to healthy men in their twenties and thirties. [Cooper et al., 1998] *No* changes in prostate size or serum prostate specific antigen (PSA) levels were detected either during or up to 25 weeks after the last dose. In another study, men treated with up to 600mg of testosterone enanthate for 20 weeks found no change in PSA values with treatment, or any correlation between the dose of testosterone and PSA levels. [Bhasin et al., 2001] So we certainly can't say with certainty that androgens cause prostate problems. If they do lead to prostatic hypertrophy, another intriguing possibility exists: the aromatization process. Teens have very high testosterone levels but very little prostate enlargement. Why? Maybe because it's not testosterone but the conversion of testosterone to *estrogen* that puts the prostate at greatest risk. [Shippen, 1998]

... *no* studies have shown an increased risk or incidence of prostatic cancer or hypertrophy with androgen use ...

Warning: this does not necessarily mean that much higher dosages, especially of highly androgenic compounds, might not adversely affect the prostate, especially in older men. While it is not known if men who have used steroids for prolonged periods will encounter more prostatic problems as they age, [Di Pasquale, 1990] "*most current medical studies show a poor correlation between testosterone levels and prostate disease of any kind.*" [Shippen, 1998 (emphasis in the original.)] Nevertheless, anyone with preexisting or undetected prostate cancer should not take anabolics, as they can cause rapid growth and the spread of existing prostate cancer. Thus, AAS users should have periodic digital exams and PSA levels checked – another reason why physicians should be involved in the use of AAS.

Anabolic Steroids and Aggressive/Psychiatric Symptoms

Picture a rabid junkyard dog, eyes bulging, mouth foaming, viciously attacking any and all passersby. That's what steroids will surely do to you, from what we read in the papers. The press frequently quotes a few misguided psychiatrists who'd have you believe that taking a single steroid tablet will instantly transform you from a mild-mannered Doctor Jekyll into a raging, psychotic Mr. Hyde. "'Roid rage" is the popular term for this juice-induced "spontaneous, highly aggressive, out-of-control behavior where the police either were called or should have intervened." [Yesalis & Cowart,1998]. Some researchers have suggested that psychiatric disorders occur with unusual frequency among athletes using anabolics. [Pope & Katz, 1988].

Don't buy into it. Most authorities regard the conclusions of these researchers with extreme skepticism. [*See* Street et al., 1996; Lubell, 1989 (Comments of Dr. James Wright and Dr. Charles Yesalis, 178)] Steroid-induced craziness is *far* from an epidemic. One review of the issue stated:

> "If ['roid rage] is real, it is relatively rare (probably less than 1 percent) among steroid users. Even among those affected, the impact of previous mental illness or abuse of other drugs is still unclear." [Yesalis & Cowart, 60,1998]

Other reviewers have noted that "Some long-time steroid users have never suffered any emotional instability, or anything more than transient physical effects" and that many steroid users describe *non-violent* feelings of euphoria, well-being and enhanced self-confidence as common effects. [Wright & Cowart, 1990] When such feelings occur, could it be because the better some people look, the better they feel about themselves? In one study to determine the psychiatric effects of AAS use on athletes, no significant differences could be found between users and non-users:

> "The fact that steroids have been used by tens of thousands if not hundreds of thousands of athletes over two decades and that behavioral effects are only recently being discovered (in small numbers) tend to support [that feelings of aggression may not be observed in the majority of steroid users]. Our findings are compatible with and complementary to those in anecdotal reports and data from individual psychiatrists." [Bahrke et al., 834-835, 1990]

A little different picture than the one the media have painted for you?

If the prevalence of 'roid rage is a media-fueled myth, what about simple heightened aggressiveness? Do steroids *cause* aggression? The most comprehensive examination of the relationship between testosterone or anabolic steroid use and aggression was conducted by Jack Darkes, Ph.D., an assistant professor of psychology and Director of Interventions, Alcohol and Substance Use Research Institute, at the University of South Florida. His exhaustive review of the literature concluded that the effects of the user's expectancy and various other factors make a one-to-one causal relationship *unlikely*, based on the literature. "The existing evidence does not support a simple relationship," he found. "There is no doubt that aggression occurs in some [steroid] users. Such aggression is real and can be harmful to users and those around them. But it is not, regardless of dose, inevitable in [steroid] users. No study reviewed reported, at any dose studied, that all participants reported aggression." [Darkes, 2000] One complicating factor is the issue of *who* takes anabolics to begin with. The literature suggests that steroid use is more likely to occur in individuals who are prone to take risks, seek excitement, and *behave aggressively*, a finding that is not surprising, given that taking them non-medically now requires breaking the law. Given anabolic steroids' popular reputation for causing aggression, such individuals might be even more drawn toward use and, once using, more likely to expect and display such effects. Their aggression likely has more to do with their *expectations* than with any direct physiological effect of anabolics. In other words, if you *expect* that anabolics will make you act aggressively, you'll be inclined to do so. Dr. Darkes has found that this model, in which individual personality and psychological differences influence drug use and its related behaviors, is consistent with findings in the steroid use literature [e.g., Bhasin et al., 2001; Yates et al. 1999]. He also suggests that the "advertising" of steroids' purported aggressive effects to the public may lead to the unintended consequence of *increasing* steroid-related aggression.

> ... if you *expect* that anabolics will make you act aggressively, you'll be inclined to do so.

Such learned expectations might also influence physiological responses linked to steroid use. For instance, increases in strength – an effect of anabolic steroid use considered to be largely physiological in nature – have been noted in experienced powerlifters who *believed* they had received steroids. [Maganaris et al., 2000] The increases largely disappeared in subjects who were later told the true nature of the treatment. The researchers concluded that, "... the beliefs of the lifters about the effectiveness of AAS appear to have been very successful at promoting an increase in their performance." Amazingly, subjects receiving placebo in a double-blind administration of testosterone reported higher levels of anger than those actually receiving testosterone. [Bjoerkqvist et al., 1994] These findings, along with other reviews of the literature on anabolics, mood, and aggression [e.g., Riem & Hursey, 1995; Sharp & Collins, 1998], suggest that *expectations* can influence both physiological and psychological responses to steroid administration.

Exactly what relationship androgens have to aggression is complex and largely speculative. Oddly, anabolic steroid supplementation (testosterone enanthate) may actually *decrease* irritability, anger, sadness, tiredness and nervousness, while increasing energy levels, friendliness, and good feelings in hypogonadal men. [Wang et al., 1995] An interesting theory about why a very small percentage of users experience aggressive behavior is that excess estrogens, not androgens, are the culprit. Because many anabolic steroids can be aromatized to estrogens, and estrogens elicit aggressive behavior [Finkelstein, 1997], "it is possible that the aromatization of anabolic-androgenic steroids in the brain may be responsible for the adverse behavioral problems observed in some steroid users." [Myhal, 2000]

> ... current evidence is not sufficient to draw cause-and-effect conclusions about adverse psychological side effects of using anabolic steroids, particularly in doses totaling less 1000mg/wk.

Not surprisingly, when psychiatric problems do occur in study subjects, there seems to be a direct correlation between dosage and prevalence of syndromes. For example, no significant psychiatric effects have been noted where the reported mean weekly dosage was 318mg (heaviest user was 620mg/wk). [Bahrke et al., 1992] Although it is likely that a small percentage of anabolic steroid users who take over 1000mg per week, "particularly those with preexisting psychopathologies, may experience adverse behavioral problems, there is no justification to conclude that the non-medical use of anabolic steroids represents a significant public health threat." [Myhal, 2000] Even in a study showing a dose-related correlation between steroid use and psychiatric effects, nearly 90% of light and moderate dosage users in this particular study exhibited *no mood disorder symptoms at all.* [Pope & Katz, 1994] "In summary, current evidence is not sufficient to draw cause-and-effect conclusions about adverse psychological side effects of using anabolic steroids, particularly in doses totaling less than 1000mg/wk." [Myhal, 2000]

What does it all mean, generally? It means that if you're a belligerent moron, steroids may make you a bigger one. That's probably to be expected. A guy who likes to throw his weight around at 200 pounds will like it even more when he weighs 250. If you have some hidden predisposition to flipping out and you take very large dosages, you're at higher risk for psychiatric problems, especially if you *expect* to have them. But don't expect juice use to be a legal scapegoat for bad behavior. Although the psychiatric effect that anabolics might have upon predisposed individuals has been tried as a defense in criminal cases [Lubell], a sampling of these cases reveals, generally, that such defenses were unsuccessfully raised. Except for very isolated instances, if you rage out, you ought to be prepared to accept the heat for it.

Anabolic Steroids and Psychological Dependence

Anabolics don't make you high. They don't make you see colors. They're not stimulants, depressants, hallucinogens, or narcotics and they don't impair your ability to operate a motor vehicle or machinery at work. It's been suggested that since testosterone fails to exhibit psychoactive properties, it does *not* meet the criteria as a psychoactive drug of abuse. [Fingerhood, et al., 1997]

> "All drugs that are subject to abuse and dependence share certain pharmacologic properties. [Jasinski & Henningfield, 1989] When given in single doses to substance abusers, they are psychoactive, producing acute changes in feeling, mood, thinking, and perception, some of which are liked. This study ... failed to demonstrate these effects for any of the three doses of testosterone." [Fingerhood et al., 62, 1997]

Nevertheless, there is some evidence that anabolic steroid use can lead to psychological dependence in certain individuals. Whether the dependence is due to chemical effects upon the brain, or simply because of the positive reinforcement occasioned by walking around with more beef than a cattle ranch, is unknown. Whatever the cause, the dependency issue may be the biggest concern about steroid use for those it affects. Stopping steroid use, especially after a prolonged cycle, typically results in a state of low endogenous testosterone levels. There can be a nasty stretch of time between the end of the cycle and the time when those lazy testicles get their shop back up and running. During this compromised period, retaining steroid-induced muscle gains can be difficult. For individuals with an inadequate sense of self, the loss of some portion of the steroid gains can be psychologically devastating to the ego. Interestingly, anecdotal reports of "withdrawal syndromes" following cessation of steroid use are mostly in bodybuilders, and are not seen in other athletes. Why might that be? Clinical studies have failed to describe "depressed moods or withdrawal symptoms following supraphysiologic doses of anabolic-androgenic steroids ... Thus, the exact cause of mood disturbances following the use of steroids in some individuals, particularly physique athletes, remains unclear." [Myhal, 2000 (citations omitted)] Again, the reports may well have everything to do with the psychology of the users themselves. Let's face it, although goals vary, if taking steroids is motivated by poor self-esteem or other skewed body image concerns and the individual sees or believes that anabolics have created his "ideal" body, then stopping use will be psychologically distressing. Such an individual is likely to continue or accelerate his use, or to start his next cycle sooner than planned. While these patterns are consistent with dependence and withdrawal, even bodybuilders who *don't* use steroids can exhibit the same patterns. For some natural trainers, missing a workout can cause distress, and a forced layoff of several days or weeks can be devastating. That's classic addictive behavior, folks.

In fact, the way some psychiatrists seem to see it, hardcore training is pathological in and of itself [e.g., Pope et al., 2000]. Harvard psychiatrist Skip Pope has devoted most of his professional life to researching steroid use by bodybuilders, and his theories have fueled many pseudoscientific anti-AAS media reports. His writings, including his co-authored work *The Adonis Complex* [Pope et al., 2000], have not only condemned AAS use, but also the psychological motivations behind bodybuilding itself. Musclemen who perceive themselves as too small are mentally ill – suffering from *muscle dysmorphia*, he contends, a sort of reverse anorexia where the patient's obsession with appearance and muscularity spins out of control into excessive exercise and steroid abuse. Women who rigidly adhere to high-calorie, high-protein, low-fat diets eaten at regularly scheduled intervals have been labeled as suffering from "eating disorder, bodybuilder type." To quote Jim Schmaltz, senior writer for *Flex* magazine, Pope and one of his cohorts "have taken a typical strict bodybuilding diet and redefined it as an eating disorder!" [Schmaltz, 2000] In jaw-dropping irony, Dr. Pope confesses to obsessive exercise himself, lifting weights six days a week for two hours a day and marking historical occasions by his workouts. [*See* "Never Too Buff," *Time*, April 24, 2000, 65] One can only speculate as to how the bizarre psychological twists of such researchers may affect the conclusions presented.

... the way some psychiatrists seem to see it, hardcore training is pathological in and of itself.

What is lacking in many studies on the psychological effects of steroids is simple common sense. This is particularly true as to withdrawal effects. Almost anyone who's achieved an impressive level of size and strength will be depressed if they regress. The more they've achieved, the more they may regress. Maybe the reason that depression is reportedly more common in steroid users is the simple fact that steroid users are more likely to develop to an impressive level of size and strength than non-steroid users. It seems somewhat obvious that it would be psychologically more devastating to go back to looking like an average Joe if you were a rock-solid 220 pounds and had the admiration of everyone in the gym, than if you were a modestly beefy 190 pounds. Individuals with weaker psychological constitutions or the proverbial "loose screws" are less likely to resist immediately resuming steroid use.

Further, as the goal of hardcore bodybuilders is not optimal muscle size, but *maximal* muscle size, dosages can become excessive. Muscular gains can become a slippery slope to abuse in some individuals. Many hardcore bodybuilders, juiced or not, really groove on the fact that others perceive them as "freaky." If you go from looking like Chris Rock to looking like The Rock, your gym peers and the girls on the Stairmasters may bathe you in adoration or incredulous silence. That's one heckuva lot of positive reinforcement to up those dosages and "wow" them even more. Many AAS users successfully use steroids intermittently and with moderation

– but not all of them. It's a sobering thought that there are some of you out there who start out on low risk, short-term cycles and ultimately end up using massive dosages for years of uninterrupted use. That's a bad thing. But the way I see it, the problem of dependence on steroids when it occurs in bodybuilders has less to do with the nature of the substance than with the psychological profile of those users. Sometimes what certain people see in the mirror doesn't reflect what others see when they look at them. The bigger the gap between the self-perception and the reality, the bigger the problem is. Is that you or someone you know? There may come a point when it's time to take a long, hard look at yourself and reevaluate your goals. Perhaps if a qualified medical professional were involved in the whole process, there would be a system of checks and balances that doesn't exist with underground AAS use. This is a chapter on the medical literature, not a lecture to those who may need it. Nevertheless, putting the legal prohibitions aside for a moment, allow me to quote a friend of mine. Bodybuilder/author Nelson Montana has a simple rule he advocates when steroid use reaches a gram of gear a week:

... the problem of dependence on steroids when it occurs in bodybuilders has less to do with the nature of the substance than with the psychological profile of those users.

> "Accept the fact that you've obtained far more muscle than you could have naturally and cut yourself off. If you try to continue beyond this point with ever increasing dosages, you may never make it back to a normal lifestyle. You may be bound for a life of dependency." [Montana, 2002]

Maybe that's advice worth thinking about?

Anabolic Steroids and Connective Tissue Injuries

Do steroids weaken tendons? It's been suggested that in conjunction with intense weight training, they can cause muscular adaptations that outpace adaptations by the connective tissues, leading to injuries. Anecdotally, numerous professional bodybuilders have torn muscles and connective tissues of the chest, arms, and knees. Pick up a copy of any hardcore bodybuilding magazine and you'll see what I mean. The reports suggest an unusual frequency and severity of injuries, often requiring surgical reattachment. But the medical literature supporting increased athletic injuries caused by anabolic steroid use is scant. [Di Pasquale, 1992] Given the number of AAS users, the number of muscle tendon ruptures is quite rare. [Street et al., 1996] Moreover, in light of the extreme degree of musculoskeletal stress imposed, it's not unreasonable to expect muscle and tendon tears in hardcore strength athletes, *regardless* of steroid use. Whether these injuries are steroid-related is as yet unknown. One animal study reported tendon degeneration, but several subsequent animal studies found no abnormalities and no decrease in tendon strength. In fact, studies show that some steroids, such as the anabolic steroid stanozolol, may actually *stimulate* collagen synthesis, which is likely to improve the health of tendons and ligaments. [Falanga et al., 1998]

There's only one study investigating the possible effects of steroids in human tendons. A 1998 British study sought to examine whether anabolics really do cause structural changes in the tendon. Specimens of ruptured human tendon from four patients were biopsied during surgical repair. Two of the subjects were anabolic steroid users and two were controls. No differences in collagen fibril ultrastructure could be seen using electron microscopy. [Evans et al., 1998] Future studies are needed to further examine this issue. Anecdotal reports of tendon ruptures in steroid users may be because the athlete's subjective sense of his own strength capabilities exceeds the tensile strength of his tendons. Another factor that may play a role is the polypharmacy engaged in by most bodybuilders. It's an open question as to what role might be played by diuretics, growth hormone or other drugs, in combination with each other or with anabolics. Lastly, there are case reports of hypogonadal athletes being more prone to injury; thus it's possible that the lifter is at increased risk for injury when coming off a cycle because of reduced testosterone and elevated cortisol levels. [Naessens, et al., 1994] Thus, by cutting back on training loads and properly reestablishing the HPTA following a cycle, the risk of muscle/tendon injury as a function of AAS use may be reduced.

... it's possible that the lifter is at increased risk for injury when coming off a cycle because of reduced testosterone and elevated cortisol levels.

Anabolics and Early Mortality

Although for many years the party line of the sports medicine community was to suggest that anabolic steroid use typically has deadly long-term consequences, there was never any proof of it. Today, many authorities concede that we really don't know much about the long-term effects of high-dose anabolic use. Massive amounts of anabolics may well have unknown long-term adverse effects. Animal studies have been conflicting, with mice given high-dose testosterone dying prematurely [Bronson et al., 1997], but hamsters given nandrolone living longer [Davis et al., 1993]. But there isn't a single reliable human study on it to be found.

When researchers have tried to look at human use retrospectively, they've screwed it up. A recent study conducted in Finland [Parssinen et al., 2000] attempted to compare 62 powerlifters, assumed to be steroid users, who competed between 1977 and 1982, to a control population of 1,000 men. While the mortality rate was higher for the powerlifters (12.9%) than for the control group (3.1%), the evidence is hardly compelling that anabolics had anything to do with it. First of all, we have no idea about what steroids (if any) the lifters were taking, and in what cycles or dosages. Further, it's been long known that larger, heavier individuals tend to have shorter life spans than thinner folks, regardless of anabolic use. Moreover, three of the eight deaths were by suicide, suggesting that some of the deaths have more to do with the psychology of the users than with steroids (a point made earlier). Aging powerlifters, like any athletes who fade from their former glory, may have a much harder time facing the advancing ravages of time. The fact that the control group was not composed of former non-steroid-using powerlifters, but rather of a general population, makes it impossible to put much stock in the study. So at this point we really don't know if anabolic steroid use diminishes life expectancy at all, or if so, to what degree. Maybe only massive quantities will have adverse effects, or maybe only prolonged usage, or maybe both.

Anecdotally, have we seen a massive die-off of elite bodybuilders from the 1960s and 1970s? Not at all. The great epidemic of cosmetic steroid deaths never came to pass. Most of the hysteria was unfounded, at least as it applied to use back then. However, let's be logical here. The dosages and cycling habits of bodybuilders thirty years ago are *very* different than those in the

1990s and today. Bodybuilders have pushed the envelope in every way possible, including the high-dose usage of ancillary drugs like growth hormone, injectable diuretics, insulin, and thyroid hormones. In 1997, a survey by Nick Evans, M.D., provided an in-depth analysis of the drug regimens of 100 bodybuilders in the United Kingdom. [Evans, 1997] The unsupervised, self-administered steroid dosages ranged from 250mg to 3,200mg per week. More than 20 different types of steroid were being used by the bodybuilders in this study, and nine out of every ten bodybuilders practiced polypharmacy, using multiple accessory drugs from a list of at least ten pharmaceuticals such as ephedrine, clenbuterol, growth hormone, insulin, thyroid hormone, and tamoxifen. The abuse of some these substances, individually or in combination with androgens and each other, may be far more hazardous than steroid use alone. This sort of complex polypharmacy may confound attempts at research, impairing the reliability of any future retrospective cohort studies on steroid use. If premature mortality is uncovered, how can we ever know what drug or combination of drugs may have caused it?

Other Adverse Effects of Anabolic Steroids

Many lay articles throw out the possibility of contracting AIDS as a possible consequence of steroid use. While it's theoretically possible that a vial of injectable steroids could be intentionally tainted with the HIV virus for whatever diabolical reasons, to my knowledge no such case has ever been reported. As a practical matter, the only way to contract the virus from steroid use would be through the sharing of needles. The ready availability of needles in most states makes needle sharing completely unnecessary. While there was an isolated case reported, no steroid user I've represented has ever reported this practice to me. From a societal standpoint, AIDS from unprotected sex presents an infinitely greater public health risk. Quite frankly, anyone who would even consider sharing needles with his gym buddies in this day and age is so irresponsible and judgment-impaired that I fear the substance of this entire chapter is lost on him.

One of the primary effects of our government's crackdown on legitimate anabolic steroids has been the expansion of a huge black market of foreign veterinary products and counterfeit substances. None of these products is made under the safety standards imposed by the FDA. Some are reportedly made under unsupervised and quite unsanitary conditions. [*See* Di Pasquale, 1995] Anecdotal reports have claimed abscesses and infections from some Mexican brands. Some products appear to be made by reliable pharmaceutical companies, but are actually counterfeit knock-offs of unknown origin. They may be contaminated with bacteria or other dangerous substances. One physician familiar with the issue said, "My colleagues at Mount Sinai Hospital in New York tell me they are treating many more athletes for side effects of counterfeit and bogus steroids than they did when reliable pharmacy-purchased steroids were available." [Allen, 1998 (Quoting Dr. Robert Price)] Prior to the current explosion of Mexican vet products, the majority of anabolics available on the black market were reportedly fakes. If the health dangers of real anabolic steroids have been overstated, the dangers of counterfeit anabolics may be understated. The problem is particularly serious because of how difficult it is to distinguish a real product from a counterfeit knock-off.

If the health dangers of real anabolic steroids have been overstated, the dangers of counterfeit anabolics may be understated.

How Reliable is the Research Condemning Steroids?

Several problems have plagued much of the past research into anabolic steroid effects. One big problem has been lack of funding. Who's going to foot the bill for steroid research? Decades of media reports about horrible steroid side effects and the enactment of the Anabolic Steroid Control Act stifled clinical interest in anabolic steroids as a therapeutic modality for a long time. Looking into the possible benefits of anabolic steroids by the big pharmaceutical companies was unheard of. Instead, what research there was focused on trying to prove adverse health effects to discourage potential users. [Myhal, 2000] If funding could be granted, perhaps the most enlightening research would be retrospective cohort studies examining the health, cancer prevalence and mortality statistics of professional bodybuilders from the 1950s, 1960s and 1970s. With studies like that, the long-term health ramifications of steroid use finally would be known and quantified. But proposals for modest grants to conduct such studies have been repeatedly *turned down*. Why? Wouldn't a strong anti-anabolics authority like the National Institute on Drug Abuse, a frequent sponsor of steroid research, be falling over itself to fund such a study? Not quite. And I think we can speculate as to why. A finding that there are generally little or *no* statistically significant long-term adverse effects of steroid use to healthy mature adult males with moderate dosages and intermittent use could be devastating to their scare tactics approach. It could rock the boat of our present national policy of criminalizing personal users of steroids. Don't expect a study like that any time soon.

... perhaps the most enlightening research would be retrospective cohort studies examining the health, cancer prevalence and mortality statistics of professional bodybuilders from the 1950s, 1960s and 1970s.

Another research barrier is that it's been considered unethical for researchers to administer the supraphysiologic dosages of anabolics necessary to simulate the use patterns of the muscle world. So, much of the literature that has reported adverse reactions associated with anabolics has come from the *medical* use of androgens. [Street et al., 1996] Most of the subjects were geriatric patients who were extremely old and sick to begin with. Are the effects of anabolics on your ancient Aunt Clara in her final days at the nursing home really relevant to a healthy elite powerlifter? When bodybuilders have been study subjects, the studies have been stuck with users *self-reporting* their unconfirmed histories of dosages and duration of use, rather than any controlled administration by the researchers. How reliable is that? Other than isolated case studies of athletes who got sick, most of these subjects were volunteers. Non-medical use of anabolics can generally be prosecuted. People who unabashedly volunteer for studies on their steroid use are probably pretty non-typical. They may be very different from people who use steroids more secretly, both in terms of psychological profile and usage patterns. Many experts in the field have criticized the reliability of this methodology.

Only in the years since the Anabolic Steroid Control Act went into effect have researchers begun to administer more substantial dosages for short-term periods, simulating the moderate-dose anabolic cycles used in the real world. [*See* e.g., Bhasin et al., 1996; Hengge et al., 1996; Bhasin, et al., 2001] These studies are generally *not* finding the serious health problems past research would have suggested. A landmark 1996 study, for example, found virtually no adverse effects when anabolic steroids were administered at a dosage of 600mg per week (about six times natural replacement dose) for ten weeks. [Bhasin, 1996] A 1999 study found anabolic steroids up to 500mg per week "appear to have minimal risk of adverse psychosexual effects in the majority of normal men." [Yates et al., 1999] Further, studies examining steroids in the context of anti-aging or age management therapies and in the treatment of HIV-related wasting disorders have been quite positive. Perhaps these findings will re-ignite the interest of Big Pharmacy to pony up some research grants. As the collective testosterone levels of America's aging Baby Boomer generation continue to plummet, it seems increasingly obvious that American pharmaceutical companies have missed the boat. Better and more publicized research demonstrating the safety and efficacy of anabolics for age management could have an explosive effect on the tiny niche market presently held by Androgel®, opening vistas of possibility for new hormonal products for aging men.

Summing It Up

While steroids can have adverse side effects, including serious ones, the scientific literature is far less conclusive about use in mature adults, particularly adult males, than is claimed by the sports establishment and government anti-drug officials. When you actually examine the studies, the findings are often substantially different from what gets reported to the mainstream media. And all too often, the research itself has been questionable at best. One major flaw in most steroid research is the failure to differentiate between *types* of anabolic steroids. Steroids are steroids, as far as the researchers' conclusions are concerned. As we've seen, nothing could be farther from the truth, particularly with respect to the effects on cholesterol, liver function, and possibly even psychological effects. Since cholesterol and liver problems result almost exclusively from C-17 alpha alkylated oral steroids, studies that generalize these effects to *all* anabolics are misleading at best.

Despite a virtually one-sided presentation in the lay press, the position that anabolic steroids are such dangerous substances to healthy adults as to warrant government enforcement tactics is surprisingly weak. The actual risk levels for mature adult males using steroids are related to various factors, such as the dosages and duration of use, the specific types of compounds administered, the existence of any preexisting pathologies, etc. It can be concluded that "[a]s used by most athletes, the side effects of anabolic steroid use appear to be minimal." [Di Pasquale, 1990] Despite over 50 years of use by athletes, "there is little evidence to show that their use will cause long-term detriment" and "the administration of moderate doses (200-300mg/week for 6 to 12 weeks once per year) of an injectable androgen, such as testosterone enanthate or nandrolone decanoate, in healthy adult males could induce positive changes on body composition and athletic performance with little or no side effects." [Street et al., 1996] Although many users are now well into middle age, we have yet to hear reports of an epidemic of steroid-related deaths. A review of the medical literature does *not* support the depiction of a serious health crisis related to anabolic steroids.

Despite over 50 years of use by athletes, "there is little evidence to show that their use will cause long-term detriment" ...

In researching an article I was writing, I once called a physician who is a frequent media spokesman about the medical consequences of steroid abuse. When he heard I was a journalist, he must have tripped over himself running to the phone. He began rattling off the many dangers of anabolics, dropping his words like pearls for me to marvel at. I fully conceded that drug-tested athletes and teenagers should be discouraged and prevented from using steroids, but began asking more pointed questions about mature adult use. I challenged his characterizations of the literature on liver function, cardiac problems, prostate problems, and psychiatric disturbances. He seemed stunned to find a journalist who wasn't simply writing down everything he said. I'm not sure a skilled cross-examiner with knowledge of the subject matter had ever questioned him. "But steroids can be dangerous for you if abused," he insisted. "Agreed," I said, "but so can tobacco and alcohol. In fact, their dangers have been *conclusively proven and seem to be considerably worse*, but mature adults aren't being arrested for using them." "Who are you, again?" he asked at one point. He grew increasingly uncomfortable, ultimately retreating to the shaky position that the true danger of anabolics is that we really don't know the long-term effects, which might be devastating. I countered, "How can a society justify a policy that locks people up – devastating their lives, here and now – for using something about which, by your own admission, we really don't know the long-term effects?" He didn't answer. I don't expect he has one.

Despite what's written here, it's likely that those within the government or the sports community with anti-anabolics agenda will resist enlightenment and continue to attempt to undermine any unbiased consideration of the case against steroids. I'll end this chapter with a true story about a call I received from a terrified Maryland man. The U.S. Customs Mail Division had intercepted a small package addressed to him purportedly containing anabolic steroids. He received a telephone call from a local detective assigned to a federal task force on drug parcels. For twenty minutes, she threatened and berated him, leaving him with the fear that he'd be under constant surveillance and might be arrested. He was a married man with a good job, and he was so terrified that he asked me to investigate whether the caller was legitimate. I was able to contact her, and the ensuing conversation was remarkable.

She proudly told me that she had arrested or helped arrest many men for personal use steroid offenses. She told me that she was a crusader, and that her work was saving lives. She launched into an impassioned diatribe on the consequences of using anabolics, reciting a list of terrible, deadly side effects. When she had finished, I commended her for her enthusiasm. I asked how she had acquired her information, and whether she had read the body of medical literature on the subject. She hadn't read a word of it. I told her I was curious to hear more about her views. She told me that steroids had killed Lyle Alzado. I asked her, "How many other steroid users have died from T-cell lymphoma?" She didn't know of any. I suggested the extremely strong probability that *something else* killed Mr. Alzado, and mentioned the associations of that form of cancer with immune disorders having no relationship to steroids at all. I then presented my own perspective on anabolic health risks in robust and extensive detail. When I finished, she seemed stupefied. I gently inquired whether some of those men she arrested might have been hurt more by *her* actions than by the effects of the steroids. Some might have lost their jobs, and some of their families may have suffered. She was silent.

She told me that steroids had killed Lyle Alzado. I asked her, "How many other steroid users have died from T-cell lymphoma?"

Looking back, it is terrifying that a person so cloaked in ignorance would be in a position to do so much harm. Even scarier, most Americans would still agree with her – but hopefully not for long.

Reference Sources

Allen, B. Steroid-using athletes and liver function. *MuscleMag International* 191 (May), 129, 1998.

Almekinders, L.C. Anti-inflammatory treatment of muscular injuries in sport; an update of recent studies. *Sports Med* 28(6):383-388, 1999.

Antonio, J. The Iron Egghead: steroid abusers. *Flex* 16 (3)(May), 240, 1998 citing *Eur Heart J* 17:1576-1583, 1996.

Antonio, J., Street, C. Androgen use by athletes: A reevaluation of the health risks. *Can J Appl Physiol* 21(6):421-440, 1996.

Bahrke, M.S., Wright, J.E., O'Connor, J.S. et al. Selected psychological characteristics of anabolic-androgenic steroid users. *N Engl J Med* 323(12):834-835, 1990.

Bahrke, M.S., Wright, J.E., Strauss, R.H. et al. Psychological moods and subjectively perceived behavioral and somatic changes accompanying anabolic-androgenic steroid users. *Am J Sports Med* 20:717, 1992

Bhasin, S., Storer, T.W., Berman N. et al. The effects of supraphysiologic doses of testosterone on muscle size and strength in normal men. *N Engl J Med* 335:1-7, 1996.

Bhasin, S., Woodhouse, L, Casaburi, R. et al. Testosterone dose-response relationships in healthy young men. *Am J Physiol (Endocrinol Metab)* 281(6):E1172-E1181, 2001.

Boccon, G.L., Dauge, M.C. et al. Prostate cancer in a 75-year-old man after four decades of testosterone androgen deprivation. *Eur Urol* 20(1):81-88, 1991.

Bjorkqvist, K., Nygren, T., Bjorklund, A.C. et al. Testosterone intake and aggressiveness: real effect or anticipation. *Aggressive Behavior 20:*17-26, 1994.

Bronson, F.H., Matherne, C.M. Exposure to anabolic-androgenic steroids shortens life span of male mice. *Med Sci Sports Exerc* 29:615-619, 1997.

Brower, K. "Anabolic steroids: Potential for physical and psychological dependence." In *Anabolic Steroids in Sports and Exercise*, edited by C.E. Yesalis. Champaign: Human Kinetics, 1993.

Charmandari E., Dittany, M.T., Perry, L.A. et al. Kinetics and effect of percutaneous administration of dihydrotestosterone in children. *Horm Res* 56(5-6):177-181, 2001.

Chen, Y., Fervenza, F.C., Rabkin, R. Growth factors in the treatment of wasting in kidney failure. *J Ren Nutr* 11(2):62-66, 2001.

Cooper, C.S., et al. Effect of exogenous testosterone on prostate volume, serum, and semen prostate specific antigen levels in healthy young men. *J Urol* 159(2):441-443, 1998.

Darkes J. The psychological effects of anabolic/androgenic steroids [On-line]. Parts I-IV, 2000. Available www.musclemonthly.com/author/jack-darkes.htm.

Davis, W.M., Long, S.F., Lin, T.L. Nandrolone decanoate reduces the premature mortality of cardiomyopathic hamsters. *Res Commun Chem Pathol Pharmacol* 81:21-32, 1993.

Dickerman, R.D., McConathy, W.J., Zachariah, N.Y. Testosterone, sex hormone-binding globulin, lipoproteins, and vascular disease risk. *J Cardiovasc Risk* 4(5-6):363-366, 1997.

Dickerman, R.D., Pertusi, R.M., Zachariah, N.Y. et al. Anabolic steroid-induced hepatotoxicity: Is it overstated? *Clin J Sport Med* 9(1):34-39, 1999.

Dickerman, R.D., Schaller, F., McConathy, W.J. Left ventricular wall thickening does occur in elite power athletes with or without anabolic steroid use. *Cardiology* 90(2):145-148, 1998.

Di Pasquale, M.G. *Anabolic Steroid Side Effects: Facts, Fiction, and Treatment*. Warkworth, Ontario: M.G.D. Press, 1990.

Di Pasquale, M.G. Does the use of anabolic steroids increase athletic injuries? *Drugs in Sports* 1(3) (August), 1992.

Di Pasquale, M.G. Black market drugs. *Anabolic Research Review* 1(1), 1995.

Duchaine, D. *Underground Steroid Handbook II*. Venice, CA: HLR Technical Books, 1989.

Eriksson, L.S., Broome, U., Kalin, M. et al. Hepatotoxicity due to repeated intake of low doses of paracetamol. *J Intern Med* 231:567, 1992.

Evans, N.A., Bowrey, D.J., Newman, G.R. Ultrastructural analysis of ruptured tendon from anabolic steroid users. *Injury* 29(10):769-773, 1998.

Evans, N.A. Gym and tonic: A profile of 100 male steroid users. *Br J Sports Med* 31:54-58, 1997.

Falanga, V., Greenberg, A.S., et al. Stimulation of collagen synthesis by the anabolic steroid stanozolol. *J Invest Dermatol* 111(6):1193-1197, 1998.

Fineschi, V., Baroldi, G., Monciotti, F. et.al. Anabolic steroid abuse and cardiac sudden death. *Arch Pathol Lab Med* 125(2):253-255, 2001.

Fingerhood, M.I., Sullivan, J.T., Testa, M. et al. Abuse liability of testosterone. *J Psychopharmacol* 11:59-63, 1997.

Finkelstein, J.W., Susman, E.J., Chinchilli, V.M. et al. Estrogen or testosterone increases self-reported aggressive behaviors in hypogonadal adolescents. *J Clin Endocrinol Metab* 82:2423-2438, 1997.

Friedl, K.E. Reappraisal of the health risks associated with the use of high doses of oral and injectable androgenic steroids. In *Anabolic Steroid Abuse*, edited by G.C. Lin and L. Erinoff. Washington, D.C.: U.S. Government Printing Office, 1990.

Friedl, K.E. Effects of anabolic steroids on physical health. In *Anabolic Steroids in Sport and Exercis.* edited by C.E. Yesalis. Champaign: Human Kinetics, 1993.

Goldman, R. *Death in the Locker Room: Steroids & Sports.* South Bend: Icarus Press, 1984.

Grunding, P., Bachmann, M. *World Anabolic Review 1996.* Houston: MB Muscle Books, 1995.

Habscheid, W., Abele, U., Dahm, H.H. Severe cholestasis with kidney failure from anabolic steroids in a body builder. *Dtsch Med Wochenschr* 124(36):1029-1032, 1999.

Hage, J. J., Dekker, J .J., Karim, R. B. et al., Ovarian cancer in female-to-male transsexuals: report of two cases. *Gynecol Oncol* 76(3):413-415, 2000.

Harding, H.R. et al. The anti-catabolic activity of anabolic steroids based on the suppression of cortisone acetate (Eac) induction of liver tryptophan pyrrolase. *VIth Pan American Congress on Endocrinology*. Mexico, 1965.

Haupt, H.A. Anabolic steroids and growth hormone. *Am J Sports* Med 21(3):468, 1993.

Haupt, H.A., Rovere, G.D. Anabolic steroids: A review of the literature. *Am J Sports Med* 12(6):469, 1984.

Hengge, U.R., et al. Oxymetholone promotes weight gain in patients with advanced human immunodeficiency virus (HIV-1) infection. *BR J Nutr* 75:129-138, 1996.

Jasinski, D.R., Henningfield, J.E. Human abuse liability assessment by measurement of subjective and physiological effects. *NIDA Res Monogr* 92:73-100, 1989.

Johansen, K.L., Mulligan, K., Schambelan, M. Anabolic effects of nandrolone decanoate in patients receiving dialysis: A randomized controlled trial. *JAMA* 281(14):1275-1281, 1999.

Johnson, C.A. Use of androgens in patients with renal failure. *Semin Dial* 13(1):36-39, 2000.

Kosaka, A., Takahashi, H., Yajima, Y. et al. Hepatocellular carcinoma associated with anabolic steroid therapy: Report of a case and review of the Japanese literature. *J Gastroenterol* 31(3):450-454, 1996.

Korkia, P., Stimson, G.V. Indications of prevalence, practice, and effects of anabolic steroid use in Great Britain. *Int J Sports Med* 18:557-562, 1997.

Llewellyn, W. *Anabolics 2002*. Patchogue, NY: Molecular Nutrition, 2002.

Lubell, A. Does steroid abuse cause – or excuse – violence? *The Physician and Sportsmedicine* 17(2) 176-185, 1989.

Matsumoto, A.M., Paulsen, C.A., Hopper, B.R. et al. Human chorionic gonadotropin and testicular function: Stimulation of testosterone, testosterone precusors, and sperm production despite high estradiol levels. *J Clin Endocrinol Metab* 56:720-728, 1983.

Maganaris, C.M., Collins, D., Sharp, M. Expectancy effects and strength training: Do steroids make a difference? *Sport Psychologist* 14: 272-278, 2000.

McNutt, R.A. et al. Acute myocardial infarction in a 22-year-old world class weight lifter using anabolic steroids. *Am J Cardiol* 62:164, 1988.

Montana, N. *The Bodybuilding Truth: Secrets You're Not Supposed to Know*. New York: 2002. Available at www.nelsonmontana.com.

Myhal, M. Lamb, D.R. Hormones as performance-enhancing drugs. In Warren, M. P. and Constantini, N.W., eds. *Sports Endocrinology*. Totowa, NJ: Humana Press, 2000.

Nakao, A., Sakagami, K., Nakata, Y. et al. Multiple hepatic adenomas caused by long-term administration of androgenic steroids for aplastic anemia in association with familial adenomatous polyposis. *J Gastroenterol* 35(7):557-562, 2000.

Naessens, G., De Slypere, J.P., Dijs, H. et al. Hypogonadism as a cause of recurrent muscle injury in a high level soccer player. *Int J Sports Med* 16(6):413-417, 1994.

Parssinen, M., Kujala, U. et al. Increased premature mortality of competitive powerlifters suspected to have used anabolic agents. *Int J Sports Med* 21:225-227, 2000.

Patel, F. The fatal paracetamol dosage–how low can you go? *Med Sci Law* 32:303, 1992.

Perry, P.J., Andersen, K.H., Yates, W.R. Illicit anabolic steroid use in athletes. *Am J Sports Med* 18(4):422, 1990.

Phillips, W.N. *Anabolic Reference Guide Sixth Edition.* Golden,CO: Mile High Publishing, 1991.

Pope, H.G., Katz, D.L. Affective and psychotic symptoms associated with anabolic steroid use. *Am J Psychiatry* 145(4):487-490, 1988.

Pope, H.G., Katz, D.L. Psychiatric and medical effects of anabolic-androgenic steroid use. *Arch Gen Psychiatry* 51:375-382, 1994.

Pope, H.G., Phillips, K.A., Olivardia, R. *The Adonis Complex: The Secret Crisis of Male Body Obsession*. New York: Free Press, 2000.

Prescott, L.F. Liver damage with non-narcotic analgesics. *Med Toxicol* 1 Supp(1):44, 1986.

Riem, K.E., Hersey, K.G. Using anabolic-androgenic steroids to enhance physique and performance: Effects on mood and behavior. *Clinical Psychology Review* 15 235-256, 1995.

Roberts, J., Essenhigh, D. Adenocarcinoma of prostate in 40-year-old body-builder. *Lancet* 2:742, 1986.

Sader, M.A., Griffiths, K.A., McCredie, R.J. et al. Androgenic anabolic steroids and arterial structure and function in male bodybuilders. *J Am Coll Cardiol* 37(1):224-230, 2001.

Schmaltz, J. Nuts to all of you. *Flex* 18(3) (May), 175-178, 2000.

Shapiro, J., Christiana, J., Frishman, W.H. Testosterone and other anabolic steroids as cardiovascular drugs. *Am J Ther* 6(3):167-174, 1999.

Sharp, M., Collins, D. Exploring the "inevitability" of the relationship between anabolic-androgenic steroid use and aggression in human males. *Journal of Sport and Exercise Psychology* 20:379-394,1998.

Shippen, E. Fryer, W. *The Testosterone Syndrome*. New York: M. Evans and Co., 1998.

Street, C., Antonio, J., Cudlipp, D. Androgen use by athletes: A reevaluation of the health risks. *Can J Appl Physiol* 21(6):421-440, 1996.

Swerdloff, R.S., Wang, C. Androgen deficiency and aging in men. *West J Med* 159:579-585, 1993.

Taylor, W.N. *Anabolic Steroids and the Athlete*. Jefferson: McFarland & Co., 1982.

Tenover, J.S. Androgen administration to aging men. *Endocrinol Metab Clin North Am* 23:877-892, 1994.

Wang, C., Alexander, G., Berman, N., et al. Effect of testosterone replacement therapy on mood changes in hypogonadal men. *J Clin Endocrinol Metab* 81(10):3578-3583, 1996.

Wecksler, M.E. Hormone replacement for men: Has the time come? *Geriatrics* 50(10):52-55, 1995.

Welder. A.A., Robertson, J.W., Melchert, R.B. Toxic effects of anabolic-androgenic steroids in primary rat hepatic cell cultures. *J Pharmacol Toxicol Methods* 33(4):187-195, 1995.

W.H.O. (World Health Organization) Task Force on Methods For the Regulation of Male Fertility. Contraceptive efficacy of testosterone-induced azoospermia in normal men. *Lancet* 336:955-959, 1990.

Wright, J.E., Cowart, V.S. *Anabolic Steroids: Altered States*. Carmel: Benchmark Press, 1990.

Yates, W.R., Perry, P.J., MacIndoe, J. et al. Psychosexual effects of three doses of testosterone cycling in normal men. *Biol Psychiatry* 45:254-260, 1999.

Yesalis, C.E., Cowart, V.S. *The Steroids Game*. Champaign: Human Kinetics, 1998.

Yesalis, C.E., Kennedy, N.J., Kopstein, A.N. et al. Anabolic-androgenic steroid use in the United States. *JAMA* 270(10):1217, 1993.

Zgliczynski, S., Ossowski, M., Slowinska-Srednicka, J. et al. Effect of testosterone replacement therapy on lipids and lipoproteins in hypogonadal and elderly men. *Atherosclerosis* 121(1):35-43, 1996.

Zmuda, J.M., Cauley, J.A., Kriska, A. et al. Longitudinal relation between endogenous testosterone and cardiovascular disease risk factors in middle-aged men. A 13- year follow-up of former Multiple Risk Factor Intervention Trial participants. *Am J Epidemiol* 146(8):609-617, 1997.

Chapter 4

MAKING A FEDERAL CASE OUT OF IT

"If we were brought to trial for the crimes we have committed against ourselves, few would escape the gallows."

— *Paul Eldridge (1888 –1982)*

What happens if you get arrested for steroids by federal law enforcement? What can they charge you with and how much prison time could you get? If you're taking anabolic steroids, or even thinking about it, you ought to know. You should know *before* you order gear online or bring some back from your Mexican vacation. You'd sure better know before you share anabolics with a gym buddy.

If you're like most people, doing jail time is your primary concern about getting busted for anything, including anabolics. That's hardly surprising. But most people don't realize that regardless of incarceration – and often even regardless of conviction – just being prosecuted for a steroid (or any other drug) offense can have a serious and lasting impact on your life.

Drew, 23, had been selling steroids for about three years. He was also taking them, and at 6'4" he was one big boy. He was a rather unsuccessful day trader of stocks and was also taking college classes part-time, hoping to return to full-time school the following semester on a college loan. A government informer [see Chapter 10] who had his own criminal charges pending against him met with DEA agents and snitched on Drew. The DEA arranged for the snitch to contact Drew on his cell phone and negotiate a juice sale. The conversation was recorded. Drew agreed to sell 90 bottles (testosterone and nandrolone) and 1,000 tablets (fluoxymesterone) for a bit over $3,700.

The meeting took place on a corner in upper Manhattan and was observed by DEA agents. As they saw Drew hand the packages to the snitch, the agents moved in for the arrest. They threw Drew to the ground, handcuffed him, and brought him to DEA offices. After interrogation, he gave a statement admitting that he had sold the informer steroids on previous occasions, but then (a bit too late) said he wanted to speak to a lawyer, and all questioning ceased. Of course, by that time they already had his incriminating statements.

Drew was brought before a federal magistrate in the Southern District of New York and released on a $50,000 personal recognizance bond with one co-signer and pre-trial supervision (a court program that monitors a defendant while his case is pending and generally requires weekly contact. While a case is pending, conditions of pre-trial release can prohibit travel outside certain areas. A client may have to surrender his passport and request specific approval from the court to travel outside the jurisdiction.) He was charged with violating §§ 812, 841(a)(1) and 841(b)(1)(d) of Title 21 of the United States Code. He faced a maximum sentence of five years in prison, but how much time would he really get? And how might the case affect the course of his life?

In most states, both state and federal laws prohibit the possession or distribution of anabolic steroids, and a person can be prosecuted under either or both. It's rare to see the same basic conduct charged in both state and federal court. It's usually one or the other. The choice depends somewhat on what agency is responsible for the arrest, and on the seriousness of the charges. If the local police arrest you for simple possession (as in a car stop), you're almost sure to be charged in state court. If your arrest arises out of an investigation by federal authorities (such as the U.S. Postal Inspector or DEA), or you are stopped by U.S. Customs at an international airport or border, there's certainly a basis to charge you in federal court. Much more often than not, however, the case will go to state court anyway. Many busy federal prosecutors have declined to handle low-level AAS cases that fall below certain quantity guidelines, although some reports say that's changing now. (A few U.S. Attorneys in Mexican border jurisdictions will take anything that comes their way). But for those AAS cases that find their way to federal court, this is the definitive treatment on the topic!

To understand steroids in the federal courts, the place to start is the United States Code (U.S.C.). It's where you'll find all the laws, called statutes, passed by our legislators on Capitol Hill. The Code is divided into Titles, each of which may have various chapters, subchapters, sections and subsections. The federal statutes contain the penalties for crimes, including steroid crimes. The statutes provide ranges and set maximum sentences.

The Code of Federal Regulations (C.F.R.) is a publication established by Act of Congress (44 U.S.C. § 1510). It represents a compilation of all the regulations issued by federal administrative agencies, such as the Food and Drug Administration and the Drug Enforcement Administration, that have "general applicability and legal effect." In other words, they have the force of law. Federal statutes furnish the authority and the limits for regulations that appear in the C.F.R. This means that the regulations on a subject should be read together with any pertinent portions of the U.S. Code.

The ranges for maximum sentences under federal law are pretty wide, and concerns about inconsistent sentencing nationwide led to the creation of the United States Sentencing Guidelines (U.S.S.G. or "federal guidelines"), initially submitted to Congress in April 1987, which impose strict parameters on judges' discretion. The federal guidelines are often the critical factor in determining what the actual length of a sentence will be.

There are federal statutes, federal regulations, and federal guidelines that impact upon the possession and distribution of anabolic steroids. You're going to learn about all of them, and see how they actually work in practice. This is pretty complicated stuff, especially when we get to the guidelines, so hold on tight.

Federal Statutes: Definitions

As we've discussed, Congress passed the Anabolic Steroid Control Act of 1990, Pub. L. No. 101-647, Sec. 1902, 104 Stat. 4851 (1990), effectively making their use criminal without a valid prescription. It did this by amending 21 U.S.C. § 812(c), which contains the initial schedules of controlled substances (revised schedules are published in the Code of Federal Regulations, Part 1308 of Title 21, Food and Drugs). Anabolic steroids are listed under subsection (e) of Schedule III. The law took effect in 1991, ninety days after it was passed on November 29, 1990, and applies across the whole country. It places steroids in the same legal class as barbiturates, ketamine, LSD precursors, and narcotic painkillers such as Vicodin. Anabolic steroids are the only hormones in the schedules.

Now that *we* know what anabolic steroids are (see Chapter 2), let's see what the *government* says they are. Under 21 U.S.C. § 802(41)(A):

> "The term 'anabolic steroid' means any drug or hormonal substance, chemically and pharmacologically related to testosterone (other than estrogens, progestins, and corticosteroids) that promotes muscle growth, and includes – (i) boldenone, (ii) chlorotestosterone, (iii) clostebol, (iv) dehydrochlormethyltestosterone, (v) dihydrotestosterone, (vi) drostanolone, (vii) ethylestrenol, (viii) fluoxymesterone, (ix) formebulone, (x) mesterolone, (xi) methandienone, (xii) methandranone, (xiii) methandriol, (xiv) methandrostenolone, (xv) methenolone, (xvi) methyltestosterone, (xvii) mibolerone, (xviii) nandrolone, (xix) norethandrolone, (xx) oxandrolone, (xxi) oxymesterone, (xxii) oxymetholone, (xxiii) stanolone, (xxiv) stanozolol, (xxv) testolactone, (xxvi) testosterone, (xxvii) trenbolone, and (xxviii) any salt, ester, or isomer of a drug or substance described or listed in this paragraph, if that salt, ester, or isomer promotes muscle growth."

It's interesting to look at how Congress drafted the definition. They chose a variety of chemicals that, other than being similar in structure and pharmacology to testosterone, are lumped together because they supposedly have one characteristic in common: *they promote muscle growth*. There's nothing explicitly in the statute about physical health risks, psychiatric adverse effects or addictive potential. Not one word. That wasn't the focus of Congress at all. *Muscle building* was the terrible evil to be avoided, so much so that it's mentioned not once but *twice*. It appears again at the end of the section, as a catchall provision for any other testosterone-related drugs or hormonal substances that share this apparently dangerous and forbidden characteristic. (The wording of the statute is consistent with the real motivation for scheduling anabolics, as revealed in Chapter 1).

Muscle building was the terrible evil to be avoided, so much so that it's mentioned not once but *twice*.

It's interesting if not alarming to note how little Congress knew about the substances being scheduled. The list contains items that are just alternate names for other listed items. Methandrostenolone and methandienone are one and the same, as are dihydrotestosterone and stanolone, and chlorotestosterone and clostebol. Formebolone is misspelled as formebulone. The list also includes at least one substance, testolactone, which reportedly has no substantial anabolic or androgenic properties. Yet in over a decade, nobody's bothered to correct the statute.

Now let's look at the subparagraph that deals with veterinary implants. Subparagraph (B) of § 802(41) provides an exemption for cattle implants, but not if they are prescribed, dispensed, or distributed for human use (see Federal Regulations below for more on cattle implants):

> (B) (i) Except as provided in clause (ii), such term does not include an anabolic steroid which is expressly intended for administration through implants to cattle or other nonhuman species and which has been approved by the Secretary of Health and Human Services for such administration.
>
> (ii) If any person prescribes, dispenses, or distributes such steroid for human use, such person shall be considered to have prescribed, dispensed, or distributed an anabolic steroid within the meaning of subparagraph (A).

Federal Statutes: Prohibited Acts

Simple Possession of Anabolic Steroids

Restrictions on controlled substances are authorized under 21 U.S.C. § 801. If you simply possess anabolic steroids without a prescription without any intent to sell or distribute, what federal law have you broken? You're in violation of 21 U.S.C. § 844, and a conviction is punishable by a term of imprisonment of up to one year and/or a minimum fine of $1,000, and prior state or federal drug convictions will up the exposure. The law reads like this:

> 21 U.S.C. § 844. Penalties for simple possession
> (a) Unlawful acts; penalties
> It shall be unlawful for any person knowingly or intentionally to possess a controlled substance unless such substance was obtained directly, or pursuant to a valid prescription or order, from a practitioner, while acting in the course of his professional practice [or except as otherwise authorized] ... Any person who violates this subsection may be sentenced to a term of imprisonment of not more than 1 year, and shall be fined a minimum of $1,000, or both, except that if he commits such offense after a prior [drug] conviction ... he shall be sentenced to a term of imprisonment for not less than 15 days but not more than 2 years, and shall be fined a minimum of $2,500, except, further, that if he commits such offense after two or more prior [drug] convictions ... he shall be sentenced to a term of imprisonment for not less than 90 days but not more than 3 years, and shall be fined a minimum of $5,000.... The imposition or execution of a minimum sentence required to be imposed under this subsection shall not be suspended or deferred ...

Distribution of Anabolic Steroids and Possession With Intent

Now, what about dealing anabolics? Distributing, dispensing or manufacturing anabolic steroids, or possessing them with intent to distribute, dispense or manufacture is a federal felony. Under 21 U.S.C. § 841(b)(1)(D), a convicted offender is punishable by up to five years in prison for steroid distribution, or ten years for a prior drug offender.

> 21 U.S.C. § 841. Prohibited acts A
> (a) Unlawful acts
> Except as authorized by this subchapter, it shall be unlawful for any person knowingly or intentionally –
> (1) to manufacture, distribute, or dispense, or possess with intent to manufacture, distribute, or dispense, a controlled substance;
> (b) Penalties
> Except as [otherwise provided], any person who violates subsection (a) of this section shall be sentenced as follows:
> ... (D) In the case of ... any controlled substance in schedule III ... such person shall ... be sentenced to a term of imprisonment of not more than 5 years, a fine not to exceed the greater of that authorized in accordance with the provisions of

> Title 18 or $250,000 if the defendant is an individual or $1,000,000 if the defendant is other than an individual, or both. If any person commits such a violation after a prior conviction for a felony drug offense has become final, such person shall be sentenced to a term of imprisonment of not more than 10 years, a fine not to exceed the greater of twice that authorized in accordance with the provisions of title 18 or $500,000 if the defendant is an individual or $2,000,000 if the defendant is other than an individual, or both. Any sentence imposing a term of imprisonment under this paragraph shall, in the absence of such a prior conviction, impose a term of supervised release of at least 2 years in addition to such term of imprisonment and shall, if there was such a prior conviction, impose a term of supervised release of at least 4 years in addition to such term of imprisonment.

So there you have it, the federal statutes on possession and sale, in black and white. But those aren't the only *federal* statutes addressing gear-related conduct. Conspiracy [21 U.S.C. § 846] may be charged in a federal AAS prosecution. The statutes addressing the *importation* of anabolics are detailed in Chapter 8, and still other federal statutes may also apply to steroid trafficking. For example, there are statutes that prohibit involving minors in the AAS trade, and that prohibit distributing to minors or near schools and parks. [See Chapter 11] There are also statutes providing for forfeiture of ill-gotten proceeds and other assets. [See Chapter 20]

Federal Regulations (C.F.R.)

The Code of Federal Regulations addresses anabolics in Title 21, Food and Drugs, Chapter II, Drug Enforcement Administration, Department of Justice. This is where you'll find the regulations that DEA has issued regarding controlled substances like anabolics. Part 1300, Definitions, sets forth the DEA's definitions concerning controlled substances. The C.F.R. mirrors the federal statute, 21 U.S.C. § 802(41), with the minor modification of combining subparagraph (A) listing the chemicals and subparagraph (B) providing a limited exemption for cattle implants into one paragraph, as follows:

> Sec. 1300.01 Definitions relating to controlled substances.
> ...(b) As used in parts 1301 through 1308 and part 1312 of this chapter, the following terms shall have the meanings specified:
>
> ... (4) The term anabolic steroid means any drug or hormonal substance, chemically and pharmacologically related to testosterone (other than estrogens, progestins, and corticosteroids) that promotes muscle growth, and includes: (i) Boldenone; (ii) Chlorotestosterone (4-chlortestosterone); (iii) Clostebol; (iv) Dehydrochlormethyltestosterone; (v) Dihydrotestosterone (4-dihydro-testosterone); (vi) Drostanolone; (vii) Ethylestrenol; (viii) Fluoxymesterone; (ix) Formebulone (formebolone); (x) Mesterolone; (xi) Methandienone; (xii) Methandranone; (xiii) Methandriol; (xiv) Methandrostenolone; (xv) Methenolone; (xvi) Methyltestosterone; (xvii) Mibolerone; (xviii) Nandrolone; (xix) Norethandrolone; (xx) Oxandrolone; (xxi) Oxymesterone; (xxii) Oxymetholone; (xxiii) Stanolone; (xxiv) Stanozolol; (xxv) Testolactone; (xxvi) Testosterone; (xxvii) Trenbolone; and (xxviii) Any salt, ester, or isomer of a drug or sub-

> stance described or listed in this paragraph, if that salt, ester, or isomer promotes muscle growth. Except such term does not include an anabolic steroid which is expressly intended for administration through implants to cattle or other nonhuman species and which has been approved by the Secretary of Health and Human Services for such administration. If any person prescribes, dispenses, or distributes such steroid for human use, such person shall be considered to have prescribed, dispensed, or distributed an anabolic steroid within the meaning of this paragraph.

Anabolic steroids (DEA number 4000) are scheduled by regulation as they are under statute under 21 CFR § 1308.13(f):

> Schedule III.
> (a) Schedule III shall consist of the drugs and other substances, by whatever official name, common or usual name, chemical name, or brand name designated, listed in this section. Each drug or substance has been assigned the DEA Controlled Substances Code Number set forth opposite it.
> ... (f) Anabolic steroids. Unless specifically excepted or unless listed in another schedule, any material, compound, mixture, or preparation containing any quantity of the following substances, including its salts, isomers, and salts of isomers whenever the existence of such salts of isomers is possible within the specific chemical designation:
> (1) Anabolic Steroids..4000

Cattle Implants

Let's talk a bit more about cattle implants, which seem to have significant interest to many nonfarmers in the muscle world. The cartridges are designed to be administered to the ears of cattle with a special implant gun. As the mode of administration was thought to limit potential human abuse, cattle implants (including Finaplix®, Implus, Revalor, Synovex, and other similar cartridges and pellets) were *excluded* from application of the Controlled Substances Act (CSA) when used on cattle. But imaginative bodybuilders have discovered a variety of methods to adapt the pellets for human consumption.

While the limited exclusion for cattle implants is within the catchall provision of the definitions regulation [21 CFR § 1300.01(b)(4)(xxviii)], it is addressed in a very broad way in another section of the C.F.R. as well. 21 CFR § 1308.26 sets forth the same limited exclusion for veterinary anabolic steroid implant products (*not* if they are prescribed, dispensed or distributed for human use) and provides an address from which to obtain an updated listing of products:

> (a) Products containing an anabolic steroid, that are expressly intended for administration through implants to cattle or other nonhuman species and which have been approved by the Secretary of Health and Human Services for such administration are excluded from all schedules pursuant to section 102(41)(B)(I) of the Act (21 U.S.C. 802(41)(B)(I). A listing of the excluded products may be obtained by submitting a writ-

ten request to the Drug and Chemical Evaluation Section, Drug Enforcement Administration, Washington DC 20537.

(b) In accordance with section 102(41)(B)(ii) of the Act (21 U.S.C. 802(41)(B)(ii)) if any person prescribes, dispenses, or distributes a product listed in paragraph (a) of this section for human use, such person shall be considered to have prescribed, dispensed, or distributed an anabolic steroid within the meaning of section 102(41)(A) of the Act (21 U.S.C. 802(41)(A)).

So, basically, cattle implants are not controlled substances as long as they're intended for animals. But when intended for humans, they transform back into controlled substances. If somebody sold an implant to another bodybuilder, he's subject to prosecution for distribution of a controlled substance. While it seems clear, there are unanswered questions as to the issue of mere *possession*. We have to speculate a bit, since there's no case law on the issue.

We often hear the term "diverted for human use." While neither the U.S.C. nor the C.F.R. use the term "divert," the word appears in the Federal Register. The DEA used it when they published their Final Rule on the topic [Federal Register, Vol. 62, No. 192, Rules and Regulations, Department of Justice, Drug Enforcement Administration (DEA), 21 CFR Part 1308, Schedules of Controlled Substances: Excluded Veterinary Anabolic Steroid Implant Products, 62 F.R. 51774 (October 3, 1997)]. The rule states:

> "The veterinary anabolic steroid implant products which are described in 21 CFR 1308.26 are excluded from application of the CSA in relation to their production, distribution, and use in animals only. If any person distributes, dispenses or *otherwise diverts* these products to use in humans, he/she shall be deemed to have distributed a Schedule III controlled substance and may be prosecuted for CSA violations." [Emphasis added]

The rule uses "otherwise diverts" and not "prescribes" as the statute and regulation do. Is the difference important? It sure could be. While nothing in any of these laws, regulations or rules explicitly says "*possessing*" these products for *self*-administration is criminal, I wonder how broadly aggressive DEA agents might construe the concept of "otherwise diverts" presented in the rule? Could a person in possession of a small quantity of cattle implant cartridges under circumstances suggesting his own personal use be charged with unlawful possession? Could the absence of the word "diverts" in the statute and regulation be a basis to challenge a prosecution? A future case may resolve these issues. (Note that state laws may vary. For example, the cattle implant exclusion in New York doesn't protect anyone "who knowingly and willfully administers [cattle implants] to himself or another person" (Public Health Law § 3306(i).])

Could a person in possession of a small quantity of cattle implant cartridges under circumstances suggesting his own personal use be charged with unlawful possession?

In the interim, other sections of the C.F.R. address various procedural issues pertinent to anabolic steroid implant products. 21 CFR § 1308.25 sets forth the process by which an application can be made to exclude a veterinary anabolic steroid implant product. Essentially, anyone seeking to have any anabolic steroid product, which is expressly intended for administration through implants to cattle or other nonhuman species and which has been approved by the Secretary of Health and Human Services for such administration, identified as being excluded from any schedule under 21 U.S.C. § 802(41)(B)(i)), may apply to the Administrator, Drug Enforcement Administration, Department of Justice, Washington, DC 20537.

Another CFR section, § 1308.33, sets forth the process by which an application can be made to exempt certain anabolic steroid products having no potential for abuse by writing to the Administrator, Drug Enforcement Administration, Department of Justice, Washington, DC 20537. Sec.1308.34 sets forth that the current list of exempt anabolic steroid products is available online at the DEA web site or by written request from DEA. Among the items on the list are various mixed androgen and estrogen esters, such as testosterone cypionate with estradiol cypionate, as well as certain low potency testosterone patches.

Other Federal and State Laws

Now here's a very important little section, almost hiding among the bunch. Sec. 1307.02 provides for the application of *state laws* and other *federal laws*: "Nothing in this chapter shall be construed as authorizing or permitting any person to do any act which such person is not authorized or permitted to do under other Federal laws or obligations under international treaties, conventions or protocols, or under the law of the State in which he/she desires to do such act nor shall compliance with such parts be construed as compliance with other Federal or State laws unless expressly provided in such other laws." *What this means, in essence, is that even if the DEA's regulations say certain conduct is permissible, that conduct may still violate other laws and you could be prosecuted for violating those laws.* You'll see a fascinating example of a conflict near the Mexican border between the DEA's regulations and Texas state law in Chapter 8.

So, we have a tangle of federal statutes and regulations outlawing various AAS crimes. If you get busted and charged in federal court, these are the laws you'll be prosecuted under. Now you know what's against the law! But as mentioned, what ultimately happens to you if you do get arrested will arguably have less to do with the statutes than with the federal guidelines. We need to tackle that topic in order to put it all together and see the system in action!

The United States Sentencing Guidelines

In 1984, Congress addressed the issue of disparities in federal sentencing by passing the Sentencing Reform Act. This Act created the United States Sentencing Commission, which it charged with the task of developing uniform sentencing guidelines in the federal courts. The intent was to achieve a measure of fairness – similar offenders convicted of similar crimes would receive similar sentences. The United States Sentencing Guidelines became effective November 1, 1987.

The USSG generally require federal judges to abide by them. The guidelines affect every stage of the process, including plea negotiations, trial strategy, sentencing, and appeals. There are 43 offense levels – generally, the more serious the offense, the higher the number of the level. The quantity of controlled substances is the major factor in determining the guideline level in drug cases. Under USSG § 2D1.1(c), a Drug Quantity Table sets forth how the quantities of controlled substances determine the level of the offense and the potential sentencing range. The Table is based on *dosage units*.

Anabolic Steroid Dosage Units

The issue, then, is what is a "unit" of anabolic steroids? Here's the formula, sometimes informally called the "steroid discount," and contained in Note G of the Drug Quantity Table in the USSG:

Oral anabolic steroids: one unit means fifty (50) tablets

Injectable anabolic steroids: one unit means a 10cc vial

What about bigger or smaller vials or ampoules? All vials of injectable steroids are to be converted on the basis of their volume to the equivalent number of 10cc vials (e.g., one 50cc vial is to be counted as five 10cc vials). Note that only oral and injectable anabolics are mentioned, opening up a variety of quantification issues in non-traditional administration situations. We can only speculate as to how items like today's blotter "paper steroids" (fifty "squares" might be one dosage unit) or unlawfully possessed cattle implants might be quantified.

The steroid discount seems to have been intended by the Sentencing Commission to recognize the large quantities that non-medical AAS users typically consume, helping to limit the potential imprisonment in federal steroid cases. However, its simplistic approach overlooks factors that might properly be considered in sentencing. For example, a 5mg tablet of Anabol is treated just the same in the dosage context as a 50mg tablet of Anadrol – despite that Anadrol is ten times more potent. A vial with 50mg of androgens per cc is not distinguished from one with 400mg per cc. Obviously, lower potency products would be possessed or distributed in higher quantities to achieve the same overall dosages as high potency products, and the accused will be unduly punished for it under the guidelines. Also, there's no distinction between harsher, more liver toxic steroids (such as alpha alkylated ones) and milder ones.

Steroid Quantities and Offense Levels

How do the units apply to the Drug Quantity Table? The more units of substance, the higher the accused falls in the guidelines. Where he starts out based on quantity is his Base Offense Level. If, for example, the accused is charged with less than 250 units, he starts out with a Base Offense Level of 6. Here's the table for Schedule III substances like anabolic steroids:

Drug Quantity Table	
Level 6:	Less than 250 units.
Level 8:	At least 250 but less than 1,000 units.
Level 10:	At least 1,000 but less than 2,500 units.
Level 12:	At least 2,500 but less than 5,000 units.
Level 14:	At least 5,000 but less than 10,000 units.
Level 16:	At least 10,000 but less than 20,000 units.
Level 18:	At least 20,000 but less than 40,000 units.
Level 20:	40,000 or more units.

Now, let's get down to the basic mechanics of federal sentencing. A USSG Sentencing Table sets forth the potential months of imprisonment for each offense level. The potential imprisonment is determined by applying the offense level to the past criminal conduct of the accused. The intersection of the offense level and the past criminal conduct provides the range of months in prison. The past criminal conduct is calculated as "points" to arrive at a "Criminal History Category." There are six Criminal History Categories, ranging from I (0 to 1 point) to VI (13 or more points).

The application of anabolic steroid quantities to the guidelines is set forth in the chart on the following page. It's simple and straightforward. For easy reference, it presents quantities not just in units, but also in actual tablets and cc's. There's no math needed. To my knowledge, it's the only chart ever constructed on the issue. Look it over carefully.

* * *

Congratulations! You now know more about federal *steroid* sentencing than most lawyers. In order to understand how an actual federal steroid sentence would be imposed, however, you'd really need to understand a good deal of the complexities of the USSG. To be sure, federal sentencing under the guidelines is *extremely* complex and would be impossible to examine comprehensively within our confines. But for those lawyers out there and assorted other brave souls, let's forge ahead to get a basic idea of how it works, using the chart to follow a simple hypothetical.

A Steroid Quantity Hypothetical

Let's say the imaginary accused gets busted in a federal case. He pleads to conspiring to sell 1,000 Mexican 10 cc vials of testosterone and 10,000 tablets of Anadrol-50. To get the dosage unit quantity, we look to Note G. We have 1,000 dosage units of injectables. We have 10,000 tablets divided by fifty, or 200 dosage units of orals. This totals to 1,200 units (1,000 units plus 200 units). Now we turn to the Drug Quantity Table. This number of units falls within Level 10. An accused with no prior arrests or convictions would have no criminal history points and therefore would be placed in Category I. The range of potential imprisonment for Level 10 with a Criminal History Category I is 6 to 12 months. For someone with a past criminal record falling in the mid-range of the categories (Category III, 4 to 6 points), the potential imprisonment would be 10 to 16 months.

Okay so far? Well, we're almost there, but it gets a bit trickier. The guidelines are further complicated by the application of upward and downward "adjustments." These adjustments are based on aggravating or mitigating factors that can increase or decrease the offense level. Examples of these adjustments include playing an aggravating role in the offense [§ 3B1.1: organizer of criminal activity involving more than five participants (+4); manager of more than five (+3); organizer of manager (+2)] or having a mitigating role [§ 3B1.2: minimal participant (-4); minor participant (-2); between minimal and minor (-3)].

An extremely common adjustment is "acceptance of responsibility" under § 3E1.1, which decreases the offense level by two (-2) or, if acceptance is "timely," three levels (-3). It is quite typical for the defendant in any federal drug case to receive adjustments of his offense level. Let's go back to our hypothetical, and assume a fairly standard downward adjustment of 2 points (-2). That brings the accused down to an "adjusted" offense level of 8. If he's got no prior record

ANABOLIC STEROID FEDERAL SENTENCING CHART

Pursuant to U.S.S.G. § 2D1.1, Note G to Drug Quantity Table

— Criminal History Category (Criminal History Points) —

Quantity (# of Units)	(Tablets) ORALS*	(cc) INJECTABLES*	Offense Level**	I (0 or 1)	II (2-3)	III (4,5,6)	IV (7,8,9)	V (10,11,12)	VI (13 or more)
less than 250 units	less than 12,500 tablets	less than 2,500cc	6	**A** 0-6 mos.	**B** 1-7 mos.	**B** 2-8 mos.	**B** 6-12 mos.	**C** 9-15 mos.	12-18 mos.
250 to less than 1,000	12,500 to 50,000	2,500 to 10,000cc	8	**A** 0-6 mos.	**B** 4-10 mos.	**B** 6-12 mos.	**B** 10-16 mos.	15-21 mos.	18-24 mos.
1,000 to less than 2,500	50,000 to 125,000	10,000 to 25,000cc	10	**B** 6-12 mos.	**C** 8-14 mos.	**C** 10-16 mos.	15-21 mos.	21-27 mos.	24-30 mos.
2,500 to less than 5,000	125,000 to 250,000	25,000 to 50,000cc	12	**C** 10-16 mos.	12-18 mos.	15-21 mos.	21-27 mos.	27-33 mos.	30-37 mos.
5,000 to less than 10,000	250,000 to 500,000	50,000 to 100,000cc	14	15-21 mos.	18-24 mos.	21-27 mos.	27-33 mos.	33-41 mos.	37-46 mos.
10,000 to less than 20,000	500,000 to 1,000,000	100,000 to 200,000cc	16	21-27 mos.	24-30 mos.	27-33 mos.	33-41 mos.	41-51 mos.	46-57 mos.
20,000 to less than 40,000	1,000,000 to 2,000,000	200,000 to 400,000cc	18	27-33 mos.	30-37 mos.	33-41 mos.	41-51 mos.	51-63 mos.	57-71 mos.
40,000 to less than 60,000***	2,000,000 to 3,000,000	400,000 to 600,000cc	20	33-41 mos.	37-46 mos.	41-51 mos.	51-63 mos.	63-78 mos.	70-87 mos.

*10 cc = 1 unit
*50 tablets = 1 unit

A = Straight probation available
B = Probation with condition of confinement generally available
C = Split sentence available

**Odd numbered levels attained by adjustments are omitted.
***While the U.S.S.G. says "less than 60,000," Level 20 should actually correspond to everything from 40,000 units and above.

(Category I), he's now looking at 0 to 6 months imprisonment. (While the Sentencing Chart on page 59 covers all steroid quantities, for the sake of simplicity it omits the odd numbered levels created by upward or downward adjustments.) Let's review the process together:

Step 1. – Note G.

1000 / 10 cc vials = 1000 dosage units
10,000 tablets = 200 dosage units

Total = 1,200 units

Step 2. – Drug Quantity Table

1,200 units falls within Level 10

Step 3. – Prior Arrests

None = Category I

Step 4. – Range of Potential Imprisonment

Level 10 + Category I = 6 to 12 months

Step 5. – Adjustments

Level 10 - 2 levels = Level 8
Level 8 = 0 to 6 months imprisonment

Relevant Conduct

Here's an interesting wrinkle about quantity, though. Two of the biggest words in federal sentencing: *relevant conduct*. The idea of relevant conduct, under § 1B1.3 of the guidelines, is that a person gets sentenced for his actual criminal conduct, not just what he's charged with. So it's not limited simply to the anabolics that a person may have sold on the day he was arrested. It's based on all his relevant past anabolics dealings, which then get included in the calculations.

The concept extends pretty far, even including reasonably foreseeable acts and omissions of others in furthering the jointly undertaken criminal activity and certain conduct that part of the same common scheme or plan as the charged offense. By permitting past criminal conduct that's "relevant" to the case to become part of the sentencing guideline computations, the quantity attributed to a steroid defendant in federal court may be much more than what he gets charged with.

Zones

Another complicating factor is that there are three "zones" applicable to the various offense levels: Zones A, B, and C. These zones permit probationary sentences, intermittent or community confinement, or split jail and probationary sentences. As the Sentencing Chart states, a defendant in Zone A is eligible for straight probation [§ 5B1.1].

Departures

Lastly, there are "departures" that allow federal judges to move upward or downward within the guidelines based upon certain aggravating or mitigating facts. The most noteworthy is the departure given to those who provide substantial assistance to the authorities. These individuals can receive a sentence *outside* the application of the guidelines under § 5K1.1 of the USSG. This section plays a critical role in the decision-making process of the defense in most drug cases. Becoming a government informer, and providing information or assistance leading to the arrest and prosecution of former friends and confederates, is rewarded by authorizing departure from the rigid parameters of the guidelines. In most narcotics cases, the obtaining of a "5K letter" from the government is a paramount goal of the defense. In steroid cases, however, the quantity discount under § 2D1.1 combined with an unusual sense of honor within the subculture of users makes cooperation less common than in other federal drug cases, but it does happen. (For more information, see Chapter 10).

Federal Sentencing in the Real World

Case #1: Drew

Want to actually work through with me a real case I handled? Let's use the USSG to determine what the actual sentence our friend Drew from New York will receive. Under the Drug Quantity Table [§ 2D1.1(c)(16)], the Base Offense Level is determined by the number of units of anabolic steroids. Now here is where it gets interesting. Under the USSG, the steroids Drew sold to the informer on the day he was arrested only make up a *portion* of the quantity to be attributed to him. Why? Relevant conduct, baby! The anabolics that he had sold in the past are added into the calculation of where Drew falls in the guidelines. Remember that Drew had been selling anabolics for about three years? Those previous sales took place between December of 1997 and February of 2000. Guess what? The total quantity from those past sales gets added into the mix. Although Drew sold a fairly small quantity (per the USSG) on the day of his arrest, his previous sales added up to an additional 815 units worth of relevant conduct. Therefore his total guideline calculation for units was between 250 and 1,000 – a base offense Level 8. Under USSG § 3E1.1(a), the offense level is reduced two levels (-2) for the "acceptance of responsibility," which brought Drew to an adjusted Level 6.

> Under the USSG, the steroids Drew sold to the informer on the day he was arrested only make up a *portion* of the quantity to be attributed to him. Why? Relevant conduct, baby!

In terms of criminal history, Drew had zero points because he had no past criminal convictions. Therefore, his Criminal History Category was Category I. After various negotiations and a physical inspection of the steroids that were recovered, ultimately a plea agreement was entered into where Drew accepted an agreement which involved a good faith estimate as to where he would fall in the sentencing guidelines. As is customary, both sides agreed not to seek any departures or adjustments not contained in the plea agreement and waived the right to appeal a sentence within the estimate. The plea agreement gives a fairly a good idea of what the range of possible sentences will be. Because Drew was at Level 6, his sentencing range was 0 to 6 months custody and the applicable fine range was $500.00 to $5,000.00. However, it's important to recognize that a plea agreement in federal court is not an agreement in the usual sense because it's only binding on the parties, and *not* on the probation department or the judge. [USSG 6B1.4(d)] It is also important to recognize that a plea agreement with the U.S. Attorney's office doesn't bind any *other* federal, state or local prosecuting authority from prosecuting Drew.

... it's important to recognize that a plea agreement in federal court is ... only binding on the parties, and *not* on the probation department or the judge.

Prior to sentence, Drew must be interviewed by the probation department, which will prepare an extensive pre-sentence investigative report making recommendations to the court as to what the sentence should be. Drew is required to meet with probation and to bring to them a variety of forms and paperwork including a detailed accounting of his finances and assets. As part of the probation investigation, he will be asked about how he got involved in the offense. It's customary for the attorney to be present or to provide a written statement from the defendant that details the crime in a brief way, but one that demonstrates that the defendant accepts his guilt and is responsible for the crime.

If either the probation department or the judge believes that Level 6 is incorrect under a factual review of the case, they can come up with a different calculation. This new calculation would need to be challenged by either or both of the parties prior to Drew's sentence. The fact that Probation comes up with a different calculation doesn't give Drew the right to withdraw his plea of guilty. There can be a substantial question as to what quantity should be included as relevant conduct. It's crucial for the accused and his lawyer to sit down and try to estimate what quantity might be attributable as part of relevant conduct *prior* to accepting a plea agreement.

The defendant and his attorney have the opportunity to review the probation department's pre-sentence report prior to the imposition of sentence, and have the opportunity to challenge or to contest anything in it by filing formal objections to the report. In Drew's case, probation's calculation of units was less than we anticipated, and nothing else in the report was particularly detrimental. Drew was looking at probation.

By statute, under 18 USC § 3561(c)(1), Drew was eligible for between one and five years of probation. Under the guidelines, the applicable term was the same because the offense was Level 6 under § 5B1.2 (note that for offense levels under Level 6, the maximum term of probation is three years). Probation ultimately recommended no custody, 2 years of probation, a $500 fine and a $1,000 special assessment – a terrific resolution in Drew's case. They additionally recommended 100 hours of community service. The fine was to be paid at $100 per month until the full $500 was paid and the 100 hours of community service would be done as directed by probation. As part of the probation conditions, drug testing was to begin, as is typical, within 15 days of placement on probation and thereafter as directed. Interestingly, probation does not routinely test for anabolic steroids even on a case involving anabolic steroids. In order to test for steroids, it is generally required that the probation officers specifically request that testing to be done. That seems to happen in fairly rare instances. Still, drug testing and probation in general is a big inconvenience. So is a felony conviction, particularly for drugs. At present, no employer is anxious to hire Drew. His college plans? Forget it for now.

The Higher Education Act (HEA) was signed into law over three decades ago by President Lyndon Johnson to open the door to a college education for students to whom it had previously been closed. It establishes federal financial aid programs such as Perkins Loans, Pell Grants, Supplemental Educational Opportunity Grants, PLUS Loans and Work-Study Programs. The Act is periodically reviewed and updated by Congress to ensure adequate funding and access to college for millions of Americans. The 1998 revision to the HEA included a new provision that blocks college opportunities to students revealing drug convictions on their Free Application for Federal Student Aid. Students must answer Question 35 of the Federal Application for Financial Student Aid (FAFSA), which asks about drug convictions. A conviction for a drug crime, including mere possession of anabolic steroids, can disqualify a student from receiving federal financial aid. The law took effect on July 1, 2000, but applies to convictions prior to that date and suspends aid eligibility for students convicted under federal or state law of sale or possession of drugs [Section 484(r) of the Higher Education Act of 1965 (20 U.S.C. § 1091(r))]. A first offense carries a one-year disqualification from the date of conviction, a second offense a two-year disqualification, and a third offense makes the student ineligible indefinitely. A student who loses eligibility can regain it by successfully completing an approved drug rehabilitation program, but may very well need to put his or her education on hold until that time.

A conviction for a drug crime, including mere possession of anabolic steroids, can disqualify a student from receiving federal financial aid.

Drew's case stands as a fairly routine way that a low level trafficking investigation can be resolved without any cooperation or the defendant becoming involved as an informer against anybody else. Drew didn't get any jail, but his future is really somewhat in the toilet. Quite a way to start out at 23 years old.

Case #2: Zach

Want to see another example of the way it works? Take Zach's case. His quantities were a bit higher than Drew's.

Zach, late 30s and in the health care industry, had never been arrested before. A government informer, looking to help himself out of his own criminal troubles unrelated to steroids, had some info from a friend of his that Zach was interested in selling gear and had recently gotten a large shipment. The snitch didn't personally know Zach, but he called him and threw around the mutual friend's name. The calls were all recorded. Zach agreed to sell 25,000 Dianabol tablets, 1,300 Anadrol tabs, and 13 boxes of human growth hormone for about $17,250. Later that day, Zach met the snitch and gave him a big box from his car trunk. The snitch wanted to see the juice, so they both got into Zach's car. That was the signal. The agents sprang out of hiding and made the arrest, which led to the search of a storage locker and the recovery of a larger quantity of various anabolics, including injectables. Zach refused questioning and requested an attorney.

Zach was charged with a violation of 21 USC § 841(a)(1), distribution of anabolic steroids. He spent 14 days in custody before he was released on bond. Under § 841(b)(1)(d), he faced imprisonment of up to 5 years, a $250,000 fine, and supervised release of at least two years.

He pled to one count of a two-count indictment. He agreed to forfeit his car and all money seized at the time of his arrest, which totaled a whopping $48,593. He now faced sentencing under the federal sentencing guidelines. How much time would Zach actually get, and how might a conviction affect his life?

Because Zach had no criminal priors, his criminal history score was zero and he was placed in Category I. All of the oral and injectable drugs together combined to 1,616.4 units, placing him at a Base Offense Level of 10 (1,000 to 2,500 units). On his guilty plea, he got a two level adjustment (-2 levels) for acceptance of responsibility, yielding an Adjusted Offense Level of 8. The imprisonment range was therefore 0 to 6 months. Zach could get no time, or up to six months. Zach saw the Probation Officer assigned to do his pre-sentence report. She interviewed his family and prior employers and found nothing but very positive information. He did very well until he was asked about his prior history of drug use. Zach admitted to using steroids for two and a half years. He also admitted to using marijuana a few dozen times over the last twenty years, cocaine six times, and methamphetamines on one or two occasions. He did not feel he needed drug counseling. The officer also found out that he had once used an alias when he lived in another state. Probation felt that the mitigating factors and aggravating factors balanced out, and recommended a middle-of-the-range sentence of three months custody and three years of supervised release. Zach served his three months in a halfway house, sharing sleeping quarters with some very shady characters. He's out now, but still under the supervision of a probation officer who keeps him on a tight leash. As a licensed worker in the health field, the felony conviction resulted in the loss of his license. Felony convictions can often do that. Members of many professions involving licensing (physicians, lawyers, dentists, pharmacists, teachers, nurses, cosmetologists, public accountants, architects, auctioneers, barbers, and licensed counselors, just to name a few) can expect a conviction to be reported to their state licensing authority, placing current employment in jeopardy. Unable to resume employment in his field, Zach is having trouble finding work and has been turned down from two jobs as a "convicted drug felon."

Zach served his three months in a halfway house, sharing sleeping quarters with some very shady characters. He's out now, but still under the supervision of a probation officer who keeps him on a tight leash.

Case #3: Grimaldi (Absconding is a Very Bad Idea...)

This case from the Eastern District of New York presented a variety of common issues in federal juice cases, and a few uncommon twists. The client had some prior steroid convictions, and also made the significant mistake of *failing to show up for sentence.* One wonderful lesson from the trenches: you're going to bump up your time considerably by failing to show up for court. The facts were as follows:

Over three days in February 1996, six registered mail parcels, all from the same return address in Spain, containing 1,120 units of gear (6,000 tablets and 10,000 one-cc vials) were seized upon arrival at JFK International. They were addressed to two different shipping and packing stores, three to each. Crecca owned the stores. A week later, U.S. Customs agents, postal inspectors and local detectives arranged for a controlled delivery. Walsh was arrested picking up the packages. Walsh rolled, and they collared Crecca the next day. Within a week, Crecca had been turned against Saunders, who owned a fitness and apparel store. Crecca taped Saunders in numerous conversations regarding Saunders' purchase of over $12,000 in juice.

When Saunders got pinched, he ratted on Grimaldi, who was the moneyman for the purchase and the ultimate purchaser. Grimaldi, an illegal European alien, lived in California. Saunders showed proof that Grimaldi had sent $7,000 by FedEx for about 1,000 amps of primo, and then had demanded his money back and threatened Saunders when he didn't receive them. Grimaldi then got busted. They were all charged with 21 USC § 846 and § 841(b)(1)(d), conspiracy to distribute and to possess with intent to distribute gear. Grimaldi's involvement was really just a two-man conspiracy between him and Saunders. Grimaldi was accountable for what he ordered—1,000 amps, or 100 units, which put him only at Level 6 in the USSG. The whole bunch took pleas. The other three each got 5 years' probation and fines (one did get a $10,000 fine).

Grimaldi, however, didn't show up for sentence. An arrest warrant was issued for him, and he was indicted for failing to appear before a court as required by conditions of release, under 18 USC § 3146(a)(1) and § 3146(b)(1)(A)(ii). Three years later, he was arrested while trying to cross the border from Mexico into the U.S. Grimaldi had a prior criminal history – several steroid charges – that put him in Category III. But here's where the Probation Department came up with a wild pitch. They said that because of his California priors for juice, they could justify a special Career Offender Adjustment which would catapult him up to a Level 17 and bump him into Category VI. Giving him -2 levels for accepting responsibility in his guilty plea, Probation figured him at Level 15, which had him facing 41 to 51 months in prison. They wouldn't back down, and defense objections were filed challenging the calculations. Luckily for Grimaldi, the judge rejected the Career Offender argument of Probation and the government, and sentenced him to 12 months custody on the steroid count and 4 months on the fugitive count. However, Grimaldi still had further problems ahead. As an illegal alien, he faced a whole new bureaucratic agency coming after him.

Criminal grounds for *deportation* exist under 8 U.S.C. § 1227(a)(2) and INA Section 237(a)(2), making any non-citizen deportable if they commit a crime of moral turpitude, multiple criminal convictions, an aggravated felony or high speed flight from an immigration check point. Further, any alien who has been convicted of a violation of any law or regulation of a state, the United States or a foreign country relating to a controlled substance is deportable. These laws apply to lawful permanent residents, individuals who have married U.S. citizens and others who legitimately possess "green cards," making them deportable despite years of law-abiding residence. Although Grimaldi's wife was an American, he was held for deportation.

In the Actual Words of the Accused...

To finish up this chapter, how about a true-life tale in the defendant's own words? This is the first of many such accounts, intended to provide a view of our steroid laws from the perspective of one who experienced their effects first-hand. This is a letter that a man named Kenny wrote to me, asking me to help in his case. I have edited it ever so slightly for brevity and to preserve anonymity, and present it with his permission in his words, as he typed them:

> *During the month of September 1998, me along with three other individuals were arrested with the charge of distribution of anabolic steroids. I was individually charged with conspiracy to distribute (steroids), only one count. I was booked and then released on $50,000 bond, three horrible days later. I thank God my parents were supportive (as they always have been). I*

accepted a plea bargain which gave me a 5 point downward adjustment in the sentencing guidelines. Three points for the plea agreements and an additional 2 for substantial assistance, which I will discuss later. I am now waiting for sentencing, which will occur in June.

I began my steroid dealing 2 years ago, via the Internet. It was a way that I found to help support me while attending graduate school. I knew it was wrong, yes, but very profitable. I tried and remained very safe with the way I conducted my business. I would visit the local bodybuilding boards and post an advertisement for about 24 hours and then remove my thread. One post 2 years ago eventually brought me a clientele of over 200 at any given time. Gross income for the first year was approx. $20,000, second (and last) year, $75,000. It paid bills and not much more. Only my girlfriend and my friend Bart knew what I did for a living.

I met Bart at the gym 2 years ago. We were just juice buddies. Nothing really in common but steroid stories and cycling theories. He also sold. He had three local guys who purchased quantity from him. So he really never needed more than a few buyers. I moved out of the city (5 miles away). Bart then followed. Bart actually moved into the same apartment complex as I did. I continuously told him that it would not be safe for him to do that because of the nature of our businesses. He said it would be fine. I knew in the back of my head that there would be problems but I chose to ignore it. All was well our last year.

Bart knew a girl, Shelly, from his old gym. We now know that Ms. Shelly was the informant. They had known each other for 6 years. Both were very good friends. Shelly introduced Bart to "her old high school sweetheart, Ed". She said that Ed (who was an undercover agent) was interested in buying some gear. Bart said sure. This was his first and last mistake. He continued to sell gear to Ed for 8 months. During EVERY buy, Ed recorded and videotaped Bart's purchases. Even Shelly was wired many times. Bart must have sold Ed a total of $14,000 worth of juice over the last 8 months. On a side note, I know how informants work and I told Bart, from the beginning, that one should NEVER physically sell to another person. I told him to stick with the mailing of the steroids. It's much safer. He never listened. Ed also wired money into Bart's bank account for the purchase of steroids. He obviously did this so that the government could legally later seize his funds in the bank account.

Bart purchased his steroids through a Malaysian source. As I did through a Greek source. Between the both of us, during 1.5 years, we probably only received 4-5 seizure notices. We did have different sources but it all amounts to how well the contents of a package are securely shipped. We never had any postal authorities knock on our doors. Well, Bart also shipped packages to his parents, who lived 2 hours away. He did this because we all know that using the same postal addy may be subjected to being "flagged." Therefore, using an alternate address is wise and that's what he did.

This is where the third party comes into the picture, his parents. They knew what he was doing but considered it a favor for him (I guess some parents really will do anything for their children including drug trafficking). It's a sad situation but true. Back to me. I would import to my PO box through my Greek connection. Never any problems. I truly stopped dealing three months prior to my arrest. Ironically, I was currently enrolled in the police academy and got out of "the business." I was tired of having to look over my shoulder all of the time. During that month in June, all 4 of us were arrested.

My two cars, computers, fax machine, and a few other items were seized. Once I was brought down to the DEA offices I did a stupid and idiotic thing. I spoke, without a lawyer. They gave me my Miranda rights but I waived them and spoke. I know, I know, never ever talk. Feds always build a case against people and speaking only solidifies their case. I wasn't thinking clearly at that time and thought that speaking would ease the situation. I have been very mature throughout this whole ordeal and will give credit where credit is due. The feds never harassed me or threatened me in any way. I feel that I was somewhat fortunate to get the respectable and decent agents who prosecuted me.

The main agent, Ed, was the one who headed the operation. Ed looks like he is 29-30. Approx. 4 years older than myself. I told them everything, as mentioned above. Generally, that I imported and sold on the Internet. Also, Shelly must have told the feds that I import because my last month of dealing I had approx. 10 packages seized, which never happens. I should have known that they were building a case. Oh, by the way, Bart and I had a warehouse. Again, at the same location (as Bart always did). Ironically the feds never knew about them. They really were sloppy with their 8-MONTH investigation. After I was booked and then released, I spoke to them again during our proffer. During that proffer, I told them about me and Bart's warehouses. I had to get that out during the proffer because I had about 20 units of steroids in my warehouse and did not want withholding that evidence to count against me.

Along with that information, I told them that Bart had $40,000 cash in his warehouse, which he did. I never snitched on anybody or turned anybody in, but I did somewhat blame Bart for this situation and gladly gave that information up to the feds. That is where the substantial assistance came in (2 point deduction). Bart's parents got out on a signature bond and both pled (parents and Bart). Now we all await sentencing and quantity amount. My lawyer (PD), told me that the feds were coming up with 5000-10,000 unit level! That is a level 14. I told my lawyer that I know during a conspiracy case that ALL involved can be responsible for each other's evidence and quantity. But I will assure you that between all of us we are not even close to 5,000 units. Completely impossible! I received the discovery last month and estimated approx. 280 units. Hardly close to 5,000. Oh, also, they even added the discovery up wrong. They weighed each product and measured them in grams, as they would coke or something. I'm beginning to believe that this may have been their first steroid case. My lawyer keeps asking them to add it up properly but they keep brushing us off. They said that they would, they just need to go back into the evidence room and re-count. I know that it would take a very long time and they are procrastinating. Regardless, that is all evidence and it all HAS to be counted properly.

One of the agents said, the other day during our plea, that the contents of one package (meaning the packages that were intercepted from me) will be counted and then be divided by the other packages to determine the approx. amount. In other words, they are finding the median by guesstimating. I don't think so because some of those packages had non-controlled drugs in them like clomid, HCG, etc. etc. I will not have them guess, when the evidence is right there. It will work in their favor if they do guesstimating work. I know that the feds have a lot of pull but evidence is evidence and it HAS to be counted.

Regardless, I feel very, very comfortable that I am sitting on a level 8. This is my first offense so I am hoping that probation is all that will come out of it. Also, the plea agreement included that they would recommend the lower range (with relation to the guidelines), which is 0-6 months. But they keep pushing for a level 14. I understand that they may be able to "guess" how many packages were coming in between the 4 of us during those 8 months. Regardless, all of us still would not even come close to a level 14. I understand that they shoot high and try to make that stick but the evidence still has to be counted and they are not doing it. That's about the gist of everything. Oh, also, when I was being interrogated, they told me not to touch my funds in my bank account (which currently has $4,000 in it). Nothing was said or signed during the plea and the funds are not seized. At this time Bart's account has been seized and forfeited but *not mine. I'm sure I have some details that were left out so if you have any further questions, I would be happy to answer them.*

The above facts, when reading, seem out of chronological order. Sorry, I've just been very busy and have not had enough time to think this through thoroughly. Please, any comments or suggestions would be great. On another note, looking back. The ONLY thing they had on ME was just the fact that the informant said I was involved. That seemed to be enough for a grand jury to indict me. Seems so wrong. A C.I. who is trying to work off charges could say anything, and that is enough for an indictment. Even if the facts are true or not. Had I not said anything, do you think I could have had a strong defense? The final report on my case should be in by Nov. 10 or so, says the P.O.

I did have a question though. The feds had seized 2 cars (Corvette, Mustang) and a 60" widescreen t.v. Upon being arrested, they pressured me into signing these items over to them. I signed the Corvette and t.v. over to the Sheriffs dept. I did not, however, sign the Mustang over. Even during the proffer the detective asked me to sign the Mustang over and my attorney (and myself) declined to do so. Of course, still to this day, he continues to ask but we are declining. They kept saying that the car was used during a drug deal. Meaning, me picking up packages at my P.O. box. Since the car was used in this action, they keep saying that it is now property of the gov't. I told them that I worked 30+ hours at the gym as a personal trainer, with moneys being paid to me under the table and that a lot of that car was paid with my working money. Not drug money. But they said, it didn't matter, it was used in the commission of the crime. I guess my only defense would be (when we go to court over it) to say that I also received my regular bill, mail, junk mail etc. etc., at the same P.O. box as I was receiving the medications at, therefore, the trip to the post office was justifiable. Also, them seizing my t.v., why was that done? The t.v. had nothing to do with "acting in the commission of the crime" and it was obviously not used to facilitate any crime. I don't get that.

Well, Kenny's television was victim to the asset forfeiture laws that permit not just instrumentalities but *proceeds* of crimes to be taken away. Anyway, I did help Kenny and his lawyer in battling the feds over the quantities to be attributed to him as relevant conduct. Kenny wound up getting a fair sentence: four years straight probation with no confinement. I spoke with him recently. Like Zach, Kenny is having a hard time landing a job, especially in the economic downturn. Every job application asks him if he's been convicted of a felony. When he answers that he has, the employers seem to have no further interest in him. He has no current prospects and no plans.

Beyond Federal Court

While most experienced federal criminal practitioners are thoroughly familiar with the guidelines, few are well-versed in their application to AAS cases. Face it: this chapter's not going to teach anybody how to defend a federal criminal indictment of any kind. However, it's a handy reference for steroid quantities under the USSG, and should give any federal criminal defense lawyer the information he needs to quickly size up and evaluate the basic issues peculiar to anabolics cases. Practitioners should also study Chapter 14, which details the factual issues relating to steroid quantities and costs.

As for the casual reader, here's what to take home from all this. The mere fact of a felony arrest, with or without a conviction, can be highly traumatic to the typical law-abiding citizen when friends, neighbors, co-workers and employers find out. The civil disabilities and practical fallout from a felony *conviction* can be devastating, regardless of whether a person serves time in jail or prison. A convicted drug offender can lose his job, and can also lose the prospects of future employment in his chosen field. The adverse effects of a conviction for steroids can impact not only the offender, but also the offender's family. Further, while it generally takes a substantial quantity of anabolics to face major prison time in federal court, most steroid cases are brought in *state* courts, where the laws are confusing and the penalties can be much, much higher. Let's turn to that topic now.

Chapter 5

STATES OF CONFUSION

"Ignorance of the law excuses no man; not that all men know the law, but because 'tis an excuse every man will plead, and no man can tell how to refute him."
–*John Seldon (1584-1654)*

Most steroid prosecutions are brought in state courts. Why? It's probably because the potential penalties can be substantially higher in state courts than in federal court. After all the time and effort of investigation and arrest, it's only sensible for law enforcers to bring the case where the best resolution for the prosecution can be attained. It's interesting to note, however, that anabolics are different from other drug cases in this way. In narcotics cases, the rigid federal guidelines can impose heavier punishments than state courts.

AAS and State Drug Laws

With the enactment in 1970 of the federal Controlled Substances Act (21 U.S.C. § 801, *et seq.*), it became necessary for states to update and revise their narcotic, marijuana, and dangerous drug laws. The Uniform Controlled Substances Act was drafted to achieve uniformity between the laws of the states and those of the federal government. A main objective of the Uniform Act was to create a coordinated and codified system of drug control classifying all narcotics, marijuana, and dangerous drugs subject to control into five schedules, with each schedule having its own criteria for drug placement, just like the federal law. While stating the prohibited activities in detail, the Uniform Act left specific fines and sentences to the discretion of the individual states. Each state has the freedom to adopt all, parts or none of the Uniform Act, as well as the discretion to set the punishments for offenses. The result? As you might guess, the drug laws of the individual states vary widely. In fact, not all states even use the term "controlled substances" to refer to restricted drug substances. As examples, Hawaii calls them "harmful drugs" and Maryland calls them "controlled dangerous substances."

Each state has the freedom to adopt all, parts or none of the Uniform Act, as well as the discretion to set the punishments for offenses.

When it comes to these drug substances, most states have laws that place them into schedules like the federal law does. Each state chooses which drugs it wants to schedule, and defines them so that everybody knows what they are. The definition doesn't have to be the same definition as under federal law, and the level within the schedule doesn't have to be the same either. Most states have laws that make selling, manufacturing or possessing with intent to sell or manufacture certain drugs a crime. But they can enact all sorts of other statutes to control drug abuse, and sometimes the result can be a maze of interconnected laws. Many states have laws as to how controlled substances may be stored or kept. Some put specific restrictions on practitioners who prescribe them. Many states have adopted laws similar to the federal statutes that enhance the punishment if a controlled substance sale occurs within 1,000 feet of a school. Some make prescribing steroids for "bodybuilding" a separate crime. Many have laws dealing with counterfeit drugs and imitation controlled substances. Some have elaborate and complex sentencing statutes, with aggravating and mitigating factors to weigh. For example, possessing a firearm along with some drugs can bump up someone's sentencing exposure on the drug charge. Some states have complicated laws as to how to calculate prison terms and parole periods, and about how concurrent and consecutive sentences are supposed to work. Some states have laws that say which sorts of prior crimes are sufficient to trigger mandatory enhanced sentencing, and laws about probation revocations, youthful offender adjudications, and a variety of other court procedures. Any of these laws might become important in a particular drug case. Of course, if all these laws were explained even for just *one* state, this chapter would be hundreds of pages long. That wouldn't really serve our purpose, which is to provide a general idea of state anabolics laws. The Appendix at the back of this book tells you exactly how steroids are defined and classified in your state, and provides some information as to what to expect from a steroid case.

The Appendix at the back of this book will tell you exactly how steroids are defined and classified in your state, and provides some information as to what to expect from a steroid case.

So, let's talk about anabolics under state laws. Anabolic steroids are defined in the federal law in 21 U.S.C. § 802(41), but each state is free to define them. Many states have followed the federal definition in whole or in part. A few have altered the definition, for better or worse. Some have scheduled substances that are not scheduled under federal law, such as androstenediol, human growth hormone (hGH) and HCG. (In the sections on each individual state in the Appendix, definitions that depart from the federal definition are explored.) Anabolic steroids are classified as "controlled substances" under federal law, and many states have scheduled them under their drug laws. Alaska and Vermont have *not* scheduled anabolic steroids as controlled substances.

How serious is it to get involved with anabolics? That depends on many factors. For starters, most states divide their crimes into felonies and misdemeanors. Felonies are the more serious crimes, generally punishable by more than a year in jail. Most states have several classes of felonies, either designated by numbers or letters, and in descending order of seriousness (i.e., Class 1 or Class A felonies are more serious than Class 2 or Class B felonies). Unlawfully selling controlled substances is almost always a felony. In New York, for example, "sell" means to "sell, exchange, give or dispose of to another, or to offer or agree to do the same." [NYS PL § 220.00(1)] Unlawfully selling a controlled substance in New York is a class "D" felony [NYS PL § 220.31] (if the substance is a narcotic, like cocaine or heroin, the crime goes up to a class "B" felony). Many states, however, don't use the word "sell" – choosing other words that pretty much mean the same thing, like "traffic," "distribute" or "deliver." However, in Kentucky, "sell" means to dispose of a controlled substance to another person for consideration or in furtherance of commercial distribution, while "traffic" means the more inclusive "to manufacture, distribute, dispense, sell, transfer, or possess with intent to manufacture, distribute, dispense or sell a controlled substance." [KRS 218A.0109(26) and (28)] In Hawaii, even "sell" and "distribute" are *not* the same [HRS § 712-1240]:

> "To distribute" means to sell, transfer, prescribe, give, or deliver to another, or to leave, barter, or exchange with another, or to offer or agree to do the same.
>
> "To sell" means to transfer to another for consideration.

Unlawfully possessing controlled substances may be a felony or a misdemeanor, as will be seen, depending on the state law and the particular circumstances. Misdemeanors are crimes punishable by a year or less in jail, and states may have classes of misdemeanors in similar descending order of seriousness. Beneath misdemeanors are "violations" or "infractions," which are non-criminal offenses. Before you think about doing juice, you should be very familiar with the laws and maximum sentencing ranges in the state you're in. You'd be a fool not to be. Say, for example, you're a New Yorker from Staten Island who goes just across the bridge for a party in New Jersey. If you think a small quantity of juice is a misdemeanor like it is in New York, you're sadly mistaken. And if you have enough anabolics for a Jersey prosecutor to think you were going to sell it, you're in even hotter water. And if you happened to be caught in a spot that was within 1,000 feet of a school, even if you didn't know it, you'd be looking at a major catastrophe! How can you know your state's laws? Again, the Appendix at that back of this book is a good place to start.

Before you think about doing juice, you should be very familiar with the laws and maximum sentencing ranges in the state you're in.

Most states, but not all, distinguish between simple possession for personal use and the more serious crime of sale or distribution. Many consider possessing a drug with the *intent* to distribute it just as serious as the act of distributing it. So, in a possession situation, the crucial issue can be whether the steroids were for personal use or for resale. The distinction can be *major* in terms of sentencing possibilities, including jail or prison exposure. How can we say if somebody's juice was intended to be sold or not? Really, a person's intent exists only in the mind. Well, what courts do is look at all the other evidence in the case, such as any records on paper or in computer files indicating prior steroid sales or any admissions that the accused might have made to the police. Perhaps the most controversial piece of evidence is the *quantity* of the steroids. If it's more than what a person might use himself, an intention to distribute may be inferred. Let me further clarify that. If it's more than what some police officer, federal agent, or prosecutor *thinks*, in what may be extremely limited experience, is more than what a person might use himself, a count of possessing to distribute will be filed. The result can be an outrageous travesty of justice. This problem merits a lot more attention and gets it, in Chapter 14.

Not all states set up their possession laws based on intention to sell. Some have set up the seriousness of their drug crimes based on *weight* of the drugs. Take Ohio for example, where possession of a small amount of anabolics is a misdemeanor but possession of a quantity equal to exceeding the "bulk amount" is a felony. "Bulk amount" for anabolic steroids is defined in Ohio as *two hundred tablets* or *sixteen milliliters of* substance. Possession of a quantity that equals or exceeds five times the bulk amount is a higher level felony, and possession of fifty times the bulk amount is a still higher level felony requiring mandatory prison. Or take Texas, which measures weight in *grams* (see Case Notes section of the Appendix).

The New York statutes have both an intent-based escalation for drug crimes and a weight-based one, but steroids are excluded from the weight-based scheme. In other states, the laws talk about *dosage units*, just like the federal sentencing guidelines do. But the states are free to define dosage units any way they want! Take Mississippi, where the greater the number of dosage units, the more prison time you're facing. But they neglected to provide any special consideration for steroids. One tablet is one unit, with no discounts of any kind. And potency doesn't matter - a 50mg oxymetholone tablet is considered exactly the same as a 2.5mg tab of oxandrolone!

Another issue is, what is "possession"? One suitable definition is written into the Missouri law's Narcotic Drug Act [§ 195.010 R.S.Mo.]:

> ... (32) "Possessed" or "possessing a controlled substance", a person, with the knowledge of the presence and nature of a substance, has actual or constructive possession of the substance. A person has actual possession if he has the substance on his person or within easy reach and convenient control. A person who, although not in actual possession, has the power and the intention at a given time to exercise dominion or control over the substance either directly or through another person or persons is in constructive possession of it. Possession may also be sole or joint. If one person alone has possession of a substance possession is sole. If two or more persons share possession of a substance, possession is joint;

That concept of "dominion and control" is very important to the issue of when you can be arrested for possession. You can possess a bottle of testosterone even if it's not actually on your person if you have the power and intention to exercise dominion and control over it. If it's in your car, house, or locker at work, that can be "possessing" it. If the locker belongs to both you and your buddy, you can both be *jointly* possessing its contents. Okay so far?

Now, some states have established *presumptions* as to possession that can be used against you. For example, Minnesota codified such a presumption as to *residences* and *automobiles*:

> Minn. Stat. § 152.028 (2001) Permissive inference of knowing possession.
> Subdivision 1. Residences. The presence of a controlled substance in open view in a room, other than a public place, under circumstances evincing an intent by one or more of the persons present to unlawfully mix, compound, package, or otherwise prepare for sale the controlled substance permits the factfinder to infer knowing possession of the controlled substance by each person in close proximity to the controlled substance when the controlled substance was found. The permissive inference does not apply to any person if:
> (1) one of them legally possesses the controlled substance; or
> (2) the controlled substance is on the person of one of the occupants.
>
> Subd. 2. Passenger automobiles. The presence of a controlled substance in a passenger automobile permits the factfinder to infer knowing possession of the controlled substance by the driver or person in control of the automobile when the controlled substance was in the automobile....The inference does not apply:
> (1) to a duly licensed operator of an automobile who is at the time operating it for hire in the lawful and proper pursuit of the operator's trade;
> (2) to any person in the automobile if one of them legally possesses a controlled substance; or
> (3) when the controlled substance is concealed on the person of one of the occupants.

Get the idea? Generally, if the bottle of test is in somebody's pocket, the charge is on him. If it's out in the open, a judge or jury is allowed to infer that whoever's near it in the room or driving the car it's found in is in knowing possession of it.

State Laws Beyond Steroids

Now, states are free to draft laws to cover other types of behavior they aim to discourage. Let's say that you decide to get enough juice to make a cycle by visiting several of your local doctors and getting a steroid prescription from each one without telling any of them about the others. Here's a statute from Hawaii [HRS § 329-46] designed to stop you from doing that:

> §329-46 Prohibited acts related to visits to more than one practitioner to obtain controlled substance prescriptions.
> (a) It is unlawful for any person knowingly or intentionally to visit more than one practitioner and withhold information regarding previous practitioner visits for the purpose of obtaining one or more controlled substance prescriptions for quantities that:
> (1) Exceed what any single practitioner would have prescribed or dispensed for the time period and legitimate medical purpose represented; and
> (2) Would constitute an offense ...
> (b) Information communicated to a physician in an effort to unlawfully procure a controlled substance, or to unlawfully procure the administration, prescribing, or dispensing of any controlled substance shall not be deemed a privileged communication.
> (c) Any person who violates this section is guilty of a crime which is of the grade and class ... for the same type and equivalent quantity of controlled substance.

Many jurisdictions make *conspiracy* or *attempt* to sell drugs punishable to the extent as actually selling them. The law in the District of Columbia is an example [D.C. Code § 48-904.09]: "Any person who attempts or conspires to commit any offense defined in this subchapter is punishable by imprisonment or fine or both which may not exceed the maximum punishment prescribed for the offense, the commission of which was the object of the attempt or conspiracy."

Many states have enacted counterfeit drug statutes, making it a crime to sell or possess fake drugs. Here's one from Georgia (O.C.G.A. § 16-13-30.1):

> (a) (1) It is unlawful for any person knowingly to manufacture, deliver, distribute, dispense, possess with the intent to distribute, or sell a noncontrolled substance upon either:
> (A) The express or implied representation that the substance is a narcotic or nonnarcotic controlled substance;
> (B) The express or implied representation that the substance is of such nature or appearance that the recipient of said delivery will be able to distribute said substance as a controlled substance; or
> (C) The express or implied representation that the substance has essentially the same pharmacological action or effect as a controlled substance ...
> ...(e) The unlawful manufacture, delivery, distribution, dispensing, possession with the intention to distribute, or sale of a noncontrolled substance in violation of this Code section is a felony and, upon conviction thereof, such person shall be punished by imprisonment for not less than one year nor more than ten years or by a fine not to exceed $25,000.00, or both.

All right, in Georgia a "noncontrolled" substance is just an imitation drug. But what about prescription drugs that are not controlled substances, like tamoxifen or clomiphene citrate? What sort of trouble goes with selling or possessing those items? Again, it varies from state to state. Here's how Delaware handles it [16 Del. C. § 4754A]:

> (a) It is unlawful for any person knowingly or intentionally to possess any drug for which a prescription is required, which is not a controlled substance or counterfeit controlled substance, with the following exceptions:
>
> (1) The possession, and transfer to a licensed health care professional by a manufacturer's representative, of drugs manufactured by the representative's employer;
> (2) The possession, compounding and sale of such drug by a pharmacist in the lawful course of the pharmacist's professional activities;
> (3) The possession and transfer of such drug by a physician or other licensed health care professional in the lawful course of the physician's or other licensed health care professional's professional activities; and
> (4) The possession, use and consumption of such drug by a person who has received the drug from a physician or other licensed health care professional who is permitted by law to dispense or prescribe such drug.
>
> (b) Possession of a drug which is not a controlled substance, in violation of this section, is a class B misdemeanor.
>
> (c) In any prosecution for "unlawful possession of a noncontrolled prescription drug," it is an affirmative defense that the drug was possessed or consumed within the residence of the defendant, that a member of the defendant's household possessed a valid prescription for said drug, that the possession or consumption by the defendant was for the purpose of treating an illness and that the drug in question was approved for use for the specific illness.
>
> (d) Any person who delivers or possesses with intent to deliver a noncontrolled prescription drug not obtained directly from, nor pursuant to, a valid prescription or order of a practitioner who is acting in the course of the practitioner's professional practice, or except as otherwise authorized by the statutes of this State, shall be guilty of a class E felony.

As you can see, state anabolic steroid laws can get quite convoluted. Further, in addition to the statutes, there are state rules and regulations affecting individuals and business entities in a variety of special situations. For example, special rules may apply to pharmacists or physicians concerning what records they must make about their controlled substance prescriptions and how those records should be kept. To address every situation would be overwhelming. The best source for information about your very particular circumstances is a licensed attorney in your own area. (The Appendices contain the applicable maximum sentences for AAS cases in every state and the District of Columbia, as well as helpful practical notes.)

At this point, however, you've got a pretty good idea of what laws juice users might run afoul of. Now let's put it into a more concrete context. How are violations of these state laws actually handled in the great machine of the criminal justice system?

Chapter 6

WELCOME TO THE MACHINE

"Justice is a machine that, when someone has once given it
the starting push, rolls on of itself."
– John Galsworthy (1867-1933)

If you've never been arrested before, the criminal justice process can be pretty intimidating. Nobody likes being handcuffed. Well, most people don't anyway. Nobody likes being treated like a criminal or potentially being left with a lasting blemish on their record. Believe me, it's best to stay the hell out of the criminal justice system. Unfortunately, not everyone does. This chapter is intended for muscleheads and other curious readers looking for a basic road map showing how the process works in most state courts. What would happen, generally, if you were to partake of a little chemical enhancement and get caught up in the state justice machine?

Investigation and Arrest

A criminal prosecution generally begins when somebody in law enforcement – such as a police officer or federal agent – decides that there's sufficient reason (called "probable cause") to believe that a suspect has committed a crime. The suspect is then arrested. The charges can be brought in either state or federal court. The overwhelming majority of steroid cases are brought in state courts, so that's our focus here. This is true even if federal authorities investigated the crime. In many federal districts, the general policy was to reject "small potatoes" cases like low quantity steroid cases (although that policy has reportedly been reevaluated recently).

... charges can be brought in either state or federal court. The overwhelming majority of steroid cases are brought in state courts, so that's our focus here.

How the officers or agents first acquire information leading to probable cause can vary greatly. The majority of steroid cases involve situations of either possession or trafficking. In many possession cases, the police may find the anabolics during a vehicular traffic stop; or Customs may find them at an international airport or border crossing; or postal inspectors may find them in a parcel sent by courier or U.S. mail. In most trafficking cases, law enforcement develops information that the accused is a steroid dealer, and an undercover police officer or confidential informer (a.k.a. snitch or rat) arranges a transaction during which, or after which, the accused is arrested. The various situations in which juicers are investigated and ultimately find themselves in police confrontations are described throughout many of the other chapters of this book. One example is the true story of Eric and Valerie, presented here.

The Rise and Fall of Eric and Valerie

Eric and his girlfriend Valerie set up a home-based, direct marketing (mail order) business in San Diego, selling "cosmetics." They were really selling anabolics, along with some of the ancillary medications used by bodybuilders, like prescription diuretics and estrogen blockers. They tried to be careful about all the details. Eric used numerous false identification cards to set up multiple private mailboxes. He kept his vehicles registered in others' names. The bodybuilders he dealt juice to didn't know his name. Valerie always used fictitious return addresses on all outgoing juice packages. Caliente Cosmetics' sales were generated through online chat rooms, classified ads in bodybuilding magazines, Internet message board postings, and through word of mouth. Business was doing well. The couple appeared to the world as another Internet entrepreneur success story.

The couple's downfall started when a purchaser in a suburban East Coast community ordered some Caliente cosmetics in his mother's name and had it sent to the home address that he and Mama shared. He miscalculated the delivery date and wasn't home when the package was delivered. Mama refused to accept delivery, and the package bounced back to the local Post Office, requiring attention. The return address was determined to be fictitious. The package was postmarked from San Diego, a primary source city for shipping drugs. Postal Inspectors were alerted, deemed it "suspicious," and began investigating. They x-rayed the package and determined that it contained ten vials of what seemed probable to be steroids. They did a computer search on Mama and determined her to be a woman in her sixties. Not your average musclehead. But they also found records that Mama's adult son lived with her.

Instead of doing a controlled delivery, the inspectors made a knock and talk visit to Mama's place and engaged her in some casual conversation. During their chat, the inspectors were introduced to Henri, Mama's beefed up son. Again, just in friendly chitchat, Henri was "interviewed" about any prior packages he might know about. The inspectors happened to mention that they could access a record of previous deliveries to his address. At this point, Henri recalled some other suspicious packages. First Henri told them that he had been a judge for bodybuilding contests, and that he had received packages in the mail containing steroids that had been sent in retaliation by disgruntled contestants seeking to discredit him. Henri must have thought his explanation sounded reasonable because the inspectors just let him keep on talking. But somewhere along the way, the story unraveled. As Mama cried beside him, Henri confessed to everything he'd ever done wrong since grade school. He let the agents open the package, revealing the gear. He provided the address to which he had mailed the cash for the anabolics. It was an address for a box #408 in a private mailbox store in San Diego.

Following the visit with Henri, postal inspectors contacted authorities in Southern California, who visited the Mail Boxes America store to which the cash had been mailed. They requested and immediately received from the store manager the registration information for the mailbox, including a photocopy of a fake California Department of Motor Vehicles driver's license that had been used to open the box. The manager, concerned about his store being implicated in some wrongdoing, eagerly confirmed that the guy in the photo had opened the box for Caliente Cosmetics, but that the mail was collected by an attractive young female. There was a high volume of mail from abroad. The agents checked out the business incorporation records for a Caliente Cosmetics, but no such business had been registered.

Meanwhile, in a rural community in Arkansas, a federal and state police task force received an anonymous tip about a suspicious package. It was enough to obtain a federal search warrant to open the package, which was found to contain over $3,200 worth of juice. The return address on the package was fictitious, but it was postmarked from San Diego. One controlled delivery later, a recreational bodybuilder named Wayne who occasionally ordered steroids for a group of his lifting buddies was handcuffed and surrounded in his kitchen.

Wayne tried to avoid cooperating, but various bodybuilding drugs were found in his refrig-

erator and the agents threatened to have both him and his wife declared unfit parents and have the kids removed to foster care. After a long talk with his wife, Wayne admitted to the agents that he had purchased the gear from a guy in California whose name he didn't know. The guy called himself Squatter. Wayne had met him through an online discussion board. Wayne said he had once talked to the guy by telephone about a delayed order, and had the number stored in his cell phone. A search of Pacific Bell records revealed that it was a prepaid cell phone purchased in San Diego. Its purchaser could not be traced.

In an effort to dig his way out of trouble and keep his family intact, Wayne showed the inspectors to his computer. He provided Squatter's e-mail address at the allegedly anonymous "shushmail.com" and printed out past correspondences, including Squatter's price list and ordering instructions. The instructions directed sending an e-mail message to Squatter and then sending cash to the Caliente Cosmetics mailbox address along with a partial e-mail address for the sender, so that Squatter would know who the order was from. Wayne would send the cash via Express Mail, and had done so on approximately eight or nine prior transactions. He further volunteered that Squatter told him that he got his steroids by international mail and also smuggled the gear up from Mexico in monthly trips, with loads of up to $50,000 at a time in a black Lincoln Navigator SUV. In addition, Wayne offered that the source had told him that he had recently also purchased a blue Cadillac Escalade.

The Arkansas task force called California to alert them. Of course, the California agents already knew about Caliente Cosmetics from the East Coast postal inspectors and the package to Mama. The California agents had already put a mail watch on the mailbox #408 to flag future deliveries; now, they stepped up the intensity and put the Mail Boxes America under surveillance. The agents observed a blue Cadillac Escalade like the one Wayne had mentioned. They watched and photographed an attractive woman enter the store, pick up mail, and drive away. Surveillance was then picked up by another agent who followed Valerie as she drove to another Mail Boxes America store. She entered the store and again departed a few minutes later with U.S. mail parcels. The agents were unable to follow her back to her home due to traffic conditions. However, a check of the tags came back to one Valerie Arroyo at an address in a San Diego suburb. A simple search of postal records confirmed that Valerie and one Eric Granger were receiving mail at the address. Driver's license photos of Valerie and Eric were obtained. A simple but illuminating search of the criminal arrest records database disclosed that Eric and Valerie had been arrested at the United States Port of Entry at San Ysidro eight months earlier with various vials of juice concealed in a factory compartment of their vehicle. At the time of that arrest, Eric was driving a black Lincoln Navigator registered to Valerie.

Later that day, the California agents paid a visit to the second Mail Boxes America visited by Valerie. The agents showed the driver's photos to the manager, who said the people shown in the pictures subscribed to a certain box #217. The box had been opened with fake identification with Eric's picture on it. The manager said Valerie mailed "a lot of parcels" at least three to four times per week, had her own postage meter, and received occasional international packages. The manager went on further to provide the store's "parcel log" for all deliveries, tracking the box number, date received, parcel tracking number, carrier and the recipient's signature.

The next day, the agents were told that several domestic letters had been received for box # 408. Agents examined them without opening them. One agent compared the bulge in the package with a dollar bill from his own pocket and suspected that the package contained a stack of U.S. currency. The activity was consistent with what Wayne described, with incoming mail con-

taining cash for orders and outgoing parcels containing juice.

Meanwhile, in an unrelated investigation in San Francisco, U.S. Customs flagged and intercepted three parcels from Lithuania that were addressed to box #217 in the second Mail Boxes America store. The parcels contained a total of three thousand tablets of methandrostenolone. Customs contacted postal agents in San Diego, who then arranged for a controlled delivery of the packages. They left a note in Box #217 for the possessor of the box, notifying that person of the parcels and advising them to see store personnel. Agents then maintained surveillance on the store. Shortly thereafter, Valerie came to the store, opened Box #217, and then requested the parcels. Upon leaving the store with the parcels she was taken into custody.

Caught red-handed with 3,000 D-bol tablets, Valerie was scared. The inspectors told her that because of her previous arrest, she would do jail time on this one. She would also be held responsible for all the steroids mailed to Wayne, they told her. They told her they knew all about her, including where all of her postal boxes were, where she used to live, how often she mailed packages, and how much money she made. They told her they knew all about Eric. They said that they knew that he was Squatter and that they had seen numerous e-mails in which he discussed steroid transactions. They also told her that he had regularly corresponded with a guy in Arkansas about how many different girls he was sleeping with. They offered Valerie one chance to save herself. Either way, Eric was going down. She told them where the other postal boxes were. There were twelve in all, each opened with a different fake identification. They presented her with a Consent to Search form, but she refused to sign it.

The agents were already in the process of drafting an application to a judge of the Superior Court of the State of California for the County of San Diego, seeking a search warrant for Eric's premises, including, but not limited to, all vehicles, garages, outbuildings and trash areas. The items sought by agents through the warrant was extremely broad including, but not limited to, steroids; paraphernalia for the use or transfer of controlled substances; controlled substance compounds or derivatives; packing material that may be used to obscure the detection of controlled substances, computers, floppy disks, papers documenting the sale or purchase, UPS, FedEx, USPS receipts and bills of lading, scales and other weighing devices, U.S. currency, fax machines, buyer lists, seller lists, address and telephone lists. Law enforcement was further permitted to freeze all bank accounts. In addition, based upon the training and experience of agents, in their application to the court they asserted that firearms should be searched for and, if found, their presence is indicative of trafficking in controlled substances because of the large amounts of cash, the value of the contraband, and the inclination of traffickers to resort to violence to resist robbery, settle disputes or thwart capture by law enforcement. The warrant further permitted agents to monitor all telephone activity in order to intercept conversations with other buyers and sellers and co-conspirators. The warrant was signed by a judge and executed by law enforcement.

Shortly thereafter, a team of ten agents from multiple agencies yelled, "Police with a search warrant!" and entered the house owned by Eric and Valerie. Some of the most important items seized pursuant to the warrant were Eric's computers and cell phone. The number of the prepaid cell phone was the number stored on Wayne's phone. The computer and cell phone not only were admissible evidence in the case against Eric and Valerie, but law enforcement officers found numerous names, addresses, phone numbers, cell phone numbers, e-mail correspondence, and e-mail addresses for buyers, distributors and co-conspirators. Eric was arrested and remanded to custody without bail because of the amount of drugs, cash and number of firearms found in the residence. The couple's assets were seized and frozen, and a civil forfeiture action was commenced seeking to take title to the house, cars, cash, and bank accounts. Welcome to the machine, Eric and Valerie.

How State AAS Prosecutions Begin

In the typical narcotics case, the police find some powder or pills in a car or in a house, or they buy a bag of it undercover, and they immediately know by their training and experience if it's a controlled substance. Unlike most drugs, which the police can identify on sight, steroids aren't readily identifiable to many law enforcement officers. Unless they have probable cause to believe a substance is a controlled drug, they may not have probable cause to arrest. So, some juice cases (a small but significant percent) include a period of delay between the recovery of the contraband and the arrest of the suspect so that the substance recovered can be tested in a laboratory. The period of delay in such cases may range from a few weeks to several months. It's not uncommon for me to receive a call from somebody who had his steroids seized but was not arrested at the time. It's usually because the police need a positive lab report in some cases to make the arrest. This is particularly common in cases where the suspect refuses to admit what the pills or vials are. Can and should a suspect refuse to talk to the police? There are few things as important as the answer to that question. You'll find out soon enough, when you get to Chapter 21, describing your rights under the famous *Miranda* decision.

After a positive lab report, there's no doubt anymore. Probable cause to arrest the suspect exists. The police have several options as to how they can effectuate the arrest. They may contact the suspect by telephone or mail to arrange a date for him to surrender at the police station, the so-called "gentleman's" approach. Or they may come and arrest him at his job, humiliating him in front of bosses and co-workers, or at his home. While they are generally not permitted to enter a suspect's house to arrest him without a warrant, they can request him to step outside. If he's apt to do so, they can then immediately arrest him, throwing him down on the lawn and handcuffing him as family and neighbors stare in disbelief.

Once a person is under arrest, he is "in custody." He's most definitely not free to leave. Resisting a lawful arrest is a crime in itself, as is escaping after arrest. The suspect is almost always handcuffed while he is transported to the station house or federal offices for a body search and the taking of fingerprints and photographs. It is during this arrest "processing" that the police or agents begin the interrogation process, designed to extract an oral or written incriminating "statement" (confession). During this process, the suspect will have little or no contact with the outside world. The process can go on for many hours if necessary. The psychodynamics of the process are crucial to understand, and it's all laid out in Chapter 22, concerning the psychology of interrogation.

Resisting a lawful arrest is a crime in itself, as is escaping after arrest.

Of course, they can't hold a suspect in the police station forever. A person arrested on a drug case has a right to request to be released on bail or bond. He has a right to be told by a judge what the charges against him are. In some jurisdictions, the accused is then brought before a "commissioner" to determine a bond amount. In others, he is brought before a magistrate or judge. How much can you expect a bail or bond amount to be? It depends on all the facts and circumstances of the case and the background of the accused. For example, does the accused have any prior arrests or convictions? Does he live in the area and have ties to the community? What is the recommendation of the investigators or prosecutor? The issue in setting bail is whether the defendant is likely to return to court for all future appearance dates. I've seen most cases of mere possession released without a bail or with a low amount. In rare cases,

I've seen people that the government viewed as major traffickers held without a bond. If the representation of a criminal lawyer has not yet been arranged, the next step in the process is to find qualified counsel.

Finding a Criminal Lawyer

Although everyone has a Constitutional right to proceed *pro se* – on one's own behalf – it's been said that he who represents himself has a fool for a client. Over the years, I've witnessed several pro se defendants try their cases with disastrous results. Navigating the minefields of our criminal justice system can be vexing even for seasoned veterans. The quaint notion that a layperson can plead his own case in a 21st Century American courtroom is woefully misguided. Don't be an idiot. No one should go to court without *professional* legal muscle.

An effective, experienced criminal lawyer is usually a veteran trial lawyer. Most respected criminal practitioners have honed their skills in courtroom battles. They are smart, tough, and articulate. They are quite naturally both intimidating and likable. They think well on their feet and work well under pressure. A 1998 study led by Georgia State psychology professor Dr. James Dabbs found that trial lawyers have higher testosterone levels than other lawyers, reaching levels similar to those of blue-collar laborers like construction workers. [J.M. Dabbs, Jr., E.C. Alford & J.A. Fielden, "Trial lawyers: Blue collar talent in a white collar world," *Journal of Applied Social Psychology*, (1998) 28, 84-94]

... most cases are resolved in plea deals struck with the prosecutor and judge. A good criminal lawyer is a skilled negotiator ...

Although criminal lawyers must be ready and able to defend their client before a trial jury, most cases are resolved in plea deals struck with the prosecutor and judge. A good criminal lawyer is a skilled negotiator with mastery of both the facts and the law, each of which can be wielded as leverage in the bargaining process.

Those who can't afford an attorney get a public defender. Some jurisdictions have institutional public defender offices while other jurisdictions rely on private lawyers who agree to take appointed cases for greatly reduced fees. Some public defenders are terrific lawyers – I know some great ones myself. All hard-working indigent defense lawyers should be commended for defending society's most downtrodden members, often for scandalously low wages. However, a paid professional is *always* the best way to go if you can afford a *good* one. While a Park Avenue or Beverly Hills doctor isn't always better than the one your HMO might give you, often in life you get what you pay for. Assuming you choose wisely.

Bar association referral services are a good source of reputable criminal defense lawyers, as are lawyer directories such as *Martindale-Hubbell* (www.martindale.com). Recommendations from trusted friends or from other lawyers can be great leads. Pay attention to where the offices are located. In suburban or rural communities, courts can be provincial domains where lawyers geographically outside the "inner circle" are ostracized. I've seen situations where adjacent counties each have their own criminal bars, with very little cross-over. A lawyer from County A will typically be less of an "insider" in County B, which can affect the very delicate process of brokering the most favorable deal possible. There's always a significant benefit to "home cooking" when it comes to choosing the right lawyer for a criminal case.

Unless you have a rock-solid recommendation, try to make appointments with at least two lawyers, and check them out online (websites can provide lots of specifics). "Interview" each lawyer in person before signing a retainer. Here are some questions to ask:

1) **How much of your practice is criminal law?** Many lawyers who handle civil matters will take on the occasional criminal case. While they may be good lawyers, they're not in the criminal courthouse every day and may not be thoroughly familiar with the prosecutors, judges and court personnel. There's nothing worse than hiring someone you thought was a criminal lawyer only to find out he or she needs directions to the courthouse. In many places, lawyers who handle mostly or exclusively criminal cases tend to have their offices near the criminal courthouse.

   Ask how long the lawyer has been in practice, and how many criminal cases she has handled. If you know the name of the judge on your case, ask if the lawyer knows that judge. *Not* because the judge might do an inappropriate or unethical favor for a buddy lawyer, but simply because a lawyer whom the judge already sees as honest and credible is likely to be listened to with an open mind. (Some clients don't want a lawyer who is too friendly with the prosecutor or judge, out of fear that the lawyer might compromise rather than aggressively push an issue and fight with her buddies. But every lawyer's primary duty is to the client, and a defense lawyer who is on friendly professional terms with the prosecutors and judges is usually a tremendous asset (provided she is respected, and not merely a push-over or "cop-out" artist). After all, most criminal cases are plea-bargained, not tried. It's human nature to subconsciously be more receptive to those we *like*, and pushy, confrontational lawyers can sometimes be at a *disadvantage*. In interviewing, ask if the lawyer is a former prosecutor (the wonderful advantage of having "played for the other side"). Ask about active membership in local, state or national criminal bar associations as evidence of a commitment to criminal defense.

2) **Who will work on my case?** Not every lawyer is in solo practice. Some of the highest-priced lawyers will dump less serious cases on junior partners or young associates. This may help to keep your legal fees under control, as the value of the associate's time may be significantly less than the value of the "name" lawyer. You may want the more experienced partner to do all the work on the case, but you may not be happy with the costs associated with it. Ask if the partner will be reviewing the associate's work, who will be doing the plea negotiating, and who will try the case if it goes to trial? Assuming an associate will be helping on the case, ask to meet him too. Feel free to ask the associate questions about his background. After all, for most people, being accused of a crime and funneled through the criminal justice system doesn't happen every day. You have every right to know all about the team that will be guiding you through these unfamiliar and sometimes treacherous waters.

3) **What are your fees and payment arrangements?** Typically, criminal lawyers either bill hourly or charge a flat fee for the whole case. Hourly billing has the advantage that you only pay for the time the lawyer expends in your defense. Sometimes a minimum fee and/or a maximum "cap" will be agreed upon. Billing rates vary widely across the country, with rates in large metropolitan areas tending to be higher than in rural areas.

Some highly regarded Manhattan and Los Angeles lawyers charge upwards of $450 per hour. Many lawyers prefer flat fees to hourly billing, and so do many clients. The flat fee is based on numerous factors, including but not limited to the seriousness of the case, the lawyer's expertise in that area, and an estimate of how much legal work and time will be incurred. Since the great majority of criminal cases are resolved through plea-bargaining, dismissal on motions, suppression hearings, etc., the flat fee usually excludes trial. The benefit of a flat fee to a client is that you know precisely what you'll owe right from the start. Many lawyers require an initial retainer of roughly half of the fee; some will accept payment plans or even take credit cards. Flat fees on criminal cases vary even more widely than hourly rates. Felonies will be more expensive than misdemeanors, and federal cases will typically be more expensive than state court cases. Obviously, price is an important factor in hiring a lawyer, but it shouldn't be the primary factor in choosing between lawyers.

4) **What do you know about anabolic steroids?** Most lawyers know *nothing* about anabolic use, although it may not deter them from delivering long-winded and wildly misinformed lectures to you about it. Their ignorance could put you at a tactical disadvantage in court. If your lawyer sees you as a typical "drug addict," she may not explore or present issues that would have been favorable to you. If your lawyer has fully bought into the anti-AAS propaganda that's been fed to the public, how can she stand up to the misinformed ranting of a rabid prosecutor or blustering judge? As a practical matter, the typical criminal lawyer will have never handled a steroid case. That's okay, as long as the lawyer – whether she is a retained lawyer or a public defender – will be willing to do lots of homework and/or hire a good expert consultant. Unfortunately, lawyers confronted with steroid cases tend to retain physicians, toxicologists or pharmacologists as consultants. Many of these so-called experts are poorly informed about non-medical anabolic usage, and the client pays the price for it. A strong, qualified expert can be crucial at the bargaining stage as well as at trial.

After the consultation, ask yourself: Did the lawyer seem willing to *listen,* not just to talk? Too many lawyers spend so much time talking you'd think they were paid by the word! A lawyer should be articulate and informative, but he should also be asking *you* questions and thoughtfully *listening* to what you have to say. Did she make you feel relaxed in your time of great stress, or did you feel rushed and anxious? The criminal justice process can be terribly intimidating, and even the mightiest powerlifter appreciates a little reassurance and some patience from his lawyer. Did the lawyer seem to genuinely *care* about you? If not, walk out. Would you want this person speaking up for you in court? Ideally, your final decision should be based upon your *comfort* and *confidence.* At a gut level, do you feel comfortable putting your trust in this person as the defender who will stand between you and the cold factory of our system of criminal justice? Do you feel completely confident in her knowledge of the law, mastery of the facts, and oratory abilities to persuade a prosecutor, judge or jury? If so, you've found the right lawyer.

Would you want this person speaking up for you in court? Ideally, your final decision should be based upon your *comfort* and *confidence.*

The Process Toward Justice

This first appearance before a judge is called the "arraignment," and it starts the prosecution. Often, it occurs within a day of the arrest if the accused is held in custody. An "accusatory instrument" is filed, setting forth the law the person is charged with violating and the facts supporting the offense. The accused is presumed innocent of the charge. The arraignment includes the advisement of rights, entry of a plea (generally, "not guilty"), and application for release on bail or bond. The prosecutor thereafter refers to the accused as the "Defendant."

In felony cases, the defendant is entitled to a preliminary hearing if he is held in custody. The function of a preliminary hearing is to ensure that a person isn't held in confinement without a basic showing that reasonable cause exists that he committed a felony. In many jurisdictions, prosecutors often avoid preliminary hearings by presenting the charges to a grand jury or by reducing the case to a misdemeanor. This is done so as to avoid the possibility of cross-examination of prosecution witnesses by the defense counsel, as the grand jury is a secret proceeding in which the accused is not permitted to see or hear the witnesses who testify against him and, thus, can't cross-examine them. If it is not already clear to you, this is the government's attempt to limit the amount of information that the defendant obtains at the early stages of the criminal procedure. In short, the less you and your lawyer know about the witnesses and evidence, the better for the government to shield confidential witnesses and evidence.

In misdemeanor cases, sometimes the defendant is arrested on a "complaint" which must later be converted into a formal accusatory "information." In felony cases, the matter must be presented to a grand jury before it can proceed to trial. A grand jury is a body of local people who will hear the prosecutor's evidence and decide if there's reasonable cause for the case to go forward. For example, in a steroid sale case, the grand jury might typically hear from the undercover agent who made the purchase and would receive a laboratory analysis of the drugs. It is fairly uncommon in steroid cases for the accused to testify in his own behalf before a grand jury. This is because the role of defense counsel at the grand jury stage is very limited. When a defendant testifies before a grand jury, his counsel's presence is permitted but he has virtually no active role. He generally cannot object to questions asked or protect the client; he is the proverbial potted plant. If the grand jury is not satisfied that there's reasonable cause to believe that the accused committed a felony, they can return "no true bill," dismissing the charges. If the evidence is sufficient, the case moves forward to an arraignment on the new accusatory instrument, called an *indictment*.

Throughout the progress of the case, the defense lawyer and the prosecutor will "conference" the case by telephone and in court. These discussions are designed to exchange information, test the strengths and weaknesses of the opposition's case, and explore the possibility of a resolution to the charges short of a trial. However, many prosecutors will play it close to the vest, withholding key pieces of information for tactical reasons. The prosecutor may make a "plea offer" to dispose of the case, or may try to induce the defendant to "cooperate" in the investigation and arrest of others. The prosecutor will take into account various factors in making an offer, most notably the seriousness of the crime and the prior criminal history of the accused, as well as the strength of the case and issues of potential suppres-

> ... it is common for years of bad and often inaccurate publicity about anabolics to taint the views of the prosecutor and judge.

sion. How the individual prosecutor assigned to the case perceives anabolic steroids can play a role; it is common for years of bad and often inaccurate publicity about anabolics to taint the views of the prosecutor and judge. The defense lawyer will conduct all necessary investigation and research, and attempt to negotiate a favorable disposition for his client. During this period, the case may appear on the court calendar and the defendant's appearance at court will customarily be required even though the case is simply *adjourned* to another day.

The defense is entitled to certain information about the case that is in the possession of the prosecution. This information may be voluntarily disclosed, or requested by the defense lawyer in papers known as *demands for discovery* and *requests for bills of particulars*. Many of the responses of prosecutors are so-called boilerplate responses that are standard forms and do not provide extensive information. Often detailed information will not be available until the pretrial hearing stage. The prosecutor will request reciprocal discovery as allowed by law. The defense will have an opportunity to view any physical evidence, such as the anabolics in question. In some jurisdictions, the defense has a right to depose witnesses. The defense may file motions challenging the case, such as seeking dismissal or suppression of evidence or review of defects in the grand jury procedure. These motions, along with the demand for discovery and request for a bill of particulars, are collectively referred to as an "omnibus" motion.

The presumption of innocence continues throughout the trial. The prosecutor must prove the case ... beyond a reasonable doubt.

If a confession was allegedly extracted, the statement may be challenged on voluntariness grounds or because of failure of the *Miranda* warnings. Suppression of the tangible evidence (i.e., the steroids) may be sought based upon a violation of the Fourth Amendment rights of the accused. If a search warrant was executed, a motion may be made to controvert the warrant. Obviously, familiarity with the issues pertinent to anabolic steroids may be of crucial importance in this process. The case may proceed to evidentiary suppression hearings in which the court decides if the jury should be allowed to hear or see the evidence. If the defense is unsuccessful in having the evidence thrown out, the case may proceed to a trial before a judge or jury. The presumption of innocence continues throughout the trial. The prosecutor must prove the case against him beyond a reasonable doubt. Each and every element of the crime must be proven. The judge or jury will render a verdict. Unless the accused is acquitted, he will ordinarily face sentencing upon a conviction a few weeks later. After sentence is imposed, an appeal may be taken to challenge the conviction or the sentence.

Overview of Plea Bargaining and Sentencing

The vast majority of cases (over 90%) do *not* go to trial. They are resolved through a variety of other means, including "plea bargaining," dismissal of the charges by a grand jury, dismissal of the case by the judge (because of a defective accusatory instrument, the suppression of evidence, or the failure by the prosecution to provide a speedy trial). In a plea bargain, the defendant gives up his right to a trial and various other rights. In return, he may be offered the opportunity to plead guilty to a lesser charge. A plea bargain is a compromise that avoids the uncertainty of a trial for both sides. Generally, the defendant gets a better deal than he would get if he went to trial and lost. Plea bargaining practices vary widely, not only from state to state but also from county to county. Some prosecutor's offices have rigid policies, sometimes spelled out in written interoffice manuals. For example, in some jurisdictions, the standard plea offer on a felony charge is a "one down" offer, so that on a class "B" felony charge the offer would be a class "C" felony. In some jurisdictions, it is common for the defense to waive a presentation to the grand jury if a plea bargain is agreed upon. In some jurisdictions, the accused must waive his right to an appeal. On misdemeanor cases, plea bargaining is often more flexible. In most cases, the judge is involved in the plea bargain, to a greater or lesser extent. In many state courts, the judge commits to a specific sentence to be imposed if a guilty plea is entered. The defendant knows exactly what sentence he will receive on the bargain prior to accepting it. In other jurisdictions, including the federal courts, the judge is not bound by the plea agreement. The sentence is only limited by laws or sentencing guidelines, and the defendant takes a chance as to what the sentence will be.

As in all drug cases, sentences in anabolic steroid cases vary widely based upon a multitude of factors: the jurisdiction, the particular judge, the background of the accused, the quantity of steroids, the seriousness of the offense, etc. Hawaii has actually codified what most judges do by discretion:

> § 706-606 Factors to be considered in imposing a sentence. The court, in determining the particular sentence to be imposed, shall consider:
> (1) The nature and circumstances of the offense and the history and characteristics of the defendant;
> (2) The need for the sentence imposed:
>   (a) To reflect the seriousness of the offense, to promote respect for law, and to provide just punishment for the offense;
>   (b) To afford adequate deterrence to criminal conduct;
>   (c) To protect the public from further crimes of the defendant; and
>   (d) To provide the defendant with needed educational or vocational training, medical care, or other correctional treatment in the most effective manner;
> (3) The kinds of sentences available; and
> (4) The need to avoid unwarranted sentence disparities among defendants with similar records who have been found guilty of similar conduct. [HRS § 706-606]

A sentence may include imprisonment, incarceration in a local jail, probationary supervision, home confinement, community service, monetary fines, surcharges or some combination. The sentence is often guided by the recommendations of the probation department. Once a guilty plea is entered, the case is typically adjourned for sentence for at least a month (sometimes a bit less if the defendant is incarcerated), during which time a presentence investigation is conducted by the probation department into the facts of the case and the character of the defendant.

A sentence may include imprisonment, incarceration in a local jail, probationary supervision, home confinement, community service, monetary fines, surcharges or some combination.

Regrettably, the pervasive misinformation about anabolic steroids can unfairly taint the judge's perceptions and result in inappropriately harsh sentencing. It is not uncommon for the report that goes to the judge to say that "documented adverse side effects [of anabolics include] cancer of the liver, jaundice, testicular atrophy, increased risk of coronary heart disease, sterility, birth defects, prostate cancer, increased masculinity in women, and increased aggressive behavior in men" (quoting an actual report). Some of these effects are legitimate, while others would need serious qualification before they could be deemed in any way accurate. The presentation of a list like this is a misleading portrayal of the actual extent of the risks to healthy adult males. Yet a steroid defendant must stand up in front of a judge who has read these reports and will rely on them in his sentence.

Alternative Sentencing Options

What sentencing options are there? It would be impossible to go through all the statutory sections dealing with all aspects of sentencing for every state. Many states have provisions requiring mandatory terms of imprisonment. However, separate provisions may provide options for "alternative sentencing," such as drug courts, drug programs or interim probation. In some jurisdictions, certain teenaged offenders are eligible to have their records sealed because of their age. State laws vary widely, but many first-time offenders are eligible, particularly in cases of personal use possession. Even for many repeat offenders, alternative sentencing options exist.

In many first-time situations, a period of probationary supervision is likely. Sometimes probation is a condition of a sentence, so that it occurs after the court case is finished. The requirements of each state's version of probation are often spelled out in great detail in its statutes. Typically, the offender is required to regularly report to the probation department offices (i.e., weekly or monthly), to submit to random or regular drug testing, to consent to home visits and warrantless home searches by probation officials, and to participate in any drug abuse counseling that probation officials deem necessary.

Most states have provisions that permit a defendant to be put on probationary supervision *before* the case is resolved, as a *condition* of its resolution. This procedure is called by different names in various states, including Conditional Discharge, Probation Before Judgment (PBJ), Pre-Trial Intervention (PTI), interim probation, deferred judgment, deferred sentence or suspended sentence. The way these procedures typically work is that, with the consent of the defendant, the court defers judgment and places the defendant on interim probation upon conditions as it may require. Upon a showing that the defendant is not cooperating with the program of probation or is not responding to it, the court may withdraw the defendant from the program, pronounce judgment, and impose any sentence authorized by law. Before taking that action, the court has to give the defendant an opportunity to be heard as to any matter relevant to the court's proposed action. Upon fulfillment of the conditions of interim probation and the payment of any fees imposed, the defendant gets discharged from probation without entry of judgment. In essence, he walks away with a clean record.

Most states have provisions that permit a defendant to be put on probationary supervision *before* the case is resolved, as a *condition* of its resolution.

For example, the District of Columbia has a provision dealing with this interim probation before judgment procedure. [DC ST § 48-904.01(e)]:

(1) If any person who has not previously been convicted of violating any provision of this chapter, or any other law of the United States or any state relating to narcotic or abusive drugs or depressant or stimulant substances is found guilty of a violation of sub-

section (d) of this section and has not previously been discharged and had the proceedings dismissed pursuant to this subsection, the court may, without entering a judgment of guilty and with the consent of such person, defer further proceedings and place him or her on probation upon such reasonable conditions as it may require and for such period, not to exceed one year, as the court may prescribe. Upon violation of a condition of the probation, the court may enter an adjudication of guilt and proceed as otherwise provided. The court may, in its discretion, dismiss the proceedings against such person and discharge him or her from probation before the expiration of the maximum period prescribed for such person's probation. If during the period of probation such person does not violate any of the conditions of the probation, then upon expiration of such period the court shall discharge such person and dismiss the proceedings against him or her. Discharge and dismissal under this subsection shall be without court adjudication of guilt, but a nonpublic record thereof shall be retained solely for the purpose of use by the courts in determining whether or not, in subsequent proceedings, such person qualifies under this subsection. Such discharge or dismissal shall not be deemed a conviction for purposes of disqualifications or disabilities imposed by law upon conviction of a crime (including the penalties prescribed under § 48-904.08 for second or subsequent convictions) or for any other purpose.

(2) Upon the dismissal of such person and discharge of the proceedings against him under paragraph (1) of this subsection, such person may apply to the court for an order to expunge from all official records (other than the nonpublic records to be retained under paragraph (1) of this subsection) all recordation relating to his or her arrest, indictment or information, trial, finding of guilty, and dismissal and discharge pursuant to this subsection. If the court determines, after hearing, that such person was dismissed and the proceedings against him or her discharged, it shall enter such order. The effect of such order shall be to restore such person, in the contemplation of this law, to the status he or she occupied before such arrest or indictment or information. No person as to whom such order has been entered shall be held thereafter under any provision of any law to be guilty of perjury or otherwise giving a false statement by reason of failure to recite or acknowledge such arrest, or indictment, or trial in response to any inquiry made of him or her for any purpose.

Where straight probation is not a viable option, other alternative sentencing options may exist. Where a judge feels that a brief period of incarceration is warranted, home detention by electronic monitoring (the ol' ankle bracelet) is a possibility in some jurisdictions. Home detention can permit an offender to keep a job he might otherwise have lost. When an offender's prior record or other aggravating factors weigh against a lenient sentence, the offender may be eligible for a brief but intense "boot camp" in lieu of a more extended term of incarceration [e.g., the "impact incarceration" of Illinois (730 ILCS 5/5-8-1.1) or "shock incarceration" of New York (NYS Corrections Law, Article 26-A)]. Even in situations where a conviction is entered, many states have provisions that permit the

Where straight probation is not a viable option, other alternative sentencing options may exist.

conviction to be expunged if the person leads a law-abiding life for a specific number of years. However, in states (like New York) that have no expungement provisions, a conviction remains on the person's record forever and can be a significant bar to future career opportunities.

Our discussion has touched upon what provisions exist on the books within each state, but the best source for what's actually happening in practice is an experienced criminal lawyer licensed to practice in and familiar with the particular jurisdiction. Not only do state laws vary, but there are variations of practice and policy from county to county within each state. Moreover, new drug treatment counseling programs arise constantly, and state laws change as well. Bottom line: while this book gives some broad information, the mechanisms by which to avoid a criminal conviction or any state's statutory prison terms should be discussed with your lawyer, who should hopefully be extremely well versed in the options including any new developments.

Our discussions in this chapter and the last one have touched upon a variety of state law provisions (see the Appendix for additional information on the most salient laws in each of the states), but the best source for what's currently happening in any specific jurisdiction is an experienced criminal lawyer licensed to practice in and familiar with that particular area. Not only do state laws vary, but there are variations of practice and policy from county to county within each state. Even within a county, individual judges often have their own quirks and sentencing policies. Just because certain mechanisms for leniency exist or are commonly utilized in some courts doesn't mean that *every* judge goes along with them. In many jurisdictions, every case is judged on its own specific facts. Moreover, new drug treatment counseling programs arise constantly, and state laws change as well.

Further, while it's been discussed earlier in the federal context (Chapter 4), merely avoiding jail or prison doesn't necessarily mean you're out of harm's way. In many states, a drug conviction even without jail can have devastating consequences. Professional licenses can be lost. Tuition assistance can be taken away. Non-citizens can be deported. A driver's license can be suspended. An AAS offender can jeopardize *present* employment as well as future employment.

Chapter 7

WINNY, WARRANTS & PROBABLE CAUSE

"Private property is held sacred in all good governments, and particularly in our own."
– *Andrew Jackson (1767-1845)*

Let's say you get arrested for a fight in a bar, and the police search your pockets and find a few tabs of Winny (Winstrol). Or you're driving around and get stopped for speeding, and the police see a Sustanon preload in your center console. Or the Postal Inspector seizes your package of gear. Or the police get a search warrant for your house because a snitch ratted. Or you get frisked by Customs at the airport. Welcome to the Fourth Amendment, my friends, which plays a part in virtually every anabolic steroid case you'll ever see.

The Fourth Amendment

The Fourth Amendment to the Constitution of the United States protects all persons in America from governmental intrusions upon their privacy, dignity, and security. It's intended to protect the rights of both the innocent and the guilty against arbitrary and invasive acts by agents of the government. It doesn't protect against the invasive acts of private citizens unless those private citizens are acting at the direction of the government. It doesn't protect specific places or property. Instead, it guards our *expectations of privacy* in places or property wherever they can be said to exist.

The protection of our privacy is not absolute. The government is allowed to interrupt the enjoyment of our privacy under certain conditions. The limits of these conditions are founded in the language of the Fourth Amendment, which is broken into two separate clauses. The first clause talks about "unreasonable searches and seizures" and the second clause deals with "warrants upon probable cause." Here's the way it reads:

> "The right of the people to be secure in their persons, house, papers, and effects, against unreasonable searches and seizures, shall not be violated, and no Warrants shall issue, but upon probable cause, supported by Oath or affirmation, and particularly describing the place to be searched, and the persons or things to be seized."

Warrantless Searches

Some people are surprised that under the first clause, we're *not* protected from searches and seizures without warrants. We're not even protected from searches and seizures without probable cause. Instead, we're protected from searches and seizures that are *unreasonable*. What's unreasonable? It depends on the situation. Inherent in the concept of reasonableness is a balance between between the government's interests and the individual's rights. Sometimes a warrant is required for a search or seizure to be reasonable. Examples might include most situations where the police want to search your house or open a piece of your mail. Under a case called *Payton v. New York* [445 U.S. 573 (1980)], a warrant for your arrest is required to enter your home to arrest you (unless you consent to let them in, or they are chasing you in hot pursuit). However, a warrant isn't always needed for a search or seizure to be reasonable. There are numerous circumstances in which a search or seizure can be quite reasonable without a warrant, or even without probable cause. These circumstances include situations of emergency or exigency. For example, the police might lawfully enter your home without a warrant if they had reason to believe that someone inside was injured and in need of immediate medical attention. If the police are in hot pursuit of a suspect, they can reasonably enter premises that otherwise would have required them to have a warrant in order to enter. A search incident to an arrest (see Chapter 9, page 123) is considered reasonable, if the search is restricted to a limited area around the arrestee. Searches of individuals entering the United States at borders don't require warrants or probable cause (see Chapter 8). Seizures and searches of cars are reasonable without warrants, and often without probable cause (see Chapter 9). Police can stop and frisk an individual on the street without a warrant or probable cause, but they do need to reasonably suspect that the person committed a crime. No warrant or probable cause is required for so-called "inventory" searches when an arrestee's car is impounded, or whenever an individual voluntarily consents to a search of his property.

Probable Cause

What's *probable cause*? Essentially, it's that a reasonable person would conclude that a crime occurred or that evidence of a crime would be found in a particular place. How would a person reach a conclusion like that? There's no specific, magic formula. In the landmark case of *Illinois v. Gates* [462 U.S. 213 (1983)], the Supreme Court articulated a *totality of the circumstances* standard to evaluate probable cause, stressing "commonsense" and "fair probability." Probable cause must exist *at the time* – it can't be bolstered by facts discovered later. The standard by which probable cause is reviewed is an *objective* one, not the subjective belief of the officer. However, in some cases an officer may use his experience to determine whether probable cause exists, such as knowing how marijuana smells or what a gunshot sounds like. For example, in *People v. Gill* [138 A.D.2d 738 (1988)], the court ruled that, "the Trooper saw the marihuana in plain view thereby giving him the requisite probable cause to arrest the occupants of the vehicle and conduct a further search." Similarly, in *United States v. Garcia-Rodriguez* [558 F.2d 956 (1977)], the United States Court of Appeals for the Ninth Circuit stated that in a valid investigative stop, the detection of marijuana odor emanating from a vehicle has been held sufficient to give rise to probable cause to search. Likewise, the observation of what apparently is contraband material in plain view within a vehicle would also give rise to probable cause for a search.

Probable cause must exist *at the time* — it can't be bolstered by facts discovered later.

In most cases, the observations of the officer – that is, what a reasonable man, knowing all of the facts within the cognizance of the officer, would have believed under all the circumstances – can establish probable cause. [*Martin v. State,* 194 So.2d 291 (1967)] For example, in *People v. Burke* [146 A.D.2d 706 (1989)], the arresting officer observed, in plain view, a clear plastic bag containing white powder that he believed to be cocaine in a vehicle which the defendant was occupying. Taking into account the totality of the circumstances (as the vehicle was parked in a manner obstructing traffic on a one-way street late at night, with the engine running and the lights on, the driver was asleep and provided mumbled, slurred responses to the police officer's inquiries, and the other occupants of the vehicle appeared to be "nervous and fidgety"), the seizure of the bag and the arrest of the car's occupants were proper.

As you can see, the police arrest people for drugs every day without lab reports. Let's say the police find a crackhead with a rock of crack in a baggie. Are they 100% sure it's crack? Of course not; it could be a piece of plaster from the wall. But if they needed a laboratory analysis in order to arrest him, they'd need to take the rock and then try to find the guy weeks later after the report came back. Nobody would ever be caught. Instead, the law reasonably allows the police to arrest him based only on *probable cause* to believe it's crack. The guy can be arrested, arraigned and held on bail all before a lab report is obtained. The same is true with anabolics. All they need is probable cause – a fair probability based on all the circumstances, including the officer's training and experience in identifying controlled substances. This can be a crucial issue in steroid cases, because not every officer's training and experience provides him with the ability to identify anabolic steroids. Obviously, if your vial is labeled "Testosterona" you may not have much of an argument. But if the case involves tablets in an unmarked container, the officer may not have a clue. Of course, if he asks you what the pills are and you tell him "steroids," he now has the probable cause he didn't have before. Don't laugh – I've seen that happen on several occasions.

Searches and Seizures

A *search* occurs when the police use their senses of sight, hearing, touch, etc., to intrude upon an individual's privacy. A search may be conducted on a person or in a place. What constitutes a search depends upon the facts. An officer who sees contraband in open view in a suspect's front yard would not be conducting a search. However, an officer moving an object to improve his or her view of it can be a search, depending on the circumstances. A search is a search, even if it happens to disclose nothing. When an officer inserts his hand into your pocket, it's a search – regardless of whether he finds any D-bol.

In *United States v. Williams* [262 U.S. App. D.C. 112 (1987)], the District of Columbia Circuit Court of Appeals ruled that a police officer did not conduct a search when he squeezed the outside of a paper bag and felt, according to his testimony, "small rolled up objects" which "felt like plastic baggies." Based on his training and experience, the officer concluded that the bag contained packages of heroin, which was confirmed when he opened the bag. The Court concluded that the officer's "plain touch" was not a search and was not more extensive than was justified by the nature of the investigation. Handling the bag left the officer reasonably certain that it contained contraband and the "apprehension of that which is already in plain view of an officer lawfully present at his vantage point does not infringe any reasonable expectation of privacy, and its exposure is not a search within the meaning of the Fourth Amendment."

Alternatively, in *Hernandez v. United States* [353 F.2d 624 (1965)], the court found a search of defendant's bags was conducted, involving both smell and touch. The government argued that the bags were not searched until they were opened. The court held that the manipulation of the bags constituted a search within the meaning of the Fourth Amendment. The contents of the bags were not exposed to the police officer's sight or smell before the bags were squeezed, forcing air out of them.

A *seizure* is a physical taking of any tangible item, and even of certain intangibles like conversations. The Fourth Amendment applies not only to seizures of property but to seizures of persons, too. A seizure is a "taking possession" of a person so that he is not free to leave. [*California v. Hodari D.*, 499 U.S. 621 (1991)] A seizure occurs when a reasonable person would have believed that he is not free to go. A completely consensual encounter which was not a seizure at its beginning can become one if, by the police conduct, a reasonable person would believe that he was no longer free to leave. Obviously, a person who is arrested has been seized. What constitutes a "seizure" in a particular case is highly fact-dependent. For example, detaining a person to question him [*Reid v. Georgia*, 448 U.S. 438 (1980)] or to ascertain his identity [*Brown v. Texas*, 443 U.S. 47 (1979)] are seizures. It is not a seizure, however, for police officers to follow a person on the street [*Michigan v. Chesternut*, 486 U.S. 567 (1988)]. Stopping an automobile and detaining its occupants is a seizure [*Colorado v. Bannister*, 449 U.S. 1(1980); *Delaware v. Prouse*, 440 U.S. 648 (1979)]. Detention of luggage for a dog sniff is a seizure [*United States v. Place*, 462 U.S. 696 (1983)], but the mere recording of serial numbers off property during the execution of a warrant for other property is not a seizure [*Arizona v. Hicks*, 480 U.S. 321 (1987)]. Interception or receiving of telephone messages by a wiretap is a seizure [*Katz v. United States*, 389 U.S. 347 (1967)], while monitoring of a beeper placed on an object moving in public places is not [*United States v. Knotts*, 460 U.S. 276 (1983)].

What the government can or can't properly search or seize in any given case is ultimately for a judge to decide. Did the police need a warrant to search what they did? Was their seizure of certain objects reasonable? If the police had a warrant, did their conduct exceed the warrant's authority? This is the stuff that criminal defense lawyers and prosecutors fight about all the time. The body of Fourth Amendment case law is enormous, and goes far beyond our scope. It's of somewhat limited practical value, anyway. Since the legality of a search or seizure is for a judge to decide, there's not too much to do about it until then. For example, under a case called *Terry v. Ohio* [392 U.S. 1 (1968)], the police can stop and frisk you on the street if they have reasonable suspicion that you committed a crime. However, they can't reach into your pockets without probable cause. If they do, and find something illegal, what are you going to do? Scream at them about *Terry v. Ohio*? Run away? Take them on, mano à mano?

A warrant is a judge's advance authorization for the government to search a particular place or seize a particular person or objects.

Challenging Searches and Seizures

The way to address an illegal search or seizure is to have your lawyer challenge it in court. Your lawyer can file a motion to exclude or suppress the evidence based upon the Fourth Amendment violation. If the prosecutor believes that the search or seizure was legally proper, he files opposition papers. The judge will generally order a *suppression hearing* to be held so that she can hear all the facts. At that hearing, the police or agents will be called to testify.

If the judge finds that the government violated your Fourth Amendment rights, the evidence produced by the search or seizure is tainted by the illegal police conduct and can't be used against you. This is the so-called Exclusionary Rule, applicable to the federal courts by *Weeks v. U.S.* [232 U.S. 383 (1914)] and held applicable to the states by the landmark Supreme Court decision in *Mapp v. Ohio* [367 U.S. 643 (1961)]. (Each state is free to enact protections greater than those afforded by federal law, but they can't do less.) So, if the police arrested you for a bar fight without probable cause, the Winny tabs they found in your pocket couldn't be used as evidence against you. (But unless you had a prescription, of course, you wouldn't get them back.)

If the battle over Fourth Amendment issues takes place in court, what *practical* information is helpful for you to know? Well, you can't control what the government is going to do to you. You can, however, control what *you* do, and that's the key to protecting your privacy interests. Your protection against the invasive acts of the government lies in maximizing your *expectations of privacy*.

Expectations of Privacy

The landmark case of *Katz v. United States* [389 U.S. 347 (1967)] established the standard for an individual's interest against governmental intrusion. To claim the protections of the Fourth Amendment against an unreasonable search or seizure, you must have a legitimate and reasonable expectation of privacy in the object or place that is the subject of the government's action. Not all expectations of privacy are equal; you may have greater or lesser expectations of privacy in various items depending on the circumstances. A guy who shares an apartment with two other guys has a lesser expectation of privacy in the place than if he lived alone. However, he would have a greater expectation of privacy in his own bedroom than he would in the shared rooms and common hallways. If a person leaves his property in open view for everybody to see, or if he discards or abandons it, he may diminish or even completely give up his expectations of privacy. In *Rawlings v. Kentucky* [448 U.S. 98 (1980)], the Court found no reasonable expectation of privacy when Rawlings stashed several thousand dollars worth of drugs in the purse of a friend, as the police were about to search him. The Court reasoned that Rawlings had never sought nor received access to the purse prior to the incident, he had no right to exclude others from the purse, and the nature of the transaction hardly supports a reasonable inference that Rawlings took normal precautions to maintain his privacy.

In *Katz*, Justice Harlan stated that the expectation of privacy, "be one that society is prepared to recognize as reasonable." In the course of the evolution of this doctrine, the Supreme Court has held that society recognizes no reasonable expectation of privacy: in movements of a vehicle on a highway [*United States v. Knotts, supra*], in activities conducted in open fields [*Oliver v. United States*, 466 U.S. 170 (1984)], in any areas easily visible from the air [*Florida v. Riley*, 488 U.S. 445 (1989)], in the public area of business [*Maryland v. Macon*, 472 U.S. 463 (1985)], in a prison [*Hudson v. Palmer*, 468 U.S. 517 (1984)], in the chemical composition of drugs [*United States v. Jacobsen*, 466 U.S. 109 (1984)], in drugs secreted in another's purse [*Rawlings v. Kentucky, supra*], or in packaging drugs at another's drug house [*Minnesota v. Carter*, 525 U.S. 83 (1998)]. The Court has found that society does recognize a reasonable expectation of privacy: in a desk and file cabinet at work [*O'Connor v. Ortega*, 480 U.S. 709 (1987)], in the taking of breath and urine samples [*Skinner v. Railway Labor Executives' Asso.*, 489 U.S. 602 (1989)], and in the home of a host by his or her guest [*Minnesota v. Olson*, 485 U.S. 91 (1990)].

Privacy in Trash

A favorite recent tactic of law enforcement is to collect the garbage of suspected drug dealers and pick through it looking for enough evidence to get a search warrant. In a recent Kansas case, local police officers tenaciously collected the suspect's garbage and carefully combed through it for five straight weeks until they finally had enough to ask a judge to sign a search warrant for the residence. The legal issue with police trash searches is whether or not the suspect retains an expectation of privacy in his own garbage, protecting it from unreasonable search and seizure. The U.S. Supreme Court addressed the issue in *California v. Greenwood* [486 U.S. 35 (1988)]. In that case, the police, suspecting drug dealing, asked the trash collectors to turn over the garbage of the residence. An examination of the garbage revealed evidence of narcotics activity, and on that basis a search warrant was obtained. The warrant was executed and drugs were recovered. Although the dissent argued that "scrutiny of another's trash is contrary to accepted notions of civilized behavior," the majority held that garbage "exposed" to children, dogs, snoops and scavengers who might pick through it retained *no privacy protections* under the Fourth Amendment.

Of course, state courts can provide greater privacy protections for their residents than the Supreme Court requires, and some have. Hawaii and Vermont, for example, have supported findings of a reasonable expectation of privacy in one's trash. [*See*, *State v. Tanaka*, 701 P.2d 1274 (1985, Hawaii); *State v. Morris*, 680 A.2d 90 (1996, Vt.) (Opaque trash bags placed at curbside for collection were protected; *Greenwood* rejected)] Some state courts have held that whether you still have privacy expectations in your garbage depends on the unique circumstances of the case. For example, the Alaska Supreme Court suggested that the analysis should consider how close the garbage was located to the dwelling, whether the dwelling was a single or multiple unit, whether the trash was removed by the police or obtained from the garbage men, and where the search of the trash took place. [*Smith v. State*, 510 P2.d 793 (1973, Alaska)] Trash bags kept next to the house or in the side yard might retain significantly more privacy protections than those at the curb under this analysis.

The public accessibility of curbside trash can raise a different issue: how do we know that what's in the can wasn't tossed in there by somebody else? A court in Illinois recently took on the issue, holding that since strangers have access to curbside trash, the existence of incriminating evidence in the trash doesn't automatically create probable cause to search the residence without some proof it was the defendant's stuff. [*People v. Burmeister*, 728 N.E.2d 1260 (2000, Ill.)]

While the courts continue to sift through the issues, there's a cautionary lesson to be learned here. Your privacy rights in your trash are limited.

Consent

The easiest way for the police to pierce privacy protections is by *consent*. Not only is a search warrant not required, but neither is probable cause. With willing consent, the police can do just about anything (within reason), because you have voluntarily relinquished your expectations of privacy. Whatever the police find, they can use as evidence against you.

Why do so many people give consent to the police to poke around their homes, mail, belongings and pockets? Police encounters of even the most innocuous types can elicit a sense of panic. The late film director Alfred Hitchcock, whose films plumbed the depths of fear and suspense, expressed only one disabling phobia: he was terrified of the police. The police may surprise you by appearing at the door: "We need to speak with you. Do you mind if we come in?" Startled and off their guard, most people can't say "no." The police can suddenly approach a person walking on the street: "Do you mind if we look in your bag?" Resistance is quickly responded to with a selection from a menu of choices, from the disarming to the oppressive.

Police officers who suspect criminal activity have a duty to gather evidence and prevent its destruction. They may be seriously concerned about their own safety, particularly if they're in the unfamiliar territory of the suspect's residence. In order to effectively do their jobs and to protect themselves, they may be both intimidating and persuasive, often simultaneously. Many people don't know that they have a right to refuse consent, or simply forget that right in the pressure of the moment. Most people are frightened that if they refuse to consent, they'll *look* guilty. So what? If they *are* guilty, they ought to be frightened about what a search would *reveal.*

The paramount issue in any consent search is whether the consent was *voluntary*. The voluntariness of consent is judged by a "totality of the circumstances" test. [*Schneckcloth v. Bustamonte*, 412 U.S. 218 (1973), *Florida v. Bostick*, 501 U.S. 429 (1991)] Each case is different, and a court's decision can turn on the tiniest factual details. The burden of proving consent rests on the government. [*Bumper v. North Carolina*, 391 U.S. 543 (1968)] There are no magic words required to express consent. It can be either written or oral. It can even be manifested just by a gesture. The FBI's *Legal Handbook for Special Agents* instructs agents to obtain consent in writing. Refusing to sign a "Consent to Search" form, but providing consent to search verbally, doesn't invalidate the search (although it may provide an argument that there really was no verbal consent). What does a "Consent to Search" form look like? Here's an example of one used in a steroid case by a township police department in Northern New Jersey:

CONSENT TO SEARCH

I,____________________________, having been informed of my constitutional rights; first, that I may require that a search warrant be obtained prior to any search being made; second, that I may refuse to consent to any search; third, that anything which may be found as a result of this search which is subject to seizure can and will be seized and used against me in a criminal prosecution; fourth, that I may revoke my consent to search at any time; and fifth, that I may consult with anyone of my choosing before I make a decision to waive my rights. By consenting to this search, I hereby authorize ______________
____________________________ and ____
(members of the XXX Township Police Dept.) to conduct a complete search of the premises or vehicle under my control described as ___________________________________
____

This written permission is given by me voluntarily and without threats or promises of any kind being made to me.

I hereby expressly waive my right to be physically present during the execution of this search.

WITNESSES Signature _________________________________

____

Date ___________________________________

____

The fact that a suspect is under arrest or in custody doesn't mean the consent is involuntary. An example is a recent case in which the defendant, under arrest for accepting the controlled delivery of a steroid package, gave consent for the agents to search a storage facility in which they recovered a larger quantity of anabolics. However, the totality of circumstances may weigh against voluntariness, such as where a suspect is on the ground, surrounded by officers with guns pointed. Must the police advise a suspect that he has a right to remain silent and a right to counsel before requesting consent to search? Most jurisdictions have held that the failure to administer *Miranda* warnings doesn't make consent involuntary (although it is a factor to consider in the totality of circumstances).

The police may request consent from a third party to search a suspect's property where that third party has the express or implied "common authority" to consent. This policy is justified by the reduced expectation of privacy that a person has in premises or property shared with someone else. The person runs the risk that the third party will consent to a search of property that is not under exclusive control. The issue arises frequently in the situation where one family member is asked to consent to the search of another's room or belongings. For example, if the suspect is not home, the police can request his mother to allow them to search his room.

Quite often, the police will assert, "Either you consent, or we'll be right back with a warrant." Such an assertion doesn't make the consent involuntary if the police have probable cause. However, consent as a result of threats, harassment or official intimidation is not consent at all. There is a difference between consent and "submission to a claim of authority." If the police assert that they have the absolute right of authority to conduct the search regardless of consent, the consent is involuntary. Of course, exactly what facts led to the purported consent can become the subject of a suppression hearing.

The "Knock-and-Talk"

A successful technique among law enforcement officers since the 1980s is the so-called "knock-and-talk." Knowing that they lack probable cause, but suspecting criminality, the officers will walk up to a suspect's door, knock, and request entry. The technique takes advantage of the elements of surprise and innate submission to authority. Once inside, the suspect is confronted with the officers' suspicions and is asked to permit them to take a look around. Although inherently coercive, these entries have been upheld by courts in many states. The knock-and-talk is standard procedure in many mail order cases where probable cause is weak or non-existent.

The knock-and-talk is standard procedure in many mail order cases where probable cause is weak or non-existent.

Note that once the police are inside, they may rely upon other concepts to justify further peeping. For example, the plain view doctrine applies because the police now are lawfully on the premises. While one officer talks to the suspect, the other may be scanning every visible corner of the room for some scrap of evidence of crime. If found, probable cause is established for an arrest, and even in the absence of consent, the area around the suspect can now be searched "incident to" the lawful arrest.

Here are the facts from an interesting case I defended in sunny southern California. My client, Ramon, was alleged to be involved with smuggling bulk quantities of juice across the border from Mexico and then mailing packages of steroids to buyers throughout the United States from a base of operations in a hotel room. The local police department had received a tip apparently from a hotel clerk that a suspicious volume of packages was being delivered to a particular room in the hotel. The police began monitoring the packages addressed to the hotel. One day, Ramon went to the front desk to collect his mail and two detectives appeared. They presented him with a domestic Priority Mail envelope addressed to his room, and advised him that complaints had been made about narcotics activity associated with the room. They said he was not under arrest, but asked what was in the package. Ramon told them that there were no drugs inside; he was just expecting some money for an apartment. They asked if he would consent to them opening the envelope right there. Caught by surprise, he assented. The package was found to contain $20,000 in cash, an airline ticket, some clear packing tape, mailing labels and other items. The detectives questioned the amount of cash and the other items, then dropped the bomb: "Do you have any drugs in the room?" Stunned, surrounded, reeling, Ramon said, "Go ahead, check it, I have no drugs." He handed the hotel key to the detectives. Once inside the room, the detectives did a visual sweep and noticed many Styrofoam peanuts used for shipping and mailing of packages. On the dresser were used Priority Mail envelopes, many unused FedEx envelopes, lots of Western Union receipts, posted notes with assorted addresses, and various shipping labels. Then bingo – amid all the clutter was a box of five hundred bottles of testosterone. Both Ramon and his roommate were arrested. A full search recovered hundreds more bottles, ampoules and tablets of assorted anabolic steroids and ancillary drugs.

Ultimately, Ramon didn't do too badly. He served 43 days in jail before being released and was sentenced to probation for 5 years to be served back in his native Puerto Rico. Still, Ramon might have quite easily avoided being arrested at all. His case presents the perfect example of how one thing leads to another. Once Ramon agreed to talk to the police, he established a precedent of cooperativeness that made it psychologically difficult to be less cooperative later on. Each further act of cooperation – consent to opening the package, answering further questions – made it more and more difficult to deny the request to search the room.

The bottom line point is: there's no way to know what if any information the police have. Probable cause? Reasonable suspicion? Just a hunch? Whether they can lawfully seize or search will be for a judge to decide. However, a basic rule of thumb: *if they have enough to search, they wouldn't be asking for consent.* Got that? If you want to maximize your privacy interests, you can do it simply: *Consent to nothing.* People who refuse to consent to give up their expectations of privacy force the government to rely only on the information that they already have. If it's not enough, no search or seizure can take place.

Confronted with a refusal, law enforcement agents will typically ask *why* consent is being withheld. The object is to keep the suspect talking. By prolonging the conversation, they retain the possibility of finding a way to persuade, cajole, threaten, bully or otherwise get you to change your mind. A person who wishes to maximize his privacy interests will simply ask, "Am I under arrest?" If not, he bids a fond farewell and sails off to other adventures. If the agents say that he's under arrest or otherwise not free to leave, he says, "I don't want to talk and I want my lawyer," and falls silent. For a fuller discussion of police interrogation, see Chapter 22.

Search Warrants

While probable cause isn't needed for many searches and seizures, it is required for the police to get a warrant. That's what the second clause of the Fourth Amendment says. A warrant is a judge's advance authorization for the government to search a particular place or seize a particular person or objects. The purpose of a search warrant is to ensure that a neutral, objective party evaluates the information that gives rise to probable cause before a search can begin.

A judge or magistrate of the federal court must approve a search warrant before a warrant may issue. An application for a search warrant can be made by telephone, fax machine, or e-mail. The police need to satisfy a judge that there's probable cause based on a *totality of the circumstances*, the standard set forth by the court in *Illinois v. Gates*, [*supra*]. They do this in a document called an Affidavit in Support of a Search Warrant, which can range from a few pages to over twenty pages. Much of it is standard "boilerplate" language used in every drug case. Typically, less than 20% of it is tailored specifically to the case. The Affidavit particularly describes the location(s) sought to be searched, such as "the brown, white-trimmed, two-story residence commonly known as 13412 17th Street West in the unincorporated village of Pierce Falls, Washington, and a 1999 Jeep Cherokee bearing Washington State plate numbers ..." and sometimes the suspect as well, such as "Mr. Richard Morelli, a white male with the birth date of April 21, 1965." The Affidavit describes, often in many pages, what evidence is sought. A very partial list might include:

> "... anabolic steroids and/or any other controlled substances; paraphernalia and equipment for the use, sale and transfer of controlled substances including baggies, tinfoil wrapping, bottles, cardboard boxes, packaging material such as Styrofoam peanuts, and bubble wrap; evidence of previously shipped packages of controlled substances such as bills of lading and receipts from UPS, FedEx, USPS and other commercial shippers; articles of personal property tending to establish and document sales of the above-referenced substances including computer hardware and software, fax machines and receipts, buyer and seller lists, and address/telephone lists; firearms and ammunition; proceeds from the sales of anabolic steroids including U.S. currency, gold, jewelry, and works of art; documents and effects tending to show dominion and control over said premises, including keys, lease, rental or mortgage agreements, utility bills, canceled mail, prescription bottles, clothing, handwriting, and identification cards."

The Affidavit will then recount the officer or agent's training and experience, including his time on the job, drug courses attended, number of arrests and investigations, and familiarity with the drug trade. While many agents will boast about being involved with many narcotics and drug investigations, I have yet to see an Affidavit stating how many of those were *steroid* investigations. It's deemed best, I'm sure, not to tell the judge about that. Many officers or detectives in local law enforcement have virtually no training or experience regarding anabolics.

In addition, many paragraphs and sometimes many pages are devoted to what "persons in the drug trade" or "drug dealers" typically do, such as possess more than one controlled substance; use their vehicles to conceal controlled substances; keep detailed records of their transactions; use computers to track their sales; keep guns and other dangerous weapons in the house; keep large amounts of cash and jewelry in the house; keep cell phones or pagers to track sales; etc. Most of this is form language used in narcotics affidavits, and some of it has little to do with anabolic steroids. Broadly worded, this section of the Affidavit will support the seizure of virtually anything in the house, as well as automobiles.

Finally departing from canned language, the Affidavit typically goes on to detail the probable cause supporting the warrant in the particular case. For example, it might describe the interception and investigation of a parcel by Customs at a particular airport. It would fully describe the package itself: "a manila envelope addressed to 'Hi-de-ho Lingerie, Richard Morelli' at 13412 17th Street West, Pierce Falls, Washington. The sender was 'Good Fortune Travel Solutions' at II Dam-Hui Rd., Prachuap Tira Khan Thailand. It contained 200 pink tablets of Methandrostenolone concealed in a stack of hollowed out white paper."

Federal and state statutes and regulations governing the time and execution of search warrants commonly require a time limit (usually 10 days) on execution, after which the warrant runs the risk of becoming "stale." Most search warrants are executed in the early morning, utilizing the element of surprise. The Supreme Court historically has had a particular loathing for nighttime searches. In *Monroe v. Pope* [365 U.S. 167 (1961)], the Supreme Court characterized them as "evil in its most obnoxious form." Consequently, many state laws require that the affidavit include a showing of cause for the need for a nighttime search. For instance, a nighttime search is more likely to be permitted when the "activities" only occur at night or the "property" could be easily moved, concealed or destroyed. [*Filgueras v. State*, 668 P2d 1172 (1983)] Also, F. R. Crim. P. 41(c)(1) states, "the warrant shall be served in the daytime, unless the issuing authority, by appropriate provision in the warrant, and for reasonable cause shown, authorizes its execution at times other than daytime."

Although the affidavit establishing probable cause is generally a document presented to the judge for approval, affidavits may be accompanied or replaced by oral testimony usually given by the officer seeking the warrant. In fact, federal law specifically permits search warrants to be issued upon oral testimony; however, the testimony must be under oath and recorded to be preserved for review. Many states permit oral testimony by rule or by case law.

Anticipatory Warrants

Where the evidence at present is insufficient to establish probable cause, an "anticipatory warrant" may be issued. Anticipatory warrants allow the issuing magistrate to grant a search warrant for the anticipated destination under the tenet that probable cause, though it does not exist at the time of issuance, will exist at the time the warrant is executed. Anticipatory warrants are recognized in the federal system and in the majority of state jurisdictions. The Second Circuit has set forth the following guidelines for anticipatory warrants in *U.S. v. Garcia* [882 F.2d 699, *cert. denied* 493 U.S. 943 (1989)]:

Where the evidence at present is insufficient to establish probable cause, an "anticipatory warrant" may be issued.

> "[M]agistrates and judges should take care to require independent evidence giving rise to probable cause that the contraband will be located at the premises at the time of the search. To ensure this degree of care is met, an affidavit must show: that the agent believes a delivery of the contraband is going to occur; how the agent has obtained this belief; how reliable the source of the information is; and what role the government will play in the delivery."

Some states explicitly denounce the use and application of anticipatory warrants, or condition the validity of warrants on the existence of probable cause at the time of issuance; these include Alabama, Colorado, Hawaii, Indiana, Iowa, Kansas, Maine and Maryland.

Sure Course

Courts have held that the validity of an anticipatory warrant to search a destination requires that the contraband be on a "sure course" to that destination. If it is not "sure," there is a strong indication by the Federal Circuit Courts that probable cause will be left wanting and the resulting warrant open to Constitutional challenge. In some circumstances, such as where vehicles are involved, sure course can require that the contraband actually arrive at the destination.

In controlled package deliveries, however, courts have held that sure course exists once the package is mailed (or deposited with a private courier) and that its temporary removal by law enforcement to conduct a controlled delivery does not remove the package from that sure course. This standard has been echoed again and again by the Court, as in *United States v. Hale* [784 F.2d 1465 (1986)], *United States v. Dornhofer* [859 F.2d 1195 (1988)], and *United States v. Dennis* [115 F.3d 524 (1997)], where the court stated, "where nothing in the record indicates that the contraband might not have been delivered to the residence to be searched, simply discovering the package in the mail stream and placing it back into the mail stream to effect a controlled delivery should satisfy the sure course requirement."

In *United States v. Hale*, the Court of Appeals for the Ninth Circuit distinguished the doctrine of sure course from the circumstances in *United States v. Hendricks* [743 F.2d 653 (1984)]. There, "the evidence was not on a sure and irreversible course to its destination; the defendant in that case was required to pick it up personally, an act which he might or might not have done if the government had not taken that decision out of his hands by attempting a controlled delivery."

Although sufficient probable cause has been found under varying and limited circumstances, the practitioner should consider questioning the validity of the factual basis upon which the affidavit in support of an anticipatory warrant is based. "All types of government-controlled deliveries are more likely to reach their destinations than other types of deliveries and, consequently, a magistrate may conduct a lesser inquiry into the sure course requirement when a request for an anticipatory warrant is based upon a government-controlled delivery." [*United States v. Dennis,* 115 F.3d 524 (1997)]

Nexus

One of the most essential aspects of a valid search warrant is the establishment of a "nexus." Both federal and state courts recognize the importance of showing a "nexus" connecting the probable cause and the place to be searched. In other words, the facts set forth in the affidavit must establish a link between the alleged criminal activity, the evidence sought, and the place to be searched. If the affidavit in support of probable cause fails to establish this relationship, the trend in the majority of jurisdictions is to find the search warrant Constitutionally lacking and warranting suppression. For instance, in *State v Goble* [945 P.2d 263 (1997)], the defendant received a package, alleged to have contained contraband, through the U.S. mails at his post office box. Finding that probable cause requires a nexus between the items to be seized and the place to be searched, the Court found this relationship lacking. Two years later

One of the most essential aspects of a valid search warrant is the establishment of a "nexus."

the Washington Supreme Court found specifically that where the affidavit provides merely the general assertions of a police officer, without a sufficient basis in fact from which to conclude evidence of illegal activity will likely be found at the place to be searched, a reasonable nexus is not established as a matter of law. [*State v. Thein*, 977 P.2d 582 (Wash. 1999)]

There have been numerous federal decisions consistent with this approach. In *Doe v. Broderick* [225 F.3d 440 (4th Cir. 2000)], the court held that affidavits must set forth the requisite nexus and found this requirement lacking where the affiant's assertions were no more than broad generalizations about the common practice of drug addicts; without more, they provided no probable cause to justify the search and seizure. In *U.S. v. Schultz* [14 F.3d 1093 (6th Cir. 1994)], the court found that although the experience and training of the affiant officer may be considered in a probable cause determination, it couldn't substitute for the lack of an evidentiary nexus. In *U.S. v. Lalor*, [996 F.2d 1578 (4th Cir. 1993)], the court found probable cause was not established where the affidavit failed to provide a nexus between the defendant's "on the street drug sales" and his home. In *U.S. v. Ramos* [923 F.2d 1346 (9th Cir. 1991)], the court found probable cause was not established where affidavit failed to provide a nexus between the discovery of narcotics in defendant's van while "on the road" and the defendant's residence.

Many states share this emphasis on establishing a nexus. For examples:

- In *U.S. v. Rosario* [918 F. Supp. 524 (D. R.I. 1996)], a Rhode Island case, the court found search warrants based on the self-avowed experience of the affiant officer invalid without any other factual nexus to the subject property.

- In *U.S. v. Rios* [881 F. Supp. 772 (D. Conn. 1995)], the District Court of Connecticut held that an officer's general statements based on his training and experience, standing alone, do not constitute a substantial basis for the issuance of a search warrant.

- In *State v. Longbine* [896 P. 2d 367 (Kan. 1995)], the Supreme Court of Kansas found that the general averments of the affiant, without more, are enough to create an impression, but fail to provide probable cause to believe that a crime is being committed or that evidence of that crime will be found at a particular location.

- In *U.S. v. Stout* [641 F. Supp. 1074 (N.D. Cal. 1986)], the District Court for the Northern District of California held that an off-the-premises arrest for cocaine possession does not provide the requisite nexus to establish probable cause for the issuance of a warrant to search the defendant's home.

- In *State v. Kahn* [555 N.W. 2d 15 (Minn. App. 1996)], the Minnesota Court of Appeals found that the nexus has not been established where the affidavit has failed to set forth evidence to connect the defendant's drug dealing conviction some eighty miles from his residence.

- In *State v. Johnson* [589 N.W. 2d 108 (Neb. 1999)], the Supreme Court of Nebraska found the general averments of the affiant with regard to the habits of drug dealers failed to provide probable cause for the issuance of a warrant where the affidavit lacked information from which it could be inferred that defendant was in fact a dealer of narcotics or that he possessed said narcotics at or near the time of his arrest.

- In *State v. Silvestri* [618 A.2d 821 (N.H. 1992)], the Supreme Court of New Hampshire held that a determination of being a "drug dealer" is insufficient to provide probable cause for the issuance of a warrant to search the defendant's home and requiring some nexus between the defendant's residence and alleged drug dealing activities in order to establish probable cause.

- In *Commonwealth v. Kline* [335 A.2d 361 (Pa. Super. 1975)], the Superior Court of Pennsylvania held that an allegation based on an assumption or supposition not supported by the facts is insufficient to support an inference of criminal activity in a premises, in spite of the fact that there are plenty of allegations alleged to relate to criminal activity of the individual who is alleged to have lived in the premises.

Why so many damned cases about nexus? It's can be *big deal* in juice cases, that's why. It's one you lawyers out there should be prepared to attack. Many steroid clients buy their gear online, and have it delivered to a private mailbox or post office box. What connects the box to the house miles away? Sometimes nothing, except unfounded speculations. As illustrated by the referenced cases, without any nexus there may not have been any probable cause to get a search warrant to raid the house. The issue of the warrant's validity then becomes "good faith."

The Exclusionary Rule and the "Good Faith" Exception

The first exercise of the Exclusionary Rule was by the Supreme Court in *Weeks v. United States* [*supra*]. It began as a judicial remedy, essentially to give effect to the Fourth Amendment (which protects the rights of persons against unreasonable searches and seizures, remember?). The purpose of the rule is mostly to deter police misconduct. It's also to protect the integrity of the courts by excluding evidence obtained in an "unreasonable" manner, in violation of your rights. This rationale first appeared in *Wolf v. Colorado* [338 U.S. 25 (1949)].

Let's say there's a Fourth Amendment violation, such as the execution of a search warrant that is later found to be defective. Is the evidence automatically suppressed? Not necessarily, because there are *exceptions* to the exclusionary rule. One exception is where it can be shown that the police had a "good faith" basis for their belief or reliance. So, once a warrant issues that is fair on its face, the fact that the magistrate may have slightly erred in the finding of probable cause does *not* necessarily invalidate an otherwise proper search. In *United States v. Leon* [468 U.S. 897 (1984)], where the police reasonably relied on a search warrant they believed to be valid, the Supreme Court held that the drugs that were discovered as a result of the search should not be suppressed. The warrant had been reviewed by several assistant district attorneys and issued by a magistrate judge, leading the officers to believe that the warrant was valid. The Court reasoned that the officers were acting on a "good faith belief" despite a subsequent finding that the warrant was defective.

If a search warrant issued by a judge contains defects, such as language that isn't supported by probable cause, the good faith exception may avoid suppression. This was the case in *Massachusetts v. Sheppard* [468 U.S. 981 (1984)], where police officers reasonably relied on a search warrant issued by a judge. The court stated that, "The exclusionary rule should not be applied when the officer conducting the search acted in objectively reasonable reliance on a warrant issued by a detached and neutral magistrate that subsequently is determined to be invalid." Of course, if there are two independently operative clauses of a warrant and only one is invalid for lack of particularity, the invalid portions may be severed so as not to require suppression of the evidence seized.

Although the Constitution encourages the use of search warrants and will go as far as validating an otherwise unlawful search if it is found that it has been executed under a good faith belief, this exception cannot cure every defect. For example, if a judge "rubber stamps" a search warrant without even reading the application, there can be no reasonable reliance on the validity of the warrant and the evidence may be suppressed. Additionally, if a search warrant fails to meet the *particularity* requirement, that is, if it lacks a "particular description" of the things to be seized required by the Fourth Amendment, then fruits of the search may be subject to suppression.

If the police go through the trouble of getting a warrant, challenging the police conduct can be difficult. The warrant can only be attacked on its face if the defense makes a "substantial preliminary showing" that the affiant (usually the officer who was seeking the warrant) made a false statement knowingly or with reckless disregard for the truth and the false statement was material to probable cause. If the defendant successfully meets this burden under what has come to be known as the *Franks* doctrine, then the evidence should be suppressed. [*Franks v. Delaware*, 438 U.S. 154 (1978)]

Execution of the Search Warrant

Even when the police are executing a valid search warrant, your right to privacy in your dwelling should be taken into consideration. You must be given the opportunity to surrender your privacy to law enforcement officials before they bust down the door. In some cases, the police may have the wrong house or the occupant may be an innocent party. This can result in the police being mistaken for intruders by a startled homeowner, who may leap out of bed and attempt to arm himself. To avoid the potential for a violent exchange between the confused homeowner and the heavily armed government agents, the Supreme Court has recognized the importance of the "Knock-and-Announce Rule" in serving these policy interests. In other words, officers are required to give some kind of notice to the occupant(s) prior to entry, typically, "Police with a search warrant!" Federal law addresses this rule by statute, as do many state courts. However, this rule is not applicable in every circumstance and it may be excused when it would have been a "useless gesture," or in the presence of other exigent circumstances.

In some cases, the police may have the wrong house ... This can result in the police being mistaken for intruders by a startled homeowner, who may leap out of bed and attempt to arm himself.

The accused or the homeowner is then entitled to a copy of the search warrant but not the affidavit in support. This does not necessarily have to be produced prior to the search and seizure, though it should be presented at some point during the search [*United States v. Hepperle*, 810 F.2d 836 (1987)]. However, failing to provide the accused with a search warrant is curable and generally not grounds for suppression. Unfortunately, police deception can occur in this context. The best-known example of this was in *Mapp v. Ohio* [367 U.S. 643 (1961)], where the police flourished a paper they claimed was a warrant but hastily retrieved it when Ms. Mapp snatched it from them. Although at trial one of the officers insisted they'd had a warrant, he later admitted it was a lie. [*See* Fred W. Friendly & Martha J.H. Elliott, *The Constitution: That Delicate Balance* 132 (1984)]

Wrapping it up

No doubt about it, Fourth Amendment issues play into almost every AAS case. Now you have an idea of the law in the area. Let's apply these principles to a variety of situations involving steroids, to examine how they figure into the war on anabolics. But first, a thought-provoking quote:

> "Loss of freedom seldom happens overnight. Oppression doesn't stand on the doorstep with toothbrush moustache and swastika armband – it creeps up insidiously ... step by step, and all of a sudden the unfortunate citizen realises that it is gone."
>
> *– Baron Lane, Lord Chief Justice of England (b. 1918)*

Chapter 8

Border Blues

"An addict is someone who does not have control over their life. You don't have that with steroids. You don't see anyone knocking over a liquor store to buy steroids."
– Hon. Paul J. Pfingst, District Attorney of San Diego County, 2000

Thanks to the Anabolic Steroid Control Act, the overwhelming majority of black-market juice is manufactured outside the United States. Since physicians are prevented from prescribing anabolics non-medically, many AAS users will attempt to sneak small amounts back across the Mexican border.

Brent made sure to wear long sleeves and long pants before heading to the border crossing. His shaved arms and legs were covered, and his shirt was bulky enough to hide his thick traps and full delts without looking out of place in the Mexican heat. He had taken off the gold barbell he wore on a neck chain and put it in his pocket, where he had a few vials of Aratest. The rest of his juice was hidden in his socks and in his girlfriend Lydia's purse. It was Saturday evening, when the crowd of tourists returning to the U.S. from a day of shopping in Tijuana might lessen the chances of a Customs inspection.

As he approached the border in his Chevy S-10 pickup, he tried to maneuver behind a large van in hopes that the van might attract attention and be diverted for secondary inspection. It would be less likely, he thought, for them to divert his truck if the vehicle before him was sent to secondary. The last few cars before the van had gone through without a hitch. Brent watched as the driver of the van answered the inspector's questions. Then the van pulled forward and went on its way. As he pulled up to the inspector, Brent could see the inspector's eyes assessing the size and thickness under his shirt. This wasn't to be Brent's day. The inspector directed him over to secondary, and the rest is an old story...

Several books and many articles have been published on the issue of gear smuggling techniques at the border, recommending what to wear, how to act, which days of the week and times are best to cross over, etc. A lot of it is simple common sense, of course. Do you really think they won't notice your shaved arms and legs and citrus beverage T-shirt that says *100% Juice*? You might as well raise both hands and yell, "Search me!" Of course, bodybuilders have resorted to some pretty extreme measures to sneak their gear past Customs. I mean, *really* extreme. Listen to me: if you find yourself in a hotel room in Tijuana thinking about trying one of these unsavory bodily methods, whatever pride or joy you once took in building your body has been sadly perverted. Skip Pope was right: go straight to a psychiatrist. Take up lawn bowling.

> Most people I see getting busted at the borders are in motor vehicles.

In my practice, I haven't seen a lot of these bizarre transport methods. I also haven't seen a lot of people busted for walking their gear across the border. That may be because few walk their gear across, or it may be that many walk their gear across but few get caught. Most people I see getting busted at the borders are in motor vehicles. They sit in a line of cars, trucks, and vans, waiting to be asked a few questions about the nature of their trip and the items they're bringing back. If the Customs inspector's suspicions are aroused, the car is directed to the secondary inspection area for a search.

Authority of U.S. Customs

The sheer volume of travelers going back and forth across our border crossings probably means that the vast majority of gear slips by unnoticed. Of course, U.S. Customs is entrusted with the authority to do all it can to interdict smuggling. If they find AAS on somebody entering the U.S., they have a range of options from simply confiscating it and collecting a fine to arresting the person and referring the matter for prosecution.

Customs has the broad authority to conduct searches of persons, their baggage, cargo, and means of transportation, authorized by Title 19 of the United States Code, sections 482, 1467, 1496, 1499, 1581, and 1582. Congress has authorized the powers of the Customs Service in 19 U.S.C. § 1582:

> "Search of persons and baggage; regulations.
> The Secretary of the Treasury may prescribe regulations for the search of persons and baggage and he is authorized to employ female inspectors for the examination and search of persons of their own sex; and all persons coming into the United States from foreign countries shall be liable to detention and search by authorized officers or agents of the Government under such regulations."

The courts have also held that this search, seizure, and arrest authority is not dependent upon either probable cause or a search warrant as is required by police officers. [*U.S. v. Ramsey*, 431 U.S. 606 (1977)] A border search must merely be *reasonable*. One reason for this broad authority is the vulnerability of our borders (including the functional equivalent of our borders, international airports) to the illegal entry of a vast amount of dangerous and prohibited items.

Customs Seizures

There are two types of seizures you may encounter at a border crossing. The first is where the law provides for forfeiture of your property; it becomes the property of the federal government, assuming that all the appropriate administrative procedures are satisfied. The second type of seizure is where your property is seized to satisfy a monetary penalty. Seizure and forfeiture may follow when there is a violation of Customs law or a related law that is enforced by Customs. Violations which can result in seizure include importing prohibited merchandise such as controlled substances, importing restricted merchandise (merchandise restricted by agencies like the EPA and FDA), importing undeclared, unreported, or smuggled merchandise or currency over $10,000, and importation of goods which aid or facilitate the illegal importation of merchandise, such as merchandise used to hide or conceal illegal goods.

When U.S. Customs Inspectors find a type of drug, quantity, or a combination of various drugs that arouses suspicions, they will ordinarily contact the nearest FDA or DEA office for advice, and will then make a final determination about whether to release or detain the article. There is no uniformity in the interdiction and enforcement of minor AAS importation cases. At U.S. land borders, the idea of equal treatment under the law is rather a joke. Many persons caught with steroids have had their contraband confiscated but were not arrested. Others were required to pay penalties to the Customs Service. The least fortunate were arrested and prosecuted, some in federal court and others in state or even local municipal courts. The situation is really a mess, with decisions apparently made with no rhyme or reason. I have personally represented individuals who reentered the U.S. with very small amounts of anabolic steroids that they did not declare to Customs. In one case, Customs agents made an arrest and then dumped the case into a tiny village court. In a different case, Customs forwarded the matter to the local U.S. Attorney for prosecution as a federal importation felony. The capriciousness of it all is startling.

Federal Importation Law

Importing anabolic steroids into the United States from other countries is unlawful under 21 U.S.C. § 960(a)(1) if the conduct falls under 21 U.S.C. § 952(b):

> "It shall be unlawful to import into the customs territory of the United States from any place outside thereof (but within the United States), or to import into the United States from any place outside thereof, any nonnarcotic controlled substance in schedule III, IV, or V, unless such nonnarcotic controlled substance —
> (1) is imported for medical, scientific, or other legitimate uses, and (2) is imported pursuant to such notification, or declaration, or in the case of any nonnarcotic controlled substance in schedule III, such import permit, notification, or declaration, as the Attorney General may by regulation prescribe ... "

An individual who knowingly or intentionally imports anabolic steroids faces imprisonment of up to five years with an additional term of supervised release of not less than two years and/or a fine of $250,000. [21 U.S.C. § 960(b)(1)(4)] Bringing even a personal use amount of juice into the United States is a federal felony.

The Personal Use Exemption

Individuals who import controlled substances without a prescription but for *medical* reasons are subject to different policy considerations from recreational drug smugglers. The confusion that surrounds the whole issue is barely understood by most lawyers, let alone the general public. The authority of 21 U.S.C. 956(a)(1) and (2) was put into place specifically to exempt certain individuals from unlawfully possessing a controlled substance for *medical reasons*. Under subdivision (1), the exemption applies to "any individual who has a controlled substance (except a substance in schedule I) in his possession

The authority of 21 U.S.C. 956(a)(1) and (2) was put into place specifically to exempt certain individuals from unlawfully possessing a controlled substance for *medical reasons.*

for his personal medical use, or for administration to an animal accompanying him, if he lawfully obtained such substance and he makes such declaration (or gives such other notification) as the Attorney General may by regulation require." The exemption was recently amended. The amendment by Congress didn't expand our rights at all. It simply *limited* the exemption. Subdivision (2) of Section 956(a) states:

> "... a United States resident who enters the United States through an international land border with a controlled substance (except a substance in schedule I) for which the individual does not possess a valid prescription issued by a practitioner (as defined in section 802 of this title) in accordance with applicable Federal and State law (or documentation that verifies the issuance of such a prescription to that individual) may not import the controlled substance into the United States in an amount that exceeds 50 dosage units of the controlled substance."

This exemption has been the topic of many online discussion board threads, with some amateur legal analysts concluding that bodybuilders can lawfully import juice any way they want as long as they bring no more than fifty units at a time. Bad advice. The exemption, even on its face, is actually of very little applicability to muscleheads. First, the exemption only applies to *land borders*, not to mail or courier delivery importations. Second, the medication must be for "personal *medical* use," *not*, my friends, for blasting up your maximum bench press or just generally slapping on some size. Third, at best, the statute only exempts the individual from the Controlled Substances Act, not from the complicated matrix of *other* federal laws (like FDA regulations, for example) or from the prosecution for violation of *state or local laws*. Fourth, the medication must be lawfully obtained and properly *declared* (which few bodybuilders seem to do, given the previously mentioned rejection of bodybuilding as a valid medical use) as required by the Attorney General's regulations. Fifth and last, since Mexican veterinary products are not for humans, they can hardly be claimed under the personal medical use exemption unless they are for an animal accompanying you. Now, might there be occasional instances of relaxed enforcement discretion where Customs inspectors allow some folks to enter with declared Mexican anabolics even though one or more of the exemption criteria aren't met? While it's been reported to me that such instances have occurred, and I'm sure that they have, only a fool would count on it. Nobody can say with certainty what might actually happen at any particular border crossing on any given day.

The DEA Importation Criteria

The Attorney General, acting through the Drug Enforcement Administration, has indeed issued regulations applying to the personal use exemption under § 956(a). Under 21 C.F.R. § 1301.26, exemptions from import or export requirements for personal medical use must meet the following criteria:

> "Any individual who has in his/her possession a controlled substance listed in [schedule III] which he/she has lawfully obtained for his/her personal medical use, or for administration to an animal accompanying him/her, may enter or depart the United States with such substance notwithstanding sections 1002-1005 of the Act (21 U.S.C. 952-955), providing the following conditions are met:

(a) The controlled substance is in the original container in which it was dispensed to the individual; and
(b) The individual makes a declaration to an appropriate official of the U.S. Customs Service stating:
  (1) That the controlled substance is possessed for his/her personal use, or for an animal accompanying him/her; and
  (2) The trade or chemical name and the symbol designating the schedule of the controlled substance if it appears on the container label, or, if such name does not appear on the label, the name and address of the pharmacy or practitioner who dispensed the substance and the prescription number, if any; and
(c) The importation of the controlled substance for personal medical use is authorized or permitted under other Federal laws and state law."

Those seem like some difficult hurdles to get over; however, it might appear that an individual who complies with these criteria may import a personal AAS supply without a hitch. Well, it's not quite so simple. Notice that under sub (c), the importation must be "authorized or permitted under other Federal laws and state law." That's in accord with 21 CFR § 1307.02, mentioned in Chapter 4, which provides for the application of *state laws* and other *federal laws*: "Nothing in this chapter shall be construed as authorizing or permitting any person to do any act which such person is not authorized or permitted to do ... under the law of the State in which he/she desires to do such act ..." Which means, as a practical matter, that some rule within the convoluted maze of laws that govern our conduct may be broken without our knowledge. Even more worrisome, it means some government bureaucrat may *think* – even mistakenly – that some rule was broken.

Prescriptions from a Foreign Physician in State Courts

An individual is in lawful possession of a controlled substance if it was obtained directly or pursuant to a valid prescription or order from a practitioner while acting in the course of his professional practice. Under federal law [21 U.S.C. § 802(21)], a practitioner is defined to include a physician who is licensed in the United States or the jurisdiction in which he practices. So, that would include any licensed physician, including a Mexican doctor. But what if the law of a particular state has a different definition?

> An individual is in lawful possession of a controlled substance if it was obtained directly or pursuant to a valid prescription ... from a practitioner while acting in the course of his professional practice.

The case against Dianne Wright [*Wright v. State*, 981 S.W.2d 197 (Tex. Crim. App. 1998)] is disturbing. A 43-year-old woman with no criminal history drove with her son from her home in Sherman, Texas to Nuevo Laredo, Mexico where she was examined by Dr. Joaquin Izaguirre Quintero, a physician fully licensed in Mexico. Dr. Quintero prescribed diazepam (Valium®) and diethylpropion (an appetite suppressant), and she filled the prescription at a Mexican pharmacy in Nuevo Laredo. Upon returning to the U.S., Wright informed Customs officials that she had prescription drugs and readily presented the medication and the documents related to them. She also signed paperwork indicating that the medication was for personal use. Customs officials had no problems with it. They stamped the documents with the notation "Cleared U.S. Customs, Laredo, Texas," and she was permitted to proceed. Twenty miles north she stopped at a border check point where her medications were reviewed. She was again allowed to proceed.

Her vehicle was later stopped in Frio County for speeding. The sheriff asked if she had any prescription medications in the vehicle. She presented the medications and documents to the sheriff. The sheriff stated that the possession of prescription Mexican medication was a felony offense. She was arrested right there on the side of the road, hauled off to court, and indicted for felony possession of controlled substances. Surely the case was immediately thrown out? No, she was ultimately convicted of the charge and sentenced to two years imprisonment, probated.

Of course, she appealed. On appeal, the State insisted that possession of foreign-prescribed controlled substances is *always* unlawful, because Texas law defines a practitioner to exclude physicians that are not either licensed in Texas or registered with the DEA. [Tex. Health & Safety Code § 481.002(39)] The Texas Court of Criminal Appeals held that under the "ultimate user" provisions of Texas law [§ 481.117(a)], it is a defense to prosecution under state law for possession of a controlled substance that: (1) the substance was obtained abroad for personal medical use directly from or pursuant to a valid prescription from a physician permitted in his jurisdiction to dispense controlled substances, and (2) the substance was brought into the U.S. in accordance with import regulations [21 CFR § 1301.26]. The case was remanded to the trial court because it was held that whether the "ultimate user" defense is established in a case is a question of fact to be decided by a jury.

Wright's case wasn't an isolated incident on the highways of Texas. Other people had already been arrested and convicted under similar circumstances. They appealed their plea-bargained felony or misdemeanor convictions for possession of scheduled drugs prescribed by foreign physicians, and got their convictions reversed [for examples, *Gaspard v. State*, 1997 Tex. App. *LEXIS* 5315; *Saulter v. State*, 1997 Tex. App. *LEXIS* 5317] – only to have the relentless prosecutor file petitions contesting the decisions on technical grounds. [*Gaspard v. State*, 2000 Tex. App. *LEXIS* 1322; *Saulter v. State*, 2000 Tex. App. *LEXIS* 1315] Luckily, the Court of Appeals for the Fourth District didn't buy it. The cases were sent back for the defendants to have their day in court. The cases were never presented to a grand jury. Instead, Frio County finally abandoned its policy of prosecuting people when their conduct fully complies with federal law. If other jurisdictions had similar policies, they have probably abandoned them as well, I would hope.

However, let the foreign steroid buyer beware. The ultimate user defense only applies if the federal regulation is complied with. The drug must be for personal *medical* use. Since the ultimate user defense is a question of fact for a jury, the particular circumstances of a case might justify letting a jury decide whether the federal law was properly met. Got the idea? Also, remember that policies and legal interpretations may vary by jurisdiction.

Importing Non-Controlled Substances

Additionally, all prescription drugs (such as Mexican versions of various ancillary medications, as well as steroids) that are not approved by the U.S. Food and Drug Administration, indicating that they do not meet the federal requirements for safety and effectiveness, may not be acceptable for importation. Customs has the discretion to confiscate foreign pharmaceuticals as "unapproved new drugs" under the Food, Drugs and Cosmetics Act. [21 U.S.C. §§ 331(d) and 355(a)] The FDA has set forth guidelines, suggesting circumstances where, in their discretion, FDA personnel may refrain from taking legal action against the importer; however, these are only *suggestions* and are not legally binding. Those circumstances are as follows:

1. The intended use (of the drug) is unapproved and for a serious condition for which effective treatment may not be available domestically either through commercial or clinical means;
2. There is no known commercialization or promotion to persons residing in the U.S. by those involved in the distribution of the product at issue;
3. The product is considered not to represent an unreasonable risk;
4. The individual seeking to import the product affirms in writing that it is for the patient's own use (generally not more than a 3 month supply) and provides the name and address of the doctor licensed in the U.S. responsible for his or her treatment with the product, or provides evidence that the product is for the continuation of a treatment begun in a foreign country.
   [See FDA web site "Traveler Alert" at www.fda.gov/ora/import traveler_alert.htm]

So even if Customs doesn't bust you, they can still take away your gear and all your other ancillary medications under the Food, Drugs, and Cosmetics Act.

A Real-life Texas AAS Case

How about an absolutely true, verified, firsthand, quite articulate account of the process from the girlfriend of a client who was arrested at a border crossing? Cool, huh? Here's the real, actual word-for-word tale, printed from an e-mail and edited only as to name:

> *When we first got to the border, we paid our toll and then drove up to the first guy. He asked us if we had any alcohol, etc., to declare and we said no, just some pottery. He placed a yellow piece of paper on the windshield of my car and told us to pull up to slot 10. When we pulled further, there were already, I'm estimating, 5-10 Customs people waiting in that area. We pulled up and they asked us to get out of the vehicle and for Jerry to open the hood and the trunk. I walked over and sat on a concrete pillar while Jerry stood on the driver's side of the door.*
>
> *The Customs guys went straight to the passenger side of my car, lifted the front seat and then popped the back inside area out enough to shine a flashlight in. He immediately thought he found something and called another guy over to have a look. This was the first place the officer looked. My dash hadn't even been looked in, nor had my trunk, our luggage, the front seats, or anything else for that matter. As soon as they pulled the stuff out, they went straight to Jerry, even though it was my car, and asked him about it. I am not sure exactly what he told them but the next thing was they had his hands above his head and was searching his clothes for items. They took him inside, and as they did so I looked at Jerry and asked what was going on.*
>
> *As soon as he was inside the officers came to me and asked if I knew what was going on and I said no, I knew nothing about what they were doing at that moment or anything about steroids they claimed to have found in my car. The officer asked me to empty my pockets and I did, nothing was in them. The next thing I remember was there were 3-4 officers standing around me, all asking questions one right after the next. For example: Do you know anything about the steroids?, Why would Jerry have them? He doesn't look like a bodybuilder, is he just getting started becoming one? It was very overwhelming and the questions didn't seem to stop. Eventually I started crying and they laid off the questioning. They asked me to have a seat by my car for a while.*

Eventually they called me in and read me my rights; that I didn't have to answer questions without an attorney etc. Nice to have known that after they already overwhelmed me with them. When they first brought me in the building, they showed me the steroids all together in one pack. They clearly didn't care that it was evidence and "tossed" it around like it didn't matter. I looked in the bag and recognized vitamin B-12. The larger bottles had had their labels torn a good bit due to the tape that was on them.

The officer then took me into one room that looked like the office and read me my rights and asked if I wanted a lawyer. I replied I have no idea what is really going on and really didn't know if I needed one. I then asked what he thought and he replied that if I didn't have anything to hide then it would make it much smoother and faster on him if I didn't and that by cooperating it would make it better for the both of us. This all began around 10:30-11:00 that morning and we didn't leave there until 8pm. At first they were going to just put a 500 dollar penalty on the car and then all of a sudden, when they realized getting that amount of money wasn't such a big deal, they said oh well, it's going to go by what your car is worth. Then one officer said 15% of the value, which he estimated at 10,995 dollars or something close to that. Jerry said he would have his bank wire him money and we would be able to get the car and I would be able to follow him to Del Rio that night.

Well at first, that was fine, one of the officers said he would take Jerry across the street (directly across) to the western union and he could get the money. But then for some reason they said, oh, no, we can't do that, now you have to find another way to get the money. Well, Jerry couldn't have money from his account wired to me so that made matters a little worse. It was going to be the next day before I could get my car out which meant I would be staying in Eagle Pass, Tx and Jerry would be going to Del Rio on his own. That evening is when I looked up the web site Jerry had somehow gotten to tell me about and contacted your emergency number.

Interestingly, Jerry wasn't a bodybuilder and nothing about him or his girlfriend would have fit a profile for smuggling. Jerry had just bought the steroids from a pharmacy not too far from the border. Pharmacy employees taped up the anabolics into a pack and hid the pack in the car. Do you suppose that those pharmacy employees had something to do with the search of Jerry's car? It's long been rumored that Mexican pharmacy workers are paid to report drug smugglers. To keep paid snitches from relaying identifying descriptions, many juice smugglers prevent pharmacy workers from seeing their vehicle and change clothes prior to crossing the border. Some wait a day to cross.

In any event, Jerry's case, and numerous others very much like it, would support the hypothesis that your friend at La Farmacia may be an undercover mole (and that's *mole* as in rodent, not as in *molé* sauce). Could somebody in Customs have shelled out a few bucks for the tip-off on Jerry? Maybe that's why Customs felt obliged to refer the case to the U.S. Attorney's Office for prosecution as a whoop-de-do felony importation indictment, when most cases with many times the quantity are routinely settled with a fine. Jerry's total quantity was only 16 vials and 40 tablets.

Forfeiture and Other Penalties

The law permits Customs to seize property and impose penalties on travelers who unlawfully import articles into the country. Under 19 U.S.C. § 1595a(b), "Customs may assess penalties equal to the domestic value of any articles introduced or attempted to be introduced into the U.S. contrary to law. Any person who directs, assists financially or otherwise, or is any way concerned in any unlawful [importation] activity ... is liable to a penalty equal to the domestic value of the article or articles ..." Illegally imported controlled substances are covered under sub (1)(B) of 19 USC § 1595a(c). "The appropriate customs officer shall determine the domestic value, at the time and place of appraisement, of any vessel, vehicle, aircraft, merchandise, or baggage seized under the customs laws." [19 USC § 1606]

"... appraised domestic value $17,000." That's a claimed value of seventeen dollars a tablet for D-bol.

The interesting issue is how they arrive at the values of the articles. Last year, I personally saw a case in which Customs placed a value on 1,000 tablets of D-bol. The client paid $450 for them – a typical price. How much did Customs appraise them for? Hope you're sitting down: "appraised domestic value $17,000." That's a claimed value of seventeen dollars a tablet for D-bol. Are they kidding? I pity the guy whose lawyer might be too lazy or uninformed to challenge such madness.

A California AAS Forfeiture

Want to see the imposition of forfeiture penalties in action? Curt was a graduate student caught with his friend jointly bringing back anabolics from Mexico in a rented van. They had exactly the following:

34 bottles of veterinary anabolic steroids (10cc each)
800 clenbuterol tablets (non-controlled medicine)

The Customs agents insisted that the clenbuterol tablets were Valium® despite Curt's protests. After being detained for seven hours, they were told by Customs agents that if they signed some paperwork they'd be allowed to leave. Curt's passenger was told he would need to pay a fine of $3,000, but the amount was reduced by a sergeant to $1,600. Curt was told because he was the driver, his fine would be more.

The "Payment in Lieu of Forfeiture" assessed against Curt was – you'd better be lying down for this one – $72,784. Can you imagine? I refused to believe it until I actually saw the papers myself. I have them in front of me right now. My office made extensive efforts to determine by what possible method they arrived at the valuation. When questioned about determining the value of seized anabolics, one high-ranking Customs official located in San Ysidro claimed that the valuation was based on a "narcotics survey of the street costs," compiled through information provided by agents based on their experiences. The value is then averaged, based on the agents' responses. She refused to divulge anything further, and vowed to oppose a Freedom of Information Act request, on the grounds that to reveal street costs would somehow compromise law enforcement effectiveness. Of course, that's ridiculous. A person should have an *absolute right* to know how the government aims to take his property from him. Knowing how property is valued is hardly spilling the beans on government secrets. If anything, it enhances government interests by its deterrent effect: if you smuggle juice back, you can be responsible for massive fines. In light of the $72,784 valuation purportedly arrived

A person should have an *absolute right* to know how the government aims to take his property from him.

at by this street costs formula, it would appear that the method is using street costs in a currency other than American dollars.

After Curt and I discussed various options, Curt sent $300 to Customs as a partial payment toward the penalty, along with a letter seeking mitigation of the amount. A month later, he was advised by Customs that the penalty should have been $5,900. Customs then reduced it to $600, applied the $300 he paid, and asked for $300 to settle it. He was never charged with any crime; case closed. Now, can you imagine if he had paid a substantial amount toward the original assessment? While Curt's case may well demonstrate an extreme example of bureaucratic incompetence, it certainly does provide a strong argument for Customs to be forced to release their secret street costs formula as a check on future abuses.

AAS at the Canadian Border

Every now and then you see a northern border AAS case. The infrequency of juice cases at our northern border makes for even more unpredictable shenanigans than at the southern border. Here's an interesting real life story of a case I handled.

> *José was a bit of a Bad Boy. He was on probation for Attempted Burglary and was prohibited from leaving New York City without permission. Nevertheless, he took a little unauthorized trip to Canada, and maybe from there to parts unknown for a week or so. He was driving back across the border from Canada with a friend and entered the primary inspection lane. The inspector at the bridge asked the usual questions. José told him that they had been in Canada three days for a stag party, but the inspector noticed "a rather large amount of luggage" and sent him to secondary. He was given the opportunity to produce any contraband before physical inspection to avoid the car being dismantled. José went to the tailgate of his Mountaineer and pulled a small bag of one hundred pink pentagonal tablets from the roof liner. "What are these?" the inspector asked.*
>
> *Here's where ignorance of Customs played a part. José told him that they were steroids. Apparently dumbfounded, the Customs inspectors pulled out a copy of the Physician's Desk Reference and tried to identify the tablets by matching them with a picture. Finding what looked like a match, they wrote up a sworn statement saying, "the Physicians Desk Reference Guide revealed the pills to be Decadron, a [sic] adrenocortical steroid." The quantity was below the threshold for the local U.S. Attorney to have any federal interest, so Customs dumped the case on the state police. José was taken into custody and brought before a judge in a little town court. He was released on $2,500 cash bail. The state police, apparently even less familiar with steroids, drafted a complaint charging felony possession, which was an error because in New York juice possession can only be a felony if it's with intent to sell. The complaint didn't even attempt to make that allegation. It charged possession of Decadron as an "anabolic steroid." Since Decadron is a* corticosteroid *(dexamethasone), not an anabolic steroid, the complaint was facially defective.*
>
> *Here's where the local prosecutor's lack of knowledge took over. When I pointed out to him that Decadron was not even a controlled substance, I could sense his concern about the embarrassing and potentially costly ramifications of a false arrest. I suggested that a timely lab report would settle everything, but if it were in fact Decadron based on the report, I would need to advise my client of his rights to sue. Concern over the issue may have dimmed the prosecutor's interest in obtaining a laboratory analysis of the tablets. Somehow, the analysis was never done. My motion to dismiss was granted without objection and José, delighted with the result, never pursued a lawsuit.*

The case is long over with. I'll never know for sure what the tablets were. Of course, foreign products wouldn't be in the Physician's Desk reference, now would they? There wouldn't be any pictures, for example, of products manufactured by the British Dispensary in Thailand. If a lab assay had been done, might it have identified the tablets as methandrostenolone, an anabolic steroid to which the Thai version is similar in size, shape, and color to Decadron? Only big, bad José knows for sure.

Resolving a Federal Court Importation Case

When an importation case is brought in federal court, what's one good way for it to play out? Let's assume it's the typical small quantity, personal use scenario. The indictment will typically include two counts: one for the felony importation under §§ 952(a) and 960(a)(1) & (b)(1)(4), and one for simple misdemeanor possession under § 844(A). Federal law permits the entry of a plea in violation of 21 USC § 844(a), a misdemeanor possession count, under the special probation provisions of 18 USC § 3607(a) and (b). A fine and special assessment are imposed, typically about $1,000. The provisions of § 3607 were enacted with the intent of providing a second chance at a "clean slate" for otherwise law-abiding individuals, permitting an accused to be placed on pre-judgment probation for up to one year. Section 3607(a) provides: "At *any time before the expiration of the term of probation*, if the person has not violated a condition of probation, the court may, without entering a judgment of conviction, dismiss the proceedings against the person and discharge him from probation" (emphasis added); subsection (b) prevents the disposition from being deemed a "disqualification" or "disability."

Anyone charged with a federal AAS felony should discuss the applicability of these provisions [18 USC § 3607(a) and (b)] with his lawyer.

Anyone charged with a federal AAS felony should discuss the applicability of these provisions with his lawyer. Believe me, not every criminal practitioner is aware of them. The lawyer should fully marshal and thoroughly present all mitigating facts to support a deferred prosecution application or a misdemeanor possession plea with pre-judgment probation without conviction. I recently negotiated a disposition under § 3607 in a Texas steroid importation case. Resolving a felony importation indictment in this manner can save a person's livelihood by avoiding a criminal conviction of any kind.

Last Thoughts

As you can see, if you're busted for juice at the border, there are a whole lot of possibilities as to what might happen. I know a guy who's not a bodybuilder and has enough of a criminal record to give him one strike left. He has nerves of steel and fairly sophisticated methods and made smuggling runs across the border on a regular basis, back and forth from California to Mexico. He worked for a pretty big player in the anabolic black market, and he never got caught. Not once.

... sooner or later he's gonna get busted. It's just a matter of time.

I can't detail his methods to you for obvious reasons, but I can tell you this: smart as he is, I predict that sooner or later he's gonna get busted. It's just a matter of time. Not every factor is within his control. A trick of fate, an inspector's whim, so many things can go wrong. I've told him so many times. I've warned him that he's going to pay a heavy price. Of course, he's not buying it. He's probably making the run tonight.

Chapter 9

FAST CARS AND ANAVARS

Here in my car
I feel safest of all
I can lock all my doors
It's the only way to live in cars.
– *Gary Numan, lyrics to "Cars"*

Car stops and searches are often chock-full of legal issues. From the perspective of Fourth Amendment privacy interests, cars, quite simply, are necessarily different. Picture this:

You're cruising the boulevard with your friends on Friday night, the radio's blaring, you're checking out the babes on the sidewalk and your car crosses the double yellow line. Suddenly, the strobe lights of a police cruiser go on behind you. You're being pulled over. Two burly uniformed police officers exit their vehicle, ceremoniously put on their hats, adjust their Sam Browne belts, and approach your vehicle, one on each side. They're large and in charge. The cop on your side has forearms like Popeye, one emblazoned with a tattoo of a pit bull.

"Do you know why I stopped you?" Okay, that's the oldest trick in the book. It's the way cops get stupid people to make an immediate admission of wrongdoing. You're not falling for that. No way.

"I have no idea, Sir," you reply. "Why?"

Pit Bull smirks, asks for the usual: license, registration and proof of insurance. You comply. You feel uneasy, helpless, and even though you won't admit it ... intimidated. His flashlight beam is in your face.

"Where you goin'?"

You reply, "Uh, uh, n-n-nowhere, just out for a ride with my bro's."

By now, a second unit has rolled to the location as backup, and two more big cops approach your car. What's this, a convention? These guys all look like they could easily push a door marked "Pull." It's disorienting, with the whirling lights, the squelch and crackling of the police radios and the speed within which a mellow time just chilling out and cruising around has turned into a confrontation with the police.

Pit Bull places a meaty paw on the butt of his Glock 9 millimeter semiautomatic pistol and growls, "Step outta the car." In his other hand is all your paperwork. You feel captive and compelled to follow his orders, or else ...

You begin to feel woozy as you step out of your car.

Pit Bull's partner moves in, strategically out of punching or kicking distance. The other two begin inspecting your car interior with their flashlights.

"Whose car is this? Where you comin' from? Where ya' going? You been drinking tonight?" Pit Bull's demeanor is uncannily reminiscent of the drill sergeant from Stanley Kubrick's film, "Full Metal Jacket," only Pit Bull's meaner and a whole lot bigger.

"You got any contraband or weapons in the car?" he demands.

Uh-oh. Your knees are trembling and you feel as though you might even lose control of your bladder. Your feeble "No" sounds like somebody else's voice.

In a true alpha male tone: "Well, then, we're gonna just search your car? No problem." It sounds more like an accusation than a request. The implication is that they're doing it no matter what you say.

"Uh, uh, yeah, no problem, no problem."

Problem. They search the car, the glove box, the trunk and they find your gym bag. They open the bag and find that vial of cyp, the darts and the bag of Anavar tablets that you picked up earlier in the day. Problem. Big problem.

Cars are inherently readily mobile, and are unlikely to stay around for the time it takes the police to get a warrant. We have lesser expectations of privacy in cars because of the strong state interest in keeping our roads safe. Also, the interior of a motor vehicle is highly visible to those outside, subject to open view. Not surprisingly, our Fourth Amendment protections in our automobiles are considerably less than in our homes. The Supreme Court recognized these differences and carved out the "automobile exception" to the Fourth Amendment, which provides that if the police have probable cause as to the vehicle, they can search it without having to bother even trying to get a warrant. [*Carroll v. United States*, 267 U.S. 132 (1925)]

Let's have some fun. Using variations on the typical traffic stop "fact pattern" above, we'll examine the various Fourth Amendment issues involved.

Reasonable Suspicion

The police can't merely stop a car and question its occupant(s) simply to get acquainted. (Some cops may refer to this as "jamming.") The police may stop a vehicle when there is *reasonable suspicion* to believe that the operator or the occupants have committed a crime. [*Delaware v. Prouse*, 440 U.S. 648 (1979)] These investigatory stops must satisfy a two-part standard. [*United States v. Cortez*, 449 U.S. 411 (1981)]:

A) First, the law enforcement officer must make an assessment on a *totality of the circumstances*, based upon probabilities. The officer must use his training, experience and common sense to make his deduction.

B) Second, the assessment of the whole picture or totality of the circumstances must raise a suspicion that the person(s) being stopped are engaged in some wrongdoing.

So, police don't need probable cause to stop a car, but neither can they stop motorists merely upon a "hunch" or a guess, or because the person fits into some ethnic profile. Of course, they can stop you for a violation of the traffic laws.

Traffic Violations

In our fact pattern, you carelessly crossed a double yellow line, violating a traffic law, and the police were therefore justified in making the traffic stop. As noted, law enforcement will almost always ask during a traffic stop: "Do you know why I stopped you?" It is very often a slam-dunk to obtaining an admission. I've also seen admissions made in court by defendants who don't have an attorney. They will often admit that they were speeding, but that they were *only* traveling five miles per hour over the speed limit. Stupid! The judge is looking for the guilty stamp and calculating the fine before the testimony's done.

Anyway, here's some common sense advice if you're stopped for a traffic violation. Always make certain that your paperwork is in order and readily available. Remove your papers from any laminations or plastic covers. Remove sunglasses if you're wearing them. When the officer approaches your car, be sure that your hands are readily visible on the steering wheel. Don't ever get out of your car and approach the officer unless directed to do so. The Supreme Court has held that officers may order the operator out of the vehicle for a mere traffic violation if the officer believes it is necessary to protect his safety. [*Pennsylvania v. Mimms*, 434 U.S. 106 (1977)] The traffic stop is one of the most dangerous parts of law enforcement and all well-trained and experienced officers approach them with the heightened awareness that they may be encountering a deadly force situation. Anything that you can do that makes their job less stressful gives you a better chance of going on your way with merely a warning.

Don't ever get out of your car and approach the officer unless directed to do so.

The police may not search an automobile incident to a stop and issuance of a traffic citation. The Supreme Court held that a search incident to a citation, instead of an arrest, in a routine traffic stop violated the Fourth Amendment when there was no arrest to justify the search. [*Knowles v. Iowa*, 525 U.S. 113 (1998)] That is, of course, unless you consent.

Consent

Here's the biggie. The issue arose in the chapter on basic Fourth Amendment concerns, and it's crucial to discuss a bit more now. While we all have a Constitutional right against unreasonable searches and seizures of our cars, we may nonetheless waive that right. The right may be waived through a grant of *consent*.

In our fact pattern, you made the crucial error of providing consent for the car search. You were merely stopped for a possible traffic violation for crossing the double yellow line, and in some states Pit Bull couldn't even ask for your consent without a founded suspicion that you were up to no good. The police had no probable cause to search the vehicle, and there was no basis to arrest and subsequently "search incident to" (see page 123) that arrest. However, once consent to a full search was granted, Pit Bull was allowed to search the entire vehicle including closed containers within the vehicle (such as gym bags, book bags, briefcases and glove box) as well as the trunk.

Why do so many people consent to searches of their cars? The most obvious reason is that they are overcome by the stress and surprise of the confrontation, and simply submit to authority. Some of the factors discussed in Chapter 22 on the Psychology of Interrogation directly apply to the initial moments of a traffic stop. In the panic of the moment, even people who should know better submit. Here's a real life example: two men, both in their 30s, were stopped for traveling 5 mph over the speed limit just outside of San Antonio, Texas. Both had backgrounds working at federal corrections facilities; one had served in the U.S. Marine Corps for nine years. Yet, when confronted by the police, they consented to a search of the car, revealing testosterone and nandrolone in personal use amounts. Asked why, they told me that the way it was presented, it seemed as if refusal to consent was not an option.

The sequence of the officer's questions also helps foster consent. After his suspicions are aroused, he asks you if there are any weapons or contraband in the car, to which you'd typically say, "No." He's now committed you to a protestation of innocence. Next he asks to search your car. Refusing to consent makes you look like a liar; nobody likes to be caught in a lie. Consenting to the search shows you have nothing to hide. On some subconscious level, you may think that if you seem unconcerned enough about the car search, the officer might say, "Well, if you really had something in the car, you wouldn't be consenting to a search, now would you? Okay, forget it, go home." Possible? Fat chance. If you're stupid enough to consent to a search of your car, it will be searched. Period.

Now, in the real world, refusing to consent doesn't always end the encounter. The reality is that if you refuse to consent, the officer is now pretty sure he's got something to sink his teeth into. He can't use your refusal against you, though. He'd like to find some other way to get into your car. Here's a true story from a Mississippi case of mine:

Don was cruising along a deserted stretch of dark highway on his way back from Mexico. He was a teacher, in his mid 30s, with a wife and family back in New Jersey. He wasn't speeding; he wasn't weaving. Hell, he knew what he had in the trunk and wasn't taking any chances.

Headlights appeared suddenly in his rear view mirror, and they were coming up fast. Red lights started whirling as the trooper's car rode his bumper. Don pulled over. The trooper who approached his window had beady little eyes.

"Do you know why I stopped you?" the trooper drawled.

"No idea, Officer."

"You didn't signal a lane change. License and registration, please."

Don handed it over, trying to look completely calm. He hadn't even changed lanes. The red lights kept whirling round and round as the trooper looked at his license. Don knew that his out-of-state tags were the reason he was stopped. Don's palms were clammy and his throat was dry.

The trooper asked where Don was coming from and going to, then asked, "Do you have any drugs in the car?"

"No," Don said, trying hard not to stammer.

"Fine, you don't mind if I search it then."

"W-w-well, I do mind," Don protested. "I'd like to be on my way, please."

The trooper's tiny eyes got even smaller. "Step out of the car."

Don obliged. The trooper shined the powerful light from his D-cell mag-lite throughout the inside of his car. "If you consent to a search of your trunk and there's nothing in there, y'all can be on your way in no time."

"I have nothing to hide, but I value my privacy. I refuse."

The trooper drew closer, frowning. He said that his county was having a problem with narcotics coming from Mexico, and that Don would need to wait while a nearby canine unit was called to the scene. Don was told that he'd be free to leave immediately if the dog didn't detect any drugs.

While waiting for the unit to arrive, the trooper began describing the dog's traits: its perfect accuracy, its great size, its viciousness, its curious habit of going totally berserk immediately upon smelling any narcotics. It's sometimes quite difficult to control the dog, the trooper said, and he'd seen the dog destroy car exteriors and even get loose and attack motorists. Far better and safer for all concerned, the trooper helpfully suggested, for Don to consent to a search before the dog arrived.

Don stood his ground. Twenty minutes later the canine unit arrived. The dog was led silently around the car twice by the handling officer. There was hushed conversation between the trooper and the canine unit officer. Don overhead the canine unit officer whisper, "Ain't got shit."

"He says, 'It's a hit,'" the trooper dutifully reported when he walked back to Don. "Give me the keys to the trunk."

"But the dog didn't bark, didn't growl, or nothing!" argued Don, dumbfounded.

"Oh, this is a different dog," the trooper smiled, as he popped open the trunk to reveal about 700cc of injectables.

Search Incident to Arrest

In 1969, the Supreme Court held in the seminal case of *Chimel* that incident to a custodial arrest the police may lawfully perform a warrantless search of the person and of the immediate surrounding area to discover any weapons that the arrestee might seek to use, or to prevent the concealment or destruction of evidence. [*Chimel v. California*, 395 U.S. 752 (1969)] This type of post-arrest search requires no probable cause or reasonable suspicion. While *Chimel* didn't pertain to an automobile, but involved an arrest in the home, the case has become an important one in the body of law on vehicle searches. A search incident to an arrest is limited to the immediate "grabbable" area of the arrestee. This area is subject to search even if the arrestee is restrained and physically unable to get to any items inside the car. The grabbable area is somewhat of a legal fiction, because the danger to the officers or the destruction of evidence has been eliminated once the suspect is removed from the car and restrained. The only restriction is that this warrantless search must generally be conducted at the *same time* as the arrest in order for it to be considered incident to the arrest.

In 1981, the Supreme Court created a rule specific to searches of automobiles incident to arrest. [*New York v. Belton*, 453 U.S. 454 (1981)] The Court delineated what is known as a "bright-line" rule that permits the search of the vehicle passenger compartment and all containers, including closed containers (and in some states, locked containers), that are within the passenger compartment following a custodial arrest. The suspect may already be removed from the vehicle, and unable to grab anything from in it. (Bright-line rules don't need to be logical, as long as they're clear.)

> A search incident to an arrest is limited to the immediate "grabbable" area of the arrestee.

Using our fact pattern, suppose you were driving with a suspended or revoked driver's license or driving while your ability was impaired by alcohol. In such circumstances, Pit Bull would be within his authority to make a custodial arrest for those crimes. Once you are out of the vehicle, handcuffed and detained in the back seat of the patrol car, Pit Bull can lawfully search the compartment of your car including an unlocked glove compartment, closed briefcase, book bag and/or gym bag. However, he may not open and search the closed trunk, hood or other areas of the car that are not within the grabbable area as described in *Chimel*. This search may be conducted out in the field while the car is on the roadside, or the vehicle may be impounded and searched later at a police impound yard.

Plain View

The constitutional limits of the plain view doctrine were set down in *Coolidge v. New Hampshire* [403 U.S. 443 (1971), modified in part by *Horton v. California*, 496 U.S. 128 (1990)]. There are three requirements: 1) there must have been a valid prior intrusion into the suspect's privacy by the officer, 2) the object seized must have been inadvertently found, and 3) the evidentiary value of the object must be immediately apparent. The plain view doctrine has been used to justify countless seizures in car stop cases. Let's say Pit Bull stops your car and sees what looks like the butt of a gun sticking out from under the seat in open view. He goes into the car to get the gun (which turns out to only be a pipe), but while he's at it he notices a clear baggie with 500 tabs of D-bol. The D-bol can be seized as evidence under the doctrine. This is pretty close to what happened to a client of mine from New York, who was busted in his car with about 280 tablets of Thai Anabol inside a black gym bag.

Probable Cause as to the Vehicle

When there is probable cause as to the car itself, such as where the police got a reliable tip that the car contains a bag of anabolics, then the "automobile exception" established by *Carroll* applies. Referring back to our fact pattern, suppose Pit Bull sees you buy some bottles of juice from a dealer in the parking lot behind the gym. He sees you pay some money and get a clear bag in return. He sees the gear and syringes, all of which he recognizes as illegal contraband. He calls for backup, and watches you get into your car, put the bag on the seat, and drive away. With the assistance of the backup unit, your car is stopped. Pit Bull approaches you with gun drawn. He has probable cause to arrest you, and also has probable cause as to your car itself, because he knows it contains the gear. He may conduct a full search of the car – everywhere the bag of juice might reasonably be, including all containers. [*United States v. Ross*, 456 U.S. 798 (1982); *California v. Acevedo*, 500 U.S. 565 (1991)] Would that include the trunk? No, because he saw you enter the passenger compartment without opening the trunk, and knew the object of his search was located in the passenger compartment. Let's say that you're arrested. Can the trunk be searched incident to your arrest? No, because it was outside your grabbable area. Of course, if your car is impounded, the trunk could be searched pursuant to an inventory search (see below).

An interesting note: when law enforcement agents apply for a search warrant for a suspect's house they often also request authority to search his vehicles. Here's a direct quote from an Affidavit for Search Warrant in a California steroid case (probably part of a basic form on all drug cases), referring to the anabolics generically as "dope":

> "Based on my training and experience, I know drug dealers will often keep all or various portions of their dope in their vehicles. This is done for several reasons. Given both the criminal nature of their business as well as their financial investment in inventory, drug dealers are always concerned about becoming compromised and losing their dope or the money derived from their drug sales to law enforcement authorities during a search. Similarly, they are also afraid of being 'ripped off' (becoming a theft victim) by rival dope dealers. Consequently, dope dealers will often hide all or part of their 'stash' (inventory) in one or more vehicles away from their residence. These vehicles include ones in the dealer's possession, for example, taken in trade or collateral for drugs, but not registered in the dealer's name. I also know drug dealers will often register cars they own in the names of others in order to avoid loss of the vehicles through asset forfeiture laws in the event they are investigated or arrested."

Keep this in mind when assessing your expectations of privacy in an automobile.

DWI Roadblocks

The Supreme Court has upheld sobriety checkpoints as being reasonable seizures under the Fourth Amendment. [*Michigan Dept. of State Police v. Sitz,* 496 U.S. 444 (1990); *United States v. Martinez-Fuerte,* 428 U.S. 543 (1976)] The primary requirement for these roadblocks is that they must be implemented through a decision by police management and conducted under management's control. There are many views as to what is constitutional, based upon state court decisions. The following are general factors to be considered as to whether a DWI roadblock will pass constitutional muster:

1) The driver receives an explanation as to the reason for the initial stop;

2) The stop is conducted pursuant to clearly circumscribed guidelines;

3) Approaching drivers are given warning of the roadblock ahead;

4) There is a legitimate display of police authority at the roadblock;

5) Vehicles are stopped on a systematic, non-random, non-discriminatory basis that demonstrates to drivers that they are not being singled out arbitrarily;

6) There is minimal detention of the unimpaired driver.

If police observe an impaired driver and place that driver under arrest, the passenger compartment of the vehicle may be searched incident to the arrest. Additionally, if any contraband is observed in open view during a DWI roadblock, the police may then search the vehicle on the basis of probable cause, or incident to a custodial arrest.

Let's take a real case I handled as an example. Burt, an AAS user, was a passenger in a car Theo was driving in Staten Island, NY. When they saw the DWI roadblock, they switched seats because Theo had a suspended license. The cops saw them do it, arrested Theo, searched the car, and found Burt's 4,000 tablets of Thai Anabol and also some syringes. Rotten luck. Burt was busted. Then in an improbable change of fortune, someone failed to write the quantity of tabs into the criminal complaint. It went to court only as a misdemeanor, not the felony possession with intent to sell it should have been. It skated past the prosecutor and judge, who never bothered to ask about the amount involved. Burt and I walked out of court with a guilty plea to Disorderly Conduct, a sealed non-criminal violation equivalent to a traffic ticket. His sentence was a $60 fine. Burt got very, very lucky. You very well might not be.

If police observe an impaired driver and place that driver under arrest, the passenger compartment of the vehicle may be searched incident to the arrest.

Non-Government Action

The Fourth Amendment protects the People against action by the government or its agents, but it does not protect the People from the intrusive actions of private citizens. Let's say that you're a student living in a dormitory at a *private* university (at a state school, the result might be different). As part of the university's anti-drug campaign, they implement a policy of randomly stopping and searching all vehicles on the campus. The policy provides that all searches are to be conducted by campus safety officers, who are employees of the university. During one of these searches, safety officers uncover a bag of Anavar tabs in your car. They confiscate the 'roids and call local, state, and/or federal police. While the search was performed without probable cause and without a warrant, it was nonetheless conducted by private actors. As long as these safety officers were not serving as agents of the government, the search would not be in violation of the Fourth Amendment. Therefore, the anabolics would not be subject to suppression at trial.

Inventory Searches

The Supreme Court has recognized the power and authority of police officers and their agents to perform a warrantless search and inventory the contents of a lawfully impounded motor vehicle. [*South Dakota v. Opperman*, 428 U.S. 364 (1976)] The Court held that such searches are reasonable and therefore lawful under the Fourth Amendment. Remember, the Fourth Amendment protects the People's right against *unreasonable* searches and seizures. Routine police inventories are justified to protect the owner's property, to protect the police against claims of lost or stolen property, and to protect the safety of police. The search may not be limited to those items in plain view and may include closed containers in the vehicle if the police department has a written policy governing such searches.

Returning to the fact pattern that started this chapter, suppose you decide to stop to hit some clubs with your buds. Unfortunately for you, you parked your car in front of a fire hydrant, and before the night is over the police tow it away and impound it. At the impound yard, the police perform an inventory of the vehicle's contents which, according to written department policy and procedure, includes a search of the trunk and all closed containers inside. The cops find the Anavars and other contraband in the gym bag in the trunk. It's a valid warrantless inventory search and you're in a world of hurt.

The Morning After

So here you are, sitting in the courthouse pens. It's morning now and you're waiting to be arraigned along with a bunch of smelly drunks and a few dudes who you don't want to even know what they did. You could have saved yourself if you had just said no when your bro's talked you into juicing. Too late for that now. You might have saved yourself tonight, too, if you'd taken former First Lady Nancy Reagan's advice and applied it to Pit Bull's request for consent: "Just say no."

Chapter 10

THE OLD BAIT AND SNITCH

"For I have sworn thee fair, and thought thee bright, who art as black as hell, as dark as night."
– *William Shakespeare (1564–1616)*

When it comes to narcotics investigations, informers make the world go round. They are the grease that keeps the wheels of the War on Drugs machine turning. The law enforcement term is always *Confidential Informant*, or *C.I.* Somehow, "informant" sounds less devious than "informer," which is the more accurately descriptive term and the one many defense lawyers prefer. But lots of people use terms like *rat* or *snitch*.

Here's Tommy's case. It happened in New York three years ago. The conversations are minimally edited from the transcripts of the audiotapes turned over to me as evidence by the prosecution.

The telephone rang and Tommy picked it up. It was Anthony, an old friend and former training partner who worked out in Tommy's basement gym a year or two before.

"Yo, Tommy, you still got any juice?"

"Juice? No, man." Tommy hadn't used steroids in over a year, since he was twenty-three. He and Anthony had once done a steroid cycle together, but Tommy was hardly working out at all lately. He was putting in long hours laying floors, and things with his girlfriend were getting serious.

"Can't you get some? I want to get huge! Come on, bro."

Tommy thought a moment. He remembered he had recently seen one bottle of testosterone cypionate in his closet. It was the last one he had from a while back. It was unopened, but he was going to just throw it out. Hey, if Anthony could use it, why not? Anthony was a good kid. "Yeah, I got something for you."

"How much you want for it?" Anthony asked. "I need it right away."

Tommy paused. It hadn't even crossed his mind. Maybe he could recoup what he paid for it. "Two hundred."

"That's too much, bro. How's a hundred and eighty?"

"Okay." Whatever. Tommy arranged to meet Anthony and dug the bottle out of his closet.

They met the next night in a parking lot they used to hang out in. To Tommy's surprise, Anthony showed up with a friend Tommy didn't know. Anthony introduced "Joey," and said that he was cool. He gave Tommy the money and Tommy handed him the bottle. Then Joey said he wanted steroids too.

"No," Tommy said, "this was just for Anthony. I don't do this."

"Yeah, but we could make some big bucks," Joey pressed. "I got guys that go crazy for this shit."

"This isn't my thing, man," Tommy answered. "This is a one-shot deal, just for Anthony. I don't sell this stuff."

Joey persisted, saying how much money they could all make. It went on for a while, but Tommy was adamant. He wasn't a dealer. He wasn't even a juicer anymore. His girlfriend would kill him if she knew he had even helped Anthony out like this.

Finally Joey gave up, and he and Anthony left. Tommy started his car. Suddenly he was blinded. Light was everywhere, with shadows moving through it. His car door opened and somebody grabbed him and threw him on the ground. Face down, his arms were pulled behind his back. Handcuffs were put on his wrists and he was dragged to his feet, thrown on the hood of his car. Everything was spinning. Lights were flashing and people were talking on radios. Somebody said he was under arrest. He was walked toward a police patrol car. Police officers were all around him; some in uniforms, others in plainclothes. What happened? Where did all these cops come from? How did they know? And where were Anthony and Joey? A sick feeling came over him as he realized ... he'd been set up by his friend for one bottle of juice ...

Becoming an Informer

How does someone become an informer? Here's the scenario as it plays out in many federal narcotics cases: Danny Doe gets popped dead to rights on conspiracy drug charges. Not steroid charges, mind you, but serious cocaine or heroin charges. He gets busted because somebody got popped and ratted him out. Danny's pretty big-time and has a record, so he's looking at doing a nasty stretch of time under the federal sentencing guidelines (USSG) if he pleads guilty or blows trial. Maybe he's held on a bond that he can't afford. The agents tell him that he can help himself if he *cooperates* with them. "Cooperation" is also a much nicer term than what it really is. After all, isn't it nice to be cooperative? It's standard for the feds to squeeze the many "small fish" they arrest into giving up their sources, leading to the arrests of bigger fish who, in turn, are squeezed to give up their sources. Fans of the HBO series "The Sopranos" will recall that the informer-as-fish analogy was used effectively to expose Tony's former crew member Big Pussy.

Any arrangement should arise from fully negotiated understandings, *in writing*, between the prosecutor and the lawyer.

It's obvious that a decision to cooperate with the government is not to be made lightly. It should not be made without extensive consultation with experienced criminal defense counsel. Far too many people immediately begin spilling their guts to the arresting agents before a lawyer is even involved. Bad idea. The agents have virtually *no* authority to cut deals. Period. Any arrangement should arise from fully negotiated understandings, *in writing*, between the prosecutor and the lawyer.

Danny meets with his lawyer and they go through the options. Danny's lawyer arranges a debriefing at the U.S. Attorney's office. Danny and his lawyer meet with the prosecutor and agents assigned to the case. Danny is given a proffer agreement for him to read and sign. It typically provides that nothing he says in the meeting will be used directly against him. There are, however, a few exceptions. He must tell the truth in the meeting. If he doesn't, the deal is off. Not only is the deal off, but whatever incriminating evidence he has told them can be used to impeach him if he later tries to falsely testify to his innocence at trial or if he offers evidence or arguments inconsistent with his statements. Also, if the information he provides leads them to other evidence separate from his statements, that other evidence could be held against him.

Perhaps most importantly, what he tells them must not be withheld from the sentencing judge and will be factored into the calculations of where he falls in the USSG.

Further, Danny must ultimately provide *substantial* assistance to get his deal. What that means, in practical terms, is that somebody else must get busted as a result of Danny's efforts, or at the least, his efforts must help convict somebody. Danny will have to name names, betray confidences, deceive people who trusted him, and maybe even testify against them in open court. He may even risk his own safety and that of his family. He must not hold back in selling out anyone he can. The more people who are arrested as a result of Danny's assistance, the better off he'll be.

What does Danny get out of all this? Under 18 U.S.C. § 3553(e) and 28 U.S.C. § 944(n), cooperators are to be rewarded. So, Danny gets a letter on his behalf from the prosecutor to the sentencing judge. This letter, commonly called a *5K letter* because its authority is under USSG § 5K1.1, will tell the judge about all the things Danny did to help arrest and prosecute his former friends and associates. Most importantly, the letter will legally permit the judge to depart from the USSG in sentencing Danny, so that even if years in prison are called for under the guidelines, Danny has a chance at getting much less time – possibly even no time. It gives the discretion in sentencing back to the judge. Most, but not all, judges bestow quite favorable treatment on cooperators, knowing their great value to a criminal justice system that heavily relies upon informers to build narcotics cases and make arrests.

Danny weighs his options, comparing where he falls in the USSG to where he might end up with a 5K letter. If he's like the substantial majority of traffickers of cocaine, heroin and marijuana facing federal time, he'll choose to become an informer. He'll tell the government everything he knows about everyone he knows. He'll tell about his drug sources and his customers. He'll tell about the neighborhood dealer and the guys who sell steroids at the gym. It will be up to the feds to choose what they want to run with.

Let's say the coke dealers are all pretty much busted already, the meth lab closed up shop, and the local weed seller cleaned up his act and went back to school. The agents will shrug and say, "Tell us more about the 'roid pushers." Of course, if Danny himself was busted for juice, he might not know much about cocaine or heroin. If he wants to cooperate, it'll probably be on AAS cases.

> It's important to know that informers work both up and down the chain.

It's important to know that informers work both up and down the chain. For example, an arrest was made of Harvey, a large-scale steroid trafficker in a western state. His primary source was located in Eastern Europe, so there were limits to what the agents could do. Instead, they worked down the ladder. Harvey ratted out his regional distributors, and then ratted out his bigger customers. One of them was Ken, my client. Harvey showed evidence to the feds of wire transfers from Ken in payment for juice. The feds looked into Ken and found that he's on federal probation for, you guessed it, trafficking in juice. They began tracing past travel and phone records to link Ken to the various other co-conspirators.

So, Danny calls his friend Ralphie and says he's got a high-rolling customer who needs some juice, and they both stand to make a few dollars. Danny sets up Ralphie just like someone set up Danny. A few months later, Ralphie's in the U.S. Attorney's office reading his own proffer agreement.

That's the way the system proceeds in most narcotics cases. To some extent, though, AAS cases are different. Although I have defended steroid clients who were set up by informers, the informers themselves were usually charged with trafficking cocaine or "club drugs" like GHB or Ecstasy or, less frequently, with trafficking steroids in *state court,* where penalties may be harsher. I have found that cooperation is less common among AAS dealers in federal court. To be sure, cooperation still takes place, but it's much rarer than in narcotics cases where the majority of defendants seem to cooperate. This may be due mostly to the lower stakes involved, as the steroid "discount" inherent in USSG § 2D1.1 (see Note G of the Drug Quantity Table or the Sentencing Chart on page 59) effectively requires enormous quantities to mandate really major prison time. Many first-time AAS defendants may figure, why cooperate if probation is a likely sentence? But the lesser percentage of federal court AAS cooperators may also be due in part to an old-fashioned "code of honor" among juicers that simply doesn't exist elsewhere in the drug world. It is interesting that although I've defended many first-timers accused of steroid trafficking in federal court, not a single one has chosen to rat out fellow bodybuilders. But this chapter is about informer cases, so let's dig up a true story of an AAS client who proffered against another AAS-involved individual.

To some extent ... AAS cases are different. Although I have defended steroid clients who were set up by informers, the informers themselves were usually charged with trafficking cocaine or "club drugs" ...

AAS Informers in the Real World

Here's a true case history about snitching. I was not involved in the case in any way, but interviewed Ronin and personally examined some of the paperwork in his case after it was finished. Ronin was given a break even though his efforts at cooperation were ultimately unfruitful.

Ronin is currently forty-one years old. He was an amateur bodybuilder and had competed at the national level. He didn't start juicing until 1989. He would get his steroids from a close buddy in Canada who was a professional bodybuilder, then bring them back across the border. Most of what he got was for personal use, as he wouldn't sell to anyone but for a few friends here and there. One of the guys he sold to was a buddy at the gym who ended up getting pinched for possession of GHB. This guy apparently agreed to work with the authorities and become an informer, to help catch "the bigger fish." He told them all about Ronin.

Although DEA generally gives anabolics a low priority, Ronin was all that the informer had to give them, so they started an investigation. The investigation went on for nearly three years! Over the course of time, they set up three buys through their informer. Finally, DEA made their move to bring Ronin to justice. The informer told DEA that Ronin would be picking up a quantity of steroids in Canada and would be crossing back over the border. They alerted Customs officials, who were ready and waiting for him. They stopped him at the border crossing and asked him to open the trunk of his car. Immediately he sensed that it wasn't a routine secondary inspection. The Customs officials found nothing in his trunk, but rather than letting him go his way, they asked him to remove his car's speaker covers. Lo and behold, there appeared 1,000 bottles of omnadren. Suddenly there were agents swarming everywhere, most of whom were from DEA.

Ronin was charged with conspiracy and distribution charges, and faced a maximum five-year imprisonment sentence. The DEA pressured Ronin to cooperate for almost two years. They wanted to use him to catch the "biggest fish." His lawyer, who had handled many narcotics cases but had never handled an AAS case, also urged him to cooperate. While Ronin resisted for almost two years, ultimately he met with DEA officials and even took a lie detector test lasting two days. He eventually betrayed his buddy in Canada. Fortunately for the guy in Canada, though, Canadian officials wanted nothing to do with the DEA or the case. So Ronin couldn't provide the substantial assistance required for a 5K letter. He was sentenced under the USSG, where his quantity placed him at a base offense level of 14. Three levels were taken off for timely acceptance of responsibility and another three based upon his efforts to cooperate (although it's unclear exactly what basis existed for this adjustment, given that cooperation didn't work out). He was sentenced at the adjusted Level of 8. Ronin's property seized and forfeited included a brand new truck, a 1985 Corvette, and the gym he owned. He also forfeited an additional $6,000 in cash. He received a three-year probationary term, but his felony conviction will be an impediment to many of his career goals.

[Ronin's quantities were allegedly substantial. To begin at Level 14, we're talking about distribution of between 5,000 and 10,000 vials of 10cc each, or between 250,000 and 500,000 tablets! The quantity calculations were based on estimates by the agents of how much Ronin had distributed over the course of his AAS dealing career (all of which is totaled as his "relevant conduct" as explained in Chapter 4). Ronin says the numbers were way off, but his lawyer never challenged them.]

Detecting an Informer

Informers are amateur undercover agents. Undercover work is by definition deceptive. The informer's true agenda, and sometimes even his identity, are extensively fabricated. It virtually always requires outright lies by its very nature. Like undercover agents, informers are allowed to use trickery and subterfuge. Even after several seasons of watching Tony Soprano and his family interact in both sophisticated and brutal ways with a variety of snitches and rats, I still hear of clients attempting to protect themselves by asking of a suspected informer prior to a transaction, "You're not a cop, are you?" Make no mistake: the informer will lie, and the courts will hold that it's perfectly permissible. Informers and undercover agents will lie, lie, lie. I once saw a case where the undercover cop allayed the client's suspicions by initiating the exchange of lengthy e-mails swearing that neither was in law enforcement.

Informers customarily record their conversations with you for use later as evidence. Telephone calls are recorded, and are often placed from the offices of the investigating agents. For meetings, the informer is generally "wired" with a device that will record the conversation. The device can be concealed on the body or in a variety of articles of clothing. Unless you are prepared to conduct a full search of an individual, you will not know whether he is wired. Even if you do search, you might not identify it.

There is, frankly, no sure way to detect an informer or an undercover agent. Many of my clients who have trafficked in gear have had their own rules of business, such as never talking about juice on the telephone, never dealing to strangers, never completing a transaction if someone unexpected (an undercover agent) shows up, etc. While some of these clients were quite sophisticated, probably more so than most readers of this book, every one of them got busted.

A different type of informer is the jailhouse snitch. He's a person who's serving time or awaiting disposition of his own case, and is looking for an opportunity to mitigate his own sentence. Despite the obvious reliability problems, many cases have been built on the testimony of jailhouse snitches. While these slippery characters are generally looking for bigger fish than typical AAS defendants, it's imperative that anyone in jail for juice keeps his mouth shut about his business until he's bailed or bonded out.

Avoiding Entrapment

Let's say you're cruising down the strip one night on the seedy side of town. You see a smokingly hot babe in a tube top and miniskirt standing on a corner. Think Brandy Dahl on six-inch platforms, or Monica Brant if you prefer. You don't know it, but she's an undercover cop on a detail to catch johns. You say a few words you regret, and you're collared. Isn't she, essentially, *baiting* unsuspecting motorists to approach her and subject themselves to arrest? Of course, she is. Might someone succumb to the temptation to commit the crime of solicitation? Oh, yeah. Is this entrapment? Not according to the many courts that have ruled on similar issues. Affording someone the opportunity to commit a crime isn't entrapment.

Simply put, entrapment refers to a complete legal defense where a person commits a crime *solely* because he was actively pressured by the police to do it. Consider the case of *Jacobson v. U.S.* [503 U.S. 540 (1992)], in which the Supreme Court held that agents may not originate a criminal design, implant the disposition to commit the act in an innocent person's mind and induce its commission so that they may prosecute it.

There are essentially two elements to the entrapment defense: 1) government inducement and 2) lack of defendant's predisposition to commit the crime. [*Mathews v. United States*, 485 U.S. 58 (1988)] Mere solicitation to commit a crime is not sufficient to support an entrapment defense, nor do lies or deceit on the part of agents support the defense; some showing of persuasion or coercion is required. [*See U.S. v Nations*, 764 F2d 1073 (1985)] In *U.S. v. Evans* [924 F.2d 714 (1991)], the court ruled that extraordinary promises were required for the entrapment defense – ones that would blind the ordinary person to his legal duties. Even if inducement has been shown, the entrapment defense fails if the person was predisposed to commit the crime. The question is whether the defendant "was an unwary innocent or, instead, an unwary criminal who readily availed himself of the opportunity to perpetrate the crime." [*Mathews, supra*] [However, if the police conduct was outrageous, the case may be dismissed on federal due process grounds despite the defendant's predisposition to commit the crime. *See United States v. Chin* , 934 F.2d 393 (2d Cir.1991).]

Each state has its own statutes and case law dealing with this issue. Under New York state law, for example, entrapment is an affirmative defense when a person is pressured by the police or their agents to commit a crime just for the purpose of arresting him, and when the methods used by the police are such as to create a substantial risk that the offense would be committed by a person *not otherwise predisposed* to commit it. This defense protects people who are not predisposed to committing a crime, but who give in only because of the nature and persistence of police pressure. It is an affirmative defense because the accused has the burden of proving it by a preponderance of the evidence. An example of a viable entrapment defense would be where an undercover agent makes repeated, persistent and badgering demands over a course of months to a person who has never sold steroids before, urging him to sell to him a quantity of steroids that had been abandoned by a former roommate.

Don't Think You're So Smart

Think you're too savvy to fall prey to a snitch? Well, let's recount the story of Kent Brown. Back in 1997, Brown was a police officer working for a DEA task force. As part of his duties, he assisted in the investigation and arrest of several anabolic steroid traffickers. Brown was well versed in police tactics. If anybody should have known every trick in the book, it was Brown. But Brown's experiences on the task force led him to question his mission, specifically with respect to anabolic steroid suspects. His experiences led him to pen a book entitled, *The Anabolic Survival Guide, a.k.a. The Steroid User's Survival Guide.* The book was a guide for steroid suspects, disclosing "inside" information Brown learned during his years in law enforcement. It went beyond the parameters of tasteful information, perhaps, by actually making suggestions as to how to best smuggle steroids across the border and various other stuff. Was Brown seen as a traitor by his former colleagues? Was a price put on his head by DEA brass?

Well, Brown himself was involved with steroids. Despite all his training and experiences working with informers, Brown was reportedly ratted out by an informer. He wound up in federal court charged with AAS dealing. It was claimed that on some occasions, he happened to be on-duty and armed with his service weapon, so the government tried to hit him with a gun enhancement under 18 U.S.C. § 924(c) for "carrying a firearm during drug trafficking."

He ended up losing not only his reputation and his job, but serving time in a federal prison – never a good place for a former cop to be. The *Las Vegas Review-Journal* printed a short piece on Brown's case in its "Nevada Briefs" (December 15, 1997) [Available online at www.lvrj.com/lvrj_home/1997/Dec-15-Mon-1997/news/6601740.html]. In it, Brown's attorney, David Houston, contended that the book influenced the prosecution of his client on steroid trafficking charges. The Assistant U.S. Attorney Ronald Rachow, denied that claim, arguing that Brown, a retired law enforcement officer with over ten years of experience, was only prosecuted for breaking the law. Houston pointed out that Brown "crossed company lines" when he wrote the book, and that he had been "warned not to write this book because of possible government retaliation." These words can be found on the first page of the introduction to the book. Brown's lawyer suggested that disclosing this type of information "crossed company lines" and that "various police agencies felt quite a sense of betrayal."

You be the judge on that one. However you make the call, the lesson to take home is that *nobody* is immune from infiltration by an informer, and that entrapment is a tough defense to prove. We started with a quote; let's end with one, too.

> "The easiest way to be cheated is to believe yourself to be more cunning than others."
> – *Pierre Charron (1541–1603)*

Chapter 11

TEENS AND TESTOSTERONE

> "MEMO TO HIGH SCHOOLS: You have a problem. Anabolic steroids are becoming the rage among teens ... They are undeterred by the risks of high blood pressure, heart disease, liver damage, cancers, strokes and blood clots and headaches and cramps and nausea and baldness and acne and sterility and increased breast size in males, shrunken testicles, stunted growth and many more."
>
> – *Doug Robinson, "No sweat? Teens are swept up in roid rage,"* Deseret News, *June 11, 2002*

> "Scare tactics don't work."
>
> – *Asa Hutchinson, DEA chief,* "Dennis Miller Live," *August 1, 2002*

I guess some journalists didn't get the DEA memo before sending out their own? Scare tactics have failed abysmally, but the media keep churning out hyperbolic drivel like this all the time. It suits them fine. Cheating Olympians and sports stars may provoke public disapproval, but the idea of our nation's teens abusing anabolic steroids is downright appalling to the public, including most parents. Journalists know this, and the problem of teen AAS abuse has received tremendous media attention.

The "scoop" that American teenagers are using steroids is still trotted out as just as much of a shocking revelation today as it was fifteen years ago. Some journalists have gone even further, such as the salacious attack on over-the-counter sports supplements entitled "Killer Bods" and published in, of all places, *Rolling Stone* [February 14, 2002, 54]. Most reporters who contact my office want to talk about the same old story: adolescent AAS usage. Most beg me to connect them with a teen user for a "juicy" interview. I presume they know what sells papers. They are disappointed, however, because the overwhelming majority of Americans – probably somewhere around 95% – who have contacted me because of steroid-related legal woes are *not* teens. This is surprising to many people because of the constant media correlation between anabolics and teens. Studies like the "Monitoring the Future" survey provide annual statistics on the percentage of teens who report using anabolics. There are no reliable statistics, however, about what percentage of AAS users are teens.

What the Stats Say

What is the percentage of teens using steroids? According to the 2001 Monitoring the Future survey [data is available at www.monitoringthefuture.org], 2.8% of 8th graders, 3.5% of 10th graders, and 3.7% of 12th graders reported using steroids at least once in their lives. Obviously, that's troubling. But as compared to the previous year, the 2001 number was *down* for 8th graders and *exactly the same* for 10th graders. The number of 12th graders who reported ever using steroids went up, but only from less than three out of one hundred to less than four out of one hundred students. Let's compare these figures to teen cocaine use. Significantly more 8th and 10th graders reported ever using cocaine or LSD than steroids, and the number of 12th graders who reported using cocaine at least once during their lifetime was 8.2% – more than *twice* the number who had ever used steroids. The number of 12th graders who reported using LSD at least once during their lifetime was 10.9% – nearly *triple* the number who had ever used steroids. And what about alcohol, which is responsible for the deaths of more than 6,000 teen drivers annually (data from the National Safety Council)? Yes, that's *six thousand* kids killed behind the wheel in alcohol-related collisions every year. The number of 12th graders who reported *being drunk* at least once was a truly alarming 63.9%, with a higher increase over the past year than the increase seen with steroids.

This is not to minimize in any way the social problem presented by teen steroid use, or teen drug use in general; it's simply to put things in perspective and hopefully put a damper on enacting more overbroad, reactionary laws. Teen steroid use is undeniably a problem, and as mature adults we ought to be doing more about it. The recent decision by the U.S. Supreme Court upholding the constitutionality of a public school drug testing policy that required all middle and high school students to consent to urinalysis testing for drugs as a prerequisite to participating in any extracurricular activities may be a step in the right direction (*Board of Education of Independent School District No. 92 of Pottawatomie County et al. v. Earls et al.*, 122 S. Ct. 2559, decided June 27, 2002). Justice Clarence Thomas delivered the 5-4 opinion of the Court, holding that the policy reasonably serves the school district's important interest in detecting drug use among its students. As such, a school does not need probable cause or even a mere individualized suspicion to require testing of students who are participating in extracurricular activities. While many schools will probably not test for steroids without some cause, the decision may have a deterrent effect on all teen drug use.

Teen steroid use is undeniably a problem, and as mature adults we ought to be doing more about it.

The Traditional Approach

Still, the threat of testing is not enough. Adolescent steroid use must be further addressed. The question is how, as mature adults, do we address it? The historical approach by the medical community and the sports lobby has been scare tactics. To quote Pat Croce, conditioning coach for the Philadelphia 76er's and Philadelphia Flyers, in his 1989 testimony before a Congressional subcommittee: "You have to scare them. You have to scare them. That is the only way...." But is it? Is scaring the pants off people the best way to stop them from engaging in undesirable behavior? Or have we "outgrown" such simplistic techniques? Government agencies like the National Institute on Drug Abuse have long favored the heavy-handed approach, and to some extent they're still desperately clinging to it. Check out www.steroidabuse.org and you'll see what they think works. Don't bet on it.

Is scaring the pants off people the best way to stop them from engaging in undesirable behavior?

Interestingly, a recent review of modern Christian teachings found that Hell has fallen out of favor. While the threat of everlasting torment in a fiery inferno was once a focal point of many sermons, today it's rarely mentioned at all. It just doesn't work anymore. Neither do steroid scare tactics, which have been beaten like a dead horse for at least a dozen years. What's happened? *More* teens are using anabolics than in 1991. Nevertheless, some of the media-friendly steroid authorities keep screeching that we need to increase teen awareness of the risks – i.e., bring Pat Croce's technique to an even higher volume. How? What's next? Further exaggerate the existing side effects, or just invent newer, scarier ones? How about leprosy, anal leakage and spontaneous combustion? Might those work?

The mentality of taking a failed approach and then doing even more of it needs to be taken behind the woodshed and shot. Scare tactics failed. They failed miserably. Why? Because in their well-meaning zeal to diminish teen use, the authorities exaggerated the dangers to such a degree that only a fool couldn't see it. Telling teens that they would drop over dead if they took a single steroid tablet inhibited only the most intellectually challenged. Most teens had already seen their friends use without keeling over, and many knew older users at the gym who were well into middle age and in excellent health. Many of yesteryear's top bodybuilding stars are doing quite well today.

Assessing the Seriousness of the Problem

So maybe, as parents, we shouldn't worry so much if our teens dabble in juice? Are steroids acceptable for teens? The answer to that question is a resounding "No." I'd worry *plenty* if it were my kids. Then again, I'd worry if my kids were even thinking about smoking cigarettes or drinking alcohol. I'd worry if my teenaged daughter were contemplating breast implants or any other type of non-necessary, purely cosmetic endeavor that subjected her to potentially serious health risks. (Of course, I wouldn't deny a mature woman from making her own informed decision about it, and I most certainly wouldn't suggest that the government should have a right to arrest or prosecute her, as they've been doing since 1991 with respect to men who use steroids.)

The most dangerous aspect of teen steroid use is probably not physiologically based at all. It's psychologically related: the potential for abuse. The teenage years are the peak period of insecurity for most of us, when we are most susceptible to peer pressure. Impatient and eager for fast results, many teens are less focused on the distant future, including possible health consequences many years ahead. Plus, there's generally a big difference in the mentality of most forty-year-olds from that of most seventeen-year-olds. There ought to be, if you've learned from life. Maturity doesn't come overnight. Teen years are often colored with a higher level of recklessness, sporadic irresponsibility, and a pervasive feeling of invincibility: "The bad stuff will never happen to me."

Impatient and eager for fast results, many teens are less focused on the distant future, including possible health consequences many years ahead.

And, of course, teens are typically less inclined to admit their use to a disapproving physician. This leads to an increased risk of health consequences by failing to monitor blood pressure, cholesterol and cardiovascular health. Further, the effects of anabolics upon size and strength are partially (and sometimes even completely) temporary. Teens seem particularly less willing to suffer these post-cycle size and strength reductions. Thus begins a vicious cycle resulting in a reluctance to ever "come off" the juice, which can lead to permanent health problems. A dangerous reliance on steroids can develop, as the only perceived way to build muscle and the only incentive to go to the gym. I've seen some young people who give up training entirely when they're not "on cycle."

Many years ago, when I was competing in bodybuilding competitions, I busted my butt in the gym year-round. About four months before a show, a young man named Josh would arrive at the gym after a long absence. He'd weigh about 175 pounds in lousy shape. Over the course of the four months, he'd go up to a ripped and ready 200 pounds, which was a lot for back then. He generally placed well at a show, but the next day he was nowhere to be found. Months would go by with no sight of him. Four months before the next show, he would return, like a swallow to Capistrano, weighing 175 again and in lousy shape, which was the way he appeared most of the year. That's no way to live.

Add it together and you have all the ingredients for disaster: a high propensity for uninterrupted usage at dangerously high dosages without medical supervision. Which raises another question: how would you even know the Sustanon you bought from Big Leo at the gym is sterile and legitimate? Even the regulars at hardcore steroid discussion boards on the Internet oppose and vigorously discourage teen use, as did the late Dan Duchaine, author of the *Underground Steroid Handbook II* (1989) and a favorite target of the anti-steroid brigade. Clearly, even in countries where they can be legally obtained without a prescription, the choice to use anabolics for physical enhancement should be made by mature, informed adults with a pre-established dedication to serious weight training. Bodybuilding writer Nelson Montana asserts his "Rule No. 1" of steroid use: "No one under the age of 24 should use steroids." His "Rule No. 2: "You shouldn't commence steroid use until natural pathways have been exhausted." He's right. Beginning lifters, those with dubious commitments to bodybuilding, or those simply seeking a substitute for hard work should never use anabolics.

... the choice to use anabolics for physical enhancement should be made by mature, informed adults with a pre-established dedication to serious weight training.

A New Approach to the Problem

So what's a parent or coach to do? There are various options. For example, I was consulted by a college student in New Jersey whose mother was cleaning his room and found steroids and syringes in his dresser drawer. Panicking, she called 911. When the local police arrived, she led them to the contraband. When he returned home from school, they arrested him on felony charges and carted him off. The judge set a bail, which the mother needed to post in cash. The mother was stupefied when she was told that she would be incurring additional costs, including significant legal fees, fines and miscellaneous court costs. She lamented that had she known what her phone call would cost her, she would have taken a different route. Few people realize what can result from bringing the police into the mix.

Of course, handling the situation as an emergency can be appropriate in certain circumstances. While the prevalence of "'roid rage" is largely a myth, some predisposed individuals can have steroid-induced psychiatric effects requiring prompt attention. Also, steroid users sometimes have periods of post-cycle depression that can be ameliorated by the administration of antidepressants. Parents need to know their children and be alert to significant behavioral changes, steroid-related or not. (If you have suspicions or concerns about possible steroid use by your teen, a good primer may be found in J.E. Wright and V.S. Cowart, *Anabolic Steroids: Altered States* [Carmel, IN: Benchmark Press, 1990], Chapter 4, "Recognizing Anabolic Steroid Use in Adolescents," 71-91.) Some steroid users may benefit from behavioral therapy or other counseling to diminish future usage, particularly where the use arises out of extraordinary low self-esteem or so-called "body dysmorphia" issues.

A study conducted by Project EAT surveyed 4,746 middle and high school students from St. Paul/Minneapolis public schools who completed surveys and anthropometric measurements as part of a population-based study of eating patterns and weight concerns among teenagers. The study concluded that, "Anabolic steroid use in adolescence is associated with poorer health-related attitudes and behaviors and exposure to socio-environmental influences encouraging weight preoccupation. Attention needs to be directed toward youth who may be at increased risk for steroid use within clinical and community-based settings." (*J Adolesc Health* 2002 Apr; 30(4):243-52.) These findings illustrate the contention that teens likely have a number of underlying reasons for engaging in steroid use. Let's face it: adolescence is a difficult and tumultuous time in our lives. A sixteen-year-old with low self-esteem and appearance insecurities may turn to steroids for a "quick fix." Far better, of course, to deal with the underlying issues.

In most situations, the first step would be to talk to the teen. The question is, how? Many teen steroid users find parents who lecture them on steroid use ludicrous on several levels. First, the parents often spout off what they've read in the mainstream media, and the kids know better. Second, teenagers tend to be sensitive to hypocrisy, and are apt to dismiss a health risk lecture from a coach or parent who smokes cigarettes or drinks to excess. (And, quite frankly, between us, they have a point. It's tough to get preachy until you clean up your own act. If your teen is using steroids, it may be a perfect opportunity to reevaluate your own poor health habits.) I've spent enough time talking to teens in gyms across the country to know that trying to scare the bejesus out of them will only serve to make us look foolish. The same will go for you if you try it. For one thing, many of these teens know more about the real health risks than you do (at least until you read this book). The approach to take, I am convinced, is one of honesty.

We can and should recite for our teens the traditional list of possible steroid side effects that are presented to all users, but we should present only the *real* risks, not some hyperbolic "Reefer Madness" version that destroys all credibility. Look, there *are* potentially serious side effects even to adults. In addition to the risks for adults, steroid use prior to puberty or in early adolescence can cause premature closure of the growth plates of the long bones, preventing the young user from attaining full natural height. Although looking good on the beach right now sounds good, even the most thick-headed teen can see the advantage in being a few inches taller a couple years from now.

... steroid use ... in early adolescence can cause premature closure of the growth plates of the long bones, preventing the young user from attaining full natural height.

Additionally, new research on animals by the experts at Northeastern University suggests that steroid use in adolescents may permanently alter *brain chemistry*, whereas the mental effects on adult users typically subside following cessation of use. Professor Richard Melloni, who helped run the study, said: "We know testosterone or steroids affect the development of serotonin nerve cells, which, in turn, decreases serotonin availability in the brain. The serotonin neural system is developing during adolescence and the use of anabolic steroids during this critical period appears to have immediate neural and behavioral consequences." (BBC News, August 16, 2002) Although this issue requires further research, this study provides support for the contention that introducing exogenous hormones to an endocrine system that has not yet fully developed can potentially have permanent and immediate consequences.

The Underestimated Value of Honesty

Still not enough ammunition for you coaches and parents? A few years ago, I overheard a nineteen-year-old college student quietly asking about steroids at a local health club I used to frequent. He weighed about 160 pounds. I only heard snippets of his gripes, but basically he was complaining about his lack of progress and was looking to boost his muscle gains with anabolics. I shook my head as I continued my own workout. When I finished my set, he asked for my opinion. What follows is what I told him. (If I had a teenaged son, it's what I'd tell him, too.)

"The way I see it, most everything has risks and benefits. That's especially true of medications, such as anabolic steroids. The choice of whether or not to take steroids involves weighing the risks against the benefits. The risks include numerous possible side effects, including the possibility of never growing to the height you should have been. Have the risks been exaggerated in healthy adult males? Absolutely. Lots of people have taken steroids and seem fine, even many years later. But a few have gotten very sick. At your age, you're a boiling pot of raging hormones. The effect of adding extra hormones on top of it all has the potential to be like throwing some gasoline onto a fire. Or maybe a health problem you may not be aware of, like a small undiscovered cluster of cancer cells, could be stimulated. We really don't know all of the long-term effects.

"Further, there's another risk that nobody talks about much. Not in the future, but here and now. That's the *legal* risk of having your ass busted. In many states, simple possession is a felony. I *know* – I've represented a slew of personal users who got jammed up. You'll be handcuffed and questioned. You'll spend a night in jail, maybe with an overly friendly guy named Bubba. You'll probably wind up needing to call your parents to bail you out, and then needing to hire a lawyer and go to court and see a judge, maybe a bunch of times. Your parents will foot the bill, and they'll never let you forget it for the rest of your life. If you're in a small town, the local papers may print your name, which happened to three teen juicers in Utah recently. You probably won't go to jail in the end. But if you're convicted of even a misdemeanor drug offense, you can lose some very important privileges including the license to drive your car and qualifying for college financial aid. Your folks will really love you for that.

... if you're convicted of even a misdemeanor drug offense, you can lose some very important privileges including the license to drive your car and qualifying for college financial aid.

"Word will probably get around about your arrest. Your teachers will see you differently, as will your neighbors. The girls at school won't think you're cool. They'll see you as a cheater. In fact, they'll attribute any muscles you have purely to the steroids. They'll disregard any hard work you may have put in at the gym. In their eyes, you'll be a lazy kid who cheated with some chemicals that made him bigger, and they will probably be right. You *didn't* pay your dues.

"You're technically an adult and can make up your own mind, but are the benefits really worth it? The way I see it, to really get the benefits you're going to need to take *more* steroids than an older guy. Why? Because your own natural testosterone levels are really high right now, as suggested by your acne. Once you take in testosterone from outside, your own natural production shuts off. It can go to zero pretty fast. You'll need a lot of juice just to get you up to where you were to begin with. An older guy, whose levels have gone down over the years, might double his natural levels by taking half of what you'd need just to break even. Studies have shown that testosterone levels of teenaged boys can jump to as high as 2,000 nanograms per deciliter of blood – about two to four times of your typical adult. How can you justify not taking advantage of the highest natural testosterone levels you'll ever have in your life? How can you justify just shutting them down? The kids who start juicing without having built any natural foundation get big fast and then get small again just as fast as soon as the cycle ends, like a yo-yo.

"If you were 200 pounds and 30 years old, I'd agree your potential for further gains after years of training might be pretty much expended. If you wanted to keep improving, I might sympathize with your dilemma. But that's not you. You haven't even scratched the surface of your natural potential. Look at you. If you need steroids to break the 160-pound barrier, take up tennis. You could easily gain twenty pounds without touching anything that might get you busted. I'll bet your training sucks, your diet sucks, and you haven't even begun to pay the necessary dues of hard work. You want fast, dramatic results? At your age, this is probably the only time in your life that you'll be able to get them without juice. Milk it for all it's worth. Revamp your training, start eating right, and stop asking people about steroids at nineteen years old."

Did I get through to him? Yes, at least for now. I gave him an exercise program and a sound nutrition plan. He's now training consistently four days each week with brief but intense workouts and heavy basic movements, hitting each body part once per week. He's also increased his protein intake to one gram for each pound of his body weight, not most days but *every* day. He's cut out the junk food, is consuming healthy fats, and is eating six small meals each day. He's making progress, and he's decided to forego juicing up and instead give his body's own resources a chance to work for him. Contrary to the views of the sports establishment's Ministry of Truth, honesty and sound reasoning can work better than scare tactics and lies.

Contrary to the views of the sports establishment's Ministry of Truth, honesty and sound reasoning can work better than scare tactics and lies.

Perhaps there's hope for more effective approaches to the problem even at the institutional level. ATLAS (Athletes Training and Learning to Avoid Steroids) is a drug prevention program designed for high school male athletes. Initiated in 1993, the curriculum utilizes a "highly scripted" hands-on-approach, with interactive activities and role-playing. A unique feature of the program is the use of an influential coach and peer leaders as facilitators in a team setting. In addition to ten 45-minute classroom sessions, there are three exercise sessions in the weight room. Regrettably, the fact that the National Institute on Drug Abuse funds the program suggests that at least a portion of it may be devoted to the same old scare tactics, which perpetuate the public acceptance of prosecuting mature adult personal users. On the other hand, the more positive aspects of the program involving diet and exercise seem to show promise. The program claims to have reduced the new steroid usage of participants by 50%. More information on the program can be found at www.ohsu.edu/som-hpsm/atlas.html.

Before concluding our look at steroids and teens, let me present my position on teen usage to the mature members of the hardcore muscle world. Obviously, I'm very much against teen juice use, and you should be, too. Someday, you may have a teen son or nephew or even a niece who'll come to you as the wise old musclehead, and ask, "What's Sustanon? Is it bad for me? Have you ever tried it?" Prepare yourself to answer those questions responsibly. If you're questioned about juice from a teen, use honest and credible arguments to *discourage* him or her from using. Many teens ask for advice from the veterans on hardcore discussion boards on the Internet, providing the perfect opportunity for mature board members to talk them out of it.

Anabolic use by teenagers is bad for them, and, quite frankly, bad for everybody. If there is ever going to be a change in public attitudes about non-medical steroid use by mature adults, it will require a Herculean demonstration of *responsibility* on the part of the muscle world. If you sell juice, despite all the cautionary admonitions in this book and against my strong advice, that's your business. If you knowingly sell juice to teenagers, you've screwed *everybody*. You'll be validating all the reasons why non-medical AAS use is criminalized, and you'll be perpetuating the lingering perception that the muscle world is some seedy subculture of immoral outcasts. If the moral guilt trip isn't enough, think about this: federal law and the laws of most states make it an enhanced crime to sell anabolics to young people or to involve minors in their distribution.

If there is ever going to be a change in public attitudes about non-medical steroid use by mature adults, it will require a Herculean demonstration of *responsibility* on the part of the muscle world.

Distributing Anabolics to Minors

Take a look at the federal statutes, such as 21 U.S.C. § 859, which says that distribution of controlled substances to persons under age 21 is punishable by doubled sentencing on a first offense, and triple for a second offense or subsequent offenses. Under 21 U.S.C. § 860, anyone who unlawfully distributes, possesses with intent to distribute, or manufactures a controlled substance in or on, or within one thousand feet of, the real property comprising a school, college, or university, or a playground or public housing authority, or within 100 feet of a youth center, public swimming pool, or video arcade facility, is subject to doubled sentencing on a first offense, and second offenders face the greater of (A) a term of imprisonment of not less than three years and not more than life imprisonment or (B) three times the maximum punishment authorized.

Employing children to distribute drugs near schools or playgrounds is also punishable by tripled sentencing. And under 21 U.S.C. § 861, the employment or use of persons under 18 years of age in drug operations is subject to twice the maximum punishment otherwise authorized for a first offense, and triple for a second offense or subsequent offenses; and the distribution of a controlled substance to any person under eighteen years of age or the use of a person fourteen years of age or younger in drug trafficking is subject to an *additional* term of imprisonment of up to five years. Now that you know, if you're still intentionally selling steroids to young people, don't call me.

Wrap-Up

Now, here's the message to pass on to teens: before you even *think* about anabolic steroids, learn everything you possibly can about training and *apply* it in the gym. Become an authority on muscle-building nutrition, and eat right consistently. Pay your dues in the gym – not for months, but for *years* – while taking advantage of the highest natural testosterone levels you will ever have. When you reach your drug-free genetic potential, you'll be shocked at how far you've come.

Chapter 12

PHYSICIANS FIGHTING FATHER TIME

"Old Age is the harbor of all ills."
– *Bion (c. 325 - c. 255 B.C.)*

Western medicine has busied itself with curing and treating specific diseases and their symptoms. The idea of focusing on enhancing *wellness* has been outside the concerns of the medical community. Doctors have accepted aging as part of nature's plan, which it clearly is. However, nature is not our friend in the long run. Nature's concern is for the survival of our *species*, not for us as individuals. Perpetuation of the species is accomplished by keeping males of breeding age in robust health. Once we've passed that age, however, nature has a rapidly decreasing fondness for us. When our offspring are pretty much self-sufficient and productive, nature becomes a backstabbing ingrate. Men become the guests who just won't leave, hangers-on at the next generation's party. Since we're using up precious resources that could be going to the young and mating, nature prefers to have us out of the way. No longer likely to breed, we are set out on the road of deterioration that leads to the grave. It can often start between age 30 and 45. Our testosterone levels drop. Our sexual desire and functioning diminish. Since we no longer need to be attractive to the opposite sex, our hair goes gray, our skin sags, our muscles shrink, our bones weaken, our teeth rot, our bellies grow. We lose hair on our heads and grow it in our ears and noses. We fall victim to an assortment of chronic and debilitating illnesses in nature's hope that one of them will get rid of us for good. For the benefit of the species, nature wants us to get very sick and die. Not a pretty picture, is it?

For the benefit of the species, nature wants us to get very sick and die.

A Brave New World of Age Management

Maybe I'm being a bit hard on nature, but it's not far off the mark. Traditional Western medicine has done little to intercede in the natural deterioration process, because aging itself is not viewed as a disease. That's beginning to change. Those progressive physicians among you have begun to explore the role of medicine in improving the vitality and longevity of the *healthy* as well as the sick. Not just in extending our life spans, but also in improving the *quality* of our lives by targeting the way we look and feel as we age.

This brave new world of medicine, commonly referred to as *anti-aging medicine,* may really be more accurately called *age management* medicine. While aging is inevitable, using medical strategies to look and feel better during the process is becoming quite popular. The model combines strategies of diet, exercise and nutritional supplementation as its foundation – three areas in which Western physicians have traditionally been less involved. More dramatic reversals of the adverse appearance changes associated with advancing age are still often addressed by cosmetic surgery procedures, such as face-lifts, eyelifts, tummy-tucks and liposuction. But the idea of using a *hormonal* approach to rejuvenating the body is becoming increasingly accepted. Testosterone and human growth hormone have become important tools in the age management arsenal.

An explosion of popular books and magazine articles on the subject of using testosterone to manage the aging process has hit the mainstream. [*See*, A. Hill, *The Testosterone Solution: Increase Your Energy and Vigor With Male Hormone Therapy* (Rockville, CA: Prima Publishing, 1997); E. Shipper & W. Fryer, *The Testosterone Syndrome: The Critical Factor for Energy, Health, & Sexuality – Reversing the Male Menopause* (New York, NY: M. Evans & Co., Inc., 1998); R. Klatz, *Ten Weeks to a Younger You* (Chicago, IL: Sports Tech Labs, Inc., 1999); J. Diamond, *Male Menopause* (2nd Edition, Naperville, IL: Sourcebooks, Inc., 1998); R. Lacayo, "Are You Man Enough," *Time*, April 24, 2000, 58 - 64; A. Sullivan, "The He Hormone," *The New York Times Magazine*, April 2, 2000, 46.] Now, here's the big surprise. "Testosterone replacement therapy" and "hormone replacement therapy" (HRT) are nice little antiseptic, politically correct ways of saying *anabolic steroid therapy*. The testosterone used for hormonal replacement is typically testosterone enanthate or testosterone cypionate – both esters of testosterone that are anabolic steroids and long-time favorites in the muscle world. Are these anabolic steroids making aging men sick? On the contrary, they seem to be making them much, much better. Enthusiasts believe that testosterone and other androgens may be the ultimate antidote for a variety of the symptoms experienced by aging men. By treating age-related *hypogonadism* (low testosterone levels) and certain sexual dysfunctions with anabolic steroids, many of the sexual and physical symptoms can be ameliorated. Testosterone replacement results in an improvement in muscle strength and bone mineral density, as well as enhanced libido and sexual functioning. Middle-aged men across the country are climbing aboard the bandwagon. In 2000, *Time* magazine estimated that four million men were on testosterone replacement therapy, mostly by self-administered injection. The reported results have generally been excellent, with few if any side effects when properly prescribed and monitored.

Enthusiasts believe that testosterone and other androgens may be the ultimate antidote for a variety of the symptoms experienced by aging men.

A growing number of open-minded doctors are successfully prescribing hormones to mature men to combat the symptoms of getting old. Some are in local family practices, some have existing dermatology or plastic surgery practices, and others have created clinics devoted specifically to the practice of anti-aging medicine. Both testosterone and human growth hormone, sometimes in combination, can have rejuvenating effects on men whose own natural levels are in decline. But while human growth hormone is *not* a controlled substance under federal law, testosterone and other anabolic steroids are scheduled.

What are the practical effects of the controlled substance status of steroids to physicians? For many physicians interested in the field of age management medicine, the Anabolic Steroid Control Act and similar restrictive state laws have had a chilling effect. Not only do physicians lose out, but so do patients. Back in 1997, one legal reviewer who examined the Anabolic Steroid Control Act concluded:

> "Many illnesses requiring managed care possibly could be eliminated with hormone treatments. This would not only trigger a social benefit but a financial benefit as well. Congress has created a barrier for the revitalizing effects of steroids for the elderly.

> By simply allowing physicians to use their professional judgment in administering steroid treatments, congressional concerns about steroid abuse would still be addressed without infringing upon the rights of the elderly to receive proper care." [J. Hedges, "The Anabolic Steroids Act: Bad Medicine for the Elderly," 5 *Elder L.J.* 293 (Fall, 1997), 320]

Why are some doctors so afraid of prescribing anabolic steroids? Many are unsure of the proper legal parameters. Others have seen or heard of physicians who were attacked or criticized for administering anabolic steroids. A physician who causes himself to appear on the radar screen of a state medical licensing board can subject himself to intense scrutiny if the authorities suspect that he is prescribing steroids for muscle building, not for the treatment of disease. An aggressive, narrow-minded medical reviewer for the board can tear into the doctor's records, page by page. An investigation can become a witch hunt, and a physician's life can turn into a nightmare. One medical board reviewer, in evaluating the practice of a physician specializing in the administration of androgens to bodybuilders whose endogenous production had been compromised by past steroid use, derided: "this practice is so far out of the realm of usual medical practice ... I asked myself whether there was possibly some new valid usage of these drugs. Looking as thoroughly as possible, by no means could I find any validity to such a practice." The physician had clearly "gone too far" in the opinion of that board reviewer.

Physicians who Prescribe AAS for Bodybuilding

Regardless of the wisdom of the policy in some cases, state and federal law enforcement authorities have prosecuted physicians who cater to *athletes*. In perhaps the most publicized case, Dr. Walter Jekot, a California physician and a pioneer in the use of anabolics in treating the wasting symptoms of AIDS, was sentenced to five years in federal prison for his practice of also prescribing anabolics to bodybuilders. More recently, a state prosecution in the Lackawanna and Luzerne counties of Pennsylvania resulted in the arrest of a physician for administering anabolic steroids to area bodybuilders who did not have a medical condition requiring them.

Even if physicians evade criminal prosecution, the laws authorize state medical licensing boards to take disciplinary action. Medical boards will institute proceedings in cases of unprofessional conduct, such as departing from the standards of acceptable and prevailing medical practice, although boards will generally not revoke licenses solely because of a doctor's practice of a therapy that is experimental, nontraditional, or that departs from acceptable and prevailing medical practices, unless it can be established that the treatment has a safety risk greater than the prevailing treatment or that the treatment is generally not effective.

Some physicians are concerned that the laws as presently written may subject them to sanctions ...

To prescribe and dispense controlled substances, practitioners are required to register with DEA and to maintain complete and accurate records of their prescriptions, generally in a single file separate from other prescriptions. This file must be readily available for law enforcement inspection. Some physicians are concerned that the laws as presently written may subject them to sanctions for the use of anabolic steroids to improve the well-being of mature men. Concededly, anti-aging medicine is impacting upon traditional endocrinology, and the standards of acceptable practice are still developing. There is a lack of consensus as to the normal cutoff level for testosterone beyond which therapy should be initiated, and whether to measure free or total testosterone. In certain cases, the line between legitimate hormonal replacement therapy and illegal dispensation of anabolic steroids may be clouded into a "gray area" – fuzzy, subjective, and open to dispute. Progressive views on the topic may be quite different from those of a conservative state medical licensing board or an ambitious state prosecutor. Cases in which physicians have been targeted appear in the Case Notes section of the Appendix. A physician in Ohio, who had his license revoked for prescribing anabolics to bodybuilders, fared far better than one in Virginia who was convicted of 17 felony counts of distribution plus other charges. A different Ohio physician was unable to use physician-patient confidentiality as a shield from the licensing board. Naturally, some patients seeking treatment for low testosterone levels are also seeking a cosmetic improvement in their muscle-to-fat ratio – something anabolic steroids can do quite effectively. What are the ethical and legal restraints for a physician in prescribing anabolics?

Medical versus Non-medical Use

It's important to understand that while aging is not considered a disease, many of its symptoms are. Physicians may legitimately treat these symptoms of aging *medically* with hormones, including anabolic steroids. The purpose of the treatment must be legitimate. It must also be medical in focus. That's because under federal regulations, anabolic steroids are controlled substances and can only be prescribed or dispensed for a "legitimate medical purpose" in the "usual course" of professional practice. [21 CFR §1306.04(a)] But what's a legitimate medical purpose?

> ... anabolic steroids are controlled substances and can only be prescribed or dispensed for a "legitimate medical purpose" ...

Some guidance in this area is provided by state laws. States can impose various restrictions on dispensing anabolic steroids, and some are more specific than the federal law. In New York, for example, the Code of Rules and Regulations § 80.67(d)(2) requires that practitioners specify on the face of each anabolic steroid prescription the condition being treated, such as "hormone deficiency." Some states have specifically legislated that bodybuilding, athletic improvement and muscle enhancement in healthy patients are not valid medical purposes, and have established criminal penalties to intimidate doctors from getting involved. As an example, look at the Louisiana Revised Statutes, Title 40, Public Health and Safety [La. R.S. § 40:1239]:

> ...C. (1) A physician, dentist, or veterinarian shall not prescribe, dispense, deliver, or administer an anabolic steroid for human use or cause an anabolic steroid to be administered under his direction or supervision for human use except for a valid medical purpose and when required by demonstrable generally accepted medical indications. Bodybuilding, muscle enhancement, or increasing muscle bulk or strength through the use of an anabolic steroid by a person who is in good health is not a valid medical purpose.
>
> (2) Whoever violates the provisions of this Subsection shall be subject to suspension or revocation of his license to practice medicine, dentistry, or veterinary medicine by his governing board.

> (3) Whoever violates the provisions of this Subsection shall also be fined not more than five thousand dollars or imprisoned with or without hard labor for not more than five years, or both.

Or check out Oklahoma [63 Okl. St. § 2-312.1]:

> A. A licensed practitioner ... shall not prescribe, dispense, deliver, or administer an anabolic steroid or human growth hormone or cause an anabolic steroid or human growth hormone to be administered under the direction or supervision of the practitioner except for a valid medical purpose and in the course of a professional practice. A valid medical purpose for the use of anabolic steroids or human growth hormones shall not include bodybuilding, muscle enhancement or increasing muscle bulk or strength of a person who is in good health ...
>
> B. The prescribing, dispensing, delivering or administering of an anabolic steroid by a licensed practitioner in violation of the provisions of subsection A of this section shall be grounds for revocation or nonrenewal of the license of such licensed practitioner to practice in this state. In addition, any licensed practitioner prescribing, dispensing, delivering or administering an anabolic steroid in violation of the provisions of subsection A of this section, upon conviction thereof shall be guilty of a felony punishable by imprisonment in the State Penitentiary for a term of not more than three (3) years, or by a fine not to exceed Ten Thousand Dollars ($10,000.00), or by both such imprisonment.

In Oklahoma, "medical purpose" is further defined in the Uniform Controlled Dangerous Substances Act [63 Okl. St. § 2-101(24)] as "an intention to utilize a controlled dangerous substance for physical or mental treatment, for diagnosis, or for the prevention of a disease condition not in violation of any state or federal law and not for the purpose of satisfying physiological or psychological dependence or other abuse."

Sometimes the restrictions are set forth in administrative rules, rather than laws, as in West Virginia's Code of State Rules on osteopathic practitioners declaring that the "administration of anabolic steroids for other than therapeutic purposes" is unethical practice. [West Virginia Legislative Rule, Board of Osteopathy, Title 24, 24-1-18, § 18.2.6.] Title 11 of the West Virginia Board of Medicine Licensing and Disciplinary Procedures has a similar restriction [11-1A-12, § 12.2(f)].

> ... anabolic steroids are okay to treat the disease symptoms of aging, but not to promote muscle growth in healthy individuals.

So, generally, anabolic steroids are okay to treat the disease symptoms of aging, but not to promote muscle growth in healthy individuals. Whether you agree with it or not, AAS therapy simply to make a healthy person get bigger, stronger or leaner (cosmetic purposes) is a violation of law and a violation of current-day medical ethics. Under today's laws and ethical standards of medicine, any mature healthy adult seeking to obtain anabolics exclusively for muscle building must resort to the black market, with all of the attendant risks.

Defining the Parameters

The parameters of proper androgen replacement therapy in the anti-aging context are not yet well defined. The American Association of Clinical Endocrinologists and the American College of Endocrinology have developed clinical practice guidelines for the evaluation and treatment of hypogonadism and sexual dysfunction in adult male patients. While these applications don't specifically address issues of age management, it is crucial for practitioners to familiarize themselves with these guidelines, which provide instructions and advice on diagnostics, dosages, administration options, side effects and contraindications. They are available online at:

www.aace.com/clin/guidelines/hypogonadism.pdf and
www.aace.com/clin/guidelines/sexdysguid.pdf

Under the hypogonadism guidelines, "Currently, men with symptomatic hypogonadism and clearly low testosterone levels (free or total, in consideration of SHBG [sex hormone binding globulin]) are potential candidates for therapy, although no specific recommendations can be given" (at 446). Many proponents recommend that elderly men with symptoms of hypogonadism and a total testosterone level <300 ng/dl should be started on testosterone replacement. But what about treating adult patients in their 30s, who might be fairly healthy or even athletic, and have only limited symptoms of age-related "disease"? Can such a patient be administered anabolic steroids to enhance his health? The answer would appear to be yes, as long as there's some component of "disease" that's being legitimately treated. The administration of anabolics *can't* be exclusively, or even primarily for the purposes of muscle building.

Many proponents recommend that elderly men with symptoms of hypogonadism and a total testosterone level <300 ng/dl should be started on testosterone replacement.

Some General Practice Guides for Physicians

How does an ethical physician treat his more youthful adult patients with androgens while protecting his license? The following list of issues and concerns was derived from reviews by one state medical licensing board and is by no means all-inclusive. It does provide, however, many of the basic considerations for practitioners interested in the parameters of the brave new world of androgens and age management.

1. Advertising and Marketing

Many physicians today advertise their services. As we've seen, a practitioner who prescribes anabolic steroids for muscle building subjects himself to criminal prosecution. Advertising hormonal treatments to bodybuilders is an invitation for the authorities to investigate. Marketing materials that mention athletes, bodybuilding, ergogenics, or muscle-building will attract attention. Even more subtle terms like "performance enhancement" may send up red flags, as will graphic depictions of muscular athletes. Of course, the higher the profile of the marketing efforts, the more likely someone in a prosecutor's office, law enforcement agency, or state licensing board will see it and become interested in taking a good long look at your patient records. Assuming everything is 100% above board, it's still not worth the hassles.

2. Physical Examination

A comprehensive physical examination is essential to properly diagnose hypogonadism and to rule out contraindications to androgen therapy. Most importantly, the practitioner must carefully examine testicular size and consistency, as well as indications of gynecomastia, abnormal hair growth and distribution, abnormal genitalia and presence of varicocele. The observations must be carefully recorded. Certain online longevity clinics that currently prescribe anabolic steroids on demand, without any physical examination of the patient, clearly violate the principles of ethical medicine.

3. Contraindications and Alternative Diagnoses

Prostate cancer remains an absolute contraindication to androgen therapy. Testing of prostate specific antigen (PSA) values is sound practice. A complete written patient history must be obtained. Failure to ascertain a history of headaches, visual changes, visual field changes, etc., could cause the practitioner to overlook a secondary cause of hypogonadism, such as a pituitary tumor. The patient's age is likely to be taken in as a factor as well, particularly if the physician is treating a large number of somewhat muscular men. A history of previous AAS abuse will also raise a red flag that the patient may be seeking non-medical steroid administration, and that patient's records will be closely scrutinized. Conventional thinking is that all use must be stopped immediately, and that continuation of the drugs by the physician is mere facilitation of the abuse.

Prostate cancer remains an absolute contraindication to androgen therapy.

4. Proper Records

The failure to make and keep detailed patient records can lead to criticism if a medical board reviewer examines the files. Even sloppy handwriting is subject to criticism, as is the failure to properly document an initial diagnosis. Comparisons can be made of the doctor's typed patient summaries to the history provided by each patient, thus ferreting out discrepancies in symptoms and complaints. It's important to note that what may appear to be discrepancies may actually be differences in patient reports. A patient may not document in writing sensitive issues like low libido or sexual dysfunction, but may orally advise the physician about them.

5. Testosterone Level Testing

Unless supported, diagnosing "hypogonadism" or tentatively diagnosing "R/O hypogonadotropic hypogonadism" will draw criticism, as will the failure to record any initial diagnosis. Total serum testosterone level is the best screening test for patients with suspected hypogonadism. If the total testosterone concentration is low, free testosterone

Total serum testosterone level is the best screening test for ... hypogonadism.

levels should be obtained. Even where total testosterone levels are well below the normal range, the practitioner may be criticized for failing to check the "free" or bioavailable testosterone levels. While low total testosterone is consistent with hypogonadism, the absence of symptoms might indicate a normal free testosterone, which is really the active hormone anyway. Obtaining multiple samples at different times of day is also most advisable. The physician's failure to note the time of day the test sample was taken may draw criticism, because slightly low LH and testosterone levels could be due to the fact that both are episodically secreted and the sample may have been drawn at nadir levels.

6. Failure to Respond to Treatment

If the patient does not respond to the anabolic steroid treatment and cannot be restored to normal physiology, other pathologies must be investigated. The possibility of a brain tumor must be seriously considered, and a physician may be criticized for failing to refer the patient to an endocrinologist.

7. Bodybuilding-style Administration

Treating patients the way bodybuilders self-administer anabolics is a great way to draw criticism upon a review of your files. If the physician's course of treatment suggests that he is merely replacing illegal drugs with legal ones, he is open to censure. Administering anabolics in cycles interspersed with HCG, clomiphene and tamoxifen may be derided as "yo-yo" therapy. This repetitive process of suppression and stimulation may be viewed as a telltale sign of the forbidden muscle-promoting purposes. Subject to even more condemnation is the concomitant administration of more than one anabolic steroid. Some medical board reviewers may view this sort of stacking as clear evidence that the physician is facilitating muscle growth rather than treating disease.

8. High-dosage Administration

Prescribing simple "replacement" dosages may be the safest way to avoid disapproval from a medical ethics board, but it may not necessarily be the best treatment for the patient. The patient's response to treatment is individualized. Restoring a patient to the low normal range may not be as therapeutic as bringing him up into the high normal range. Prescribing clearly supraphysiologic dosages, while surprisingly safe based on recent research, would be a red flag to a medical board reviewer that the true purpose of the therapy was for the illegal and unethical purpose of bodybuilding.

Restoring a patient to the low normal range may not be as therapeutic as bringing him up into the high normal range.

The currently accepted way to treat a patient with a history of self-administering anabolics is to help the "addicted patient" withdraw from using them. This is typically accomplished by cessation of all use, and in some cases by the use of HCG to stimulate LH and FSH production to help normalize testosterone levels. In some cases, testosterone replacement therapy may be indicated, but dosages must be to treat the medical problem of hypogonadism, not to facilitate continued cosmetic usage.

One Model for Age Management

An example of a hormone replacement clinic that has designed a sophisticated protocol for the use of AAS in age management is the Cenegenics® Medical Institute, located in Nevada [www.888younger.com]. Cenegenics focuses on middle-aged patients interested in optimizing their hormone levels to feel younger. A substantial percentage of Cenegenics patients are physicians themselves, and the institute does not accept healthy bodybuilders seeking muscle-building applications of anabolics. Before any patient is accepted for treatment, a comprehensive evaluation is conducted to rule out contraindications and to determine the specific hormonal deficiencies to target. Cenegenics uses a variety of hormonal modalities, including human growth hormone and anabolic steroids. When using AAS therapy, the goal of the therapy is to bring the patient into the top one third of the normal range. Alan P. Mintz, M.D., president of Cenegenics, firmly believes that this is the range where maximum therapeutic benefit can be achieved without adverse effects. The focus is on health optimization, not maximum muscle building. However, the side effect of Cenegenics therapies, according to Dr. Mintz, is a significant muscle gain and fat loss in most patients. Pretty good side effect, I'd say.

The Future of Non-Medical, Physician-Prescribed AAS Use

Is there a legitimate argument to allow cosmetic, non-medical AAS use to occur with FDA-approved products under careful medical supervision instead of with contaminated black market veterinary drugs in the bathrooms of gyms? Yes, I believe that there's a *compelling* argument in that regard. Regrettably, the mainstream medical view currently clings to the judgment that *all* non-medical use of anabolics is *abuse*. The assertion that anabolics can be responsibly and ethically administered purely to improve cosmetic physical appearance is considered taboo. Many sports medicine practitioners, conditioned to associate non-medical steroid use with athletic cheating, might find the very suggestion tantamount to heresy. Of course, as long as these archaic views are maintained, cosmetic AAS use will continue to be more risky than it needs to be, and beneficial applications will go unrealized.

Anabolic steroids have a place in medicine, and can greatly enhance the physical well-being of many patients. As the benefits of male hormonal therapies for anti-aging become more widely known, perhaps both the general public and the medical community will reevaluate their negative perception of anabolics. If the elderly who are suffering from the ravages of aging are taking steroids and feeling and looking better without physical harm, haven't we judged these hormones too harshly? Perhaps the age management applications will pave the way for consideration of broader non-medical uses. If that occurs, maybe the pharmaceutical industry will begin to step back into the market that it had largely abandoned back in the 1980s. The success of Viagra® proves that there's a massive market of

If the elderly who are suffering from the ravages of aging are taking steroids and feeling and looking better without physical harm, haven't we judged these hormones too harshly?

American men seeking reinvigorating drugs. Anabolic steroids would seem to offer far more than erection-only drugs. The time may well be ripe for the pharmaceutical companies to escalate their research efforts in this area, and to gear up for a re-education campaign targeting not only the general public, but also the mainstream medical community.

Chapter 13

SOLDIERS ON STEROIDS

"He stood, a soldier, to the last right end,
A perfect patriot and a noble friend."
– *Ben Jonson, British dramatist, poet (1572-1637)*

While the prevalence of AAS use in the armed services is unknown, what is clear is that the punishments may exceed those that a defendant might receive under civilian law. It's important to recognize that people in the armed services, particularly those living in the communal environment of a military base, have lesser privacy interests than those in civilian society. The law has recognized the military's need to maintain good order and discipline through its own unique justice system.

The military has several systems to deal with steroid offenses; some are administrative and some are judicial. A steroid charge, even for minor personal use, can result in a court-martial proceeding, or being discharged from the military with a less than honorable discharge, or losing a hard-earned retirement.

Military personnel (servicemembers) may be tried in state court and still be tried by the military. Double jeopardy does not prevent a state prosecution and a federal prosecution for the same offense because they are two different sovereigns. However, since military courts are federal, one could not be prosecuted in civilian federal district court and also in a court-martial for the same offense.

Nonetheless, if a servicemember were prosecuted in either civilian federal or state court, the military could initiate administrative separation or discharge proceedings and the individual's military service could be terminated. These administrative proceedings may be described as the military's way of firing employees. Each branch of the service has extensive regulations governing how these proceedings are to be conducted. Depending on various factors, such as the length of service and the type of discharge the military wants to give the servicemember, there are varying degrees of due process afforded, such as the right to an adversarial hearing before a board (similar to a jury in civilian courts).

Drug Charges in the Military

Title 10 of the United States Code deals with the armed forces. Under Subtitle A, Part II, is Chapter 47, the Uniform Code of Military Justice. The possession, use, and distribution of anabolics are governed by Article 112a of the UCMJ. Article 81 deals with conspiracy. While violations of these articles subject one to a possible court-martial, they also potentially subject one to the administrative discharge procedures discussed above. Article 112a reads in part as follows:

§912a. Art. 112a. Wrongful use, possession, etc., of controlled substances

(a) Any person subject to this chapter who wrongfully uses, possesses, manufactures, distributes, imports into the customs territory of the United States, exports from the

United States, or introduces into an installation, vessel, vehicle, or aircraft used by or under the control of the armed forces a substance described in subsection (b) shall be punished as a court-martial may direct.

(b) The substances referred to in subsection (a) are the following:
  (2) Any substance ... that is listed on a schedule of controlled substances prescribed by the President for the purposes of this article.
  (3) Any other substance ... that is listed in schedules I through V of section 202 of the Controlled Substances Act (21 U.S.C. 812).

It is typical for a servicemember charged with certain anabolic steroid crimes to be additionally charged with conspiracy under 10 USCS § 881:

§ 881. Art. 81. Conspiracy
Any person subject to this chapter who conspires with any other person to commit an offense under this chapter shall, if one or more of the conspirators does an act to effect the object of the conspiracy, be punished as a court-martial may direct.

Punishment Options

How a case involving the possession or use of anabolics is handled varies from base to base. A decision will be made by the Staff Judge Advocate and the unit commander to determine how to proceed. On some bases, virtually every case is referred for court-martial proceedings. On other bases, depending on the unit commander and strengths or weaknesses of the case, the servicemember may face an administrative discharge, which may be: a) a discharge that is other than honorable; b) a general discharge, which is under honorable conditions; or, c) an honorable discharge. On yet others, the service-member may be offered to accept a non-judicial punishment pursuant to Article 15 of the Code of Military Justice, permitting resolution of the case without formal court-martial proceedings. Article 15 affords the possibility of being retained rather than discharged from the service. There is no authority to discharge the servicemember directly as a punishment at the Article 15 proceeding; however, a guilty finding may result in the military initiating the administrative separation process. At the very least, the servicemember may be compelled to attend drug abuse counseling.

A decision will be made by the Staff Judge Advocate and the unit commander to determine how to proceed.

The procedure undertaken by the unit commander may be based upon any number of factors including the history of the servicemember, the severity of the offense, and the way in which it was discovered. A serviceman with a poor history who was overheard admitting his drug use to others will likely be treated more harshly.

Expectations of Privacy (Getting Busted)

It's important to discuss expectations of privacy for servicemembers. Servicemembers' medical records are property of the U.S. military, and as such, there is no expectation of privacy and/or doctor/patient confidentiality. According to Military Rule of Evidence 513, there is a patient/psychotherapist relationship; however, there is no such privilege to the servicemember who is treated by a medical doctor. As you may be aware, civilians have a confidential relationship with their physicians which provides that the physical condition, records, notes, history, X-rays, nurses' notes, emergency room records, ambulance call reports, and all statements made in the furtherance of treatment are confidential. As such, a civilian medical doctor shall not discuss or disclose the patient's prior illegal steroid use unless the patient has waived the privilege. This privilege does *not* exist for those in military service. In fact, according to the U.S. Navy regulations, the medical doctor would actually have *an obligation to report* this violation (although I haven't heard about this happening in practice).

Servicemembers should also be aware that, depending upon their unit commander, they can be *drug tested* at any time. In fact, the unit commander may invoke a policy that all servicemembers are to be tested when they return from leave. The point is that it's all within the commander's discretion.

What about expectations of privacy within the barracks? Even though there is an expectation of privacy within the barracks, they may be searched. If the unit commander has a policy of inspecting the barracks for the "health and welfare" of the servicemembers, a search may be conducted. But this must be according to a policy, although it need not be written, and the military has the burden of proving by a standard of *clear and convincing* evidence that the search was for health and welfare purposes. If the military does not meet that burden of proof, any evidence found during that search may be inadmissible at a court-martial. However, the evidence shall still be admissible at an administrative proceeding. Additionally, if probable cause is established (see Chapter 7), the unit commander may sign a "search authorization" permitting a search to be performed. It is important to note that there is no judge involved in this process. The unit commander will most likely consult with his/her attorney in this decision — the staff judge advocate — but the commander has both the authority and the power to sign the search authorization.

If the unit commander has a policy of inspecting the barracks for the "health and welfare" of the servicemembers, a search may be conducted.

Upgrade of Discharge

If a servicemember receives less than an honorable discharge, it can have consequences throughout his or her future civilian employment career. The servicemember may seek an upgrade of the discharge by applying to the Discharge Review Board within a 15-year statute of limitations from the date of the discharge. If the servicemember loses at this board and is within the Department of the Navy (Navy and Marine Corps), he/she may proceed to the Board for Correction of Naval Record (BCNR). He/She can make an application to the BCNR within a three-year statute of limitations from the date of discharge. If not made within the three-year statute of limitations, the applicant must then apply and show good cause as to why it was not made within that time frame.

Each branch of the service has its own board; within the Army it is the Army Board for Correction of Military Records. A starting point for those interested in seeking a discharge upgrade would be to visit the web site at *www.VA.gov.*

Case Examples: Personal Use

The military juice cases with which I have been involved demonstrate that the armed forces aren't looking the other way when it comes to steroids, even in situations of simple personal use. Take the tale of Arnie, 45 years old, with 24 years of dedicated service to the U.S. Air Force and an unblemished career. For the first time in his life, he made the terrible mistake of ordering ten vials of Deca from the Philippines. When U.S. Customs snagged it and sent him a seizure letter, he e-mailed the source requesting a refund. Instead, as is often the case, the source sent a replacement package. When Arnie went to his base P.O. Box to collect his mail, he was busted walking out by a squadron of agents from Customs, DEA, Postal Inspection Services, and the Office of Special Investigations (OSI). They threw him to the ground, handcuffed him, tossed him in their car and took him to the base security office. They interrogated him for three hours, keeping him handcuffed throughout. He was repeatedly told he was not under arrest while also being told that he had to make a confession and submit to a urine test before being allowed to leave. He was suspended and faces an uncertain future.

... the armed forces aren't looking the other way when it comes to steroids, even in situations of simple personal use.

Or take the case of Tom, a sergeant in the Air Force, late 30's, with a 19-year exemplary career as a troubleshooter for Air Force computer hardware and software equipment. Customs agents in San Francisco found a small envelope from Thailand containing 318 tablets of methandrostenolone addressed to one "Peter Harmon." The DEA was contacted, an investigation was conducted into who lived at the address, and Tom was identified. Air Force administrators were notified, and about two weeks later a California State Superior Court judge signed a warrant to search Tom's residence and car. The warrant specifically stated that the search could only be initiated if either "Peter Harmon" or Tom accepted delivery.

The envelope was prepared with fluorescent powder for use in a controlled delivery, which was conducted the next day. A Postal Inspector disguised as a letter carrier delivered the envelope. When Tom answered the door, the inspector asked if Peter Harmon lived there. The exact conversation is in dispute, with the feds claiming that Tom falsely identified himself as Peter Harmon (who was actually a former occupant of the address). In any event, Tom accepted the delivery. Two minutes later, a total of ten agents burst through the door to execute the warrant and conduct the raid. Prior to their dramatic entrance, Tom had written, "Does not live here, wrong address" on the package. He was nonetheless handcuffed and given his *Miranda* warnings, which he invoked. The agents ransacked the house, top to bottom, and searched his cars and even his garbage. Not much was found, except a handful of vials and some additional pink tablets. These were seized, along with his computer, about twenty syringes and "body building supplements in powder and pill form." Now here's where military procedure differs from the typical civilian arrest for juice.

The standard practice of military investigators in a steroid delivery case is to obtain an Authority to Search and Seize, permitting them to seize a urine sample from the suspect. In the Air Force, that's an AF Form 1176. Tom gave some urine, and the sample went to the UCLA Olympic analytical lab. It came back nearly two and a half months later, positive for methandienone (methandrostenolone) metabolites, 19-Norandrosterone and 19-Norethiocholanolone.

Tom was charged with violating Article 112a of the Uniform Code of Military Justice for his use of methandienone. He was offered to dispose of the case with a non-judicial punishment pursuant to Article 15. This permitted resolving the case without formal court-martial proceedings. He accepted the deal, and the issue was then whether or not he would meet the criteria to allow him to be retained in the Air Force. The "Retention Criteria and Consideration" are outlined in AFI 36-3208, *Administrative Separation of Airmen*, paragraph 5.55.2.1:

5.55.2.1. A member found to have abused drugs will be discharged unless the member meets all seven of the following criteria:

1. Drug abuse is a departure from the member's usual and customary behavior.
2. Drug abuse occurred as a result of drug experimentation (a drug experimentor is defined as one who has illegally or improperly used a drug for reasons of curiosity, peer pressure, or other similar reasons).
3. Drug abuse does not involve recurring incidents, other than drug experimentation as defined above.
4. The member does not desire to engage in or intend to engage in drug abuse in the future.
5. Drug abuse under all the circumstances is not likely to recur.
6. Under the particular circumstances of the case, the member's continued presence in the Air Force is consistent with the interest of the Air Force in maintaining proper discipline, good order, leadership, and morale.
7. Drug abuse did not involve drug distribution. For the purposes of this paragraph, drug distribution means the delivery to the possession of another. Distribution does not occur with the transfer of the drugs from one person to another while such persons are engaged in the mutual use of drugs, except that individuals who obtain, or arrange for obtaining, the drugs used by others are involved in distribution. Delivery means the actual, constructive, or attempted transfer of the drugs, whether or not there exists an agency relationship.

Tom's work performance reports were exemplary and his letters of character were stellar. He was called "a pillar of strength" in one letter. Another read, "To watch [Tom] assume command is exciting. Leadership is one of [Tom's] strongest qualities. If you're wrong, he's going to tell you that you were wrong, and if you're right he'll defend you to the end. Either way, he'll stand behind you through it all. You can feel the admiration his troops have for him." His civic and charitable involvements were numerous, including volunteer work for a battered women's shelter and the local humane society. Tom met all the criteria for a waiver of administrative discharge except, arguably, one. At issue in his case was whether his possession of multiple units of anabolic steroids (enough for one steroid cycle) could be construed as *recurring incidents* of abuse. The continuation of Tom's distinguished career hung on the determination of that issue.

My involvement in the case was to present the proposition that an anabolic steroid cycle was a "one-time" experiment, not a series of recurring incidents of abuse. Individuals who experiment with anabolics are involved in an entirely different process than those who experiment with crack or heroin. Realistically, experimenting requires *experiencing* the effects. Anyone curious enough about the effects of crack or heroin could experiment with the substance by consuming some of it at a single sitting and then experiencing the effects shortly thereafter. This isn't possible with anabolic steroids. Anabolics have no immediate effect. They're not hallucinogenic, stimulating or tranquilizing. Experiencing their effects takes several weeks to a few months. Experimenting with anabolics by taking one tablet would be like trying out a new birth control method by taking one pill. One-time experimentation with steroids is most fairly construed as a continuous process that lasts from the *inception* to the *conclusion* of a cycle. It should also be noted that because of the difference in the timeliness of effects, those experimenting with hard drugs typically purchase and possess the amount that can be consumed in a sitting, while those experimenting with anabolics purchase and possess the amount needed for the *whole anticipated cycle*. Tom was lucky. My arguments were accepted as logical and convincing (and properly so), and he was permitted to continue his dedicated service to our country. Still, I was troubled by Tom's case. How misguided is our military that they would be more inclined to retain someone who smoked crack or shot up heroin, even once, as opposed to a dedicated American like Tom?

One-time experimentation with steroids is most fairly construed as a continuous process that lasts from the *inception* to the *conclusion* of a cycle.

Not every case works out as well as Tom's. The following case note describes a case I had no involvement with. It was decided by the United States Air Force Court of Criminal Appeals:

United States v. Diamond
ACM 33605, 1999 CCA LEXIS 227 (A.F.C.C.A. Aug. 12, 1999)

> Senior Airman J. Diamond was convicted of conspiracy to import steroids, making a false official statement, and wrongful use, possession and importation of anabolic steroids under Articles 81, 107, 112a of the Uniform Code of Military Justice, 10 USC §§ 907, 912a. His sentence resulted in a bad-conduct discharge, 95 days confinement, and a reduction to the class of E-1.
>
> Diamond's case is noteworthy because he believed that the prosecutor's emphasis on his duty status with security forces substantially prejudiced him and aggravated his sentence. In particular, Diamond argued that his punishment was more severe than one that would be given to an ordinary civilian because of the prosecution's argument that law enforcement officers must set an example and uphold the laws and regulations they promulgate. The introduction of the fact that Diamond graduated second in his class from the Utah Police Academy in 1996 and was chosen as a full-time officer on the Clearfield Police Department was only meant to heighten his punishment.
>
> The Court disagreed with Diamond, affirming his conviction, and held that he would have received the same sentence irrespective of the statements regarding his occupation.

Arrests for the personal use of steroids are not limited to the Air Force. I've received calls from members of several branches of the military, most recently from Jeff, a Navy serviceman on the East Coast, who was returning to base when his car was searched, revealing needles. He was arrested and immediately tested for anabolic steroids. The case is pending.

Case Examples: Distribution

So far, we've talked about personal juice use. Distribution situations are looked at with extreme prejudice by the armed services. Servicemen caught trafficking in anabolics can be subjected to punishments far in excess of those permitted under the federal sentencing guidelines. A case in point is the story of a soldier we'll call Sergeant Timothy Davidson, whose case was referred to me on appeal after his conviction at trial. Davidson was an Army Ranger and Desert Storm veteran with an exemplary career for nearly 20 years. A devoted powerlifter, Davidson's personal use of anabolics, friendship with a lifting buddy named Mickey Rizzo, honesty with military investigators, and bad legal advice led to disastrous consequences.

Rizzo was a civilian competitive bodybuilder who dealt gear on the side. Local police knew about it and arranged for a confidential informer to purchase $3,000 worth of steroids from him (allegedly 8 bottles of testosterone propionate and 11 bottles of nandrolone decanoate). The deal went down in a parking lot of a doughnut shop. The snitch was wired to record the transaction. When he gave the prearranged signal, the words "This is enough to get massive on," the police knew the transaction was complete and busted Rizzo. Another 5 bottles of Deca were found in Rizzo's car.

Rizzo quickly caved in and agreed to rat on his friend Davidson. Rizzo spilled his guts about how he and Davidson would get their juice supply by sending money orders to a friendly Mexican veterinarian, who in turn would send the steroids across the border via taxi (supposedly the taxi driver would wait until one of his friends was on duty before attempting to cross). An unidentified person would meet the taxi driver, box the steroids up, and send them to Rizzo or Davidson via ground mail.

Rizzo claimed that on one occasion, at Davidson's request, he went to Mexico himself to bring back a supply. The veterinarian wrapped the bottles of steroids in plastic bags and had them taped to the inside of the trunk of a taxi. After leaving the clinic, the driver dropped off Rizzo a block from the border so that he could walk across. The taxi then met him on the other side, took him to get packaging materials, then to FedEx to mail the box, and then to the airport to return home. Rizzo made himself sound like a lackey for Sgt. Davidson, although the truth may well have been quite the reverse. The Record of Trial suggests that Rizzo would say anything to lessen his own sentence.

Rizzo made himself sound like a lackey for Sgt. Davidson, although the truth may well have been the reverse. The Record of Trial suggests that Rizzo would say anything to lessen his own sentence.

Davidson committed the damning error of making admissions to investigators. Then on the advice of his military lawyer, he entered a guilty plea to some of the charges and went to trial on others. Rizzo testified against his former friend, making all manner of outrageous and unsupported claims. Regrettably, military defense counsel "played possum" and conducted no cross-examination whatsoever.

The prosecution's so-called experts, one of whom was completely unqualified, plied the jury with hyperbolic and misleading comments without defense objection or rebuttal. Both the testimony of the prosecution witness and the statements of the prosecutor herself on summation hammered away at the point that steroids cause liver tumors – remarks that inflamed, frightened, and prejudiced the jurors. Such statements were *wholly misleading* because the allegations against Davidson *exclusively* involved testosterone esters and other injectable steroids that have virtually *no* liver toxicity. [See Chapter 3] These sorts of comments should never have been permitted, and demonstrate the dangers presented by uninformed defense counsel.

Davidson was convicted of conspiring to import and distribute Mexican steroids to other bodybuilders and sentenced to a term of imprisonment of *six years*. How would he have fared in civilian court under the quantity calculations of the federal sentencing guidelines? There was ample testimony from which to make the calculations. According to the testimony, he imported about $38,000 worth of steroids over the course of five years. Based upon the Mexican pharmacy prices alleged in the Record of Trial, his cost averaged about $2 or $3 per cc of juice. This computes to roughly between 13,000 and 19,000 cc's – or 1,300 to 1,900 federal dosage units. The drug quantity table places this amount at *Level 10* (out of 43 total) in the guidelines, even after the application of guideline adjustments based on the specific facts of the case. In a non-military federal court, Davidson would have faced a guideline imprisonment sentence of *six to twelve months* and would have been eligible for a sentence of only *probation* with some initial home confinement. Even somebody with a *horrible* criminal history would have faced a guideline imprisonment sentence in civilian court of only between *two years* and *two and a half years.* His appeal is pending.

Davidson is not alone in his draconian treatment by the military courts. Here's a case I found from the United States Navy-Marine Corps Court of Criminal Appeals:

United States v. Miller
01047, 1998 CCA LEXIS 433 (N-M.C.C.A. Oct. 6, 1998)

R. Miller, an E-1 Private of the Marine Corps, was convicted of conspiracy to import anabolic steroids into the United States, importing anabolic steroids into the United States, possessing anabolic steroids with the intent to distribute them, and distributing anabolic steroids, in violation of Articles 81 and 112a of the Uniform Code of Military Justice. His sentence included confinement for five years, total forfeiture of pay and allowances, and a dishonorable discharge.

Despite an argument by Miller that his sentence was too severe because he was not the principal player in the importation of steroids into the United States, the Court held that Miller's conspiracy with others to import a large quantity of illegal drugs (in excess of $15,000), his service as a financial conduit between the purchaser and the supplier, his accompanying the supplier to Mexico, and his personal delivery of 100 tablets of a Russian anabolic steroid to a former Marine unquestionably warranted a dishonorable discharge. It is important to recognize that the Court treated the nature and severity of Miller's offenses as strictly as it would a principal importer, in order to prove that even a minor role in the distribution, use, and possession of anabolic steroids can have the harshest of consequences.

Want more? Here are a few other military cases to check out:

U.S. Court of Appeals for the Armed Forces
United States v. Hall
No. 01-0418, 2002 WL 832773 (C.A.A.F. May 2, 2002).

Airman J. Hall, a weight lifter, offered to connect his dorm mate, an Air Force Security Policeman, with a source to obtain steroids. The dorm mate reported the unsolicited offer to an agent of the Office of Special Investigations (OSI), which arranged for a controlled buy. The transaction took place off base, where the dorm mate purchased the steroids with $120 in prerecorded money. As the dorm mate and Hall approached the base, the dorm mate signaled the OSI agents. OSI surrounded the vehicle, ordered both men out, and handcuffed them.

Hall was convicted by the general court-martial of two specifications of assault, failure to obey an order, and wrongful distribution of a controlled substance in violation of Article 112a, UCMJ, 10 USC § 912a. The United States Air Force Court of Criminal Appeals affirmed, and the United States Court of Appeals for the Armed Forces affirmed, holding that the military judge's error in excluding testimony in support of the defense of entrapment was harmless in the court-martial of an accused charged with wrongful distribution of steroids, where the accused's own testimony established his predisposition to facilitate the transfer of steroids, and testimony was corroborated by the accomplice's testimony and uncontested portions of the undercover agent's testimony.

Hall was sentenced to 12 months imprisonment and a reduction to the lowest enlisted grade.

United States v. Horton
ACM 34128, 2002 CCA LEXIS 183 (A.F.C.C.A. Jun. 25, 2001).

Senior Airman J. Horton was originally convicted by general court-martial of wrongfully using and distributing anabolic steroids, wrongfully using 3,4 methylenedioxymethamphetamine (ecstasy), and wrongfully using cocaine. Horton was sentenced to a bad-conduct discharge, confinement for 30 days, and reduction to E-1. However, prior to authentication of the Record of Trial, the physical evidence relating to his use of cocaine had been tested and shown to be lidocaine, which is not a controlled substance under Article 112a of the Uniform Code of Military Justice.

Upon a rehearing, despite the removal of the cocaine charge, the convening authority refused to reduce the original sentence. Horton's anabolic steroid charge was deemed so severe that even the removal of his cocaine charge did not affect his sentence. On appeal, Horton unsuccessfully argued that the ecstasy charge should be dropped because the record showed no evidence that the tablets he ingested were ecstasy. The court rejected Horton's argument and affirmed, because there was nothing in the record inconsistent with the guilty plea that Horton knowingly and consciously ingested ecstasy. By pleading guilty and admitting to the use of ecstasy, Horton waived a trial of the facts.

United States Navy – Marine Corps Court of Criminal Appeals
United States v. Mount
NMCM 98 01202, 1999 CCA LEXIS 243 (N-M.C.C.A. Aug. 19, 1999).

E-2 Hospitalman Apprentice M. Mount was convicted of conspiring to import anabolic steroids, conspiring to introduce marijuana, the wrongful importation and introduction of marijuana, and the wrongful importation, possession, and distribution of the anabolic steroid Sustanon in violation of the Uniform Code of Military Justice, Articles 81 and 112a. Mount was subsequently sentenced to confinement for three months and granted a bad-conduct discharge.

On appeal, Mount argued that a military accused couldn't be convicted solely on the uncorroborated testimony of an accomplice if that testimony is self-contradictory, uncertain, improbable or implausible. The Court rejected this argument, holding that the accomplice's testimony was neither self-contradictory nor implausible in light of Mount's confession. Mount's second major argument was that his sentence was inappropriately severe in comparison to the sentence of his accomplice, who did not receive a punitive discharge. The Court responded that a court-martial is free to impose any legal sentence that it determines appropriate. The general rule is that the appropriateness of an accused's sentence is to be determined without reference or comparison to other cases. Only in very narrow circumstances has sentence comparison been recognized. Even if the cases being compared meet the closely related threshold requirement and the sentences in the two cases are highly disparate, the sentence will still stand if there is a good and cogent reason for the disparity. In Mount's case, his sentence was not highly disparate from that of his accomplice, but even if it was, Mount's guilty plea and acknowledgment of responsibility for his offenses satisfied the good and cogent reason test.

United States v. Harrington
NMCM 99 00517, 1999 WL 450683 (N-M.C.C.A. Jun. 23, 1999).

The case of P. Harrington, an E-5 Sergeant of the U.S. Marine Corps with 11 exemplary years of service and an unblemished disciplinary record, demonstrates that an experienced and well-respected noncommissioned officer of the Marines will not receive a more lenient sentence, but rather the harshest of penalties. Harrington was convicted of wrongfully attempting to distribute anabolic steroids and three specifications of wrongfully distributing steroids in violation of Articles 80 and 112a of the Uniform Code of Military Justice. He was sentenced to a bad-conduct discharge and one year confinement for his actions.

Harrington attempted to distribute a significant quantity of anabolic steroids to a person who turned out to be an agent of the Naval Criminal Investigative Service (NCIS). After arrangements were made for delivery of the substances from Harrington's on-base quarters, those quarters were searched by NCIS agents and the steroids were recovered. This case clearly illustrates the idea that an individual in a position of power and influence, who knowingly distributes illegal drugs, must be punished more severely than an ordinary civilian because he tarnishes the order and discipline necessary in the military forces.

Last Words

In closing, it's important to understand that nothing good will come from getting caught using anabolic steroids in the military. If you get caught, even for simple personal use, take it extremely seriously, because the military will. Even if you're lucky enough to avoid a court-martial proceeding and not do a single day in custody, your career in the military is likely to be ruined and as discussed above, this can have far-reaching consequences for future civilian employment. You may be dishonorably discharged and lose your retirement and benefits. Even if you're successful at avoiding discharge, the Article 15 will remain on your record to haunt you for the rest of your career. According to Terri R.Z. Jacobs, Esq., an active judge advocate in the Marine Corps Reserve who practices military law in private practice: "The military justice system, including the various administrative procedures available to commands to deal with suspected steroid use, can be complicated. If a servicemember becomes involved with any of the judicial or administrative proceedings that could result in loss of a military career, I highly recommend consultation with a current or former judge advocate who has substantial experience in navigating these waters." Good advice, don't you think?

Chapter 14

AAS Numbers for the Criminal Justice Community

"There are three kinds of lies: lies, damned lies and statistics."
– *Mark Twain (1835–1910)*

So, you're a member of the criminal justice community and you've got your first AAS case. Maybe you're a defense lawyer, or maybe you're a police officer, federal agent, prosecutor, or judge. You're likely to be confronted with issues of steroid *numbers*, such as the calculation of dosage units, the street costs of particular anabolics, or the quantities of anabolic steroids that users could personally consume. Fair enough, I can help you in this chapter. Like statistics, the AAS numbers I've seen used in courts aren't always very accurate.

Threshold Legal Issues

Most criminal defense lawyers and prosecutors will be fully familiar with the common factual and legal issues in car stops, border searches, and confidential informant cases. Many lawyers are less familiar with cases that originate from Internet transactions or arise out of domestic or international mail seizures. There are chapters in this book devoted to these issues, including the Fourth Amendment implications.

There are a variety of threshold legal issues when approaching an AAS case, and both prosecutors and defense lawyers need to be aware of them. Under what laws will the matter be prosecuted? If it's a state case, refer to the Appendix if you are unsure as to the statutes and general plea disposition policies in your state. Obviously, practices and policies can vary at the county or local levels. If it's a federal case, check out Chapter 4 to get a full understanding of the statutes, regulations and sentencing guidelines that apply in anabolic steroid cases. Lawyers on both sides must be prepared to determine the quantities that might be attributed to the accused, including all relevant conduct under the USSG. These quantities must be applied to the Drug Quantity Table to assess the potential sentencing range that the individual is facing. Remember that regarding "units," in the case of anabolic steroids, one "unit" means a 10 cc vial of an injectable steroid or fifty (50) oral tablets. All vials of injectable steroids are to be converted on the basis of their volume to the equivalent number of 10 cc vials (e.g., one 50 cc vial is to be counted as five 10 cc vials).

One of the biggest barriers to the just resolution of AAS cases is misinformation. Years of misleading press statements and poorly researched reports about anabolic steroid side effects have distorted these hormones in the general public perception and tainted the attitudes of those in the criminal justice system. The defendant in any steroid prosecution is likely to be viewed through this distorted lens. Based upon what they have heard or read, many lawyers, prosecutors and judges see no reason to distinguish the relative dangers of "hard drugs" like cocaine and heroin from the inherent risks of hormones like anabolic steroids. Indeed, media reports of violent 'roid rage tales have provoked some jurists to view anabolic steroids as an even greater social menace than narcotics. This mindset can result in harsher treatment in both possession and distribution cases than would be imposed by a more enlightened criminal justice system. There's extensive information contained in this book designed to foster a more accurate and objective assessment of AAS defendants, particularly those charged with personal use possession.

Most AAS users are wary of those in the legal system, and with good reason. They see themselves as being unfairly painted with the same broad brush as heroin junkies and cokeheads. But unlike those addicts, most muscle builders see their steroid usage not as an impediment to their productive aspirations, but as a tool for achieving them. The well-meaning defense lawyer who starts out by making judgmental statements, referring to the charges as a "narcotics case," or by insisting on drug treatment before even inquiring about the client's use patterns is risking being seen as the enemy. I've spoken to AAS defendants who didn't hire a lawyer because the lawyer started out in one of those fashions. Some steroid clients do indeed need drug counseling or psychotherapy, but it's not necessarily a given and it's a bad way for a defense attorney to start the initial consultation. Further, many physique enthusiasts who use anabolics are astonishingly well informed about the health hazards associated with AAS use. While a lawyer can pontificate to a coke or heroin user about how those drugs can ruin his health, the extent of the risk isn't so clear with steroid use. It's impossible for a lawyer to effectively lecture a client when the client knows much more than the lawyer does. A lawyer shouldn't pretend to be knowledgeable when he's clueless. Reading Chapter 3 regarding the real health risks of anabolics can be tremendously helpful.

Identification of Controlled Substances

A threshold issue for law enforcement agents who confront a possible AAS case is the proper identification of which items are controlled substances and which are not. While the inability of many law enforcement agents to identify anabolic steroids has resulted in some offenders averting an arrest, the *misidentification* of *non*-controlled substances as anabolic steroids has resulted in the erroneous arrest of individuals. Most AAS users self-administer not only controlled substances, but also a variety of non-controlled substances (see Chapter 2). I have seen cases where the police have seized ancillary non-controlled medications like insulin, Arimidex® (anastrozole), Nolvadex® (tamoxifen citrate), or Clomid® (clomiphene citrate) under the mistaken belief that the substances were controlled. Drugs like clenbuterol and human growth hormone (hGH), for example, are mildly anabolic but neither is an anabolic steroid nor a controlled substance under federal law. At the state level, human chorionic gonadotropin (HCG) and growth hormone are controlled in some jurisdictions, but not in others. As long as police officers are uncertain as to which anabolic or ancillary substances are controlled and which are not, the potential for the arrest of innocent individuals continues. The problem can be quite significant for the officer in the field. The glossary contained in the Appendix to this book should prove helpful in many cases.

When a case is brought to court, it's incumbent on both the prosecutor and the defense lawyer to quickly ascertain whether the substances seized are in fact controlled substances, particularly in a situation where bail is set and cannot be posted. Sometimes, it's a mixed bag: some substances are anabolic steroids, while others are ancillary medications or even currently over-the-counter products such as prohormones or herbal preparations. Failure to promptly sort the controlled substances from the non-controlled substances may result in a significant mistake as to the total quantity of steroids. I've seen many instances where inappropriately high bail amounts were imposed because of errors in this regard. For example, what if 500 tablets were recovered in an AAS arrest, but 300 are really tribulus terrestris (a legal, over-the-counter bodybuilding herb), 150 are tamoxifen, and only 50 tablets are anabolic steroids? You get the picture. The actual amount of AAS's can impact upon substantive issues as well, such as whether the accused intended to distribute the steroids. It can also affect sentences that are quantity-based (such as in federal court). Defense counsel must be prepared to carefully review the accusatory instruments and all police documents (and conduct his own research) regarding the identity of the substances recovered to avoid improper charging or overcharging.

Quantity and the Intent to Distribute

In many state courts, the difference between simple possession of drugs and possession with intent to sell or distribute drugs is tremendous. Traffickers are viewed as deserving of substantially heftier punishment than personal users. In cases where there is no direct evidence of AAS sales, the intent to traffic can be inferred from the circumstances. The possession of a particularly large quantity of drugs has traditionally been a basis upon which to infer or presume that the possessor was a dealer rather than a personal user. The crucial issue is whether or not the quantity is inconsistent with a personal use amount. It's common to see a steroid offender prosecuted as a *dealer* based *merely* on the quantity recovered from a search of his home or car, and without any other evidence of distribution. In the past six months, for example, I've seen two car stop cases in New York where possessors of Thai Anabol, in the amounts of 207 tablets and 280 tablets, were charged with possession with intent to sell without any other evidence of such intent. In one of the many cases generated by the Maryland State Police, Tim was charged with possession with intent to distribute steroids when his mother accepted a controlled delivery package containing 100 Anadrol tabs, two bottles of testosterone cypionate, three bottles of nandrolone and two bottles of Winstrol. The house search recovered an additional 300 D-bol, 100 Winstrol tabs, a bottle of Finaplix and twenty syringes. This is an extremely typical example of a situation where the variety of substances combined with the total quantity was viewed by law enforcement as inconsistent with personal use.

However, such an inference is not always warranted. Mistakes occur because of the extensive experience state and local law enforcement authorities have with "street drugs" cases, where possession of even fifteen or twenty individually packaged units of product (such as cocaine or heroin) implies an intent to sell. The implication is based on the fact that narcotics users tend to purchase and possess only enough for an immediate "high." However, many AAS users purchase their drugs with significant and often meticulous advance planning. Uncertain about future supply availabilities, most AAS users will purchase a sufficient quantity of steroids and ancillary medications to prevent running out of anabolics in the middle of a cycle. AAS users who purchase their steroids by mail order tend to do so in volume, both because of price discounts and because of an interest in limiting the risk of package seizures by making less frequent orders. Some AAS "pack rats" will stockpile enough anabolics to complete a series of cycles each lasting many weeks or months. Since steroid cycles typically involve the stacking of different oral and injectable preparations of varying androgenic-to-anabolic ratios, it's not surprising that law officers can view a heavy personal user's home as a major distribution warehouse. It's not uncommon for them to exclaim, "He's got a whole pharmacy in there!"

What and How Much Do Bodybuilders Use?

What sorts of quantities do non-medical users, particularly bodybuilders, actually consume in their cycles? Most physicians are extremely poor sources of such information. Because steroids are controlled substances and may not be prescribed except for a few medical purposes, the majority of physicians know almost nothing about them. Those endocrinologists who are familiar with them are mostly limited to knowing about their *medical* uses, not the *non*-medical self-administration by the muscle community. The standard medical dosage for hormone replacement – 100mg per week – is totally irrelevant to (and ineffective for) bodybuilding use.

The athletes themselves, on the other hand, have amassed their own body of underground anecdotal evidence derived from their observations of themselves and their peers, or from "underground" treatises on self-administration of steroids. The medical community itself recognizes this truth:

> "Athletes using anabolic steroids today have a sophisticated pharmacologic knowledge base for using these agents that surpasses that of the vast majority of physicians ... Today, it appears that the experts on anabolic steroid use in athletic competition are not medical clinicians but the athletes [themselves]." [Perry, et al., *see* Chapter 3 references]

The following anonymous postings, reproduced here without grammar and usage editing (but with some substance clarifications), were copied from a popular Internet discussion board in response to a posted question of "What's everybody using?":

> 6 weeks. just started 2nd. 1500mg primoteston [testosterone] /600 deca. 4 weeks off, then 6 weeks again. 1500mg primoteston/anabol 50mg/day/ deca 600 wk. another 4 weeks off, then 6 weeks on again. 1500mg primoteston/ 100mg day tren/ 40mg anabol. 5 weeks off then, then finally 6 weeks on. winny tabs 150 mg/day (waiting to hear from you guys how toxic)/ deca 600mg wk/ halo [fluoxymesterone] 30 mg/day (5 weeks)/ t-3 [Cytomel] 175mcg/day.

* * *

> Just started 750mg a week (Sustanon), 400mg T-200 [testosterone], 75mg Fina [trenbolone] EOD [every other day], 100mg of ... winny a day for first two weeks, then taper off injects in 10 weeks and use 50mg Winny last four weeks.

* * *

> I now use: 750mg ICN enanthate (rules!);250 paki sust;200mg deca;75mg methandriol (2x wk);150mg a50 day;1/4 arimidex EOD; 1 clomid EOD. In 6wks switch the a50 to 50mg dbol day; 500mg sust AND 500mg ICN; 75mg fina ED every day]; stay on same deca and methandriol. Last 3wks use prop; fina; primobolan.

* * *

> about to start 1000mg omna 800mg deca 60mg D-bol all for 8 weeks

* * *

> 1250 omna 100 drol 100mg susp ed clomid and armidex eod
>
> * * *
>
> Just thought I'd start out on ... Cyp 1000mg/week Nan300 600mg/week Dbol 40mg/day Good start, say 6-8 weeks
>
> * * *
>
> Down to just 500 mg deca/week now. Will take 4 weeks off in December then back on with 50mg D-bol 1000 mg Aratest [testosterone] and 500 mg deca. Probably add some winny and clomid in at the end.
>
> * * *
>
> 1250 mg/wk Aratest, 250 mg/wk Miro-Depo, 150 mg Tren EOD, 600 mg EQ/wk.

The content of these postings confirms that bodybuilders use substantial dosages and multiple products to achieve their aims. While those who posted these messages were anonymous, their claims are consistent with information reported to me by hundreds of bodybuilders with whom I've personally consulted. The numbers are also corroborated by information contained on countless bodybuilding Internet sites, in various magazines such as *Muscular Development, MuscleMag International,* and *Rx Muscle* (available by subscription through www.rxmuscle.com), and in books such as *Anabolics 2002* by William Llewellyn [Patchogue, NY: Molecular Nutrition, 2002] and the infamous *Underground Steroid Handbook II* by Dan Duchaine [Venice, CA: HLR Technical Books, 1989].

I recently contacted a trusted former client and a veteran juicer for their "expert" input on the issue. They were gracious enough to provide me with the following chart, broken down for newer users and veterans, showing the typical weekly or daily (ED is "every day") dosages for various anabolics. A user stacking numerous different agents would likely use the lower end dosages of each product, while somebody stacking only two products would likely use the higher end.

— TYPICAL DOSAGES —

AAS	Beginner-moderate	Experienced-ambitious
Testosterone	200-750mg/wk	750-3,000(+)mg/wk
Deca	200-400mg/wk	300-1,000mg/wk
EQ [boldenone]	150-300mg/wk	300-1,000mg/wk
Primobolan	100-200mg/wk	300-1,000mg/wk
Winstrol	50mg 2-3x/wk	100-200mg/ED
Anadrol	50mg/ED	100-250mg/ED
D-bol	20-40mg/ED	40-150mg/ED
Anavar	10-20mg/ED	20-50mg/ED
hGH	2-6iu/ED	5-20(+)iu/ED

By all accounts, significantly supraphysiologic doses and multiple preparations are the norm, with a wide spectrum of dosages and cycle lengths ranging from the very conservative to the exceedingly dangerous.

A Sampling of AAS Cycles

At the most conservative end is the following basic beginner's cycle (complete with the web site's commentary as to "expected results") taken from a popular bodybuilding web site. It is a simple eight-week cycle combining an oral steroid with an injectable in a pyramid-type structure (dosages increase, level off, and then decrease):

Week	Testosterone	Dianabol (dbol)
1	200-250mg	20 mg per day
2	200-250mg	25 mg per day
3	400-500mg	30 mg per day
4	400-500mg	35 mg per day
5	400-500mg	35 mg per day
6	400-500mg	30 mg per day
7	200-240mg	20 mg per day
8	200-250 mg	15 mg per day

"Expected Results: This cycle will give good mass and strength gains for any first timer or novice steroid user. More experienced users will most likely not experience the gains they would want from doing this cycle. If someone doing this cycle eats right and trains very hard they can expect gains from 10-25lbs. Everyone is different so gains vary a lot. Most people I have talked to that have used this or very similar cycles to this one, have gained a min. of 15lbs. This cycle is a very good first time mass cycle for someone wanting to bulk up." [Quoted from web site]

In my experience, around 500 to 600mg per week is most typical of non-competing, more "casual" steroid users, although 750mg per week is very common too. While these dosages obviously exceed medical replacement dosages, they are not necessarily dangerous if medically supervised. A landmark 1996 study stunned many in the medical community when it found virtually *no* adverse effects when anabolic steroids were administered at a dosage of 600mg per week (about six times natural replacement dose) for ten weeks. [Bhasin, et al., 1996, see Chapter 3 references] Interestingly, with all the media attention given to anabolic steroids, this very *positive* study received suspiciously little popular press.

Examples of two other novice to intermediate level cycles are reproduced on the following page (with commentary taken from the web sites), taken from another very popular hardcore web site. These cycles include stacking 600 to 800mg of injectable testosterone esters weekly along with nandrolone, trenbolone, or oral steroids, and various ancillary medications as well. Based upon my experience, this type of polypharmacy is much more typical than the simple cycle above. Where methandrostenolone is used, it is used at 25 mg per day (five tablets daily), which is quite common when stacked with other anabolics.

"Once the educated decision has been made to use steroids, an appropriate cycle can be designed. Even a cycle for a beginner should utilize at least one gram of steroid per week. This can be an extremely effective dose for both beginner and intermediate bodybuilders but has almost no side effects if designed properly. Listed below are two very simple examples of cycles of this magnitude."

Cycle 1- Lasting 8 weeks

Weeks 1-6:

600 mg test cypionate or enanthate per week
400 mg deca per week
50 mg clomid per day
5000 IU of HCG during week 4

Weeks 7-8:

600 mg test propionate per week taken in divided doses of 200 mg EOD
350 mg of winstrol per week taken in divided doses of 50 mg per day
50 mg clomid per day continuing for 3 weeks after the cycle

Cycle 2- Lasting 6 weeks

Weeks 1-3:

750 mg of Sustanon per week
175 mg of methandrostenolone per week taken in divided doses of 25 mg per day
50 mg of clomid per day
250 mg of cytadren EOD
5000 IU of HCG during week 3

Week 4:

800 mg of cypionate or enanthate
175 mg of methandrostenolone at 25 mg/day
50 mg of clomid per day
250 mg of cytadren every day

Weeks 5-6:

600 mg propionate per week taken in divided doses of 200 mg EOD
350 mg of trenbolone acetate taken in divided doses of 50 mg every day
50 mg of clomid per day continuing for 3 weeks after the cycle

The following advice is from Bill Roberts, one of the more recognized non-medical authorities on "anabolic pharmacology" and the use of steroids for athletes:

> "Someone who is already 40 lb. more muscular than he could achieve naturally, and who wishes to add still more for the purposes of competitive bodybuilding, will simply find no use from a recommendation to use 500 mg/week of Sustanon. At best such a dose might allow him to maintain what he has, instead of slowly losing muscle while off drugs. Such an athlete will probably not achieve his goals with less than a gram per week of injectables, stacked with at least 50 mg/day of orals. And he may need more than this. He is already far beyond what he could attain naturally, and more yet will not come easily."

The One Gram Per Week Rule

Based upon my conversations with countless steroid-using bodybuilders of all levels, the belief that one gram (1,000mg) of anabolic steroids per week is the benchmark for serious anabolic effects has been long accepted. This dosage would require, for example, four Sustanon 250 ampoules per week. Such weekly doses were being reported in the medical literature even in the more conservative 1980s: "Doses reportedly used by athletes for a cycle of use lasting 6 weeks or more can exceed 1 gram per week" [C.E. Yesalis, R.T. Herrick, et al., "Self-Reported Use of Anabolic-Androgenic Steroids by Elite Power Lifters," 16 *The Physician and Sportsmedicine*, (1988), 91-100]. However, today the rule is frequently interpreted as a gram of *testosterone* per week, or very close to it, in conjunction with other androgens. For example, Dave Palumbo, a hardcore national level competitor and the Editor-in-Chief of *Rx Muscle Magazine*, advises as follows in his Internet Q&A column:

> Q. How should I stack Sustanon 250 and Anadrol 50?
>
> A. Take 750mg-1000mg per week of the Sustanon and 1 Anadrol 50 (50mg) per day for 8 weeks then taper off very slowly.

The total weekly dosage of orals and injectables would be 1,100 to 1,350mg. However, bodybuilding dosages are not always limited to one gram of testosterone per week. Many AAS users take *considerably* more. Whether such massive dosages are safe or effective is irrelevant for the moment; the point is that many muscle builders do believe that such amounts are required, and administer accordingly. This "megadose" behavior extends to oral steroids as well. For example, oxymetholone, an orally active 17-alkylated androgen, is used at very high doses, typically 150mg/day in conjunction with other androgens. Methandrostenolone is also used heavily (see applicable section later in this chapter).

A few steroid "gurus" have advocated frighteningly high dosages. Representative of such theories is an article entitled "Steroid Cycling for Bodybuilders" which was taken from a popular hardcore bodybuilding web site. The dosages recommended for an "elite" level athlete are up to a whopping *4,000mg per week*. Based on the ten-week cycle suggested, the amount of testosterone esters alone would be in excess of 26,000mg for the cycle. Further toward the dangerous end of the spectrum, it is widely rumored that professional bodybuilders today routinely take a combination of oral and injectable steroids totaling 5 to 10 grams per week. Ten grams would be one thousand times replacement dose. Some medical authorities claim to have documented such dosages. [*See*, A. Wroblewska, "Androgenic-anabolic Steroids and Body Dysmorphia in Young Men," 42 *Journal of Psychosomatic Research* 3, (1997), 225-234. "Successful body-builders, through stacking and pyramiding, can take over 1000 times the clinically recommended dose of AAS."] Some researchers have reported even higher dosages, although I am personally highly skeptical about the high-end dosages referenced. [*See,* F. Murad, & R.C. Haynes, "Androgens." In A.G. Gillman, L.S. Goodman, et al., (Eds.), *The Pharmacological Basis of Therapeutics* (7th ed., MacMillan: New York, 1985), 1440-1458, reporting that *daily doses* can range up to 2,000mg equivalent of testosterone per day.]

Street Prices of Anabolic Steroids

Sometimes the prosecution will base intent to distribute charges on the argument that the high *value* of the steroids found in the defendant's possession is inconsistent with personal use. The position may be based upon estimates of current street prices of anabolics reported by Customs or other law enforcement agencies. How these estimates are arrived at is sometimes a bit of a mystery, and they are frequently substantially off the mark. Sadly, sometimes neither the prosecutor nor the defense lawyer is knowledgeable enough to challenge them. As a guide for criminal defense practitioners, prosecutors and judges, I reviewed the sales prices of numerous AAS dealers and conferred directly with many sellers and buyers to obtain an up-to-date black market price list. As can be seen, bulk prices can be significantly lower than gym prices. Internet prices will vary, often coming in at the low end of the retail range for moderate quantities. It is the attractive pricing that makes many AAS users brave the risks presented by online steroid purchasing.

STREET COSTS:

Price Listed:	Gym	Retail high/low	Bulk high/low $3-5000+
T200 Test enanthate 10ml	$60-150	$45-80	$20-35
Sustanon 250 1ml	$15-25	$10-20	$5-9
Test Suspension 20ml	$200-300	$150-275	$100-200
Deca 200ml 10ml	$100-200	$80-150	$50-80
Deca 200ml amp	$15-25	$8-15	$5-10
EQ 50mg 50ml	$150-200	$75-100	$50-75
EQ 200mg 10ml	$100-175	$75-125	$50-75
Primobolan 100mg 1ml	$15-30	$12-20	$7-12
Winstrol 50mg 20ml	$180-250	$150-200	$120-175
Winstrol tabs 2mg 100tabs	$125-150	$100-125	$85-120
Anadrol 50mg 100tabs	$250-400	$200-300	$140-200
D-bol 5mg 100tabs	$80-150	$45-100	$25-40
Anavar 2.5mg 100tabs	$150-200	$100-125	$75-95
hGH 126iu kits	$600-1,000	$500-750	$400

Methandrostenolone: An Example of the "Intent to Sell" Problem

A frequent example of the "intent to sell" problem arises in cases involving low dosage oral tablets, such as methandrostenolone. For example, a very big guy in Nassau County, New York, was recently charged with intent to sell for possessing less than four hundred tablets in his car. In a northern California case I worked on, prosecutors insisted that receiving a package of one thousand methandrostenolone tablets by mail proved an intent to sell, despite that one thousand tabs was the *minimum* quantity that could be ordered from that particular Thai source.

Methandrostenolone (called methandienone in Europe) is a moderately androgenic oral steroid that became quite famous in the 1960s when it was manufactured by Ciba pharmaceuticals under the brand name Dianabol®. While the brand was discontinued many years ago, "Dianabol" or "D-bol" is still the popular appellation for all methandrostenolone tablets. No longer manufactured by U.S. drug companies, the drug is imported from countries where it is still made lawfully. For several years, the British Dispensary in Thailand manufactured the most common brand. Called Anabol, each pink, pentagon-shaped tablet contains 5mg of methandrostenolone. The product is commonly ordered and imported directly from Thailand in tubs of 1,000 tablets. Prices vary, with foreign import prices lower than domestic resales. A good ballpark figure is $400 to $650 for a tub of a thousand tablets. (Note: This product is commonly counterfeited, although experienced users can usually detect fakes. Counterfeits may contain little or no active substance.)

Consistent with most AAS use patterns, typical bodybuilding dosages of methandrostenolone range widely. For example, in the conservative eight-week beginner's cycle described earlier, the daily dosage was six (6) or seven (7) tablets during the four heaviest weeks in the pyramid-type cycle. As written, a total of two hundred and eighty-eight (288) tablets are required for just the one beginner's cycle. Another popular online steroid guru who publishes a "layman's guide" to steroid use advises using methandrostenolone in a ten-week, pyramid fashion, starting at four tablets a day and working up to ten, then working back down to four. The total number of tablets used would be exactly 492.

Most serious male users I have interviewed average five to up to ten tablets per day (25mg to 50mg), although heavy users sometimes consume more and national level or professional bodybuilders may consume substantially more. Additionally, some beginners who lack the requisite knowledge as to the dosage necessary to achieve their goals may decide to use quantities that far exceed what the average steroid novice would need. Female users typically use two tablets per day, or risk potential virilization effects.

It is crucial to recognize that each Anabol tablet contains a *very tiny amount* of active anabolic steroid product. To put it in context, let's make a comparison. The closest steroid cousin to methandrostenolone is oxymetholone, another orally active 17-alpha-alkylated androgen, which is manufactured in the United States by Unimed under the brand name Anadrol-50. The two steroids are similar in structure and effect, and can be used somewhat interchangeably in structuring steroid cycles. Although methandrostenolone would not generally be used at a 1:1 ratio with oxymetholone, a comparison is generally instructive as to relative potencies. A single Anadrol-50 tablet provides *fifty* milligrams – ten times the amount of an Anabol tablet. Typical daily dosages of Anadrol-50 are one to three tablets for bodybuilders. Actually, this is one of the rare instances of athletic steroid use where the non-medical dosing is *lower than* the recommended safe medical dosing (even for women). The package insert for Anadrol-50, available online at www.anadrol.com, states:

Dosage and Administration

The recommended daily dose in children and adults is 1-5 mg/kg body weight per day. The usual effective dose is 1-2 mg/kg/day but higher doses may be required, and the dose should be individualized. Response is not often immediate, and a minimum trial of three to six months should be given. Following remission, some patients may be maintained without the drug; others may be maintained on an established lower daily dosage. A continued maintenance dose is usually necessary in patients with congenital aplastic anemia.

So a 220-pound (100 kg) anemic patient would need 100 to 200mg per day to get the *low end* effective dose, which equates to two to four tablets daily. Since one Anadrol-50 tablet a day is equivalent in milligram potency to *ten Anabol tablets daily*, the more conservative medical dose of Unimed's oxymetholone would theoretically equate to *between 20 and 40 tablets daily of 5mg methandrostenolone tablets.* Note further that the minimum trial period recommended by the manufacturer is three to six months of administration – much longer than the typical bodybuilder's cycle of uninterrupted use.

In actual practice, surprisingly high dosages are firmly supported by the formal scientific literature regarding non-medical use of methandrostenolone. One study confirmed that it has been administered by bodybuilders in doses of twenty *tablets* (100mg) per day. [G.R. Hervey, I. Hutchinson, A.V. Knibbs, et al., "'Anabolic effects of methandienone in men undergoing athletic training," *Lancet*, 2, (1976), 699-702]

Another study in the medical literature noted that doses up to 300 mg per day (*sixty tablets daily*!) have been reportedly used by some muscle building enthusiasts for several years. [D.L.J. Freed, A.J. Banks, et al., "Anabolic steroids in athletics: Crossover double-blind trial on weightlifters," *British Medical Journal*, 2, (1975), 471-473] Although a regimen of this amount could be extremely hepatotoxic and dangerous, it's possible that some reckless national level and professional bodybuilders may employ dosages not too far off these numbers (and, because of the criminal status of their anabolic use, probably won't seek medical monitoring).

In my experience, a regimen of between 25 and 100mg daily would be most consistent with typical hardcore steroid users. Postulating one three-month cycle or two six-week cycles, for example, at 10 tablets (50mg) daily, a total of nine hundred (900) tablets would be required (most likely pre-purchased as a single tub of 1,000 tablets).

What Does It all Mean?

(Well, what it *doesn't* mean, for any AAS users reading this, is that mega-dosing on massive quantities of juice is a good idea. It's not. Some of the guys using at the high end of today's outrageous dosage ranges will get very, very sick. Just because they're stupid doesn't mean you should be.)

What it does mean, and the reason why presenting this information is so crucial, is that bodybuilders use steroids in more substantial amounts and *purchase* steroids in more substantial amounts than most players in the criminal justice community realize. If you're a law enforcement agent, prosecutor or judge, you may find the information presented here to be helpful in future cases. If you're a defense lawyer with a client improperly charged with trafficking, you are cautioned never to blindly rely on the government experts as to personal use quantities or as to costs. Always research the accuracy of such assertions. If they are off base, you may wish to make the information in this chapter part a well-crafted presentation to the prosecutor and court. An expert affidavit applicable to the specific facts of the case can be a very persuasive addition, yielding fantastic case resolutions. Just one example: a Public Defender's office in the San Jose, California area recently contacted my office on a case involving methandrostenolone in a fairly substantial amount. Although the client was indigent and cost was a critical problem, I was able to secure a reasonably priced expert within the local area to provide expert testimony on the issue. The strategy was a smash hit, and the client consequently obtained a highly successful result that had been previously unavailable.

(Of course, if you're a bodybuilder who's being wrongfully prosecuted for intending to traffic, this chapter should be immediately presented to your lawyer. The unique issues related to quantity and costs are among many ways that anabolic steroid cases are different from "typical" drug cases. Work closely with your lawyer and be sure that he is thoroughly versed on the issues. With a fully educated and prepared attorney in your corner, you stand the best chance of getting a fair shake in court!)

Chapter 15

Failing the Drug Test Q & A

"If we're looking for the sources of our troubles, we shouldn't test people for drugs, we should test them for stupidity, ignorance, greed and love of power."
–P.J. (Patrick Jake) O'Rourke, U.S. journalist (b. 1947)

No book that ventures to be an authoritative source on the subject of anabolics could be complete without a discussion of drug testing. After all, it was panic over the failures of drug testing in competitive sports that caused the creation of the Anabolic Steroid Control Act. At the 1988 Olympic games in Seoul, Ben Johnson ran the 100 meters in 9.79 seconds and became the fastest human ever. The media frenzy that surrounded his subsequent positive test for steroids ushered in a new era in which militant anti-doping organizations cornered the market on popular opinion. For many years, they have convinced an unquestioning American public that what's best for the tiny minority of serious competitive athletes is best for everybody else. Even today, the recent flap over steroids in Major League Baseball has imbued the anti-doping lobby with the audacity to demand that various over-the-counter supplements be banned for all Americans in furtherance of their own agenda.

Without question, testing for performance-enhancing substances will continue in organized sports. But as mentioned previously, most AAS users are *not* competitive athletes. What most non-competing bodybuilders don't know is that *they* have the potential to be drug tested for steroids in a variety of contexts, and that there are several reasons why they might *fail* the test even without prior AAS use.

Q: Who Can Be Tested?

A: Anyone who works in government employment can be subject to a drug test, particularly those in sensitive positions. Most commonly, law enforcement agencies do not test for anabolics in the pre-employment drug screen or during the course of their employment. However, if there is some suspicion, which may be based upon facts and circumstances, an admission, or even an informer's tip, the officer or agent may be subject to testing. Some federal law enforcement agencies perform a pre-employment polygraph examination (lie detector test) and specifically ask about illegal use of anabolics.

If anabolics are found in the possession of anyone in the armed services, they will be compelled to submit to immediate drug testing. Also, if a package of anabolics addressed to a servicemember is intercepted, that person will be compelled to submit to a drug test (see Chapter 13).

Criminal offenders who are under the supervision of a probation department are regularly given drug screens, and may be subjected to a urine test for anabolics. I receive lots of calls from former juicers who are being placed on probation and who are wondering if steroid testing will be routinely performed. They are often concerned that because of the long periods that some anabolics remain in the body, past steroid usage may cause a positive test although they haven't used any anabolics while on probation.

Obviously, I can't speak to the policies of the probation department of every county in every state in the country. I can tell you that in the federal and state matters that I have handled, I have yet to see a probationer who was ever given a urine test for juice as part of routine testing, even, curiously enough, if the crime for which he's on probation involved steroids. However, I *have* seen a number of probationers steroid tested where the probation officer was given some *reason to suspect* steroid use. The probation officer may request that the laboratory test for steroids by checking a box that is typically on the testing form. What constitutes a "reason to suspect?" That varies individually, I suppose. While it may be unlikely that a probationer will be juice tested, it seems rather foolish to take the chance, doesn't it?

I have seen a number of probationers steroid tested where the probation offi-cer was given some reason to suspect steroid use.

There are a number of persons and or/entities that may require testing: employers, parole officers, police departments, health insurance companies, the military, and as of recently, high school athletic departments. Recall that in cases involving testing by private employers, there is no government action and therefore no violation of the Fourth Amendment right against an unreasonable search and seizure. A recent Supreme Court decision has upheld the constitutionality of the drug testing of teens who participate in extracurricular activities at *public* school (see Chapter 11).

Q: What Is Testing and Who Determines What's Illegal?

A: "Testing" is a phrase used to describe the detection of illegal or, in the case of sport, performance-enhancing drugs. The federal government ultimately determines the list of illegal drugs, although many regulations follow the International Olympic Committee (IOC) and the newly formed World Anti-Doping Association (WADA).

The IOC publishes a list of "prohibited and restricted" drugs to which many doping programs within the U.S. adhere. It is important to note that a number of the drugs on the IOC list, such as prohormones, are perfectly legal supplements as of this writing (visit www.SteroidLaw.com for future changes in the legal status of prohormones). However, if the drug testing protocol that you are subjected to follows the IOC framework, as many do, you could potentially suffer from disciplinary measures following the use of a perfectly legal food supplement!

The IOC prohibited and restricted drugs fall into three main categories: 1) short or immediate-acting stimulants and beta-blockers (ephedrine, caffeine, clenbuterol), 2) anabolic agents, and 3) masking agents (drugs that may affect the ability to detect other drugs being tested for). As of October 2002 there are twenty-eight IOC accredited labs throughout the world, with the U.S. laboratory based at UCLA School of Medicine. Although the IOC has traditionally been seen as the world leader in doping regulation and testing procedures, it is shortly going to pass the mantle onto the World Anti-Doping Association (WADA). The universal World Anti-Doping Code (World Code) is scheduled to take effect at the beginning of 2004 and is intended to ensure harmonization of anti-doping efforts "across all sports and governments." The primary objective is supposedly to "protect the *Athletes'* fundamental right to participate in doping-free sport..."

Although non-competitors reading this chapter may think WADA will not impinge on them, the truth may be very different. WADA wants to exercise control over *your* rights and freedoms as well. This is because the proposed WADA World Code (Draft Version 2.0, accessible at www.wada-ama.org) may require national governments, including the U.S., to alter their drug laws to conform to WADA's rules. If the elected governments do not conform to the World Code, the penalty will be isolation from international sporting competitions, including the Olympic games! Section 6.1 of the proposed Code requires governments to commit to "[p]ublic anti-doping policies, laws and regulations conforming with the *Code*." (Of course, it also requires "financial support" for the anti-doping agenda from all governments. [Section 6.3]) The problem with altering our American laws to conform to WADA regulations is that these regulations aren't necessarily in line with our current laws and constitutional rights.

WADA wants to dictate the "production, marketing and distribution of food and drugs." [Section 6.8] The proposed Code states that any elected government must change its laws to:

> "... restrict availability including importation, exportation, distribution, and manufacturing of Prohibited Substances ... and methods" and to "prohibit Trafficking of Prohibited Substances ... and Prohibited Methods." [Comments to Article 6]

Of course, "prohibited substances" go *way* beyond our current list of controlled substances. It's conceivable that the U.S. government could be forced to make the possession of many currently legal food supplements, such as prohormones and ephedra, illegal on the say-so of WADA. The proposed World Code could destroy the protections of DSHEA, affecting *all* of us. Also included as prohibited substances are non-controlled drugs under federal law like hGH, HCG, and insulin, as well as (in men) tamoxifen and clomiphene. WADA even seeks to regulate "professions, such as doctors and pharmacists, who contribute to sport." [Section 6.6] Sports are wonderful, but what about the rights of the rest of us?

... the U.S. government could be forced to make the possession of many currently legal food supplements, such as prohormones and ephedra, illegal on the say-so of WADA.

Q: What Types of Samples Are Taken?

A: The test procedures will normally begin with the collection of a urine specimen; however, in other limited instances a hair or blood sample may be required. Urine is generally the method of choice for steroid abuse detection as it is relatively cheap, non-invasive, and can detect steroid breakdown products (metabolites) for long periods after the initial administration.

Blood samples are now becoming more commonplace in some Olympic sports, although their use is generally limited to detecting compounds such as EPO, which is not excreted in the urine. The use of blood in the detection of steroid abuse is very limited, due largely to the rapid metabolism of steroids within the bloodstream. For instance, oral stanozolol is completely metabolized, and therefore undetectable, after only 8 hours within the bloodstream. Conversely, the metabolites of the same stanozolol tablet can be detected in the urine for up to 14 days!

Some work has been done on the detection of steroids within hair. This technique is, however, relatively expensive ($150-$300) and is to a certain degree invasive. It should also be pointed out that some religions, such as Sikhism, do not permit hair to be cut. Because of this, hair sampling may be seen as racially biased and was one of the considerations used by the IOC when deciding not to use this approach in their anti-doping policy.

Q: How Are Urine Samples Taken?

A: Although many procedures are used for urine sampling, most organizations or companies tend to model their procedures on those of the IOC.

In a typical IOC sampling procedure, one or two "Independent Sampling Officers" (ISO's) approach the chosen individual and request a urine sample to be provided. The sampling officers then remain with the individual at all times until the sample is voided. This is to prevent the individual from taking some action that might mask a positive result. One such action that has been widely reported is where an individual is catheterized and their bladder flushed and then filled with clean urine. When the individual is ready to provide the sample, they are required to remove sufficient clothing so the urination can be clearly viewed by the sampling officers. This is to prevent clean urine being dispensed from a hidden catheter or other delivery device.

Normally, a volume of 75ml is required; this sample is then tested for pH and its specific gravity. These two tests help determine whether the sample undergoes any chemical or physical changes during transportation to the laboratory. Such evidence has been used in a number of cases to demonstrate bacterial activity. This is important; as it has been shown that bacterial activity may result in changes in the testosterone/epitestosterone (T/E) ratio within the sample (this ratio is used to determine exogenous testosterone use).

After collection, the 75ml sample is normally split equally into two separate containers, thus creating an "A" sample and a "B" sample. The bottles are then sealed in front of the person being tested. The sampling officer then notes any medication or products that the individual is taking at the time of the test and any anomalies that have occurred during the sampling process. The person being tested is also given the opportunity to note any points he or she may feel are important. It is crucial that anyone giving a urine sample takes this process seriously, especially when you consider false positives can arise from illness, prescription medications, pregnancy, eating certain foods and the use of perfectly legal food supplements. As such, you should always place as much information on the appropriate sampling form as possible!

It is crucial that anyone giving a urine sample takes this process seriously ... false positives can arise from illness, prescription medications, pregnancy ... certain foods and ... food supplements.

Once this process is completed, the sample is placed in a sealed bag and sent to the laboratory for analysis. Most testing programs require some form of chain of custody, although in most cases this consists of little more than a FedEx slip. A full chain of custody can be very useful in the defense of a positive result, as it can often show mishandling of the sample. In particular, it may highlight any extended periods when the samples are not refrigerated, thereby exposing the sample to potential bacterial growth.

Q: Who Will Do the Testing?

A: Anyone with a mass spectrometer in their garage can test urine samples for steroids. Despite this, it is unlikely that any testing program would risk using a non-accredited laboratory. Accreditation normally comes from an independent governmental or internationally recognized organization, such as the IOC or the International Standards Organization (ISO). Accreditation is normally dependent upon the laboratory's ability to identify steroids within spiked samples provided by the accreditation organization. Other factors such as security, data storage and general traceability of samples and data are also taken into consideration during the accreditation process. Accreditation is normally performed annually to confirm continuing good laboratory procedures.

Q: What Does the Laboratory Look for in Urine to Identify Steroid Use?

A: When a steroid is injected or ingested, the molecule has to move from the injection site or gut to the receptor sites located within cells throughout the body. A thin layer of fat, known as a lipid membrane, surrounds all cells within the human body. For the steroid molecules to pass through this membrane they must be in a fat-soluble form (i.e. dissolved in fat). As these steroids are fat-soluble they are also water repellent or hydrophobic. This makes it difficult to excrete steroids directly into the predominately aqueous urinary system. As such, the body metabolizes steroids into different forms or "metabolites." Metabolites may go on to perform other functions in the body or may be excreted into the urine. As very little "free" (fat-soluble) steroid is ever excreted in urine, testing methodologies normally depend on the detection of water-soluble steroid metabolites.

A good example of this is the anabolic steroid nandrolone, which is metabolized in the body into three major metabolites: 19-norandrosterone (19Na), 19-noretiocholanolone (19Ne) and 19-norepiandrosterone (19Nea).

As the amount of free nandrolone excreted in urine is minimal, the testers rely on detection of one or more of the water-soluble metabolites: 19Na, 19Ne and 19Nea. If one or more of these metabolites is detected in concentrations of 2ng per ml of urine or greater, it's assumed that the individual has undertaken illegal use of the parent molecule, nandrolone.

Q: How Is the Urine Sample Analyzed?

A: Various analytical options are available for analyzing steroid metabolites, but generally a process known as Gas Chromatography Mass Spectrometry (GC-MS) is used. GC-MS is a two-step process, where GC separates the sample into its constituent parts and MS provides the exact molecular identification of the compounds. Compounds are separated by GC and are then introduced, one at a time, into a mass spectrometer. As the sample constituents enter the MS, they are bombarded by electrons, which cause the compound to break up into molecular fragments. The fragmentation pattern is reproducible and characteristic, and is considered the "molecular fingerprint" of a specific compound. GC-MS is considered to be the most definitive method for confirming the presence of a drug in the urine. Selective ion monitoring has been used to improve the GC-MS results. This procedure is the most costly, averaging approximately $200 per sample to test.

Q: Is the Method Foolproof?

A: What is, in life? The testing procedure is complicated and can be spread out over two or more days. Consequently, mechanical and human errors have occurred. It is always important to have an expert review the data from any positive test and not simply assume the testing procedure is infallible.

Q: What About Detecting Natural Androgens?

A: For certain synthetic steroids, simply their presence (or the presence of a metabolite) in a urine sample is considerable evidence of a doping offence. However, when a steroid occurs naturally within the human body (endogenously), its presence in a urine sample cannot be used as evidence of steroid use. Two naturally occurring steroids that have created significant detection problems are testosterone and nandrolone.

The presence of these compounds can be identified in urine using standard GC-MS techniques. However, as these steroids are produced endogenously, their presence alone does not provide sufficient evidence that steroids products have been taken. Due to this, a number of controversial strategies have been adopted in order to determine whether the origins of these steroids are natural or synthetic (exogenous).

Nandrolone is chemically very similar to testosterone, and its metabolites are normally excreted in rather low quantities. Because of this the IOC has set a threshold limit, stating that levels above a given concentration are deemed to be indicative of a doping offense, while concentrations below this level are believed to be from endogenous production. This may seem relatively simple until you realize that no published scientific research has conclusively determined what the levels of natural production in a human body should be. It is clear that the levels set by the IOC (2 ng of metabolite per ml of urine) are normally higher than the average person's natural production; however it isn't clear if this is true in all cases. The human body can certainly excrete nandrolone metabolites in the urine at significantly higher levels than the 2 ng threshold. Pregnant women may excrete metabolites at a level of 10 ng per ml of urine or higher. For this reason, an accredited laboratory will regularly perform pregnancy tests, often without permission, on any urine they deem suspicious. Females also have to be careful when taking a number of contraceptives, which may (and have) resulted in false nandrolone positives. In particular, the drug norethisterone is well known to produce false nandrolone positives. It is possible that other contraceptives or medications may also result in false positives but the research simple has not yet been done.

Q: What Is the "T/E Ratio" Test?

A: Although the levels of nandrolone are variable within the human body, testosterone concentrations are so variable that it's impossible to even attempt to set a threshold level to identify a positive result. So, testosterone abuse has been traditionally identified by looking at the ratio of testosterone (T) to epitestosterone (E). The principle behind this method rests on the fact that an enzyme converts T to E. The amount of this enzyme is constant and limited, and as a result only a fixed amount of T can be converted to E in a given time. If an individual injects T, the limited enzyme will now convert a smaller portion than normal of the overall T to E. The result of this is to increase the ratio of T to E. When this ratio reaches 6 to 1 it is assumed that this level becomes "suspicious".

... testosterone abuse has been traditionally identified by looking at the ratio of testosterone (T) to epitestosterone (E).

Due to the variability of the human body, it is well known that humans can exceed the 6 to 1 ratio without having administered a T-based product. As a result, further evidence is normally required to prosecute such cases. The IOC states that:

> "In the case of T/E higher than 6, it is mandatory that the relevant medical authority conduct an investigation before the sample is declared positive. A full report will be written and will include a review of previous tests, subsequent tests and any results of endocrine investigations. In the event that previous tests are not available, the athlete should be tested unannounced at least once per month for three months. The results of these investigations should be included in the report." [Olympic Movement Anti-Doping Code Appendix A, Article I]

In the case of the IOC, they depend on a number of subsequent urine samples (over a period of three months) to show a consistently high ratio or a medical investigation to turn up an androgenic tumor before clearing an athlete. The problem with this approach is that we do not fully understand the potential causes of naturally high T/E ratio. So, there's been significant effort to develop a new test that doesn't rely on T/E ratios.

A new test recently recognized by the IOC will, it is hoped, remove some of the ambiguity surrounding the T/E test. This test is known as Stable Isotope Ratio Mass Spectrometry (SIRMS), and can distinguish between endogenous and exogenous T. The principle of this technique rests on the carbon atoms that make up the T molecule. According to British sports doping expert Dr. Simon Davis, who has successfully defended a number of athletes (including Olympics medalists) against positive results and is involved in ongoing research to improve the validity of the testing procedure, these atoms come in two forms, carbon with a mass of 12 (^{12}C), and carbon that contains an extra neutron resulting in a mass of 13 (^{13}C). As the ^{13}C is heavier than a standard carbon atom, it is known as an "isotope." (This term should not be confused with radioactive isotopes, as the addition of a single neutron results in a nonradioactive or "stable" isotope.) As the atoms within the T molecule come from the food we eat, the ratio of ^{13}C to ^{12}C in the molecule will be the same as the average $^{13}C/^{12}C$ ratio of ingested food. Synthetic T is normally derived from plant materials and thus has a very different isotopic ratio signature to natural T. When synthetic T is injected it will alter the $^{13}C/^{12}C$ ratio of the T and any breakdown products derived from it; however, it will have no effects on the $^{13}C/^{12}C$ ratio of any T precursors. The new test takes advantage of this by taking a T precursor, such as cholesterol, and comparing its $^{13}C/^{12}C$ ratio with the T $^{13}C/^{12}C$ ratio. If the two ratios differ significantly, the T must have been derived exogenously.

Q: What if I Fail the Test?

A: Individuals who fail a drug test may challenge the results on a number of fronts: collection errors, interruptions in the so-called chain of custody, lab error and mishandling, a false positive for a legitimately consumed product, or even intentional manipulation of the sample and results. Sabotage of the results is one of the least likely effective challenges.

A variety of possible contaminants in food, drink and nutritional supplements may cause a false positive on a drug test. The most widely publicized have been over-the-counter prohormone products. Prohormones are precursors of certain androgens that are legally sold for oral consumption as a dietary supplement. Androstenedione is a prohormone that the body can convert to testosterone (and vice versa). Oral androstenedione supplementation very briefly increases blood levels of testosterone, and can affect the T/E ratio. Also, the urinary metabolites formed after ingesting certain illegal anabolic steroids are also formed after ingesting totally legal prohormone products. Particularly, the 19-nor products, legal and over-the-counter prohormone supplements, have been implicated in numerous false positives for the anabolic steroid nandrolone.

... the 19-nor products, legal and over-the-counter prohormone supplements, have been implicated in numerous false positives ...

According to Patrick Arnold, organic chemist, president of LPJ Research, and the man who may be referred to as the "Father of Prohormones" because he researched and developed androstenedione for commercial availability as a dietary supplement, many of these products sold in the United States originate in factories that also produce anabolic steroids. As such, the same equipment and machinery is used in the manufacturing process, resulting in possible if not likely cross-contamination during production. Such cross-contamination could result in a false positive for an anabolic steroid based on the innocent consumption of legal prohormone products.

Can simple food consumption cause a positive result for steroids? Believe it or not, people who consume pork from non-castrated male boars may show high levels of nandrolone in urine samples. A team of Portuguese scientists at the National Laboratory of Veterinary Investigation published their findings in the January/March 2002 issue of the Portuguese Journal of Veterinary Sciences. Their study referred to a previous investigation by a team from Nantes University. People who had consumed 300 grams of liver from non-castrated pigs were tested by the team at Nantes and their urine samples all showed unacceptably high levels of nandrolone. The Portuguese team concluded their report by stating that the consumption of pork from such non-castrated animals can lead to serious consequences for those who face a test for anabolics.

There are other reports that positive results have occurred after the consumption of chicken that has been injected with anabolics. It has been reported that positive results for clenbuterol have occurred when animals treated with clenbuterol have been consumed.

Q: How Long Do Anabolic Steroids Stay Detectable?

A: When persons are aware that they potentially face a test for anabolics they may prepare for it by using masking agents in an attempt to obscure the test results. However, the use of these compounds can be interdicted by no-notice testing. The NCAA and NFL have short-notice (1-2 days) programs, whereas the United States Olympic Committee approved the implementation of a no-notice program. There are many methods that may be employed by those who have notice of an impending test. Some are effective, while others are merely myths. However, I will not go into them in detail because this chapter is not intended as a "how-to manual."

... detection times may vary from as little as two days, as in the case of testosterone undecanoate (Andriol), to twelve months, as in the case of nandrolone decanoate (Deca-Durabolin).

Anabolic steroid detection times may vary from as little as two days, as in the case of testosterone undecanoate (Andriol), to twelve months, as in the case of nandrolone decanoate (Deca-Durabolin). The following is merely presented as an overview of possible time frames for the detection of some of the more common anabolic steroids. (See the Glossary for profiles of many of these substances.) It should be noted that many of the testing dates for injectable steroids may be highly variable due to injection volume and injection technique.

48 Hours

Clenbuterol (although not a steroid it is anabolic and banned in sports)
Testosterone undecanoate (Andriol)

One Week

AquaViron (testosterone water suspension injection)
Human Chorionic Gonadotropin (HCG)
Most oral prohormones

Two Weeks

Testosterone propionate
Mesterolone (Proviron)
Nolvadex
Most oral steroids including: Oxandrolone (Anavar, Lipidex); Oral stanozolol (Winstrol-V) Methandienone/methandrostenolone (Dianabol, Anabol, Anabolex, Bionabol) Oxymetholone (Anadrol-50, Anapolon, Hemogenin) Fluoxymesterone (Halotestin, Stenox)

Four to Five Weeks

Trenbolone acetate (Finaplix, Finaject, Finajet (no longer in production), Trenbol 75)
Methenolone enanthate (Primobolan Depot) (injectable)
Testosterone blends (Sustanon, Sostenon, Sten, Durateston, Omnadren)
Testosterone enanthate
Testosterone cypionate

Two Months

Injectable Stanozolol (Winstrol)
Formebolone (Esiclene)
Drostanolone propionate (Masteron)

Four to Five Months

Boldenone undecylenate (Equipoise, Equi-gan, Ganabol, Maxigan, Ultragan, Pace)

Twelve Months

Nandrolone Phenylpropionate (Durabolin, Anabolin, Equibolin-50)
Nandrolone Decanoate (Deca-Durabolin, Deca-Durabol, Turinabol Depot, Norandren).

Conclusion

Athletes of all countries who use drugs or OTC supplements to cheat in sports should be punished. But the rest of us Americans should think long and hard before we relinquish further freedoms to meet the demands of global special interests.

"I believe in ... sports. But I do not believe in them if they degenerate into the sole end of anyone's existence."
– *Theodore Roosevelt (1858 – 1919)*

Chapter 16

Cyber-Security

"Anonymity is a shield from the tyranny of the majority ... It thus exemplifies the purpose behind the Bill of Rights, and of the First Amendment in particular: to protect unpopular individuals from retaliation – and their ideas from suppression – at the hand of an intolerant society."

– *U.S. Supreme Court Justice John Paul Stevens*

Since it went online, the World Wide Web has become a catalyst for the exchange of information. This exchange includes bodybuilding information, and more particularly, discussions about bodybuilding drugs, how to use them, and how and where to obtain them. What was once limited to hushed conversations in the gym among a small group of hardcore lifters has grown to worldwide proportions because of the 'Net. But it isn't just talk going on. The Internet has become a medium for all kinds of commerce; steroids are increasingly being bought and sold in cyberspace. One reason that these discussions and transactions have grown to such an extent is the anonymity and security measures that the Web offers, like screen names, remailers, encryption, and dynamic IP addresses. While discussion and commerce have expanded, so has law enforcement's interest in them and their methods of interdicting criminal activity.

William, a 33-year-old New York resident, used the Internet to purchase anabolics from overseas. A package of 100 Thai Anabol was flagged, and Customs thereafter recovered a total of 600 more tablets that had been shipped in packets of 100. The police did a controlled delivery of two packages, then executed a raid on his home. They seized his computer and arrested him. He was charged with felony possession of a controlled substance with intent to sell. The case seemed likely to be resolved with a misdemeanor and no jail time until the police examined his computer and found correspondences in his e-mail program indicating he had been selling steroids in substantial volume. The District Attorney refused to offer a misdemeanor plea based on this newly discovered evidence on William's computer.

In recent years, the *majority* of anabolic steroid arrests can be traced back to online activities – frankly, it's an *overwhelming* majority. Incriminating trails of cyber-activities have led both to the identification of otherwise unknown suspects by law enforcement and to the successful collection of evidence against previously identified targets. Cyber-juicing has gotten people busted. Most of the guys getting collared are buyers, not sellers. Somebody will be busted for cyber-juicing within a day or two of your reading this, I'm sure. But today, he's figuring he has nothing to worry about. His state-of the-art, brand-spanking-new, over-clocked, water-cooled, modded, Pentium IV computer is behind a firewall. He has just installed the latest stealth software program and his overall security methods would make the infamous Kevin Mitnick* seem like a newbie. He's thinking he's a ghost. Think again.

* *Kevin David Mitnick was at the time a 31-year-old computer programmer from Los Angeles, California. Dubbed by some as "America's Most Wanted Computer Outlaw," Mitnick eluded police, U.S. Marshals*

and the FBI for more than two years, after disappearing while on probation for his 1989 conviction for computer and access device fraud. His downfall was a 1994 "hack" into the computers of Tsutomu Shimomura in San Diego, California. Less than two months later, he was tracked down after a cross-country electronic pursuit. On February 15, 1995, Mitnick was arrested by the FBI in Raleigh, North Carolina.

The Basics of Cyberspace

The Internet is simply a collection of networks that are all interconnected. There's no centralized point on the Internet where all the traffic can be monitored. When you connect to a web site, your traffic goes through several Internet "carriers" known as Internet Service Providers (ISPs). ISPs are private companies that provide Internet services. When one "dials-up" the Internet through a modem, or accesses it through a DSL (Digital Subscriber Line), cable modem, or DSS (Digital Satellite System), you go through your local ISP.

Bodybuilders may find the Internet of interest for many reasons (including checking out the web sites of the hottest fitness chicks), but the following are primary: e-mail, discussion groups, discussion boards, and file transfers.

Internet mail is "e-mail," or electronic mail, faster by several orders of magnitude than the U.S. Mail, which is scornfully known by Internet regulars as "snail mail." Internet mail is not unlike a fax in some regards; it's electronic text and global in scope. E-mail can also send software and certain forms of compressed digital imagery as file attachments.

The discussion groups, or "newsgroups," are a world of their own. This world of news, debate, and heated argument (commonly referred to as "flame wars") is generally known as "USENET." USENET is comprised of an enormous mingling crowd of gossiping, sometimes trash-talking people with a voracious appetite for news and information. USENET is not so much a physical network as a set of social conventions. In any case, at the moment there are more than 2,500 separate newsgroups on USENET, and their discussions generate millions of words of typed commentary each day. Naturally, there is a vast amount of talk about fitness on USENET, but the variety of subjects discussed is enormous, and it's growing larger all the time. One of the biggest and best meeting places for those serious about diet, training, supplements, and anabolics is *misc.fitness.weights*. This is an un-moderated, no-holds-barred discussion group, so be warned: the language and content can be rough. USENET also distributes various free electronic journals and publications.

Some web sites offer "discussion boards" for such topics as training, gossip, nutrition, and anabolic steroids. Much like newsgroups, discussion boards are open to nearly anyone with an Internet connection. Some offer free registration allowing users to post and participate, requiring only a "screen name" and a password. These boards are sometimes moderated by an administrator or by trusted, long-time members. They may delete objectionable material at their discretion but for the most part will encourage candid and open discussion among members. These boards have become the overwhelming favorites, as they are user-friendly and easy to navigate.

"File transfers" allow Internet users to access remote machines and retrieve programs or text. Many Internet computers allow any person to access them anonymously, and to simply copy their public files, free of charge. This is no small deal, since entire books can be transferred through direct Internet access in a matter of minutes. Internet file-transfers are becoming a new form of publishing, in which the reader simply electronically copies the work on demand, in any quantity desired without any fee.

All right, with the basics covered, let's get down to business. Just how secure is cyber-security?

Your Computer Is Vulnerable

The connection of a private network to the Internet can expose your critical or confidential data to malicious attack from anywhere in the world. Not just from the government, but from hackers of all kinds. Everyone who connects a computer to the Internet must be aware of these dangers, their implications, and how to protect private data and critical systems. Firewalls can protect both individual computers and corporate networks from hostile intrusion from the Internet – intrusion that could compromise confidentiality or result in data corruption or denial of service. Most people don't use firewalls, and few people understand them.

A firewall may be a hardware device or a software program running on a secure host computer. In either case, it must have at least two network interfaces, one for the network it's intended to protect, and one for the network it's exposed to. A firewall sits at the junction point or gateway between the two networks, usually a private network and a public network such as the Internet. The earliest firewalls were simply routers. The term firewall comes from the fact that by segmenting a network into different physical subnetworks, they limited the damage that could spread from one subnet to another – just like firedoors or firewalls would prevent fire from spreading from one room to another. Okay so far?

> Firewalls can protect both individual computers and corporate networks from hostile intrusion from the Internet ...

There are two methods by which firewalls deny access to intruders. Either a firewall may allow all traffic to pass unless it meets certain criteria, or it may prevent all traffic from passing unless it meets certain criteria. The type of criteria used to determine whether traffic should be allowed through varies from one type of firewall to another. Firewalls may be concerned with the type of traffic, or with source or destination addresses and ports. They may also use complex rule bases that analyze the application data to determine if the traffic should be allowed through. How a firewall determines what traffic to let through depends on which *network layer* it operates at.

Packet filtering firewalls work at the network level of the OSI model, or the IP layer of TCP/IP. They are usually part of a router. A router is a device that receives packets from one network and forwards them to another network. In a packet filtering firewall, each packet is compared to a set of criteria before it is forwarded. Depending on the packet and the criteria, the firewall can drop the packet, forward it or send a message to the originator. Rules can include source and destination IP address, source and destination port number, and protocol used. The advantage of packet filtering firewalls is their low cost and low impact on network performance. Most routers support packet filtering. Even if other firewalls are used, implementing packet filtering at the router level affords an initial degree of security at a low network layer. This type of firewall only works at the network layer however, and does not support sophisticated rule-based models. Address Translation (NAT) routers offer the advantages of packet filtering firewalls but can also hide the IP addresses of computers behind the firewall, and offer a level of circuit-based filtering.

What does all this mean? It means that without the use of a firewall, a user's networked computer or one connected to the Internet could be accessed by someone remotely. That access could be for any number of reasons. It could be a private hacker looking to explore your hard drive, install Trojan horse programs and viruses, and/or corrupt your programs. Or maybe the feds have a certain curiosity about you.

It's crucial to understand that firewalls offer limited protection. A firewall cannot prevent individual users with modems from bypassing the firewall altogether when dialing into or out of the network. Employee misconduct or carelessness cannot be controlled by firewalls; policies involving the use and misuse of passwords and user accounts must be strictly enforced. These are management issues that should be raised during the planning of any cyber-security policy, and cannot be solved with firewalls alone.

The arrest of the Phonemasters cracker ring brought these security issues to light. Although they were accused of breaking into information systems run by AT&T Corp., British Telecommunications Inc., GTE Corp., MCI WorldCom, Southwestern Bell, and Sprint Corp., the group did not use any high tech methods such as IP spoofing. They used a combination of social engineering and dumpster diving. Social engineering involves techniques not unlike those of a confidence trickster to fool people into revealing sensitive information. Dumpster diving or garbology, as the names suggest, is nothing but poking around through a company's trash. Obviously, firewalls can't be effective against either of these techniques.

Your Web Surfing Can Be Monitored

Your computer's IP address uniquely identifies your computer and is most-often stored by every web site you visit. This information can be bought and sold between web sites and linked to your real world information to create a comprehensive profile of your personal data, including everywhere you surf. Not what you'd want, is it? Could be embarrassing, perhaps?

Anonymizer is the first and one of the most well-known services to allow web surfing to be done anonymously by hiding your IP address from the site that you're visiting. When you view a page through the Anonymizer service, the software is designed to modify or remove JavaScript and other HTML tags that could cause your browser to make a direct connection to the site you're viewing, which would defeat the anonymity of the service. When the user of Anonymizer visits a site, the Anonymizer IP address is seen, not the user's.

Of course, anonymous web surfing services won't help you if your computer is seized in a raid.

There are some very good Anonymizer-type sites that also encrypt the URL so that even your ISP and, if you're surfing the Web at work, the IT people at your company can't read your URL. While Anonymizer only hides your IP information from the sites you visit, if you use a product or company that encrypts your URL, your own ISP can't tell where you've gone either.

Of course, anonymous web surfing services won't help you if your computer is seized in a raid. Your web surfing adventures will be saved in your history unless you delete them.

Your E-mail Is Open to Inspection

It's important for all Internet users to understand that basic e-mail offers no privacy, and can actually be read by many people other than the recipient. Unless the e-mail is "encrypted," almost anyone can read your e-mail if they are determined. The Internet Service Provider (ISP) may keep a copy on its computer, copies of e-mail sent from a networked computer (such as at work or school) are most likely maintained, and all of the Internet computers the e-mail goes through on its way to the recipient can keep a copy. The administrators of all these computers can read your e-mail if they choose to, and they can send it to anyone they want. The FBI may intercept e-mail and scan it for interesting words or phrases.

Here's something scary. Anyone who can intercept e-mail can alter its content, and anyone can send e-mail that looks as if another sent it. Working within the Public Key Infrastructure (PKI), a user can obtain a digital certificate (Digital ID). A Digital ID provides an electronic means of proving your identity online, the same way that a passport or driver's license does in face-to-face interactions. The digital certificate consists of a private key (that only the user has) and a public key (that the user sends to people so they can verify the user's identity). The user can digitally sign his/her e-mail and encrypt the contents. Automatically, an encryption program will calculate a complex mathematical value (called a "hash") based on the exact content of the e-mail message, and will then encrypt that value to the user's private key. The recipient of the e-mail will then use his/her encryption software and the sender's public key to automatically make the same calculation. If the calculations match (the recipient's software automatically will use the sender's public key to re-create the encrypted hash), that is proof that the message has not been altered in any way (no spaces or letters have been added, deleted, changed, etc.). And since only the user has the private key that encrypted the hash value that was now decrypted with the public key, this indicates that only the user could have sent the e-mail. So when encryption says that the signature is good, that proves that the message is both unaltered (integrity), and from the sender indicated (identity).

It's best to look at it this way; sending e-mail without encryption is like sending a postcard through the mail – anyone can read it. Encryption is like putting the letter in an envelope and sealing it, thereby obscuring its contents from curious readers. The real weakness in encryption is in allowing someone access to your private key and your pass phrase. Why would somebody do that? The most likely scenario is that the holder of the key and pass phrase gets popped by law enforcement, and in an effort to gain favorable treatment for himself, he turns them over. Once they are turned over, authorities can access the content of all of your communications. Not just what you've sent to others, but what others have sent to you.

The real weakness in encryption is in allowing someone access to your private key and your pass phrase.

Any time authorities seize your computer, they will have access to your private key. Where they run into trouble is when it is kept on an encrypted drive. No one can read your encrypted e-mail even with your private key until they get your pass phrase. That is much easier said than done. As long as you use proper password building rules, such as substituting numbers and special characters, pass phrases are very hard to break. An example of proper password building may be as follows: "r1ckc0ll1n5kn0w5b35t," rather than merely "rickcollinslegalmuscle."

PGP, an abbreviation for "Pretty Good Privacy," is a public key encryption program originally written by Phil Zimmerman in 1991. Over the past few years, PGP has acquired thousands of adherent supporters all over the globe and has become the standard for encryption of e-mail on the Internet. PGP is available for many different operating systems, including Windows, Unix, MS-DOS, OS-2, and Macintosh. Some people using the latest PGP programs believe they're using the best form of encryption available. In reality, only PGP version 6.5.8 or earlier are the versions that Zimmerman was still involved with, and are *open source code*. Later versions not affiliated with Zimmerman are not open source code. It's possible that the developers of these later programs have written a "backdoor" into the program so that prying eyes might have a way into your e-mail without knowing your pass phrase. In that case, your privacy might be simply an illusion.

Your Web-Based E-mail Isn't Really Anonymous

There are hundreds of web-based e-mail services – including Hotmail, Yahoo, Excite, Pobox, and too many more to list here – that apparently offer anonymity. In actuality, very few do. The only ones that appear to offer security, such as Hushmail and Ziplip, will only do so if *both* users have accounts on those systems. In each of these cases, the user is allowed to create a pseudonym to be used for messages. Unfortunately, through sign-up procedures, logging, and message headers, it is ridiculously simple to determine the user's ISP, and even that person's true identity.

As a user, it is your responsibility to know that your Internet anonymity is only as secure as the service's privacy policy. You should always familiarize yourself with the usage and privacy policies of any e-mail or Internet service you consider using. In fact, many e-mail providers are actually quite helpful to the Government. Consider the case of *U.S. v. Maxwell,* [45 MJ568 (1995, AFCCA)] wherein America Online anticipated that a warrant would be issued regarding certain e-mails, and programmed software that automatically extracted the information that the FBI was seeking. When the warrant was executed, AOL officials turned the e-mails over immediately.

When using Hushmail or Ziplip, prudent users will still use PGP in conjunction with these systems. It takes only seconds to use both, and offers most likely the best security possible, short of going to the extreme of accessing the account from the public or college library, opening a Hotmail account there, and only using the account from that location.

Not All Re-mailers Are Alike

A re-mailer is a computer service that privatizes your e-mail. High-quality re-mailers are in sharp contrast to the average Internet Service Provider, which is terribly anti-private. Almost every ISP can monitor, store, and share your web wanderings and e-mail with many so-called "authorized persons" without your knowledge. Until the late 1990s, a re-mailer allowed you to send electronic mail to a USENET newsgroup, or to a person, without revealing your true name or e-mail address to the recipient. Today, web-based re-mailers permit you to send e-mail using your real name, if you so desire, while protecting your e-mail records from disclosure to your Internet Service Provider and anyone else.

People might use the expression "anonymous re-mailer" in reference to all re-mailers. This is actually misleading. A *pseudo-anonymous re-mailer* is basically an account that is opened by the user with a re-mailer operator. This means that the operator and his assistants will know your true e-mail address. Your privacy is as good as the re-mailer operator's integrity and motivation to protect your records. In actuality, a court could issue a subpoena compelling a pseudo-anonymous re-mailer operator to reveal your true identity. The advantage of most pseudo-anonymous re-mailers is that they are user-friendly. If you can send e-mail, you can probably understand pseudo-anonymous re-mailers – but the price you pay for ease of use is less security.

Truly *anonymous re-mailers* are a different animal. They provide much more privacy than pseudo-anonymous re-mailers. However, in general, they are much harder to use than their pseudo-anonymous counterparts. There are basically two types of anonymous re-mailers. They are "Cypherpunk re-mailers" and Lance Cottrell's "Mixmaster re-mailers." If a user is seeking maximum privacy, the message should be sent through two or more re-mailers, as well as using PGP encryption software. If done properly, the user can ensure that no one (re-mailer operator or anyone else) can read both the real name and the message. This is the true essence of anonymity. In practice, nobody can compel an anonymous re-mailer operator to reveal the identity of the sender of a message, because the operator has no idea who the sender may be.

If a user is seeking maximum privacy, the message should be sent through two or more re-mailers, as well as using PGP encryption software.

For most low-security tasks, such as responding to personal ads, pseudo-anonymous re-mailers with pass code protection are undoubtedly safer than using real e-mail addresses. However, the potential for weaknesses is almost always present. Here are some possibilities to consider:

A. The person who runs your e-mail system might intercept your secret messages to and from the re-mailer;
B. The re-mailer could possibly be a government sting operation or a criminal enterprise designed to lure unsuspecting victims;
C. Hackers' abilities are seemingly limitless. It's possible that civilian or federal agents have hacked into the re-mailer and they can read your messages at will;
D. It's a possibility that federal agencies collect, scan, and store all messages, including pass codes, into and out of the re-mailer;
E. If you use a United States-based re-mailer, a U.S. judge could subpoena the re-mailer's records.

Carnivore Program May Be Watching You

Carnivore is a sophisticated new wiretapping and/or eavesdropping program that scans a user's e-mail. The FBI euphemistically refers to it as a "diagnostic tool." According to the FBI's Carnivore web site, in recent years they have encountered an increasing number of criminal investigations in which the criminal subjects use the Internet to communicate with each other or with their victims. Because many ISPs lacked the ability to discriminate communications to identify a particular subject's messages to the exclusion of all others, the FBI designed and developed Carnivore. The Carnivore "device" provides the FBI with a "surgical" (the FBI's term) ability to intercept and collect the communications that are asserted to be the subject of a lawful court order, while ignoring those communications that they are not authorized to intercept. The FBI asserts that this type of tool is necessary to meet the stringent requirements of the federal wiretapping statutes.

The Carnivore device is not unlike commercial "sniffers" and other network diagnostic tools used by ISPs every day. "Sniffers" are Internet wiretap programs that are used widely in order to debug problems on the Internet. For example, if you notice that you cannot get to *www.steroidlaw.com*, then engineers somewhere are putting sniffers on the wire in order to locate the problem.

Previously, an "application for interception" had to be performed as follows: under Title III, the application must receive the authorization of a high-level Department of Justice (DOJ) official before the local United States Attorney's offices can apply for the order. The Interception Order must be filed with a federal district court judge or with other courts of competent jurisdiction. Therefore, unlike typical search warrants, federal magistrates are not authorized to approve such applications and orders. Further, interception of communications is limited to certain specified federal felony offenses.

Applications for electronic surveillance must demonstrate probable cause (see Chapter 7) and state with particularity and specificity: the offense(s) being committed, the telecommunications facility or place from which the subject's communications are to be intercepted, a description of the types of conversations to be intercepted, and the identities of the persons committing the offenses that are anticipated to be intercepted. Applications must indicate that other normal investigative techniques will not work or are too dangerous, and must include information concerning any prior electronic surveillance regarding the subject or facility in question. Court orders are limited to 30 days and interceptions must terminate sooner if the objectives are obtained. Judges may (and usually do) require periodic reports to the court (typically every 7-10 days) advising of the progress of the interception effort. This circumstance assures close and ongoing oversight of the electronic surveillance by the U.S. Attorney's office handling the case. An application for an extension of the order may be submitted to the court (consistent with requirements of the initial application) and, if supported, may result in an extension for a period of up to 30 days.

However, under the USA Patriot Act passed in October 2001, agents may now install Carnivore by obtaining an order from a U.S. or state attorney general, without going to a judge. After-the-fact judicial oversight is still required.

The Achilles heel to Carnivore is encryption. Carnivore will not detect encrypted files. However, where there is a will, there is a way. *Magic Lantern* is just one in a series of enhancements to the Carnivore project which falls under the umbrella project name of Cyber Knight. The FBI envisions one day using Magic Lantern to record the secret key a person might use to scramble messages or computer files with encryption software. In addition to possibly defeating encryption, Magic Lantern could largely resolve an important shortcoming with the FBI's existing monitoring technology – the "key logger system." This system has required in the past that investigators sneak into a target's home or business with a so-called "sneak-and-peak warrant" and clandestinely attach an electronic device to the target computer.

In contrast, Magic Lantern could possibly be installed over the Internet by using a ruse. Law enforcement could deceive a person into opening an e-mail attachment or by exploiting some of the same weaknesses in popular commercially available software that allow hackers to break into computers. It is unclear whether Magic Lantern would transmit keystrokes it records back to the FBI over the Internet or store the information to be seized later in a raid. If they were to use a program of this kind, it could potentially be a highly effective way to bypass any encryption impediments. In this regard, the FBI will essentially have the keys to the house and have complete access to anything that individual is doing. Magic Lantern would essentially watch when the user employs PGP encryption. Once initiated, the program would then log the pass phrase used to start the program, thereby giving agents the wherewithal to decrypt e-mail.

The difference between Carnivore and Magic Lantern is that the latter targets one suspect at a time. However, the former does not and could potentially be overbroad in practice and thereby "sniff" packets of data to and from those who are not the target of investigation. All of these raise Fourth Amendment issues which are clearly beyond the scope and intent of this chapter, which is to educate the reader about how unsecure the 'Net can be.

Your Hard Drive Is a Collection of Lots of Data

In addition to what is floating around in cyberspace, many times the surveillance and evidence obtained by law enforcement has been from computer hardware and software, including hard drives. Nearly all search warrants authorize law enforcement to search for evidence indicative of the transfer and sale of controlled substances. In addition, it will authorize a search for all articles of personal property tending to establish and document the sale – including but not limited to: computers, laptops, floppy disks and memory sticks – and to open or download and forensically examine all computer software and programs seized pursuant to the warrant. Some people go so far as to use a program like E4M or Bestcrypt to create an encrypted hard drive. These programs work by creating a file which, when opened by a pass phrase, opens a "virtual drive" that looks exactly like an actual hard drive. However, most folks don't seem to use these programs.

You may think that a deleted item actually disappears from your hard drive, but this is not necessarily so. It can be retrieved or reconstructed by law enforcement agents with evidence retrieval programs like Encase. Few people use secure deletion programs like Evidence Eliminator every time they use their computers. Consider the case of *Commonwealth v. Copenhefer* [587 A.2d 1253 (1991)]. In that case, the defendant was convicted based on a ransom note recovered from his hard drive that he had deleted and thought had disappeared. He was sentenced to death.

Many times, unbeknownst to the user, there's a great deal of damaging evidence contained on a computer's hard drive. The temporary Internet folders file can contain a history of web pages visited. I've seen countless cases where the computer was seized during the execution of a search warrant, and the information retrieved from it was devastating to the client.

Cookies are short pieces of data used by web servers to help identify web users and track their web habits. Some cookies last only until the user closes his/her browser; they are then destroyed. Other types, known as persistent cookies, have an expiration date and can remain on the hard drive until that date expires or the cookie is deleted manually. The popular concepts and rumors about what a cookie can do have reached almost mystical proportions. No files are destroyed or compromised by cookies, though they may allow your web browsing to be traced. The Web is not based on persistent connections to servers; therefore, cookies are used to track sessions for most any web service that requires a login. If you disable cookies, most web services with logins will not work.

You can prevent any cookies from being sent to your system using the browser options. In Internet Explorer 4.0, choose the View, Internet Options command, click the Advanced tab and click the Disable All Cookie Use option. In Netscape 4.0, choose the Edit, Options command, click on Advanced and click the Disable Cookies option. After that, no cookies will be stored on your system. You will need to turn cookies back on if you want to use any online services that require them. You can also choose the option to prompt you before accepting a cookie, but at many sites you will be continually closing the warning dialog box.

If you are using earlier versions of Netscape or Internet Explorer, you can require that the browser warn you before accepting a cookie, but it cannot block all cookies. However, be aware that at a busy shopping site, acknowledging all the warnings can become tedious.

Preventing your browser from accepting cookies does not make you an anonymous user; it just makes it more difficult to track your usage. More difficult, but *not* impossible.

Summing It Up

Does it all sound pretty paranoid? After all, the FBI has bigger things to worry about than your annual juice cycle. And hopefully they're working hard on them. Many Americans have no problem with the government using sophisticated spying technologies to protect us from international terrorists who use the Internet to exchange their villainous communications, or from predatory pedophiles who lure children into danger. In fact, I'd wager that the vast majority of the muscle world would *applaud* that. But bored and restless agents from other government branches may have more time on their hands to think about you and your juice. I've already seen plenty of situations where compromised Internet anonymity or incriminating hard drives have factored into the evidence in an AAS case. In some situations, it's made the difference between getting busted and going free. In others, evidence of other steroid dealings discovered via the computer have either bolstered the prosecutor's case or incited the judge to go heavier on the sentence. In still other situations, employers or vindictive estranged wives have been able to use stored computer information against somebody who never saw it coming. Look, the importance of every American's individual privacy is integral to the Constitution. As noted by Justice Stevens at the beginning of this chapter, so is anonymity.

Chapter 17

Online Pharmacies

"A computer lets you make more mistakes faster than any invention in human history – with the possible exceptions of handguns and tequila."
– Mitch Ratliffe, *Technology Review.* April, 1992

Not a week goes by that I don't get a call from somebody interested in the legalities of buying steroids online. Quite often it's the prospective purchaser, who's heard rumors on Internet discussion boards of various exemptions or loopholes that might allow him to lawfully score a personal use quantity. Sometimes he'll have stumbled upon a foreign online pharmacy that assures him that it's perfectly legal to do so. Or sometimes the call I receive is from an ambitious dot-com entrepreneur who sees the proliferation of online longevity centers and wants a piece of the action.

Categories of Online Pharmaceutical Suppliers

Let's start at the beginning, and talk generally about who's selling prescription drugs online. We can divide the online pharmaceutical suppliers into four categories:

1) Underground sources
2) Foreign pharmacies
3) "Invisible doctor" clinics
4) Legitimate pharmacies

We can dispense with underground sources right off the bat. Legal? Come on, you're kidding, right? These sources are typically individuals trafficking drugs under a shield of Internet-enabled anonymity. The majority of people I see getting busted for gear are as a result of these types of online transactions. It's not usually the sellers who are being arrested, mind you, but the *purchasers*. Check out the many examples in the chapters to follow.

At the other end of the spectrum, there are legitimate Internet pharmacies out there. These entities meet the licensing and registration requirements of their home state and of all states to which they dispense medications. The National Association of Boards of Pharmacy (www.nabp.net) has a program called the Verified Internet Pharmacy Practice Sites™ (VIPPS™) program that provides a VIPPS seal of approval for online pharmacies that are legitimately operating via the Internet, and that have successfully completed a rigorous criteria review and inspection. Since these sites will not write prescriptions, unless you've already got one you're out of luck. So much for them, for the purposes of our inquiry.

How about foreign pharmacy sites? They're all over the Web. Some of these entities may be real pharmacies located in jurisdictions with relaxed laws on the dispensation of drugs. But most are simply underground sources that, because they're physically located beyond the reach of American law enforcement authorities, can operate more openly. None of these sites require a prescription. If you order and receive drugs from them, you will not be in lawful possession. Some of these companies promise to package your order discreetly, so as to avoid detection by American authorities. Others take the opposite approach, and claim that they are legitimate under American laws. Some of these entities will actually include a prescription for you in the package they send, along with the medications. Such a prescription is *invalid.* If a prescription is invalid, the medication is not legitimately possessed.

Unapproved New Drugs

Separate and apart from the validity of the prescription is the legality of the product itself. The FDA is the agency having jurisdiction over prescription medications. Their interest is not as to the propriety of the prescription, but as to the product itself. In order to import any prescription drug, the importation must be in accordance with the Food, Drug and Cosmetic Act. Adulterated or misbranded drugs are prohibited under 21 U.S.C. § 331(a) and (c) and § 381(a). *Unapproved new drugs* are prohibited under 21 U.S.C. § 331(d) and § 355(a). What are these "unapproved new drugs"? Just about anything you might want to import, actually. For example, if a product is available in the U.S., a foreign version of it is not approved. While the FDA has a guidance that permits the exercise of "enforcement discretion" in personal use situations involving drugs that do not present an "unreasonable risk," do not exceed a three month supply, and are being supervised under the treatment of a U.S. physician, the drugs are must be for a serious condition "for which effective treatment may not be available domestically" – and even then they are still technically illegal and may be confiscated. It's important to know that this guidance does *not* apply to controlled substances, which fall under the jurisdiction of the DEA, not the FDA.

What are these "unapproved new drugs"? Just about anything you might want to import, actually.

Longevity Clinics Online

Now, what about online clinics that offer prescription medications for longevity or anti-aging purposes? Are they legit? Well, we've already discussed the issues surrounding the proper and ethical parameters for prescribing androgens [see Chapter 12]. Let's focus here on the broader issue, which has to do with the fact that the relationship between the clinic and the patient exists only in cyberspace. The patient and the clinic may be separated by thousands of miles; they may even be located in different countries. How can a doctor treat a patient she's never met?

The online clinic may provide an "invisible doctor" who prescribes the medications without actually seeing the patient. Many of these clinics have sophisticated online procedures that are designed to mimic an office visit. Patients send medical information via the Web to the online clinic, where an unseen physician reviews the information and ships the medications directly to the patient's residence. Inexplicably, some of these outfits will require a blood test to be taken, but will prescribe and ship the pharmaceuticals *before* they even receive the results.

The American Medical Association has taken the position that prescribing medications without a physician-patient consultation is *unethical.* State medical boards generally agree that prescribing drugs without physically examining a patient falls far below the acceptable standard of medical care. And with good reasons. How can a physician properly diagnose a patient without a face-to-face physical examination? How can a physician discuss treatment options and determine with the patient the best course of treatment? How can follow-up evaluations be effective without a physical examination? And how can a physician know whether the patient is really who he says he is without face-to-face interaction? For example, the media have reported abuses where online pharmacies unwittingly issued prescriptions and shipped Viagra® to children and pets. The AMA has stated that it would assist the Federation of State Medical Boards (FSMB) in developing state laws to address invisible doctor clinics, and encourages state medical boards to investigate doctors who prescribe drugs for cyberpatients they have never seen.

How can a physician properly diagnose a patient without a face-to-face physical examination?

Government Regulation of Cyber-Prescribing

Since some of these entities seem to have been operating for quite a while, it's sometimes suggested there's little risk of legal repercussions. Why aren't they all out of business by now? Our legislators and law enforcement authorities were unprepared and overwhelmed by the explosive proliferation and variety of online pharmaceutical suppliers. They're still attempting to play "catch up" and to clarify their positions on the many issues that exist. In the near future we can expect the development of new laws, regulations and hopefully clear-cut enforcement policies. In the meantime, though, state governmental authorities haven't been sitting on their hands.

Generally, the regulation of pharmacies and supervision of physicians has been a state function. States have the duty to ensure that pharmacies maintain proper facilities to store medications and qualified personnel to safely dispense them. Under the majority of state laws, prescribing medications to patients outside the state in which the physician is licensed is considered the unlicensed practice of medicine. For example, a physician in New York who prescribes and dispenses medications to a patient in California may have engaged in the unlicensed practice of medicine in California. He could be subjected to prosecution in California for practicing medicine there without a license. He could also face disciplinary proceedings by the medical board in New York for his unethical conduct of practicing medicine outside his licensing. This might occur because the California medical licensing board reports his conduct to the New York board.

The Osteopathic Medical Board of California ordered a physician to shut down two online sites through which he sold Propecia®. He was using an online questionnaire in lieu of a good faith physical examination. The Washington Medical Quality Assurance Commission charged a physician with unprofessional conduct for similar conduct with respect to Viagra®, as did the medical board in Illinois with respect to an Illinois practitioner. An Ohio physician was criminally charged after prescribing drugs on the Internet without physically examining the patients. Colorado, Maryland and Wisconsin have also taken action against physicians for prescribing on the Web.

Various state Attorneys General have initiated lawsuits against online entities for improper online prescription sales. For example, the Attorney General of Kansas filed a suit against several online pharmacies and physicians, obtaining temporary restraining orders to prevent them from selling pharmaceuticals over the Internet. This was after state investigators were allegedly able to obtain prescription-only medications without a prescription or a physician consultation. These actions allege that the defendants are engaging in the unauthorized practice of medicine and pharmacy and are violating state merchandising laws by selling prescription drugs to consumers without proper state licensure or registration. The Illinois Attorney General's office sued four companies for online prescription sales, alleging violations of state consumer fraud and medical regulation laws by selling prescription drugs without proper licensing. The New Jersey Attorney General sued numerous online pharmacies for illegally selling prescription drugs. The Attorney General of Arizona sued a Nevada-based online pharmacy because prescriptions were written by doctors unlicensed in Arizona and who didn't physically examine the patients. The Missouri Attorney General obtained a permanent injunction against a Texas-based Internet pharmacy, and the Pennsylvania Attorney General obtained injunctions against Arizona-based companies.

State legislators are taking action to prohibit Internet prescription sales. The Nevada state legislature, for example, has enacted statutes to address illegal Internet pharmacies. Under NRS § 453.3638, selling prescription drugs via the Internet is a category C felony for individuals operating from within Nevada and for individuals outside the state who knowingly prescribe to Nevada patients. Under NRS § 453.3643, Nevada practitioners are expressly prohibited from prescribing medications unless they have physically examined the patient within the past 6 months when they suspect an illegal Internet pharmacy will fill the prescription. Out of state practitioners are similarly prohibited with respect to Nevada patients.

The folks on Capitol Hill are also involved. Representative Ron Klink of Pennsylvania introduced the Internet Pharmacy Consumer Protection Act (H.R. 2763) to amend the Food, Drug and Cosmetic Act by requiring Internet pharmacies to post the name of the principal practitioner, the address and telephone number of the principal business location and the states in which the pharmacy and its consulting physicians are licensed to practice. Failure to comply with the requirements of the law would empower authorities to shut down the enterprise and impose sanctions.

Controlled Substances Online

So far we've been talking about prescription drugs. Anabolic steroids are, of course, prescription drugs. They're also controlled substances. The DEA doesn't care where you get your Propecia® or other prescription medications. That's for the FDA to investigate. But once a controlled substance is involved, DEA jurisdiction kicks in. Online pharmacies that sell controlled substances are a big concern for them.

> Like the AMA, DEA views the invisible doctor scenario as *not* constituting a legitimate doctor-patient relationship. Physicians engaged in this type of practice with respect to controlled substances are unlawfully dispensing these drugs, and are subjecting themselves to criminal sanctions.

First of all, in order for a local pharmacy to start processing controlled substance prescriptions, it must be registered with the DEA. Internet pharmacies are held to the same responsibilities. The physical location of the pharmacy that actually stores and dispenses the controlled substances to be processed by the Internet site must be registered with DEA (as well as licensed by the state in which the pharmacy is located and the states where patients will be located).

Could an entrepreneur set up a legitimate online longevity clinic and pharmacy to prescribe and dispense controlled substances like anabolics? Yes, provided that the entity conformed to all legal and ethical requirements. For example, the pharmacy would need to be registered with DEA and with all applicable states, and a system would need to be created wherein each and every patient would have a physical examination by a physician. Few entrepreneurs are likely to conform to the rules.

Instead, many of these entities lack face-to-face contact between patient and physician. Like the AMA, DEA views the invisible doctor scenario as *not* constituting a legitimate doctor-patient relationship. Physicians engaged in this type of practice with respect to controlled substances are unlawfully dispensing these drugs, and are subjecting themselves to criminal sanctions. In practice, however, many of the sites involved in this practice are located outside the U.S., and the physicians associated with them may also be outside American jurisdiction. The DEA recognizes that effective actions against these illegal suppliers are hampered by a variety of factors, one of which is that these suppliers, who often operate through "evaporating" web sites, are very hard to locate and identify. Even if identification is possible, the practical and jurisdictional problems of trying to go after faraway, overseas entities can be insurmountable. So these sites will likely continue to operate.

Online Prescriptions: The Risks to the Consumer

What about the consumer who purchases an AAS prescription through one of these sites? Since the invisible doctor scenario is bogus, any prescriptions issued pursuant to this situation are *invalid*. An invalid prescription is not a lawful one. So the consumer who obtains anabolics under this relationship is not in lawful possession of the controlled substance and faces the risk of prosecution as if he had no prescription at all. The "three month supply" enforcement flexibility of the FDA for prescription drugs does *not* apply to controlled substances. The exemption authority under 21 U.S.C. § 956 and 21 CFR § 1301.26 for up to fifty dosage units of controlled substances only applies to *land borders*, not mail importations. Unless you're registered as an importer, you can be arrested and prosecuted for ordering juice online.

An invalid prescription is not a lawful one.

Sounds harsh, doesn't it? Well, DEA concedes that the ordinary consumer may somewhat reasonably believe that prescriptions obtained through the websites in this category are legal. They've indicated that a large-scale public information campaign should necessarily precede any actions taken against the consumer. Hopefully, they'll stick to that position. However, anybody who purchases anabolics through one of these outfits is risking legal consequences.

The Bottom Line

In sum, I hate to be the bearer of bad news, but the prospects of getting gear legally over the Internet are slim to none. There are all sorts of ways of getting jammed up. For example, my firm represented a woman who ordered Valium® (a controlled substance) from a web site that did *not* require a prescription but seemed quasi-legit. She in fact did have a legitimate medical need for it, and had previously been prescribed the medication by a doctor. When she accepted the delivery of the package, she was arrested and charged in state court with possession of a controlled substance. The web site was actually a sting operation orchestrated by the U.S. Postal Inspector's office, which arranged the controlled delivery of the parcel. While it is highly questionable whether limited government resources are wisely expended in operations like this, it is likely that we have not seen the last of them.

The much more typical way of getting yourself jammed up would be having the AAS package you've ordered online get snagged by law enforcement authorities en route. That's the topic we're heading into straight away.

Chapter 18

THE PACKAGE IS ON ITS WAY

"This is the Night Mail crossing the Border,
Bringing the cheque and the postal order."
– *W.H. Auden (1907-1973)*

The DEA decided a while back that their resources were best spent on the interdiction of narcotics – meaning hard drugs. Every once in a while they'll bust a few low-level juice dealers or even a hapless personal user just for deterrent effect, but only anabolic steroid trafficking of the highest magnitude really interests them much. You see, back when anabolics were first scheduled as controlled substances, DEA started putting some effort into enforcement. Not throwing themselves into it, mind you, but seriously testing the waters. Between February 1991 and February 1995, DEA initiated 355 anabolic steroid investigations resulting in over 400 arrests and over 200 convictions. [C.E. Yesalis and V.S. Cowart, *The Steroids Game* (Champaign, IL; Human Kinetics, 1998), 107] While one Miami gym owner got eight years in prison, DEA brass came to a disappointing conclusion: federal judges were going too easy on AAS traffickers to make it worth the DEA's while.

The frustrations of federal law enforcement were expressed in June of 1995 when DEA's Office of Diversion Control held a "Conference on the Impact of National Steroid Control Legislation." Presenting their observations since enactment of the Anabolic Steroid Control Act of 1990, they lamented that the guidelines hampered their ability to fight trafficking. Urging that convicted steroid offenders be subject to longer imprisonment, they called for amendments "so that steroids are treated as seriously as any other Schedule III drug." Ironically, this is the same agency that had *opposed* scheduling steroids at all just a few years earlier!

Enter the Postal Inspectors and Customs Service

While DEA really has very limited interest in AAS cases anymore, the U.S. Customs Office of Field Operations and the U.S. Postal Inspection Service are completely different. Now that the anthrax scare has scaled down for the moment, these guys are looking for something new to do. In the War on Drugs, compared to the busy DEA, the Postal and Customs guys are practically sitting on their hands. Steroid cases are the best thing that's happened to them. The Internet has created a veritable explosion of international commerce, which lends itself perfectly to the importation of products like juice that are readily available throughout the world but heavily restricted in domestic manufacture. Last year, investigations by the U.S. Postal Inspectors led to the seizure of more than 288,000 units of steroids. (U.S. Postal Inspection Service, *2001 Annual Report of Investigations, Illegal Drugs and Trafficking*) That's a lot of gear, but that's just the report of the Postal Inspector, not U.S. Customs, which is involved in a lot more AAS seizures. Last year, U.S. Customs agents made 8,724 seizures, up 46 percent

Last year, investigations by the U.S. Postal Inspectors led to the seizure of more than 288,000 units of steroids.

from 1999 and up eight-fold from 1994. AAS busts are a godsend to these agencies, which can easily rack up some decent arrest numbers to justify a bigger budget next year. Accordingly, they have every incentive to get a peek into your package in the hopes of snagging a collar out of it.

> *Doug was a clean-cut computer technician in his late 20s, married with two children and living in Connecticut. Doug worked out hard and intermittently used juice. He didn't trust the dealers at the local gym. The last thing he wanted to do was get caught and charged with a felony. He had a lot to lose. The lure of the Internet called to him. He went online to explore the possibility of connecting with a steroid source. He used various techniques to conceal his identity, such as using the computer terminal at his local library. Feeling secure in his anonymity, he found a steroid source apparently located in far-off China. He reached out to the source, using encrypted messages for all of his communications. The source offered an extremely reasonable price for a variety of anabolics, including some exotic, custom stuff. The source assured that the package would be mailed discreetly, in several different small packages, decreasing the likelihood of close inspection. To prevent the creation of a paper trail, Doug was told to wire the funds, in advance. Doug was advised to open a private mailbox in which to receive the gear. Doug followed the instructions he was given.*
>
> *A few days later, Doug went to the box after work to collect his prize. Instead, he found a piece of correspondence from the Department of the Treasury. Apparently, U.S. Customs had intercepted and seized his package, and had found it contained steroids. The letter told him he could contest the seizure, or he could waive his rights in the package. The envelope included a form for him to sign and mail back. Doug didn't know what to do. He contacted his source and complained. His package had been seized and now he was in trouble. He was out several hundred dollars. The source assured him everything would be made right. Several days passed. Doug went to the box after work one day, and was greeted by two federal agents. One said he was from U.S. Customs. He had a package in his hands addressed to Doug. The package appeared to have been opened and resealed. He asked Doug if he was expecting anything in particular. Doug said, "No." The agent asked if he could open the package. Uncertain but intimidated, Doug agreed. To Doug's horror, the contents of the box were not a refund of his money, but instead a replacement shipment of the anabolics he ordered. Things went downhill from there.*

Of course, there's a legitimate governmental interest in identifying and confiscating illegal materials in the mail. "Inspectors" for the Postal Service aren't like the Hanes underwear inspector or Laverne and Shirley, standing on an assembly line watching packages pass by. They are federal law enforcement special agents trained to investigate and interdict crimes involving the use of the U.S. Postal Service, including mail bombs and child porn. They carry badges and firearms and have arrest powers. We may not even mind so much if they go a little overboard sometimes, as long as they're doing something praiseworthy like seizing some mailed obscene materials from the creep who's been hanging around your kids' middle school. But for our own letters and packages, we very much *do* mind if Big Brother starts poking around. We seal our personal correspondences in envelopes expecting them to be kept private. Our right to that privacy seems fundamental.

The balancing between the government's interdiction interests and our privacy rights in our letters and packages has created a body of Fourth Amendment jurisprudence made up of cases, statutes and regulations. Let's see what we've got.

Domestic U.S. Mail

As previously discussed in Chapter 7, the Fourth Amendment protects against unreasonable searches and seizures of those things in which there exists a *legitimate expectation of privacy*: our "persons, houses, papers and effects." [*Katz v. United States*, 389 U.S. 347 (1967)] Implicit is our privacy interest in the personal letters and correspondence – the papers and effects – that we send to others and they send to us. In 1878, the U.S. Supreme Court in *Ex parte Jackson* [96 U.S. 727 (1878)] held that letters and sealed packages in the United States mail are as fully protected as if they were kept in the sender's own house, and can only be opened and examined pursuant to a search warrant based upon probable cause. But the Court distinguished between "different kinds of mail matter – between what is intended to be kept free from inspection, such as letters, and sealed packages subject to letter postage; and what is open to inspection, such as newspapers, magazines, pamphlets, and other printed matter, purposely left in a condition to be examined."

... the U.S. Supreme Court ... held that letters and sealed packages in the United States mail are as fully protected as if they were kept in the sender's own house ...

Congress followed up by authorizing the creation of different classes of mail, protecting only the *highest* class from warrantless searches: "The Postal Service shall maintain one or more classes of mail for the transmission of letters sealed against inspection. ... One such class shall provide for the most expeditious handling and transportation afforded mail matter by the Postal Service. No letter of such a class of domestic origin shall be opened except under authority of a search warrant authorized by law ...". [39 U.S.C. § 3623(d)]

The Postal Service protects the type of mail intended for actual or personal correspondence: *First Class Mail* (including *Priority Mail*) and *Express Mail*. Periodicals (formerly Second Class Mail), Standard Mail (formerly Third Class Mail), and Package Services (formerly Fourth Class Mail) are *not* protected from warrantless inspection. (*See* www.usps.gov for definitions, rates and fees.)

Domestic Mail Protected from Warrantless Search

Protected	*Unprotected*
First Class Mail	Periodicals
Priority Mail	Standard Mail
Express Mail	Package Services

As part of their routine, postal inspectors have a "drug-smuggling profile" to help identify suspicious mailings. The court-approved profile includes: size and shape of the mailing; heavy wrapping in tape with an attempt to seal all openings; hand printed or written labels; unusual return name and address; unusual odors coming from the package; fictitious return address; package sent from or to a "source city or a destination city" for illegal drugs. [*U.S. v. Hill*, 701 F. Supp. 1522 (D. Kan. 1988); *see also U.S. v. Daniel*, 982 F.2d 146 (5th Cir. 1993)]

Obtaining a Warrant to Open a Protected Package

Protected mail that is suspicious mail can be *temporarily detained – but not opened* – for investigation if inspectors have a *reasonable suspicion* of criminal activity and the packages aren't detained for an unreasonable time. [*U.S. v. Van Leeuwen*, 397 U.S. 249 (1970)] Investigation may include shaking or feeling the outside of the mailing, x-raying it, researching the identities or addresses of the designated sender or recipient, or subjecting the mailing to a drug-sniffing dog. A dog-sniff test does not require probable cause or a warrant. [*See U.S. v. Place*, 462 U.S. 696 (1983)] However, as of this writing, no canine unit in America has been trained to detect anabolic steroids.

... as of this writing, no canine unit in America has been trained to detect anabolic steroids.

If the investigation uncovers facts that raise suspicion to the higher level of probable cause, the inspectors will prepare an affidavit in support of an application for a *search warrant* to open the package. This is typically done by preparing a form called an Application and Affidavit for Search Warrant and presenting it to a federal magistrate. Note that if contraband is found in the protected package and a decision is made to do a controlled delivery, a *second* warrant will be requested. Typically, this will be a search warrant for the suspect's residence, and it will be conditioned upon the suspect taking possession of the package under controlled circumstances (under surveillance). This second warrant will typically be presented to a state court judge, not a federal judge.

The Application for a warrant to open the protected package will be captioned something like this: "In the Matter of a Search of a Priority Mail parcel approximately 12 ½" X 9 ½" X ¼", addressed to C. White, 2251 Belton Vista Drive, Houston, TX 77000, bearing a return address of B.G., 231 17th Street, East Meadow, NY 11500." The postal inspector will attach an affidavit stating the weight of the package, the Post Office from which it was mailed, the date it was postmarked, and the facts supporting probable cause. Once signed by a magistrate, the warrant permits the mailing to be opened and the contents examined. Where investigative circumstances require, delays of up to 72 hours between the detention of suspicious mailings and the approval of a magistrate have been upheld as "not unreasonable." [*U.S. v. Aldaz*, 921 F.2d 227 (9th Cir. 1990)]

So let's be clear here. Protected mail and packages in the United States Postal Service mail system are prevented from being opened *without* a warrant, not protected from being opened at all. Can a warrant be obtained? You bet your striated glutes it can if there's probable cause, and I've seen numerous situations (most recently in Michigan) where postal inspectors were able to convince a judge to sign a warrant on information that's a bit, well, "iffy."

What happens if the feds have enough to strongly suspect juice in a protected domestic package in the U.S. mail, but *not* quite enough to get a warrant to open it? They can do a "knock-and-talk" with package in hand, and more likely than not they'll get a collar out of it. But not always. Here's what they did to Jack, a college student in a Southern university.

> *Jack answered a knock on his door to find two gentlemen in suits from the U.S. Postal Service. They had a package addressed to him, and asked if they could come in. Caught off guard, Jack let them into his foyer. They asked for consent to open the package and produced a form for Jack*

to sign. Jack told them that he did not order the package and that he did not want it. They said, "We know there are illegal drugs inside this package." Jack said the package could have a bomb or anything else in it and since he didn't want any part of it, he most certainly wouldn't have them open it in his house. They growled, "You're in deep trouble. We know you ordered this package. If you work with us in building evidence against the guy who sent it, you'll be off the hook." Jack said he had no interest in doing any such thing because he did not order the package and wanted nothing to do with it. "We can just get a warrant to open," they hollered. "Get out of my house, please," Jack said firmly. At this point, they looked at their feet for a while, took the package and left. It's the last Jack saw of them.

Private Courier Packages

The Fourth Amendment protects against unreasonable searches and seizures conducted by the *government* and those acting in conjunction with it. It does *not* generally protect against the actions of *private parties*. The illegal seizure of evidence by a private party will not be attributed to the government when the private party turns the evidence over to the government. [*See Coolidge v. New Hampshire*, 403 U.S. 443 (1971); *Burdeau v. McDowell*, 256 U.S. 465 (1921)] Whether the privacy invasions by the employees of a private carrier are accidental or deliberate, or are reasonable or unreasonable, because of their private character they do not violate the Fourth Amendment. [*U.S. v. Jacobsen*, 466 U.S. 109 (1983)] Searches by private carriers have been upheld as private, not governmental. [*U.S. v. Young*, 153 F.3d 1079 (9th Cir. 1998); *see also U.S. v. Koenig*, 856 F.2d 843 (7th Cir. 1988)]

... courier companies like UPS and FedEx do not handle U.S. mail and their conduct is *not* restricted by the statutory protections.

While domestic First-Class or Express Mail cannot be opened without a warrant signed by a judge and based upon probable cause, courier companies like UPS and FedEx do not handle U.S. mail and their conduct is *not* restricted by the statutory protections. As private parties, they reserve the right to inspect packages tendered for transport according to their own policies. [*U.S. v. Young*, 153 F.3d 1079 (9th Cir. 1998); *U.S. v. Souza*, 223 F.3d 1197 (10th Cir. 2000)] UPS has a standard policy, for example, of inspecting packages insured for more than $1,000 to ensure proper packing. [*See U.S. v. Parker*, 32 F.3d 395 (8th Cir. 1994)]

Courts have held that those who use private couriers simply have a lesser expectation of privacy in their packages:

> "... [T]he most dangerous aspect of trafficking in narcotics lies ... in the distribution. This is especially true where the drugs have been consigned to a third person for shipment. During that period, the principals have relinquished all control over items which could lead to their arrest. Should the drugs be exposed, and if their nature as contraband is immediately apparent, they must know that their arrest will follow. Their privacy interest then is dependent upon two factors: the risk of exposure and the incriminating appearance of the contraband. ... [T]he possibility that Federal Express would for some purpose open the package, be it for reasons of security, an accident, or damage, is a risk that must, or at least should have been considered by [Defendant] when he decided to

use their services. ... That decision could only serve to reduce his subjective expectation of privacy in the parcel consigned." [*U.S. v. Barry*, 673 F.2d 912, 919 (6th Cir. 1982)]

The court decisions in private carrier seizure cases generally provide the details of how the suspect came undone. Usually a package is opened because it is damaged, odorous or leaking, or because it is suspicious to the shipper's employees due to its appearance. Other cases have involved citizen "tips" about illegal contents [*U.S. v. Martin*, 157 F.3d 46 (2nd Cir. 1998)] and identification of the package by DEA officials during drug parcel interdiction training at the carrier's facility [*Souza, supra*].

In *U.S. v. Jacobsen, supra*, FedEx employees saw a damaged package and opened it pursuant to a written company policy regarding insurance claims (although a post-trial affidavit indicated that they might have opened the package because it was suspicious, not damaged.) While examining the contents, they cut the end of a suspicious looking tape tube and observed a white powdery substance concealed within eight layers of wrappings. They summoned a DEA agent, who removed a trace of the powder, subjected it to a chemical test and determined it was cocaine. The Supreme Court held that a DEA agent's field test, although exceeding the scope of the private search by the carrier, was not an unlawful "search" or "seizure" requiring a warrant before doing so. The decision was based on the grounds that the privacy interest in the package had already been largely compromised, and that a chemical test that merely discloses whether or not something is a controlled substance, and no other arguably "private" fact, diminishes no legitimate privacy interest.

International Mail and Packages

While domestic First Class Mail is expressly protected, incoming *international* mail is different. In 1977, the Supreme Court in *U.S. v. Ramsey* [431 U.S. 606 (1977)] resolved a legal conflict among the Circuit Courts as to whether the Fourth Amendment prohibited the opening of incoming international letter-class mail without probable cause or a search warrant. The case involved a sack of mail from Thailand that was being inspected at the General Post Office in New York City, where international airmail landing at Kennedy Airport is taken for routing and customs inspections. A customs officer spotted eight "rather bulky" envelopes. Aware that Thailand is a country known as a source of narcotics and feeling something in the envelopes other than plain paper, he weighed them and found them to be substantially heavier than normal mail. He opened them and found heroin.

> ... it makes no difference that an item is *mailed*, not carried, across the border. Neither probable cause nor a warrant is required.

The Court's analysis relied on the Fourth Amendment's "border search" exception. The acceptance of border searches without a warrant or probable cause has a history rooted in English statutes dating back centuries, grounded in the right of the sovereign to protect its borders against inbound contraband and to collect duties on inbound freight. Even before the adoption of the Fourth Amendment, such searches at traditional land borders have been considered "reasonable" merely by the single fact that the person or item in question had entered into our country from outside.

In applying the border search exception to incoming mail, the Court in *Ramsey* found that it makes no difference that an item is *mailed*, not carried, across the border. Neither probable cause nor a warrant is required. But the Court noted that Congress has expressly authorized customs officials "to search any trunk or envelope" only if based upon "reasonable cause to suspect" a violation of law, [19 U.S.C. § 482] and that regulations allow international mail that appears to contain matter in addition to, or other than, correspondence, to be opened by customs only with reasonable cause to suspect the presence of merchandise or contraband. [19 CFR § 145.3(a); authorized by 19 CFR § 145.2] Further, customs is generally restricted from the warrantless opening of any sealed mail which appears to contain only correspondence [19 CFR § 145.3(b)] and is prohibited from reading any correspondence without a warrant authorizing that action. [19 CFR § 145.3(c)] The Court was satisfied that these extra safeguards adequately protect Constitutional rights in personal correspondence from outside the country, and upheld the search as valid.

Since *Ramsey*, the border search exception has been expanded to searches of persons and things *exiting* the United States (exit searches) [*see U.S. v. Des Jardins*, 747 F.2d 499 (9th Cir. 1984), *vacated in part on other grounds*, 772 F.2d 578 (9th Cir. 1985); *U.S. v. Udofot*, 711 F.2d 831, (8th Cir. 1983)] and to searches significantly removed from the actual border crossing in time or distance under the so-called "extended border" doctrine [*see U.S. v. Alfonso*, 759 F.2d 728 (9th Cir. 1985)]. The extended border search doctrine has been applied to exit searches of *outgoing* international mail even 3,000 miles from the border. [*See U.S. v. Cardona*, 769 F.2d 625 (9th Cir. 1985); *U.S. v. Whiting*, 781 F.2d 692 (9th Cir. 1986)]

> ... the border search exception has been expanded to searches of persons and things *exiting* the United States ...

Who in government can conduct searches of the international mail? Only an official from an agency specifically authorized to conduct such searches. It has been held that the U.S. Customs Service, Border Patrol and Coast Guard are so authorized; the F.B.I. and Office of Export Enforcement are *not*.

How are international drug packages seized? The largest international mail facility in the nation is JFK International Airport in New York. With 120 international flights arriving every day, the volume of incoming mail is huge (over 30 million pieces of mail each year). An interview with John McCormick, branch chief of U.S. Customs at JFK airport ("Illegal Arrival," *ZDTV.com*, August 18, 2000), described the process of identifying and seizing illegal drugs. First, suspicious packages are profiled and segregated by inspectors. Some are subjected to canine sniffs, and others are x-rayed in a holding room called "the cage." After being tested, processed and assigned a seizure number, a drug package is routed to the vault, where it is stored while a decision is made about what to do with it. The inspectors then notify the Customs investigators about each day's drug seizures (usually about 50) that could possibly be prosecuted. Decisions are made as to which packages will be resolved with seizure notices and which ones will become controlled deliveries (see Chapter 19).

Package Seizures and Seizure Notices

Let's say you're one of the unlucky ones, and the Postal Inspector or Customs identifies your package as containing a controlled substance and seizes it. Maybe it leaked or smelled funny or otherwise looked suspicious. Maybe they x-rayed it, and saw the pills and ampoules. Now they have two options. They can either confiscate your package or they can deliver it under controlled circumstances in order to arrest you. If they choose to confiscate, they will let you know that they have the item by sending you a letter. This correspondence, commonly called a seizure notice or seizure letter, informs you that the feds have the package. The letter advises you of your rights and remedies to challenge the seizure and try to claim the parcel. While there are several variations, here's a typical example of a seizure notice from the U.S. Customs Service:

Dear Sir/Madam:

The records of this office indicate that you may have an interest in Winstrol Depot, Profasi, Serno Disolvent, Ventolase and a Ceramic Figurine seized by the U.S. Customs Service, Port of Louisville, Kentucky on August 23, 2002. The property was seized under the provisions of Title 19, United States Code, Section 1595a(c) as it was determined to be in violation of Title 21, United States Code, Section 952. The medication, a controlled substance, was illegally submitted for entry into the United States. The ceramic figurine was used to facilitate the importation of the medication.

The domestic value of the medication was determined to be under $250.00.

Under the provisions of Title 19 United States Code, Section 1618, you may petition for relief from the above liability. The enclosed Notice of Seizure and Information for Claimants explains your options with regard to the remission of the forfeiture of seized property. If you wish to petition for relief from forfeiture, you must provide an express agreement to defer judicial or administrative forfeiture proceedings until completion of the administrative process. Completion of the enclosed Election of Proceedings form will provide this express agreement.

Your petition for relief must be received within 30 days from the date of this notice and should be filed in triplicate at the following address ...

Sincerely,

____

The Election of Proceedings form looks like this:

ELECTION OF PROCEEDINGS
FORM AF-POST

NOTE: READ THE ATTACHED "NOTICE OF SEIZURE AND INFORMATION FOR CLAIMANTS" BEFORE YOU FILL OUT THIS FORM. THIS FORM MUST BE COMPLETED AND RETURNED WITH YOUR PETITION OR OFFER. IF YOU DO NOT COMPLETE AND RETURN THIS FORM, WE SHALL PROCEED TO FORFEIT THE PROPERTY ADMINISTRATIVELY, REGARDLESS OF WHETHER YOU FILE AT PETITION OF OFFER.
TO: CUSTOM FINES, PENALTIES AND FORFEITURES OFFICER.

I understand that property in which I have an interest has been seized by the U.S. Customs Service, under Case No. .

Check ONLY ONE (1) of the following choices:

[ ] **REQUEST THAT THE CUSTOMS SERVICE CONSIDER MY PETITION OR OFFER ADMINISTRATIVELY.** That document is attached. By making this request, I understand that I am giving up my right to (1) begin administrative forfeiture proceedings immediately, as provided by title 19, United States Code (U.S.C.), section 1607 and title 19, Code Federal Regulations (CFR), section 162.45, or (2) Immediate referral of the case to the U.S. Attorney for court action as provided by 19 U.S.C. 1608 and 19 CFR 162.47. If administrative forfeiture has begun, it will be stopped until my petition or offer is considered. However, I understand that at *any time* I can request, in writing, that you begin administrative forfeiture proceedings, and you will continue to consider my petition or offer. I also understand that at *any time* I can file a claim and cost bond with you, and Customs consideration of my petition or offer will stop and the case will be sent to the U.S. Attorney for court action

[ ] **REQUEST THAT THE CUSTOMS SERVICE BEGIN ADMINISTRATIVE PROCEEDINGS TO FORFEIT THE PROPERTY.** Please immediately begin the posting of the notice of seizure and intent to forfeit the property, and consider my petition or offer, if any. I understand that within 20 days of the first publication of the notice, I can request that you send the case to the U.S. Attorney for court action.

[ ] **REQUEST THAT THE CUSTOMS SERVICE REFER THE CASE FOR COURT ACTION**. Please immediately refer the case to the U.S. Attorney for a court decision. I am filing/will file a claim and cost bond with you.

Signature ______________________ Date ______________________

You can, of course, challenge the seizure. However, unless you have a lawful basis for possessing the controlled substances, such as a valid prescription, you won't get far. In fact, your attempts to claim the package may backfire. Identifying yourself to the U.S. Attorney as the person who ordered the juice and intended to receive it could quite probably get you busted.

You can accept the confiscation and forfeiture by checking the box, signing the form, and mailing it back. Or, instead, you can do nothing. The notice provides that if you simply ignore it, they will proceed with administrative proceedings to forfeit the property anyway. After 20 days, you will have forfeited any interests you may have had in the parcel. You won't get it back. Then again, you also won't be volunteering to be busted or signing anything that might be better not to have on record. The majority of people who call me to report that their packages were seized don't sign or return the letter, and it's the last they hear of it ... until the next package.

A government record is made of every seizure. Various bits of identifying information are entered into a nationwide database for future reference. This information includes your name and address, the return address, and in international mailings, the country of origin. While return addresses are often fictitious, the use of the same fictitious address in the future will trigger an alert on the package. Information on the country of origin is useful in identifying source trends and so-called "hot" countries. Federal authorities can place a watch on your address or flag your name for future deliveries. In the majority of cases I've handled where controlled deliveries were conducted, the target had previously received a seizure notice under the same name or designated to the same address. Remember Doug, the hero of the true tale that started this chapter? There was a mail watch on Doug's box because of the previous seizure. Sadly, Doug's miscommunication with his source over the rectification of the seized package resulted in his arrest and prosecution.

Federal authorities can place a watch on your address or flag your name for future deliveries.

How "Big Brother" Is Watching

When your international package is seized by customs, your name and address is stored in a database. That same database might also contain the name and location of Post Office boxes you've set up under that name, any orders you might have placed for cattle implants, any tickets, prior convictions, or other seizures you are connected with. This is just the beginning. The reality is that most people have no idea what information the government has access to or can cross-reference. For instance, Customs officials might refer to a system known as TECS II, the Treasury Enforcement Communication System. This system is available to the IRS, Customs, the Secret Service and the U.S. Mint, and contains records of seizure information, parcels, prices, license plates, and names and addresses, among other information. This information is compiled primarily by input from various agencies and information gathered through interviews and investigations. The High Intensity Drug Trafficking Areas (HIDTA) are areas nationwide, designated by the Office of National Drug Control Policy (ONDCP). In order to address the drug trafficking in these areas, a variety of information systems and software are utilized. For instance, Autotrack products gather information from public sources and produce personal profile information, such as addresses, phone numbers, relatives, and real estate on those associates.

But this is just one of the many sources available. In New Mexico, for example, the New Mexico Investigative Support Center (NMISC) currently has the following databases available: Internal Database System, Treasury Enforcement Communication System (TECS) II, Private Aircraft Enforcement System (PAES), Automated Commercial System (ACS), National Criminal Information Center (NCIC), National Law Enforcement Teletype System (NLETS), INS Central Index System (CIS), Commercial Drivers License Information System (CDLIS), New Mexico Taxation and Revenue Departments Customer Information Control System (CICS), Inspection Selection System (ISS), DEA Narcotics and Dangerous Drugs Information System (NADDIS), New Mexico Criminal Justice Information System (CJIS), FBI Field Office Information Management System (FOIMS), AutoTrack, PhoneDisk, Internet, Information America, Texas Household Drivers Report (HDR), and Albuquerque PD Computer Offense Program System (ACOPS). As you can see, there is an exhaustive list of resources from which even state law enforcement authorities can draw. The feds have even more juice (excuse the pun). More information can be accessed at the United States Department of Justice web site, www. usdoj.gov/dea/foia/foiatoc.html.

Looking from the Other Side

I've seen a few hundred cases that were slight variations on the true tale that started this chapter. To detail each one would be more repetitive than helpful. What is helpful, though, would be to look at the process from the *other* side, which can be done by examining the applications and affidavits that cops draft up to get judges to sign search and seizure warrants. Here's what led to a controlled delivery in Maryland:

> *Customs Special Agent Jameson of the Mail Division was working a detail at Dulles International Airport and came across a suspicious courier parcel addressed to "L. Bates" in Maryland. There was no sender's address. He opened it (it was an international package, so he didn't need a warrant, remember?) and found "200 dosages of Clenbuterol." The parcel was seized, a warning letter was sent out, and the name and address were entered into the Customs computer database. Two weeks later, Special Agent Henderson of Customs was working at Dulles and was alerted to a package addressed to "Larry Bates" at a different address – a private mail box – but in the same county. This one had a return address from the United Kingdom. Henderson opened the package, finding fifteen vials of Sustanon and one vial of Ketamine, also a Schedule III drug. Henderson checked the courier records and Express Mail records of parcel deliveries to the address in question, as well as parcel records coming from the U.K. address. There were numerous previous parcels to the private mail box, all from the U.K., and all of the same size and weight as this one. He contacted the Maryland State Police (MSP). The MSP did a motor vehicle check on Larry Bates and found out his race, height, weight, date of birth and registered vehicles. The MSP also did a criminal background check. The MSP told Special Agent Henderson that they would be interested in doing a controlled delivery of the package, and requested that the parcel be forwarded to them through Customs officials in Maryland.*

You'll notice that Larry's package containing clenbuterol got only a warning. Clenbuterol is not a federal controlled substance, although it is on the Customs alert list and is subject to immediate confiscation and seizure. His second package earned a controlled delivery, probably because there was already a record of the first one. The fact that there was some ketamine in the parcel surely didn't help. While only a Schedule III drug, ketamine is a hot target right now and you're really asking for trouble if you have some tossed into an AAS package. I should make clear, though, that the vast majority of AAS cases I've handled have involved *only* anabolic steroids and non-controlled ancillary bodybuilding medications. I can think of no steroid cases that involved heroin, only one steroid case that involved cocaine, and only a small minority that involved marijuana or Ecstasy.

> ... the vast majority of AAS cases I've handled have involved *only* anabolic steroids and non-controlled ancillary bodybuilding medications.

Worry about the Other Guy

Now here's something not many guys think about. Maybe there's no watch on your address, but there could be a watch on the address of the *sender* of a package to you. If he's under surveillance and mails a steroid package to you, that package may be intercepted and delivered to you under controlled circumstances. You could get jammed up even if it isn't gear. Look at what happened in this Michigan case:

> *Teddy in California was under surveillance by the Postal Inspector as a suspected steroid dealer. Bill in Michigan ran a bodybuilding supplement business. When Teddy sent a UPS overnight package to Bill using a false name and old address, local Michigan police were notified. They seized the package, which was found to contain $4,000 in cash. While there was insufficient evidence to charge Bill with any offense, the police suspected wrongdoing and refused to release the package to either Teddy or Bill. Bill got a local lawyer to fight for his money, but the anticipated legal fees favored a compromise with the local police, allowing them to keep part of the money.*

All sorts of ways have been devised to try to evade Customs seizures. While most foreign shippers use small flat envelopes on the theory that they will attract less attention, sources have hidden juice in every conceivable container, including hollowed-out books and paper stacks, ceramic statuettes, videocassettes, stereo speakers, and locked boxes. Imaginative shippers have used cold cream bottles to submerge the amps right into the cream, or even put tablets into vitamin bottles and resealed the bottles. The problem, of course, is that if the inspectors go through the hassle of getting at them, the amps or tabs themselves would provide probable cause to get a warrant for a raid.

Perhaps an even more ingenious method that's been used has been to package injectable steroids in alternative containers likely to contain oil, such as aromatherapy oil bottles. An inspector who examined the product, although suspicious, might not have probable cause to get a warrant to raid the house after a controlled delivery. The only way to get probable cause might be to lab test the oil. The testing would likely take at least a few days and maybe longer. If the person awaiting shipment was tracking the package via the courier's online tracking service, he might know not to accept it long before the controlled delivery arrived (depending on the reliability of the courier's system). Of course, suspicious Customs investigators could always just do a knock-and-talk with the package, and most likely obtain incriminating admissions. Also, once Customs was wise to the method, it would be useless after that, and it's unlikely that a source would be able to keep switching his packaging to stay ahead of the feds. Even the so-called paper products of recent popularity are not foolproof. Feds learned long ago what blotter paper looks like because it was once used for LSD. All things in life are fraught with risk.

Playing Bad Odds

What percentage of mailed AAS parcels are identified and seized? Nobody can say. The government won't tell us, especially if the number is quite low, because it might undermine the deterrent effect. I see a lot of cases of mail seizures and controlled deliveries, but I naturally don't know about all the packages that make it through. Clearly, the heightened privacy protections in domestic U.S. postal mail make it harder to open domestic mail. While many clients have told me that they feel domestic First Class mail is pretty safe, I've seen situations where the police have gotten a warrant and opened a parcel. International mail, by all accounts, is more risky. Based on the number of controlled deliveries of international packages I've seen, I have to say that ordering gear from overseas, especially repeatedly, is almost begging to be busted.

... I have to say that ordering gear from overseas, especially repeatedly, is almost begging to be busted.

Former clients of mine with extensive personal experience in these matters tell me that due to the overwhelming volume of mail arriving from daily from outside the U.S., the number of parcels that make it through unmolested is astonishingly high. But look at it this way: even if 90% get through, that means out of ten guys who order, one will get bagged! Or, since most juicers proceed to make multiple purchases over time, if a guy makes ten purchases he's almost certain to get busted! That might very well be you!

Chapter 19

CONTROLLED DELIVERY Q & A

"Someone is coming to get you:
The mailman ... enters with a letter on a tray
Whose message is to change everything..."
–John Ashbery, U.S. poet (b. 1927)

If a package is identified as containing a controlled substance, the authorities can conduct what the government calls a "controlled delivery" of the package. That sounds nice, doesnt' it? A "controlled delivery." It's one of those bloodless government terms that sound benign enough, as if it were a function that a calm, kindly mailman might perform. It's actually anything but. First, a band of government agents will lie in wait, covert operatives playing a cat and mouse game until you make the horrific mistake of accepting your mail. Then, like a plague of locusts, they'll descend upon the sanctity of your home, ransacking it from roof to basement.

These paramilitary tactics have evolved in order to fight the War on Drugs, and are no doubt necessary in dealing with dangerous cocaine dealers. But I've seen far too many of these operations targeted at hapless personal AAS users. We're talking eight to ten government agents spending their day at the taxpayers' expense sifting through the house of some otherwise law-abiding musclehead for some vials of hormones while his wife and kids are held hostage. The government may claim that they're only going after the big fish. False. Maybe that's what they're trying to do, but they certainly aren't doing it very well. I've seen quite modest amounts of gear deemed worthy of the costs and efforts of controlled deliveries and raids in numerous confirmed cases: 20 tablets and 10 vials (North Carolina); 300 Anabol tablets (Grand Rapids, Michigan); 20 vials of testosterone (Lansing, Michigan); 150 Anabol tablets (Cincinnati, Ohio); 10 Sustanon bottles and 150 Winstrol tablets (Texas); 13 testosterone vials and 200 D-bol (North Dakota) and many, many others. In fact, I'd estimate that the *majority* of controlled deliveries I've seen have involved quantities that are consistent with personal use. Further, of all the controlled deliveries I've seen, only a tiny percentage has been to a teenager or a competitive athlete – the two classes targeted by steroid criminalization. The people being targeted for government raids are mostly cosmetic AAS users in their 30s.

Some state authorities appear to be more into going after juice cases than others. Texas and Michigan seem to produce a high number of calls to my office. But the most active of all is Maryland. It's either the juice capital of America or the anti-juice capital of America. Either the volume of AAS packages destined for the jacked-up population of Maryland is so outrageously out of control that authorities quite reasonably just *have* to do something, or the Maryland State Police really have a massive vendetta against juicers and way too much time on their hands. I've seen more low-level AAS cases in Maryland than anywhere else in the country. I don't know why.

Here's a controlled delivery story from Maryland. I'm reproducing it in the client's own words, just as he sent it to me by e-mail, with only a couple of minor but necessary identity changes:

I was washing my car at approximately 11:00 a.m. when the postman approached with a package. He asked if the address was 1628 and I answered yes and took the package. I set the package down in the garage area and continued to dry my car off. At this time unmarked vehicles swarmed the driveway, a tall male got out the car closest to me and asked if I was [name]. When I answered yes he immediately handcuffed me and said I was under arrest for possession of narcotics and they had a warrant to search the premises. He then proceeded to walk me into the garage area while other agents entered the house. Moments later they came back out and said, "We're clear."

I was then escorted into the house and sat down in the kitchen. I asked to see the warrant and the tall male informed me that it was not my property, and my parents would see it when they got home. They did not have a warrant at this time because phone calls were being made to see if they had it yet. Also, other agents were complaining about the process of getting a warrant, saying that it took too long to get a hold of the judge in many cases. I was questioned about the contents of the package that was delivered and told them I didn't know. It was labeled as PC software, so I told them it probably was. I received packages quite regularly, and explained the return address didn't sound familiar but I do sign up to receive free items quite often. An officer then showed me two packages that had been stopped by Customs and asked what I knew about them, and I told him I knew nothing about them. They asked me if I had any drugs in the house and I told him I had some capsules of DNP, an abbreviation for 2,4 dinitrophenol, a legal pesticide. I showed two agents where the DNP was located, and told them I also had some white pills that I could not identify.

I was then walked back into the kitchen. One agent began asking me for general information (name, address, phone # etc.) but he was interrupted by a female officer because she wanted to read me my rights. Other agents were searching the yard and other rooms in the home. The officers again began to question me about the package, trying to intimidate me. At this time a female officer opened the parcel and inside were twelve ampoules of Sustanon 250. They asked me what they were and by reading the label I was able to tell them the Sustanon looked to be testosterone. I was told I was a "low man on their totem pole" and they hadn't been very busy lately. They said if the drugs were for someone else, I should call that person and they would arrest him instead of me. I also was questioned about some old friends and they said they could make things a lot easier on me if I would sign up to be a confidential informant and help them make a few busts. I was also questioned about who was growing pot in the area. I told them I didn't know because I got myself out of that life many years ago.

At this time another female officer was left to "baby-sit" me while the officer who was questioning me went to search the vehicles including a 1993 Dodge that it was later discovered was not on the search warrant. At one point an agent came out and said, "We have a whole pharmacy back there." They continued to badger me into cooperation and tell them about the drugs and it was at this time I invoked my Miranda rights. The tall male that made the arrest said my mother was on her way home. Not much more was said and a little later the agents brought out two large paper bags, a desktop computer, and a rifle from my room. When an officer asked if I should stay until my mother arrived, the tall male explained that he did not really call her. No one was notified of my arrest during this search and I was not able to call a lawyer when I requested, which I thought I had the right to do as an American citizen. The arresting officer even told me a lawyer couldn't do anything except tell me to sit there and cooperate. He said I would have an opportunity to do so at the detention center.

Anyway, controlled deliveries of anabolics are something we'll need to deal with. So let's talk about the issues that come up most frequently when people ask me about the topic.

Q: What's the deal with signing for a package? Is it, if you sign, you're guilty, but if you don't, you're off the hook?

A: I've heard some people say that. A bit too simplistic to be true, don't you think? Forget it; here's the real deal.

The object of a controlled delivery is to get you to take possession of the package. There are two reasons for this. First, once you accept the package of contraband, you can be arrested for possessing it. There's probable cause that you've committed a crime. Second, before delivering the package to you, the agents will have usually obtained a search warrant to raid your house. However, the warrant is often an *anticipatory warrant,* meaning that it can't be executed until you accept the package (*see* Chapter 7 for more on search warrants). So, the agents need you to accept the package in order to raid your house. The anticipatory warrant, however, won't specify *how* you must accept the package. In other words, I've never seen a judge explicitly require that the target sign for the package. You just have to accept delivery. But the agents must be able to prove it.

This is where the signature comes in. Your signing for the package removes any argument that you didn't accept it. It's proof, right there in your own handwriting, that you took possession of the package. Hell, you signed for it! Could a prosecutor prove that you accepted possession of the package *without* your signature? Of course she could, but it won't be quite as clean or easy. Something printed in black and white that's signed is always very persuasive in court. Especially when it's supported by the undercover agent's testimony about the *conversation* that took place. "Does Johnny Johnson live here?" You said, "Yes." "Are you Johnny John-son?" You nodded. "Will you accept this package?" You said, "Of course!" and looked really excited when you looked down and saw the return address from China. So, signing is not the key here. *Accepting possession* is the key, and signing is one very effective way of proving acceptance.

> Your signing for the package removes any argument that you didn't accept it. It's proof, right there in your own handwriting, that you took possession of the package.

Signing for a package is still the most typical way of accepting possession. Here's another true-life story from Maryland. Vincent was a self-employed landscaper supporting two children. He was 34 years old and had once been a competitive body builder. One day, the postal inspectors seized a domestic Express Mail package at the Baltimore Air Mail Facility that contained a suspected controlled dangerous substance. It was being shipped to an address in Maryland. The feds couldn't open it without a warrant, but they x-rayed it and presented enough cause for a magistrate to sign a search and seizure warrant (Warrant #1) to open the package. The package was found to contain a total of 63 bottles of testosterone, stanozolol, and various other anabolics. The inspector ran an autotrack computer database check on the address and identified Vincent as the resident. A motor vehicle check was then done on Vincent, local police were contacted, and a controlled delivery was arranged.

A mail carrier appeared at Vincent's door one day. Vincent signed for a package and took it inside. After the package was accepted, the agents obtained a search warrant to raid the house (Warrant # 2), which they had arranged in advance to get very quickly. Moments later a platoon of local and state law enforcement agents raided his house. The package had not been opened. A small quantity of anabolic steroids was recovered from inside the house as well as $4,500 in cash and numerous Postal Services mailing receipts and packaging materials. The case was somewhat weak as to the intent to distribute, but Vincent fixed that. Under pressure, Vincent signed a confession admitting distribution to between 20 and 30 people.

Could acceptance of possession be proven in other ways? Absolutely. There's no magic formula here. The issue is determined by looking at all the facts and circumstances of what you did and what you said. Take the conversation we just described, for example, where you admitted that you were "Johnny Johnson." You said you were the person intended to receive the package, and you explicitly stated that you would accept it. Will the absence of a signature magically protect you from a search and raid? Not on your life! Will it protect you from a conviction in court? Not necessarily, but we'll talk more about that later.

Will the absence of a signature magically protect you from a search and raid? Not on your life!

Let's say you're a cagey rascal and you decide you're going to refuse to sign, but try to accept the package verbally. A real courier wouldn't give it to you if a signature was required, but let's say this undercover agent courier would. Have you avoided an arrest, a ransacking of your house, and the seizure of all sorts of incriminating evidence? Of course not, because you've accepted the package. What's more, your suspicious behavior will be used against you in court as evidence of your knowledge of the illicit contents of the package — why else would you refuse to sign? Get it?

I've seen a number of cases where the target gets a funky feeling about the delivery guy and rejects the package. At that point, the undercover courier will do everything possible to get the package into the target's hands, with or without a signature. It's the only way to execute the raid.

In one desperate case, the courier blew his own cover and flashed a badge. He summoned his partner, and the two asked to step inside to talk about the package. They told the target he was in a lot of trouble. The target told them he had no idea what was in the package and that they most certainly could *not* come in his house. The conversation continued on the lawn. The agents said the package, sent from Thailand, contained suspected drugs, and asked the target if they could open it right there. "Do what you want, it's not my package." The agent opened it, and inside were 500 Anabol tablets. The agent looked them over carefully and said, "My mistake, these are okay. You can import a personal use supply. I'm sorry, here, you can take them." He tried to hand them to the target. Nice try. The target told the agent to stick the tabs where the sun don't shine and avoided an arrest and raid by the eight other agents skulking in wait just off the property.

Q: But if there's no signature required and I just accept the package and don't open it, how can they prove I knew the contents?

A: Well, all they need is *probable cause* — a pretty low standard – to collar you; then you're in the system. That's bad in and of itself. To *convict* you, the government needs proof *beyond a reasonable doubt* that you knowingly and intentionally possessed a controlled substance. But again, it can be based on all the facts and circumstances. In *U.S. v. Lucus* [1998 U.S. App. LEXIS 30634], the defendant was convicted by a jury and argued "on appeal that the government produced no evidence showing beyond a reasonable doubt that he possessed the drugs knowingly. The thrust of his argument is that there was no direct evidence of his mental state other than his own testimony, in which he stated that he did not know that the package contained drugs until the agents told him so." His conviction was affirmed, with the Seventh Circuit holding that "the government may prove its case through circumstantial evidence that invites the trier of fact to draw inferences, so long as those inferences are reasonable." In that marijuana and cocaine case, the circumstantial evidence included the actions of the defendant, who appeared nervous and suspicious and questioned the undercover agent about the delay in delivery and lack of Federal Express markings on the van, as well as the finding of three boxes of Ziploc bags in the defendant's garage.

Conversely, in *People v. Patello* [41 A.D.2d 954 (1973)], the evidence proved *insufficient* to support the jury's conviction. The defendant came to the door and was asked by the mail carrier to sign his name to a postal receipt to acknowledge delivery of two packages sent in care of a friend. Upon signing his name, he was arrested. One of the packages was opened immediately thereafter in defendant's presence and found to contain hashish. The defendant denied having any knowledge of the contents of the packages, but admitted to receiving previous packages from his friend, in his care. The totality of circumstances failed to establish that the defendant had any knowledge that the packages contained a controlled substance.

Q: What if I receive a package in somebody else's name?

A: Most mailed drug packages use fictitious names. Every federal agent is well aware of it. That's why they conduct various checks on the residents of the address prior to the controlled delivery. They already know who lives there, and who their target is among the various residents. Even if the package was addressed to a real resident of the house, your wife, let's say, they'd know from motor vehicles records that at 5'7" and 275 pounds, *you* are the juicehead for whom the package is intended. They'd direct the controlled delivery to you.

But let's say the name on the package doesn't match up with the address, and the agents figure you're just using a fictitious name like most everybody else does. Let's say it's the name of somebody real who doesn't live there, like the class nerd in high school, or it's a made-up name. If your name's not on the package, the agents will likely want to make you physically accept the package in a face-to-face encounter with an undercover agent posing as a courier. The courier will ring your bell and ask, "Are

If your name's not on the package, the agents will likely want to make you physically accept the package in a face-to-face encounter with an undercover agent posing as a courier.

you Johnny Johnson?" showing you the name on the package. What are you going to say? If you take possession of the package by misrepresenting that *you're* Johnny, that's mighty strong evidence that it's *your* package. Right? But if you say you're *not* Johnny, and it's really a legitimate delivery, you can kiss the package good-bye. Oh, you could be sneaky and say, "No, but Johnny's a friend of mine. I'll accept the package for him because he's away in California." While even a legitimate courier might question you about why Johnny is using your address, let's say the phony courier gives you the package, you take it inside, and you get raided. The agents will want to know all about Johnny. If he's a real person, they'll investigate him to better pin the blame on you. If he's fake, you're a liar. If you keep your mouth shut, they'll bust you and let your lawyer try to convince the prosecutor or a jury that you're taking the rap for your imaginary friend.

A Georgia Court of Appeals case, *Perkins v. State* [244 Ga. App. 412 (2000)], illustrates this point. Again the totality of the circumstances was taken into account. The packages were delivered via a controlled delivery. When the defendant was asked to sign for them, he explained that the name on the packages wasn't him and the person whose name it was would be back at 3:30. Since the packages didn't require a signature, the undercover delivery agent dropped off the packages on the porch at 3:00 pm. The defendant was later seen bringing the packages inside the house and acting suspiciously, such as performing what one deputy called a "heat check": "the recipients of [contraband] packages often leave the residence immediately after the package is delivered to perform a 'heat check' – i.e., 'to check and see if they're being observed, if they're being followed, if they're under surveillance ... They'll just drive around with no particular place to go.'" At trial, "Agent Shelton testified that he had been involved in 50-100 controlled deliveries of contraband, and that in 99 percent of the cases the packages were addressed to a fictitious person. Agent Bertsch testified that he had been involved in more than 50 controlled deliveries, and that he had never seen a true name on a package. Deputy Hester testified that he had been involved in more than forty controlled deliveries, and that in no more than three cases had the package been addressed to a real person." When considered in the totality, the court held that the evidence at the very least created a "grave suspicion" that the defendant was the intended recipient and was aware of the contents of the packages. Obviously, writing a fictitious name on the package proved detrimental in this case.

Q: Am I protected by using a Post Office Box or Private Mail Box (PMB)?

A: Lots of guys have their anabolics delivered to post office boxes or private mail boxes, partly because they think it makes it less traceable to them, partly because they think it's harder to accomplish a controlled delivery in such a place, and partly because they think it prevents a search of their house. Let's talk about each.

In one of the few cases of mine involving a teenager, Evan was a 19-year-old Canadian kid who was helping a friend in upstate New York to distribute juice packages in return for free supplements. He went to the friend's post office box to pick up a package. Seeing a tag in the box advising that there was something waiting at the desk, he walked out nervously, paced around a while, then went back in. He presented the tag, signed for the package in his friend's name, and walked out with the gear. He was under surveillance the whole time. Postal inspectors and local police grabbed him as he walked out the door with the package of 100 vials and 500 tabs. He had the key to the box in his pocket, the package in his hand, and he'd used somebody else's name to get the package. He quickly cracked under interrogation, and was charged with a felony in state court.

To open a box, you almost invariably need to show picture identification, a copy of which is customarily kept on file. If the postal inspectors or Customs seizes a package, they can quite easily determine who opened the box by contacting the post office or mail center manager. Once they have your name and address, they'll be quickly able to access a wealth of data about you through motor vehicle and criminal background checks. What's more, they can check courier and postal records for previous packages to use, and even find other boxes you may be renting elsewhere. I've seen some clients open boxes using false identification. Aside from being a crime in itself, that's not going to stop further investigation. If they suspect you're using a false identity, they can do a bit of surveillance and ultimately find out where you live and who you are.

Is it harder to do a controlled delivery at a post office or private mail center? Not really. It does require more patience, but they have to get a rough idea of when you're most likely to be able to receive the package, and then set up surveillance and wait. It's actually probably easier for the surveillance team to avoid being spotted in a commercial area than lingering around your rose garden. Look, all they have to do is get the package into your hands. It doesn't really matter all that much where. I've seen many controlled deliveries effectuated at post offices or mail centers. Sometimes the agents just watch the suspect pull it out of the box, but more often a note is left in the box indicating some problem with the parcel, which must be picked up at the desk. The suspect will be arrested once he takes the package out of the building. Would the case be stronger if they waited to arrest until the suspect *opened* the package? Surely, but extracting an incriminating *admission* from the suspect is just as good or better, and the agents get one of those in the overwhelming majority of cases. (Please, don't forget to read Chapter 22!)

> ... all they have to do is get the package into your hands. It doesn't really matter all that much where.

Can the agents search your house if the package is delivered to a PMB? It depends. The issue is one of nexus, or link, between the two locations. Most often, the police will seek a search warrant *before* they deliver the goodies. If the designated address to receive the package is a house, there's no problem. If it's a PMB, the judge has to decide whether the suspect's receipt of the package at the box provides probable cause that he has juice in his house. (This topic was covered in Chapter 7 on search warrants.)

Q: What if the package is coming by regular domestic mail?

A: So you'd be tipped off if somebody showed up trying to hand you the package, right? Well, the way authorities have traditionally handled this would be to send a postcard or make a telephone call to the designated recipient, saying that the package was slightly damaged in the mail and would require a waiver to be signed. The package would be said to be waiting at the Post Office for pick-up. When the target claimed it, he'd be busted. Of course, this method isn't very time effective. Sometimes a call would be placed claiming the package was leaking, and needed to be picked up right away or the authorities would be called. These methods are still popular in some areas.

More recently, law enforcers have been using technology to get the job done. The problem with a controlled delivery via regular mail is that it's tougher to refute the innocent possessor defense: "Hey, I just scooped all my mail from my box. I don't know anything about this!" Without a signature or any verbal statements, it's harder to prove that your acceptance of possession was intentional rather than a mistake or accident. Some judges might not sign a warrant to raid the house if the package is going to be delivered by regular mail. Here's the solution that law enforcement found: they wire the package to signal when it's opened. When someone opens a package, that's pretty good evidence that he's the one who ordered it and knowingly intended to possess its contents, right? It might even be stronger evidence than signing for it.

When someone opens a package, that's pretty good evidence that he's the one who ordered it and knowingly intended to possess its contents, right?

Take a real case from Florida, for example. Sam was a bear of a man, 39 years old and married for fifteen years and living on the west coast of Florida. One day, three packages of gear from Israel were intercepted at JFK International Airport by Customs. Two days later, the Customs in New York forwarded the three packages to Customs in Florida. The agents shopped the case to the U.S. Attorney's Office, but the case was declined for prosecution for falling "within the blanket declination guidelines" for the District. So they offered it to the locals for state prosecution, and a deal was struck. When the packages arrived in Florida, they were inspected by a combination of agents from Customs, DEA, Postal Inspection Services and local police. A full background check was done on the resident of the designated address. Postal authorities determined that the address had been receiving six to seven overseas parcels every two weeks for the past several months. A controlled delivery was planned. Two of the packages would be wired with AT-4's (electronic signaling devices). An application for an anticipatory warrant was drafted, brought to the State Attorney's office for review and approval, and then to a local judge for his signature. The next day, a team of agents took up surveillance positions around Sam's neighborhood. An undercover mail carrier delivered the mail to the whole block, including Sam's gear. When Sam came out and collected his mail, the agents prepared for the raid. Within minutes they had their signal, and they swarmed the house yelling. "Police with a search warrant."

Several jurisdictions have begun using small electronic signaling devices, typically AT-4's, to confirm that a target has opened his package. No part of the device is visible unless the package is opened. When opened, the wires break. The device makes no audible sound but transmits an alert signal to a remote receiver manned by the agents. These devices can be used in cases where face-to-face deliveries might spook the target, or even as additional proof in face-to-face deliveries. The application for the search warrant will request authorization to execute the raid once the signal goes off. An AT-4 can make the difference between a botched operation and a successful raid. Not every jurisdiction yet has access to the devices, but it's likely that this is the wave of the future.

Some authorities in Washington State have been successfully using AT-4's in AAS cases. They used one recently on Robby, 34 years old, married with two children, and gainfully employed as a machinery assembler. He ordered some D-bol and Winny from an online source. He had gotten one Customs seizure notice about two weeks earlier. For whatever reason, he'd signed it and mailed it back. Regardless, his address was flagged. Three packages from Thailand were intercepted at the San Francisco FMU/ Daly City Airmail facility. Package one had 200 tablets total of D-bol and Winny; package two had 199 D-bol tabs; and package three had 209 Winny tabs. All were concealed in stacks of hollowed-out white paper. Customs got the local police on board and wired a package for delivery with an AT-4 transmitter. Pre-raid surveillance was set up, the delivery was made and Robby signed for the package. When Robby opened the package, he saw a little black device. Panicking, he took out the batteries and ran out to his car. He was stopped by the raid team, who took him back to the house and searched, seizing everything connected with bodybuilding including his Schwarzenegger book. They found 19 Sustanon preloads in his garbage. Robby waived his rights, admitted four previous Internet juice orders, and was even pressured into saying that 600 tablets is more than one person could use. (The deputy prosecuting attorney refused to plea bargain the case below a felony level for months, but ultimately accepted a letter I provided as a consultant in the case that the quantity of tablets recovered were indeed very consistent with one man's personal use. Robby got a misdemeanor plea and a one year suspended sentence.)

Q: What if the package isn't opened?

A: If the judge specifically conditions the execution of the raid on the AT-4 signal, obviously law enforcement has a big problem. In a pending case, the AT-4 installed in the package failed to signal some three hours after the target's wife took it into house, and over two hours after the target had arrived home. Prevented from executing the warrant without an opened package, they decided to attempt a knock-and-talk. Had the target and his wife refused to invite the agents in, it is unclear what would have happened. If the agents couldn't find another alternative, perhaps no case could have been built. The contraband would have remained inside. What would have happened to it? Would a judge have authorized a new warrant, based on the acceptance of the parcel without its opening? We'll never know. In this case, the target and his wife all too typically let them into the house. They signed written waivers of their *Miranda* Rights. They were then separated and independently questioned. They completely incriminated themselves. The husband has been arrested and indicted, and the information on his computer has fueled further investigations.

Another option might have been for the agents to contact the judge for a new warrant, since, after all, there's now probable cause to believe that the drugs are in the house. Or they could have done a few trash searches over the next few days.

It's important to recognize, though, that even without a signature, any verbal statements, or any indications that the package is opened, you're still not out of the woods. Let's say a judge agrees to sign an anticipatory warrant that allows a raid as soon as you take the package out of your mailbox after a delivery by regular mail. A phony postman delivers all the mail to the whole block, and a team of agents keeps your box under surveillance until you pop out to get the mail. Once you take it inside, they can execute the raid. Now, they can ransack your home, and whatever they get as a result can be introduced against you. That includes any contraband they find, but it also includes *any evidence linking you to the package*, even if it's not in and of itself criminal. Like papers or notes, perhaps, or a computer with incriminating e-mails. Since the overwhelming majority of juicers still keep gear in their house even when ordering steroids through the mail, what's found in the search can make an otherwise flimsy case pretty strong.

Q: What if I write "Return to Sender" and put it by the door?

A: Okay, we have to talk about this. I don't know when this started, but it was recommended in a 1998 book on steroid import methods. Now it's become pretty standard practice. I've heard claims that this is the magic bullet that stops law enforcement in its tracks. Write "Return to Sender" on the package as soon as you accept it and then put it by the front door like you don't want it. When the raid team comes crashing in, you'll have a built-in defense: "Hey, I refused the package! Get out of my house!" Your brief possession can be claimed as a simple mistake. Sounds good, especially in this uncertain age of mail bombs and anthrax letters, doesn't it? Sometimes it can be.

Here's a real-life example. Bill was in the health care field, married with three children (including twins). A Priority Mail package from England in his own name arrived. He accepted it in a cursory way, and a half hour later a team of agents with a search warrant swarmed his house. The package was sitting unopened with "Return to Sender" written on it. The house was searched and a tiny quantity of steroids was found. He denied knowledge of the contents of the package (which contained 1,000 D-bol). The agents took his computer, the steroids from his house and the package. He was never charged. Six months later, his lawyer contacted the local prosecutor to obtain an agreement not to prosecute. The prosecutor consented, and a full year after the raid Bill's computer (now obsolete) was returned. In Bill's particular case, the fact that the package wasn't opened and was apparently rejected may have been a helpful factor in the excellent resolution. However, it's crucial to note also that Bill's conduct in accepting the package was not patently inconsistent with its subsequent rejection, and that Bill never admitted ordering the package. Bill was lucky, because the fact that a small quantity of juice was found in the house certainly could have pushed this case in the other direction. Some prosecutors might have gone forward on a borderline case like this.

Clearly, "Return to Sender" worked for Bill. But depending on the situation, it could actually be quite *damaging* to your defense, a complete backfire! It depends on all the circumstances, and not all the circumstances are within your knowledge or control. Let's flesh out a scenario. Say the doorbell rings. You answer it. It's Mr. Courier Service with a package for you. He asks if you're the person whose name is on the package, right? Of course he does, otherwise he shouldn't give it to you. Let's say your name is on the package. You respond that you are, in fact, that person. He now says, "Sign here."

Clearly, "Return to Sender" worked for Bill. But depending on the specific situation, it could actually be quite *damaging* to your defense ...

You have two choices at this point, and you can't know which is right because you can't be sure if the delivery is legit or not. You can say, "Hey, no, wait, I wasn't expecting anything. I don't want it." In which case, you will have avoided taking possession of the package (but will probably be visited shortly thereafter by two agents for a knock-and-talk, as described in Chapter 7). You will have also lost your gear. If you keep rejecting packages, you'll eventually be steroid-free (which, after reading some of these chapters, may not seem like such a bad idea, huh?).

Or, you can accept the package. Accepting the package is like ringing a bell. Once it's rung, you can't un-ring it. You're now in possession of the package. You accepted it knowingly and voluntarily. But now in the course of five minutes you make a mad dash for your felt marker and scribble your rejection of it just in time for the knock on the door. Does that *really* support the inference that your acceptance of the package was an accident or mistake? Or does it imply that you're a crafty devil who's using a deceptive tactic to thwart the investigators? How, they will ask, did you know that you didn't want it without opening it? What new information struck you, like a bolt of lightning, in the seconds between your very willing acceptance of it at the door and your mad scramble to disconnect yourself from it moments later? Let me let you in on a little secret: law enforcement has been aware of the "Return to Sender" ploy for quite a while. The agents might even get away with testifying at trial that writing, "Return to Sender" on a package and putting it near the door is a hallmark of drug traffickers who use the mail. There's an argument, isn't there, that your curious conduct suggests a *guilty knowledge* of the contents, don't you think? Might not a persuasive prosecutor get a jury think so?

And this is all assuming that the raid yielded nothing. If anything was found that *connects* you to the package or to AAS use in general, you've got a bigger problem. Not only does juice in the house form the basis for an independent charge of criminal possession, but it further supports *the inference that your acceptance of the package was no mistake*! Got that? Lastly, the viability of an innocent mistake defense assumes you've made *no incriminating admissions*, which may be quite an unrealistic assumption. Despite all my suggestions in articles and magazines over the years, almost everybody still spills their guts under pressure. Maybe you should memorize Chapter 22 when you get to it.

Not only does juice in the house form the basis for an independent charge of criminal possession, but it further supports *the inference that your acceptance of the package was no mistake*!

Q: How can I properly refuse a package?

A: This odd but truly excellent question was posed to me recently by a big buddy of mine from the Midwest. Let's assume that you're innocent and as pure as the driven snow, and that a mail carrier or private parcel courier shows up at your door with a package. In these dangerous times, it's perfectly reasonable to be wary of a parcel from an unrecognized address. If it's from another state or a foreign country, and you don't know anybody or do business with anybody there, unless you like taking unnecessary risks it might not be a good idea to take it. That would be particularly true if it's in somebody else's name. What would any reasonable person do? If it isn't in his name, he wouldn't take it, right?

He'd say, "I'm not 'Danny Deltoids,' so this package isn't mine. I won't accept it. Take it away." Under *no* circumstances would he touch it or sign for it. Simple, huh?

And if the package *is* in the person's name? What then? Well, I know one guy who, for whatever reasons, knew he didn't want to accept a package. When the doorbell rang, he came to the door, looked at the package and quickly said, "I didn't order anything from China. It's not mine. Take it back. I'm on the phone. See ya." It turned out to be an attempted controlled delivery, and the undercover courier tried to throw the package in his door, but he pulled the door closed before he could. Now the agents had a terrible problem, because the warrant they had said they could only execute it *after the suspect accepted the package* (as is typical). They were forced to try a knock-and-talk, but he said, "Go away!" without opening the door. Surely, they were going to ask him why he would refuse a package that had his name on it, unless he *knew* that it contained contraband. That might have been tough for him to answer, so he never came to the door. Eventually they left and never came back.

Q: Can I be subpoenaed to testify against the source of the package?

A: Yes. Just recently, I've seen a few cases where the recipient has received a federal grand jury subpoena to testify against a domestic source located many states away. In both cases, a controlled delivery was attempted but, for one reason or another, the case against the recipient was weak or compromised and no arrest was made after the raid. Presumably, local authorities were weighing their options. In the meantime, authorities in the jurisdiction from which the source was conducting business were looking to make a big case against him. The subpoena currently going around commands the recipient's physical appearance and for him to "provide any and all notes, documents, memoranda, correspondence, and other documents of any kind relating to your purchase of anabolic steroids." An accompanying letter states, "You have been subpoenaed to testify as a witness for the United States Government" and provides a map to the courthouse and travel and lodging reimbursement information. *It is absolutely imperative for anyone receiving a grand jury subpoena like this to contact an experienced criminal lawyer immediately*. Qualified counsel can find out the nature and parameters of the prosecutor's interest in you and advise you accordingly. The concept of *use immunity* (basically, that your testimony can't be used against you but evidence obtained independently of your immunized testimony *can* be a basis to prosecute you) and the potential application of your privilege against self-incrimination must be discussed between you and your lawyer as they apply to the particular facts of your situation. Disregarding or ignoring the subpoena can have severe and adverse consequences.

An accompanying letter states, "You have been subpoenaed to testify as a witness for the United States Government" ...

Q: What can I expect from the raid?

A: The police have a job to gather evidence. Allowing a suspect to calmly ruminate over his options is counterproductive to that goal. Immediately asserting dominance and instilling fear makes it more likely that a suspect will quickly hand over contraband and admit his guilt. Aggressive police conduct during a raid is an effective and often necessary tool. In case you haven't gotten the picture from the many real world examples of intimidating confrontations with the police, let me personalize it for you, here and now. I'm doing this not to scare you, but to *prepare* you. Let's pretend you're the target. Hypothetically, here's the way it's going to go down.

You've just accepted a package from a mail carrier. Maybe you've signed for it; maybe not. Maybe you write, "Refused. Return to Sender" on it; maybe you actually open the package. In any case, you're in possession of the package of gear. There's a knock on the door. "Police with a search warrant! Search warrant! Search warrant!" You open the door and get bowled over by a tidal wave of armed federal agents and local police conducting themselves like military commandos. There's screaming and hollering and footsteps sounding all over the house. You can't see too much because your face is buried in shag carpet and there are two agents on top of you, twisting your arms behind your back and slapping cold metal handcuffs onto your wrists.

You're yanked to your feet, thrown down onto a kitchen chair. The intruders may seem to be multiplying, swarming over every part of the house. They're in your face, shouting at you. You're outnumbered, feel violated, and are overwhelmed with a sense of powerlessness. They begin ransacking your home. They throw the package on your lap. They tell you that you're going down, big time. Tell us where you stash your steroids, they demand, or we'll be camped here for a week and take this house down to the studs. Your wife, children, father, brother, etc., have been held hostage in another room, sequestered out of sight. The situation is terrifying. You feel completely violated. They are tearing through your personal papers, throwing your effects around, demanding answers from you immediately.

More than anything else, you want this horror to end. It seems to go on and on. How far will they search? How long? What condition will your house be in? Will all the neighbors gather? How can you subject your family to this humiliation? If you give them the steroids, so what? They'll find them anyway. It will only take an extra two hours of sitting handcuffed in this chair, with all the screaming and harassment. You know it's all pressure tactics. They'll keep pumping up the pressure to get you to incriminate yourself, give up the evidence, and cooperate with them against others. It's simple psychology. They negatively reinforce unwanted behavior, and positively reinforce desired behavior. If you don't cooperate, they're combative and accusatory. Give them a little, they lighten up.

At some point, after you've been worn down, one agent will take the lead in addressing you. He may allow you some small consideration, such as giving you a drink or making your family more comfortable. These small gestures will seem tremendous. He will ask you a few innocuous questions, opening a dialogue. He'll seem to understand, and call you by your first name. He'll stand out like a life preserver in a raging, stormy sea. Instinctively, you will want to reach out to that "kind keeper," so different from the others. He may say, "Look, from this point on, you can only help yourself. So why don't you just talk to me about how you got involved with steroids? Talk to me and we can stop this circus. These other guys are crazy. I know you're not a bad guy." You'll like him, at least compared to the others. He's offering you to make it all stop. Hey, *anything* would be better than this, right? It's just some steroids anyway. They've got me cold, you think.

There are a million justifications you can think of. So you talk to him. And soon enough, it *will* stop. Why? *Because he got what he wanted.* He made his case against you. There's no reason to continue. And you got what you wanted too, an end to your immediate problem.

Of course, you may have given yourself an even bigger problem. By talking to him, you may have given the prosecution the strongest evidence against you in the case: a confession. I've seen countless cases both as a prosecutor and as a defense lawyer where the prosecution might not have been able to proceed at all but for the suspect's own words.

I won't be at your house when the raid comes. No lawyer will. You'll be on your own. How you handle the confrontation in your home will have a major, sometimes dispositive effect on what will happen to you in court. Before you waive your Fifth Amendment privilege and Sixth Amendment right to counsel, are you really sure you want to do that? If you want to use certain information you have to get yourself a better deal, that's your choice. The issue is, when? The only one with authority to cut you a deal in court is the prosecutor. If cooperation's the route you're looking to go, shouldn't you be talking to her? And shouldn't that only be *after* you've hashed out your options with a seasoned defense lawyer who knows all the ins and outs? Think of it as a transaction, like buying a car. Will you get a better deal walking into a dealership cold, where ten salesmen pressure you in your moment of utmost vulnerability — or later, with a professional negotiator by your side? Think about it.

How you handle the confrontation in your home will have a major, sometimes dispositive effect on what will happen to you in court.

Chapter 20

KISS YOUR ASSETS GOODBYE

"When a strong man, fully armed, guards his castle, his property is safe. But when one stronger than he attacks him and overpowers him, he takes away his armor in which he trusted and divides his plunder."

– *Bible: New Testament, Luke 11:21.22*

What if you lived in an oppressive state that employs an elite force of jack-booted, heavily armed, Nomex-hooded and ballistic-body-armor-wearing storm troopers who are sworn to uphold the laws, as cruel as they may be. Further imagine that a platoon of these storm troopers, using a battering ram, burst into your home at dawn. You leap from your bed, confused and bleary-eyed from sleep. You resist being subdued and restrained, and are sprayed in the face with oleoresin capsicum (a powerful eye and skin irritant), shocked with a stun gun, and struck with a baton. Once done, other troopers storm your home in search of any perceived evidence of criminality, finding a small quantity of anabolics. You're arrested and charged with a crime. As if the indignities and terror of the raid weren't enough, now the *real* horror starts. Zealous prosecutors lay claim to your computers, laptops, cash, cars, and even your house itself. Then your bank accounts are frozen, leaving you unable to pay your bills. Once the property is seized, heartless government lawyers start a civil lawsuit, seeking to legally and permanently take all this property from you. What's worse, you're now compelled to pay to the court *ten percent of the value of your own property* as a bond, and prove at trial how your property is *not* the proceeds of a crime or the instrumentality for the completion of one. That's right – you have the burden of proof! You are entitled to hire a lawyer to defend you, but your money has been seized and you have no way of paying one ...

That would be one helluva dream, huh? The kind a bodybuilder wakes up from in a cold sweat at 3 a.m., after having eaten one too many burritos on his off-season cheat night. Sure, this nightmare is an exaggeration. But just how far-fetched is it? We've already seen that police raid tactics can be pretty aggressive. And what's all this crazy talk about taking away property? This is America, after all.

Well, you're in for a bit of an education.

What is Asset Forfeiture?

There are two types of asset forfeiture: 1) criminal asset forfeiture; and, 2) civil asset forfeiture. Most often, asset forfeiture is used in cases involving drugs. The present federal laws are the result of a trend that had begun more than thirty years ago in an attempt to expand the authority of law enforcement at the height of efforts to combat drugs and terrorism. The fundamental distinctions between these two forms of forfeiture, criminal and civil, have both practical and legal significance for the government's ability to impose forfeiture and the procedures by which such a forfeiture action can be accomplished.

1) Criminal Asset Forfeiture

In 1970, Congress enacted the first federal *criminal forfeiture law*, the Racketeer Influenced and Corrupt Organizations (RICO) statute. Enactment of the Continuing Criminal Enterprise

(CCE) statute followed in 1984. Unlike civil forfeiture, criminal forfeiture was justified as a punishment imposed upon a criminal based upon an *in personam* proceeding directly against an individual offender for his misconduct, not to an inanimate object through legal fiction. In contrast to civil forfeiture laws, which are premised on a taint theory, criminal forfeitures are premised on a *punitive* theory. It's all about punishment.

In contrast to civil forfeiture laws, which are premised on a taint theory, criminal forfeitures are premised on a *punitive* theory. It's all about punishment.

Criminal forfeitures are authorized under 21 U.S.C. § 853. This section subjects to forfeiture that person's property which is either directly or indirectly the proceeds of that violation, or the property used or intended to be used to commit or facilitate that violation.

Criminal forfeiture requires that the owner of the property first be convicted, that is, found guilty of the crime "beyond a reasonable doubt." A forfeiture proceeding may then follow conviction, at which the government must show by either a preponderance of the evidence or beyond a reasonable doubt that the defendant acquired such property during the period of time of the violations for which the defendant was convicted.

The federal government, however, has not used RICO and CCE as frequently as had been anticipated, largely in part because the statutes rely on criminal convictions and require the government to prove its case "beyond a reasonable doubt," rather than simply showing probable cause, as with civil forfeiture.

2) Civil Asset Forfeiture

In 1970, Congress also enacted the Comprehensive Drug Abuse Prevention and Control Act. This Act empowered the government to use civil forfeiture against property used or acquired in violation of federal drug laws. Civil asset forfeiture involves a civil lawsuit brought by the government seeking to obtain legal title to real or personal property, when it is proved to be the proceeds of a crime, or the instrumentality for the commission of a crime.

Seizure occurs when the government and/or or its agents take the property. *Forfeiture* means that the legal title is transferred to the government. Civil asset forfeiture may be pursued under federal or state jurisdiction. The lawsuit seeks a civil remedy in the nature of transferring title from one to another. Because is not a criminal proceeding, the action is governed by rules of civil procedure and civil rules of evidence. Additionally, civil rules for appellate procedure apply. This chapter provides a general overview of the civil asset forfeiture proceeding.

Seizure occurs when the government and/or or its agents take the property. *Forfeiture* means that the legal title is transferred to the government.

Most states model their civil forfeiture laws on the Uniform Controlled Substances Act, or an amended version of it. The Uniform Act makes subject to forfeiture: (1) all controlled substances manufactured, distributed, dispensed, or acquired in violation of the Uniform Act, (2) all raw materials, products, and equipment used in manufacturing any controlled substances, (3) all property used as containers for controlled substances, (4) all conveyances used to transport controlled substances, and (5) all books, records, and research products used in violation of the Uniform Act. The Uniform Act was designed to complement the federal drug legislation and to achieve uniformity between the participating states' laws. The idea was to create an interweaving of federal and state law enabling all levels of government to more effectively combat the drug trade. The National Conference of Commissioners on Uniform State Laws was most concerned with halting the interstate – as well as the international – flow of drugs. At least twenty-nine states and the District of Columbia have enacted the Uniform Controlled Substances Act or an amended version of the statute.

If a state does not have its own forfeiture laws and it seeks to acquire assets, the local agency must involve the federal government in the investigation and have the property forfeited under federal law. This involves a request that the federal government "adopt" the forfeiture. Consequently, it will be considered a federal forfeiture and the state or local government can only enjoy proceeds if it applies for an equitable share. While a state case is presented as an example of how unfair a forfeiture action can be, an analysis of each state's procedure is beyond the scope of this book.

The civil forfeiture lawsuit is commenced on the basis of what is known as *in rem* jurisdiction. *In rem* means that the *property* – the thing itself – is the subject matter of the lawsuit, not a person. The court will obtain jurisdiction (the ability to hear the case) on the basis that the property is present in that forum. Jurisdiction over a person is referred to as *in personam*, or personal jurisdiction.

All forms of civil (*in rem*) forfeiture can be traced back to Biblical origin. Early English common law required that the Crown be compensated for the loss of life of one of its subjects caused by an inanimate object or animal (the deodand). The deodand was forfeited to the king and was applied to pious uses. As a result, civil forfeiture of property does not rely on the successful criminal prosecution of the property owner, and in fact, the innocence of the owner of the property subject to forfeiture has almost uniformly been rejected as a defense. The concept has at its roots a legal fiction that objects can be "guilty" of wrongdoing. Congress adopted this belief in 1789.

According to the DEA, to ensure that criminals do not benefit financially from their illegal acts, certain crimes are subject to forfeiture to the government. The DEA says that since drug trafficking is a crime of greed, asset forfeiture is an effective weapon because it removes the profit from such illegal activities. Its position is that asset forfeiture can also financially disable drug-trafficking organizations. This is accomplished by preventing international drug traffickers from using their wealth to purchase the very best state-of-the-art weaponry and communications equipment, thereby making it more difficult to thwart law enforcement. According to the Department of Justice, without civil forfeiture:

> "The United States would be virtually powerless to act when the criminal profits and other property of foreign criminals are found within our own borders and when criminal operatives are able to evade arrest. Without civil forfeiture, our ability to fight international crime would be crippled." [U.S. Department of Justice, Annual Report of The Department of Justice Asset Forfeiture Program 9 (1991)]

Federal Civil Forfeiture Procedure

The matrix of federal statutes governing civil forfeiture is contained in a number of sections of the United States Code. In drug cases, the government pursues civil forfeiture under the Controlled Substances Act. A civil asset forfeiture action may be brought pursuant to 21 U.S.C. § 881 (forfeitures) and 18 U.S.C. § 981 (civil forfeitures).

No property may be seized unless the government meets the standard of "probable cause," the same standard of proof required to arrest a person or secure a warrant to search a person's home (see Chapter 4). Evidence showing probable cause must rise above the level of mere suspicion but need not amount to a preponderance of the evidence. The field office of the seizing agency makes the probable cause determination on a case-by-case basis. The seizing agency must have a search warrant to seize and forfeit, or the warrantless seizure must meet one of the recognized exceptions to the Fourth Amendment's warrant requirement. Once probable cause is established, the burden of proof formerly shifted to the owner/claimant who had to establish by a preponderance of the evidence that the property was "not guilty." This has been changed by the Civil Asset Forfeiture Reform Act of 2000 (see below). Property is seized only when there is probable cause to establish that it may be a tool for, or the proceeds of, illegal activities such as drug trafficking, organized crime, or money laundering. Clearly, the intent was to bust guys like Tony Soprano, Paulie Walnuts and the rest of the crew.

The government only has to suspect that the property is being used in connection with some activity that is either illegal or claimed to be illegal. The property can be seized at any time, before or after an arrest or indictment. Prior to reform, *the owner had to pay a nonrefundable bond of ten percent of the value of his own property.* Note that this still may be the case in state actions. To best represent their interests, owner/claimants will require an attorney and have to pay attorneys' fees. What's worse, with protracted litigation those fees can be quite extensive, and the money that may have been used to pay the attorney may also have been seized. It's a Catch-22. The property that may be seized can include cash, motor vehicles, a business, land and even the person's home. Property that may be seized and for which there is no property interest is set out in 21 U.S.C. § 881, and includes but is not limited to: all controlled substances, paraphernalia, raw materials, chemicals, conveyances, vehicles, firearms, books, records and cash. Notice of the intent to seize must be served pursuant to Federal Rule of Civil Procedure 4.

Once seized and forfeited, the property may be destroyed, retained for official use, or sold. Proceeds from sale pay all expenses of the forfeiture proceeding, and any surplus is forwarded to the Treasurer of the United States for deposit in the general fund of the Treasury.

When the lawsuit concerns real property, the government may file what is known as a *Notice of Lis Pendens* with the county clerk in which the real property is located. A *lis pendens* establishes what is commonly referred to as a "cloud on title." This means that, when filed with the county clerk, it will be on record that there is a claim and dispute regarding the title to that property. Therefore, if a potential purchaser of that property performs a title search they will be put on notice and will be highly unlikely to accept imperfect title. Pursuant to 18 U.S.C. § 1985, the filing of a *lis pendens* and the execution of a writ of entry for the purpose of conducting an inspection and inventory of the property shall not be considered a seizure.

Sometimes, in the most egregious cases, the owner was not aware that a tenant, family member or even a stranger was using drugs on their property. Other times, just having the property, such as a large amount of cash, is sufficient for seizure. Cash is especially vulnerable, since paper money often has traces of cocaine or other drugs.

Forfeiture in Action: a State Case

Take, for example, the recent state case of Kareem. Kareem merely made weekly overnight visits to his parents' home in Farmington Hills, Michigan. He had no ownership interest in his parents' home, motor vehicles or bank accounts. The SUV he drove was leased.

Kareem attends Michigan State University as an undergraduate. He buses tables at a college hangout in East Lansing. On the weekends, he drives back to his parents' home to help around the house and enjoy some home cooked meals. After school and work is done, he likes to blow off steam and hit the weights at Gold's gym. Workouts improve his self-image, health, and make him more physically attractive to the cuties on campus. He supplements his workouts with protein drinks and modest cycles of anabolics.

In the summer of 2002, Postal Inspectors intercepted a parcel that was addressed to Kareem at his parents' home at 1500 Pontiac Avenue. The return address on the package was confirmed as being fictitious. A previous package having been seized by Customs Inspectors, the Postal Service was now engaged in an ongoing investigation into Kareem's parents' address for drug trafficking. The inspector applied for and was granted a search warrant to open the package.

The inspector opened the package and discovered the following: 20 bottles of testosterone propionate, 35 bottles of Sustanon 250, 5 bottles of Ganabol, 5 bottles of trenbolone acetate, 5 bottles of cypionate and 15 bottles of nandrolone decanoate. The inspector repacked the parcel, along with an AT-4 electronic transmitter. The inspector then applied for and was granted a search warrant to retrieve the package following a controlled delivery at 1500 Pontiac Avenue.

The next day, police officers from the elite Bureau of Special Operations (SWAT team), working in conjunction with the postal inspector, traveled to Kareem's parents' home.

The postal inspector, dressed as a U.S. Postal Service letter carrier, pleasantly delivered the parcel to the home at approximately 2:00 p.m. Kareem wasn't home, but his father Kumar was. Kumar answered the door, exchanged pleasantries with the letter carrier, signed for the package as requested, and took it in the house. Kareem called his father shortly after the delivery, and told his father that the "vitamins" he had ordered were the wrong ones, and that the package needed to go back. He told his father to write, "return to sender" on it and place it outside the home on the doorstep.

Meanwhile, officers monitored the electronic transmitter. After approximately 2 hours, no signal was sent. The raid team began to lose patience. Finally, they decided to execute the raid. They burst through the front door and swarmed the residence, warrant in hand, to retrieve the package. One officer threatened to blow Kumar's head off if he moved.

With Kareem's mother Winnie and his father shocked, screaming, crying and restrained at gunpoint on the living room floor by six special operations officers, other agents proceeded to sweep and clear the remainder of the residence. In a rear bedroom, which police were told Kareem uses, they found a syringe, an empty vial of testosterone cypionate and 15 pink tablets in plain view on a dresser. Police officers then secured the premises while applying for another warrant to search the premises for further evidence of controlled substance sales, use and/or possession.

Pursuant to the execution of the second warrant, which was based upon plain view observations of the gear, police recovered further evidence of anabolic steroids, a ledger which they asserted lists AAS transactions, a green pouch with $5,400 in cash, an envelope with $5,000 in cash, and bank transfers from Kareem's mother's account at Midwest Bank One to Thailand Merchant Bank.

Police officers then proceeded to Grand River Avenue and served a search warrant upon Midwest Bank One, which resulted in the seizure of Winnie's account, totaling more than $40,000, and another $20,000 in cash which was in a safe deposit box. This was Kumar and Winnie's "nest egg."

The following day, the county prosecutor served a Notice of Seizure and Intent to Forfeit upon Kumar. The notice identified the seized property as the cash, bank accounts, Kareem's leased

SUV, Kumar's and Winnie's cars. It even listed Kumar's pride and joy, the thing he has worked his whole life for, his modest suburban house. Interestingly, while no narcotics were ever found at any time, the notice states that the property is being held for narcotic forfeiture purposes pursuant to Michigan Compiled Laws Annotated (MCLA) § 333.7521.

Where does that leave the family today? If Kumar, Winnie and Kareem want to challenge the seizure and assert their interest in their own property, they must now file a claim with the county prosecutor's office. And they had better get a move on, because they have a mere 20 days to do so from the date of service of the notice. Their failure to do so within the statutory time frame will essentially result in judgment in favor of the government on default, and an administrative forfeiture of the property. Homeless, emotionally and financially devastated; they will be compelled to somehow hire an attorney to represent them in the civil action, as well as one to defend them in the potential criminal case. Moreover, Michigan law requires that a ten percent bond be paid. Under Michigan law, the government now has four months to commence the forfeiture action which Kumar, Winnie and Kareem must defend if they want their property. They are required to prove by a preponderance of the evidence, in a court of law, that the property was not the proceeds of a crime or the instrumentality for the commission of one. Now here's the kicker: *NO CRIMINAL CHARGES HAVE BEEN FILED YET!* What's worse, even if criminal charges are filed and they are ultimately tried and acquitted, they may still lose the forfeiture action. Take note: there are different standards of proof in criminal cases as opposed to civil cases. Even if not proven guilty beyond a reasonable doubt of the criminal charges, Kumar, Winnie and Kareem may fail to prove *by a preponderance of the evidence* the lack of criminality associated with the property. Even completely *innocent*, they could lose *everything*. If this doesn't make you angry yet, check yourself for a pulse.

"A Modicum of Sanity ..." Federal Reform (CAFRA)

The U.S. Supreme Court had criticized the federal civil forfeiture law, saying that prosecutors had been allowed to confiscate the assets of innocent people long before criminal trials were commenced. The critics of the law also included the National Association of Criminal Defense Lawyers, of which I am a life member, the American Civil Liberties Union, and the National Rifle Association, among others. After years of complaints, Congress passed the Civil Asset Forfeiture Reform Act (CAFRA). It was signed by President Clinton on April 25, 2000, and became effective August 23, 2000. The Act was the culmination of the joint and competing efforts of a host of advocates and detractors recognizing the need for an overhaul of the American civil forfeiture process. The chief proponents were John Conyers (D. MI), Orrin G. Hatch (R. UT), and Patrick J. Leahy (D. VT); however, no single proponent of reform was more vocal and persistent than the Chairman of the House Judiciary Committee, Henry Hyde (R. IL).

However, bringing some degree of sanity to the federal system of civil forfeiture ... that had been widely criticized by the judiciary, academic commentators and the media, required compromise.

Notwithstanding Congressman Hyde's passionate and persuasive call for change and the resulting Act that has become synonymous with his name, the compromises necessary to pass the bill may have, perhaps, created a less than perfect remedy for the perceived unfairness attributed to civil forfeiture actions in this country. A modicum of sanity was the mission of Hyde, the acknowledged father of Civil Asset Forfeiture Reform Act (CAFRA). However, bringing some degree of sanity to the federal system of civil forfeiture, a system that that had been widely criticized by the judiciary, academic commentators and the media, required compromise.

While the Department of Justice and federal prosecutors were busy driving stakes through the hearts of organized crime figures, money launderers and drug traffickers, too many innocent owners of property like Kumar and Winnie were caught up in a net that was cast far too wide.

Prior to reform of the federal law, property could be seized and subjected to civil asset forfeiture proceedings without any opportunity to establish a hardship. CAFRA addresses this inadequacy with 18 U.S.C § 983(f), which provides for the release of a claimant's possessory property provided the property is not contraband, cash, and/or evidence likely to be used in a crime. Essentially, the court will be called upon to balance the interest of the government with the property owner's interest. The court must look to factors such as the owner's ties to the community and the severity of the hardship (e.g., homelessness, loss of profits). Mitigating factors must be balanced against the likelihood of weakening of the government's case or releasing instrumentalities that facilitate a criminal enterprise.

This new reform can provide a great deal of relief to owners who would otherwise be displaced from their homes and businesses while somehow endeavoring to defend against a civil forfeiture action and possible criminal action. This provision makes a move toward basic fundamental fairness with minimal loss to the government.

Shifting the Burden of Proof

Prior to the enactment of CAFRA, property owners had very little protection against federal civil asset forfeiture. For the government such actions were like taking candy from a baby, because the burden of proof essentially rested with the owner, who had to show by a preponderance of evidence that the property should not be forfeited. As a practical matter, the Government had a preliminary burden to establish, by mere probable cause, that the property should be forfeited, at which point the real burden shifted to the claimant.

The House Judiciary Committee took note of the fact that the law required that the government prove very little, but rather compelled the owner to prove disprove guilt.

CAFRA has remedied this by now imposing upon the government the burden of proving, by a *preponderance of evidence, that the property should be forfeited.* Congressman Hyde and other members of Congress were advocating a much more stringent burden of proof – by "clear and convincing evidence" – but this effort fell victim to compromise. Additionally, CAFRA no longer permits the government to use hearsay in proving its case.

For the government such actions were like taking candy from a baby, because the burden of proof essentially rested with the owner, who had to show by a preponderance of the evidence that the property should not be forfeited.

Notwithstanding the fact that CAFRA is a compromise, the burden of proof shift represents a major step in the direction of fairness.

Time Limitations

Prior to CAFRA, the federal government was not pressured much to meet administrative deadlines, other than a general requirement that notice be served upon the owner promptly. Once served with notice, the owner was compelled to post a cost bond in addition to filing a claim for the property. However, government policy was most often to provide notice of intent to start a forfeiture action within 60 days of seizure. The exceptions were where such notice would jeopardize a criminal investigation, or risk the concealment or destruction of evidence, and/or danger to witnesses and informants. Nonetheless, some forfeiture notices did not fall within the self-imposed 60-day period and did not fall within the recognized exceptions, but satisfied the promptness provisions of the statute.

Pursuant to CAFRA, the government *must* give the owner notice within 60 days of the seizure or upon identifying the property's owner. However, the Act also provides for the safeguarding of the aforementioned exceptions by permitting the government extensions to the 60-day notice requirement. In order to invoke the extension, the government must file a written application to the court seeking an order, known as a *motion,* making the request and setting out the basis why the court should grant the relief requested.

Once served with notice, the Act provides that the owner must file a claim within 30 days, but the cost bond requirement has been completely abolished. Another rigorous deadline placed on the government by CAFRA is that the government must actually file a civil forfeiture complaint within 90 days of receipt of the owner's claim, or forfeiture will be permanently barred. The limitation periods set forth in CAFRA establish firm deadlines and rein in the government from abusing the due process rights of owners. The government still retains the ability to delay notice in those in which it is deemed necessary. However, that delay must be substantiated and applications for an extension must have judicial approval as well. As such, these provisions may be viewed as establishing more fairness.

Damages

Prior to CAFRA, the government was generally exempt from tort claims arising out of their wrongful seizure and possession of an owner's property in connection with civil forfeiture actions. Pursuant to CAFRA, the Federal Tort Claims Act is amended to provide for compensation to victims of forfeiture where their property was seized for the purposes of forfeiture and the claimant was not convicted of a crime giving rise to that forfeiture.

While the possibility for abuse may exist, the Act sets forth a clear a departure from the almost absolute government immunity of the past.

Court and Attorney Fees

CAFRA provides for court-appointed counsel for indigent owner/claimants provided that the following requirements are satisfied:

1) The indigent/owner makes a "good faith" claim and is already represented by court-appointed counsel in the related criminal case; and,
2) The subject of the forfeiture is the indigent owner/claimant's primary residence.

Moreover, non-indigent claimants may be entitled to court and litigation costs provided they "substantially prevail" in the civil forfeiture action. However, the term "substantially prevail" is entirely ambiguous. In using the term "substantially prevail," the legislators let courts to make a discretionary but reasoned decision on whether reimbursement satisfies the standards of justice.

Innocent Owner/Claimant Defense

CAFRA provides for an innocent owner/claimant defense. What is unique about CAFRA is that it created a uniform innocent owner defense applicable to all federal civil asset forfeiture statutes. The new law establishes that an innocent owner's interest in property shall not be forfeited under any civil forfeiture statute.

Innocent owners fall into two possible categories: pre-existing owners and after-acquired owners. In the case of the pre-existing owners, they must establish by a preponderance of evidence that they are innocent owners. After satisfying this initial burden they must prove:

1) They are "in fact" the rightful owner of the property; and,

2) They had no knowledge of the alleged unlawful activity associated with their property; or

3) Upon learning of the activity they did all they could reasonably be expected to do to prevent it. In so doing, the owners are not required to place themselves or others not engaged in the unlawful activity in danger.

In the case of after-acquired owners, they must establish:

1) They are "in fact" the owner of the property; and,

2) They are bona fide purchasers for value; and,

3) At the time they acquired the property they did not know or have reason to know that the property is the proceeds of criminal activity.

The innocent owner defense provisions of the Act make the civil forfeiture less draconian. The amendments regarding after-acquired property do not pose a significant obstacle to the defense and stand to prevent sham transactions where criminals transfer the property to third parties merely with the intention and purpose of thwarting forfeiture. Furthermore, the definition of "bona fide purchaser for value" has been broadened to include property acquired by inheritance or probate.

The Future of the Oppressive State?

CAFRA provides the impetus for change in American civil asset forfeiture law, particularly in its application involving a personal use supply of anabolic steroids.

The passage of the Act was only possible through a compromise of conflicting and competing interests. As such, the legislation offers some benefits to law enforcement, which was necessary to gain the support of the Department of Justice. In this respect, it may be easier for prosecutors to gain forfeited property after criminal convictions. It also establishes a new procedure for federal courts to enforce the forfeiture judgments of foreign nations, which is contained in 28 U.S.C. § 2467. Additionally, it gives the government greater access to financial records to facilitate forfeiture in cases where assets may be held in foreign accounts. As with any compromise, each party walks away with something that is less than they wished for. This is the essence of CAFRA. Not every deficiency and inequity of federal civil asset forfeiture has been addressed; however, considerable improvements have been made for owners/claimants.

Nonetheless, some of the more criticized and controversial problems in civil asset forfeiture remain untouched. The whole concept of *in rem* forfeiture and the punishment of the "thing" belie the Constitution. To ignore that the deprivation of one's property is a form of condemnation and punishment to the individual is illogical and unconstitutional. CAFRA has not changed this underlying premise behind civil asset forfeitures, despite the merits of the Act. For now, we can take some solace in the fact that the CAFRA has brought at least a "modicum of sanity" to the federal civil forfeiture system. But bear in mind, while the U.S. attorney for the federal district may refuse to prosecute the case, state prosecutors across the country may do so, as in Kareem's case. As for Kumar, Winnie and Kareem, their lives remain in a state of uncertainty.

Chapter 21

SILENCE IS GOLDEN

"It is a common delusion that you make things better by talking about them."

– *Dame Rose Macaulay* (1881–1958)

Ernest Miranda was a career criminal whose accomplishments included various minor sex offenses, burglary, driving a stolen car across state lines, and an arrest for armed robbery. (Thank God he wasn't a bodybuilder, or steroids would be blamed for all of it.) In March of 1963, Miranda was arrested in his home and taken to a Phoenix police station, where he was put into a line-up and viewed by a rape victim. She couldn't be sure which man was her attacker. "How did I do?" Miranda asked the police as they took him to an interrogation room. "You flunked," they lied.

Although Miranda was certainly no stranger to the criminal justice system, it didn't take the police long to get a written confession out of him, which he signed. At the top was a typed paragraph saying that Miranda's confession was being made voluntarily, without threats or promises of immunity and "with full knowledge of my legal rights, understanding any statement I make may be used against me." But it didn't specifically say what those rights were. The officers admitted at trial that Miranda was not advised that he had a right to have a lawyer present. Miranda was convicted of rape and kidnapping. The case went all the way up to the United States Supreme Court [*Miranda v. Arizona*, 384 U.S. 436 (1966)]. Chief Judge Warren wrote the opinion, holding:

> From the testimony of the officers and by the admission of respondent, it is clear that Miranda was not in any way apprised of his right to consult with an attorney and to have one present during the interrogation, nor was his right not to be compelled to incriminate himself effectively protected in any other manner. Without these warnings the statements were inadmissible. The mere fact that he signed a statement which contained a typed-in clause stating that he had "full knowledge" of his "legal rights" does not approach the knowing and intelligent waiver required to relinquish constitutional rights.

The *Miranda* Warnings

The *Miranda* decision reaffirmed that confessions must be *voluntary*. It also established a new legal principle. It held that the prosecution can't offer certain statements of the accused unless procedural safeguards are used to protect the privilege against self-incrimination. What kind of procedural safeguards? A series of cautionary advisements would have to be administered before questioning a suspect in custody. These advisements, known to every television detective series viewer since the late 1960's, have come to be called the "*Miranda* warnings." They go like this:

- You have the right to remain silent.
- If you do say anything, what you say can be used against you in a court of law.
- You have the right to the presence of a lawyer prior to and during any questioning.
- If you cannot afford a lawyer, one will be appointed for you if you so desire.
- If you choose to talk to the police officer, you have the right to stop the interview at any time. (This last one often gets short shrift.)

So, if the police give you your *Miranda* warnings, you have a choice. You can either *invoke* your rights or *waive* them. If you invoke your right to silence, the police must *stop* questioning you, at least for a good while. [*Michigan v. Moseley*, 423 US 96 (1975)] If you request a lawyer, your protection is even greater because they can't question you further unless you reinitiate the conversation. You can invoke your right to remain silent or you can ask for a lawyer immediately. You can do *both* – and why not? If you waive your rights, the police might grill you for hours. Who has the time for that?

Do the police *always* have to give the *Miranda* warnings? No, they don't. The rule of *Miranda* applies only to *custodial interrogation*. The two elements – custody and interrogation – must coexist for the warnings to be required. If it's either one without the other, the warnings aren't required.

Custody

Let's talk about custody first. If you're *not* in police custody, the warnings are not applicable even if the police question you. What does "custody" mean? Custody generally means that a reasonable person, innocent of any wrongdoing, would feel that he or she was "not free to leave." The place doesn't matter: it can be at your home or job, at the Postal Inspector's office, in a police car, on the street, or wherever. The standard is an *objective* one. Among the factors to consider are whether the person's presence is voluntary, whether the person was told he was under arrest, whether he was allowed access to food and drink, whether he was allowed contact with his family or friends, and the atmosphere and length of contact with the police. Obviously, *Miranda* doesn't apply if you're questioned over the phone. It doesn't apply if at the time of the questioning, a reasonable person innocent of the crime would feel free to leave.

Custody generally means that a reasonable person, innocent of any wrongdoing, would feel that he or she was "not free to leave."

Let's say you're walking down a street in your town one evening and the police drive up in a patrol car. They stop and ask you if you live in the neighborhood. They ask for your name and address. They ask for identification and where you're going so late at night. Not showing identification and not answering pedigree questions such as your name and address can, in some circumstances, result in an arrest (in some scenarios, not answering a question like what you're doing in the area can lead to a loitering charge).

But they don't stop there. As you answer their questions, they ask further ones. The encounter is uncomfortable. You feel intimidated. Their attitude intentionally implies that you have no choice but to answer their questions. It might not even occur to you that unless the police have probable cause or reasonable suspicion, you have the right to excuse yourself and simply walk away. As their suspicion builds, they may ask more questions, you may give more answers, and before you know it they may have developed enough cause to arrest and handcuff you then and there – maybe in a case of mistaken identity, no less! Without the information you so graciously provided, they might never have had any basis to arrest you at all. You will have effectively talked your way into an arrest! Now, what about the fact that they failed to start out by giving you the *Miranda* warnings? Doesn't that count against them? Sorry, my loose-lipped friend, but unless a judge finds that you were *in custody* when you flapped your gums, everything you said will come back to bite you at trial.

Interrogation

Now let's talk about the second requirement for *Miranda* to apply: interrogation. Basically, that's asking questions (except for pedigree stuff like name, address, etc.). Also, questioning during an investigative traffic stop has been held to not require *Miranda* warnings. [*Berkemer v. McCarty*, 468 U.S. 420 (1984)] But otherwise, if you're in custody and they're going to question you, they have to give the warnings. If you're not going to be questioned, even if you're in custody, the police don't have to give you the warnings. Got that? Let's say they arrest you for a crime, bring you to the precinct, and start fingerprinting you. They're not asking you any questions, so there are no warnings given. But you're nervous and embarrassed, and you mention that you've never done anything like this before and you're really sorry you did it. Can they use your heartfelt expressions of remorse *against you* as admissions of guilt? You bet, my loquacious friend. If you start talking *spontaneously*, they can write every word down and stick it to you in court. No questioning, no *Miranda* needed.

If you're not going to be questioned, even if you're in custody, the police don't have to give you the warnings.

The same goes if they talk to *each other* about you, such as, "This guy is going to be doing some major time, huh, Charlie? He's too stupid to help himself." If you peep up about the case, it's all against you. Look at what happened in *Rhode Island v. Innis* [446 U.S. 291 (1980)]. Innis was arrested for a shotgun robbery. En route to the precinct, two officers engaged in conversation with each other about the fear that the shotgun was probably in the vicinity of a school for handicapped girls, and that one girl might find the gun and accidentally fire it, killing herself. Innis interrupted them to blurt out the location of the shotgun. The Supreme Court held that the safeguards of *Miranda* don't apply if a person's spontaneous statement isn't foreseeable. Sometimes, though, the police can go so far, such as in dumping evidence in front of a suspect after he's invoked his rights, that it becomes the *functional equivalent* of questioning.

Failure to Give the Warnings

Okay, here's the big question. *What happens if the police don't administer your rights?* The case gets thrown out, right? Wrong! The warnings are necessary only if the police interrogate you and want to use any of your responses as evidence against you in court. If they fail to give you *Miranda* warnings, the remedy is that nothing you say in response to the questioning can be used to convict you. Your statements are excluded, or "suppressed" because of the *Miranda* violation.

In addition, under a doctrine known as the "fruit of the poisonous tree," if the police find evidence derived as a result of an interrogation that violates *Miranda,* that derivative evidence is also inadmissible at trial. For example, if you tell the police where you keep your AAS stash in response to questioning that violates *Miranda,* the police will not be able to use the recovered gear as evidence (unless the police can prove that they would have inevitably discovered the steroids without your statements, or that they found out about them from an independent source). However, if the police question you without the warnings and improperly elicit statements, then leave but come back much later and question you anew *after* giving the warnings, statements from the second questioning (and derivative evidence) will be admissible if it is sufficiently "attenuated" from the first – that is, separated by a pronounced break in time or a change in location.

Do some interrogators fail to administer the warnings and then lie about it in court? A few, no doubt. One former detective once told me that a standing joke among certain of his colleagues was that the first time a defendant should hear his rights is when you testify at trial that you gave them to him. Hopefully, that sort of stuff is very rare. But whether the interrogator administers the warnings or not, the rights themselves are guaranteed.

Protecting One's Rights Under *Miranda*

Should a person in custody waive his rights and answer to police interrogation? If you were in any way connected to criminal activity, the almost universal advice of experienced criminal defense attorneys would be to *keep quiet.* In fact, many defense lawyers advocate this approach in almost *all* situations, on the theory that you may not even know you were involved in a crime and could talk yourself into an arrest by opening your mouth. What you say can provide the "missing ingredient" to lock you up. For example, let's say you had picked up a package at the post office for a friend, and it turns out to be juice. What exactly did you know about the contents? Wouldn't it be better to answer *no questions* beyond pedigree ones, and let a lawyer's advice control later on?

Let's assume you've decided that it's absolutely not in your best interests to answer police questions. How do you protect your rights described by *Miranda*? If you're not under arrest, you can simply ask, "Am I under arrest? If not, I'd prefer not to stay and talk to you. I'm leaving now." If the officer replies that you're not free to leave, then you should remain and leave it the courts to decide whether holding you there was proper. Still, you should not answer questions.

Most often, though, you won't get a straight answer as to exactly what your custodial status is. You may be answered with other questions, such as, "Why? If you did nothing wrong, what are you afraid of?" or "Why not get it over with now, rather than have us continue our investigation and have to come to your home or job?" Like a good blackjack dealer, the investigator's job is to make it seem eminently reasonable to stay at the table. They may attempt to convince you that only a guilty person would remain mute or demand a lawyer, and that you'd be best to take advantage of their offers to help you. They will explain in a way that may seem earnest that staying and talking is in your own best interests. That's their job. They're crime fighters. If you've committed a crime, they're against you. However they may personally feel about it is irrelevant. They are sworn to enforce the laws. They have that interest in mind; you have yours.

Assuming that you want to avoid the possibility of self-incrimination, you should be polite, maybe even thank them for their time, but leave as fast as you can. Fly, fly away, and don't incriminate yourself by your own words. In nearly twenty years of practicing criminal law, I can't remember a situation where it benefited a guilty person to answer police questions prior to speaking with a lawyer. You can simply invoke your Fifth Amendment privilege by saying, "I have nothing to say," "I want to remain silent," or "I don't want to talk to you." Even better, invoke your *Sixth Amendment* right by saying, "I want a lawyer right now." Then shut up. If you're under arrest, just sit there. If you're not, immediately scram. A few clients of mine have actually said something like, "Gee, I'd like to chat with you, officer, but on the strictest advice of my lawyer, I can't say a word. Here's his card. Call him; he's a crackerjack. He'll explain everything."

In nearly twenty years of practicing criminal law, I can't remember a situation where it benefited a guilty person to answer police questions prior to speaking with a lawyer.

Be prepared: the appearance of a lawyer in the mix may make the police appear to be very unhappy. They know that lawyers generally have one function at the pre-arrest and arrest stages: to stop their clients from talking. Once a person invokes his Sixth Amendment right to counsel, the invocation preempts further questioning. They hate that. Some detectives might be so angry that they'll continue to interrogate even after invocation of the rights, but a person has the absolute right to stick to his guns and keep waiting for his lawyer.

The importance of an inculpatory statement in a case is huge enough to make Mr. Olympia Ronnie Coleman look tiny. Since many juice prosecutions for possession hinge upon the suspect's knowledge of the contents of the package, a statement can be the key piece of evidence. Sometimes without it, there can be a weak case ... or no case at all. The statement, however, need not be a full confession. Many are the sad souls who made the mistake of thinking a denial on the ultimate issue was enough. For example, I've had numerous clients who vigorously denied any knowledge of the contents of a controlled delivery package, only to then admit to prior steroid use and even to previous steroid mail orders. (Sometimes the agents falsely say that they've identified previous suspicious parcels going to the address.) They overlook the fact that their admissions about prior steroid-related activity tend to incriminate them notwithstanding their denial.

Since many juice prosecutions for possession hinge upon the suspect's knowledge of the contents of the package, a statement can be the key piece of evidence.

In one pending case in Kansas, the police executed a search warrant on my client's house and recovered a very small amount of anabolics. The most damaging piece of evidence was not anything physical. It was his admission to the police that he had made a few dollars on gear that he picked up for his gym buddies. Suddenly, by his *own words* alone, he had elevated himself in the mind of the prosecutor from a personal juice user to a gym dealer. All because he opened his mouth, and for no other reason. Was his mistake unusual? Not a chance. The file cabinets in my office are *bursting* with very similar cases.

We all know the *Miranda* warnings. We all know our Constitutional rights. It's generally bad to incriminate ourselves. So why are there so many confessions? Doesn't it seem odd to you? Most people *don't* invoke their rights. Huh? Why is that? A study conducted in Salt Lake City, Utah, in 1994 found that 84% of suspects did *not* invoke their Constitutional rights during custodial questioning. [P. G. Casell and B. S. Hayman, "Dialogue on *Miranda*: Police Interrogation in the 1990s: An Empirical Study of the Effects of *Miranda*," 43 *UCLA L. Rev.* 839, (1996)] Why are so many people doing so much yapping? How do the police get people to admit what they did, even after they've been administered the warnings?

The police must have some pretty good techniques of getting people to confess. They have to, otherwise many crimes including brutal murders and savage rapes might go unsolved. The police catch the bad guys to protect the rest of us. Is it really so bad if a detective applies a bit of pressure or even trickery in getting some soulless predator to admit where he buried his child-victim's body? Many people are just fine with that.

There's a problem, though, if the techniques are so good that they can get people to confess to crimes they *didn't* do. Take the New York Central Park Jogger case of over a dozen years ago, where a 28-year-old jogger was brutally beaten and raped. Five teenagers were convicted of the crime after they were questioned by police and confessed. They served prison time. Sounds like justice was served, right? Except that now it seems like they didn't do it. A convicted rapist-murderer has confessed that *he*, not the boys, did the crime. And DNA tests reportedly back up his story. If the teens were actually innocent, how could such a thing happen? The next chapter explores the reasons. This is where it gets *really wild* ...

Chapter 22

THE PSYCHOLOGY OF INTERROGATION

"I'm not against the police. I'm just afraid of them."
– *Alfred Hitchcock (1899-1980)*

Interrogation tactics have changed over the centuries. Gone are the days of the rack, rubber hose beatings, or hours under hot lights. Few suspects are hit in the head with a telephone book anymore. Statements extracted by torture, food and sensory deprivation, or brutality are not *voluntary*. Involuntary statements are *inadmissible* in court. Such statements are thrown out, along with any "fruit" derived from the tainted statements. Law enforcement techniques have had to evolve over the years. Today, most law-abiding citizens would like to think of the police as being fair in their questioning of suspects. After all, law enforcers are the guardians of our security from the local to the international level. They are the heroes who keep our families and homes safe from those who have sworn to destroy our way of life. In this age of international terrorists, sexual predators, serial snipers, and assorted criminal dirtbags, we need them now more than ever, that's for sure.

Modern Interrogation Methods

If medieval methods are no longer accepted ways of extracting a confession, why do most suspects today still *waive* their rights, and proceed to talk to the police without an attorney? Why do so many clients come to see me *after* they've spilled their guts to the police? What techniques are employed by modern law enforcement that so effectively extract incriminating statements?

The modern practice of in-custody interrogation is *psychologically* rather than physically oriented. It was concern over present police practices, as documented in various police manuals and texts, which prompted the Supreme Court to institute the rules set forth in *Miranda v. Arizona*. The Court specifically cited various interrogation guides, including F. Inbau & J. Reid, *Criminal Interrogations and Confessions* [Gaithersburg, MD: Aspen Publishers, 1962, currently available as 4th Ed. 2001], and C. O'Hara, *Fundamentals of Criminal Investigation* (out of print, 1956; 7th Ed. to be released January 2003), which advocate the psychological stratagems to employ during interrogations. Law enforcement interrogators are trained in a variety of tactics, enabling them to switch approaches if one isn't working or in order to constantly keep the suspect off balance. Let's not forget that these tactics were developed to succeed in getting even the most jaded and uncooperative rapists and murderers to incriminate themselves. As a society, we seem to be pretty okay with these methods in that context. But these are the same techniques employed in questioning somebody about his possession of a few packages of juice.

The police manuals instruct that the "principal psychological factor contributing to a successful interrogation is privacy – being alone with the person under interrogation." [Inbau, *supra*, 1] The efficacy of this tactic has been explained as follows:

> "If at all practicable, the interrogation should take place in the investigator's office or at least in a room of his own choice. The subject should be deprived of every psychological advantage. In his own home he may be confident, indignant, or recalcitrant. He is more keenly aware of his rights and more reluctant to tell of his indiscretions or criminal behavior within the walls of his home. Moreover, his family and other friends are nearby, their presence lending moral support. In his own office, the investigator possesses all the advantages. The atmosphere suggests the invincibility of the forces of the law." [O'Hara, *supra*, 99]

Obviously, not every interrogation can wait until the suspect can be brought to an interrogation room, euphemistically referred to as an "interview" room by law enforcers, at the station house. For example, in controlled delivery cases, interrogation may begin immediately upon execution of the search warrant. Successful interrogation can be crucial in controlled delivery cases, particularly as to knowledge of the contents of a package that wasn't opened upon receipt. But to whatever extent possible, the police will use the spatial layout of any room in which the questioning will take place in order to maximize the intimidation and stress levels. The suspect typically will be seated with his back to the door, instilling apprehension and uncertainty. Sometimes a piece of furniture will initially separate the interrogator from the suspect, creating a sense of personal space that the interrogator will later invade at a crucial moment. The interrogator will establish control over the situation from the outset. Friends or family will be removed. A sense of isolation sets in. The suspect is alone to face his inquisitors.

Let me address you, the potential suspect. You may be bright and educated. You may have 21" arms with veins like garden hoses. You may be the most massive, jacked-up juicehead in the gym facing off against an interrogator with a pacemaker and arms like spindles. You may even be a police officer yourself, facing an investigator from Internal Affairs. It doesn't matter. In the crucible of interrogation, you are woefully outmatched. He is in a position of power; you are in a position of weakness. He's been instructed in the psychology of persuasion; his tools are patience and perseverance. He's been taught specific methodologies to elicit information. He is the hunter and you are his prey. Unlike the inquisitors of old, he will employ techniques of such subtlety that you will be unaware of them until it's too late.

You may be bright and educated. You may have 21" arms with veins like garden hoses ... It doesn't matter. In the crucible of interrogation, you are woefully outmatched.

Establishing Trust in the Interrogator

The processing associated with an arrest requires that conversation take place between the suspect and the interrogator. At a minimum, pedigree information such as name, address, and date of birth are necessary for the suspect to disclose. Other pieces of information, such as past addresses, employment information, and names of relatives and their contact data, are requested as part of the standard paperwork of an arrest. Thus begins a give-and-take verbal interaction between suspect and interrogator. In a purported effort to make the suspect feel "more comfortable," the interrogator will begin to offer some small talk during the process. "You live on Maple Street? Isn't that the one after Oak Street, the one with the school? Is that the school you went to?" Or, "You're a computer technician? I'm having trouble with my laptop. What could be wrong with it?" Conversation will begin to flow. "Do you want something to drink?" It's all part of the interrogation process, calculated to ultimately lead to an incriminating statement or full-blown confession.

An interrogator trained in psychological manipulation begins by establishing an initial rapport prior to initiating any sensitive questioning. If a bond of mutual interests can be established, a sense of trust can be created. The interrogator will begin calling the suspect by his first name, then follow by feigning interest in the suspect's hobbies or activities. Obviously, in juice cases, this is often achieved by the investigator professing to have an interest in bodybuilding or fitness. He may pretend to have a friend or family member who is a serious bodybuilder. In an actual case from southern California, a detective told "stories of how his wife used to date [a former Mr. Olympia runner-up] and injected him during this time." He may say the suspect looks just like his cousin who is also a bodybuilder. He may ask for diet or training advice, or take note of a suspect's strongest body part and ask what exercises he does for that. He will fool the suspect into thinking that they have a lot in common. Bodybuilders generally love to talk about bodybuilding, and most will take the bait. Remember, the more you talk about *anything* the better it is for the interrogator.

If a bond of mutual interests can be established, a sense of trust can be created. He may ask for diet or training advice ... the more you talk about *anything* the better it is for the interrogator.

Of course, once a suspect starts talking about bodybuilding, the topic will inevitably go toward muscle-building drugs. The interrogator will feign genuine interest, maybe even asking about side effects and safety issues. The conversation will have a "just-between-us" quality, encouraging honesty. Since the suspect already committed himself to truthful answers on some subjects, it's now harder to lie about others. It also becomes more difficult to invoke the right to silence, after having shared a bit of quality time together. The suspect now *trusts* his interrogator.

The interrogator may employ the strategy of "self-disclosure." He will pretend to reveal certain truths about himself. "You know, Joe, when I was a kid, I thought about taking steroids. Lots of my friends did," or even, "I once tried steroids, Joe. It's true. I understand where you're coming from." Of course, these "revelations" are completely invented and are merely designed to make it easier for the suspect to make an admission. This strategy takes advantage of the overwhelming wave of relief that typically comes when the suspect perceives the interrogator as "someone who understands." The interrogator may not ask the suspect directly about his sale or possession of anabolics in the case. He may work up to it slowly, first by asking about steroids in general, then about whether the suspect has ever tried them. "Come on, look at the size of you. Nobody gets like that without steroids, Joe."

Reading the Cues

During the questioning, the interrogator will closely monitor the suspect's body language, facial expressions, and other verbal and non-verbal cues. Verbal cues may include talking in a higher-pitched voice, speaking more slowly, taking longer to start answering a question, and making more frequent speech errors. Fidgeting, leg-shaking, finger-tapping, and gaze aversion are all carefully observed.

Researchers have found that an honest (and *innocent*) suspect, when questioned, tends to be helpful, expects exoneration, displays resentment towards the guilty party, and appears both spontaneous and sincere. A deceptive (and guilty) suspect provides less helpful information, shows inappropriate concern about being a suspect, lacks response spontaneity and sincerity, and uses both guarded and clearly edited verbal responses. Emotionally, the guilt of dishonesty or the fear of detection can initiate a stress reaction that activates the sympathetic nervous system into a "fight or flight" mode. Intensely cognizant of the apparent cues of his nervousness, the suspect will try to restrain them all. Usually he'll fail, sometimes by *overcompensating* and appearing stiff and artificial. Sometimes, the interrogator will point out the telltale signals of guilt; drawing the suspect's attention to them can elicit a confession. Interestingly, rehearsing the interrogation in advance may assist in the effectiveness of deception by allowing a suspect to cognitively play it out, although a canned speech that sounds rehearsed is a dead-giveaway of dishonesty. For more information on this general topic, *see* A. Vrij, *Detecting Lies and Deceit: The Psychology of Lying and the Implications for Professional Practice* [John Wiley & Sons, 2000].

The emotional attitude of the interrogator also plays a role in the interrogation. Interrogation manuals instruct the police to display an air of total *confidence* in the suspect's guilt. Guilt is to be posited as a fact, fully established. The interrogation is presented as merely the process of confirming the details about what the police already know. For example, the interrogator may ask *why* the suspect committed the crime, as if the only remaining issue is the motive. "Look, we both know what happened, Joe, I'm just trying to figure out why." The interrogator may begin making suggestions as to the reasons for the crime, incorporating into his suggestions facts about the suspect he has already learned. "Look, Joe, I know how much you want to turn pro. You're doing what you have to do to make it in bodybuilding, that's all." By supplying the excuse for the commission of the crime, the interrogator offers the bait of rationalization. Of course, the interrogator doesn't really care what reason the suspect gives for committing the crime as long as he admits that he did it.

Interrogation manuals instruct the police to display an air of total *confidence* in the suspect's guilt. ... The interrogation is presented as merely the process of confirming the details ...

Minimizing the Offense

This approach can be extended into an extremely effective technique called "minimization," that downplays the moral seriousness of the offense. "It's not like this was hard drugs, Joe. If it were, I wouldn't be talking to you. It's just steroids. Help me wrap up this paperwork and we can all move on," or, "I know you're not a dealer, Joe. We both know that. This was personal use. Help me to help you, Joe." The interrogator may minimize the legal consequences, too. "Nobody goes to jail for this, Joe. What's important here is that you learn from this. The judge will see that." Of course, not every judge does see it that way. Maybe the suspect has some prior convictions or maybe the quantity of steroids was exceptionally large or maybe the judge just has some quirky distaste for muscleheads.

Of course, if the suspect then admits, for example, the knowing possession of the anabolics for personal use, the interrogator will not necessarily relent. If there are any facts suggesting that the suspect was distributing anabolics, even if it's just the possession of a large quantity, the next goal would be to explore fully the personal use theory in an effort to develop factors that might be inconsistent. "But, gee, Joe, that sounds like a lot of steroids for yourself. Most guys share steroids with their gym buddies. There's nothing really wrong about that, Joe. But I have to know, okay?"

Theme Development

During the process of *theme development*, the interrogator will toss out various scenarios that the suspect may be attracted to. If the suspect appears to be listening to the interrogator, the interrogator will know he is on the right track. "Anyone can make a mistake, Joe. Do you think everyone deserves a second chance?" An innocent person might reject this theme, but a guilty person would not. If the suspect appears to reject this theme, the interrogator will move on to another one. "I'm not saying you did this, Joe. But if you did, it's going to eat at you. Don't you have something to tell me, Joe?"

Theme exploration can go on for long periods, as the interrogator assesses the suspect's receptivity to various offerings. "Judges like to hear people say they've learned a lesson from their mistakes, Joe. I know you'll never do this again. Can I tell the judge that about you, Joe?" If the suspect continues his denial, he will be met with persistence, offering different "ways out." "Look, Joe, we both know what happened. If I thought you'd done this thing before, I wouldn't be here. I want to help you. If you tell me this was your one and only time, I'll write it up that way." The art of this technique is in the ability to make the suspect believe, despite his better judgment and every ounce of common sense, that it is in his own best interests to confess the crime to his inquisitor. Sometimes the suspect will have a family member or close friend in law or law enforcement, and will tell the interrogator that this person advised him to never talk to the police without a lawyer. The job of the interrogator is to sell the idea that somehow this one unusual, particular, unprecedented, once-in-a-lifetime situation is *different*. Of course, it isn't.

The art of this technique is in the ability to make the suspect believe, despite his better judgment and ... common sense, that it is in his own best interests to confess the crime to his inquisitor.

Cooperation Overtures

It's extremely common for the interrogator to urge the suspect to *cooperate* against his confederates, in return for a promise of leniency. He will state that he is less interested in the suspect than in the suspect's associates, particularly his supplier(s). That's probably true, in the grand scheme of things. But right now he's also very interested in getting a confession. If the suspect manifests some interest in this theme, the interrogator stands to reap a double benefit: a confession from the suspect and the potential for other arrests.

While the subject of cooperators is more fully discussed in another chapter, a few obvious observations must be made here. First, if you were looking to strike a deal, wouldn't the bargain be more to your advantage if a skilled and experienced criminal lawyer negotiated it? Second, be advised that only the prosecutor, *not* the cop or agent, has the authority to make a binding plea agreement. Third, don't forget that you can't cooperate without first *waiving your rights* and talking about your criminal conduct. Assuming you do want to cooperate, wouldn't it make sense to make that choice only after having fully discussed it with an attorney, who could also discuss the pros and cons of the prerequisite waiver of your right to silence?

Assorted Techniques

Various other manipulation techniques assist the interrogator. It has been reported that some interrogators will stuff a file folder with various unrelated papers and write the suspect's name on it. The folder is then used to suggest the large volume of evidence against the suspect. Some interrogators will punctuate periods of conversation with long periods of silence, which can become so psychologically discomforting that the suspect will engage the interrogator into further conversation. Others will break the suspect down by repeatedly throwing him off balance, such as by alternating intervals of complimentary remarks ("You must bench a ton") with insults ("You must have balls like raisins"). If the suspect has children in the home, it's not uncommon for interrogators to suggest that the children may be taken away to foster care because of the suspect's steroid involvement. The psychological stress produced by these effects can make the suspect's priorities change from preserving his rights to stopping the intense discomfort of the situation.

Simple behavioral modification techniques can be employed during questioning. One such method is to positively reinforce desired responses and negatively reinforce undesired responses. The lab animal that is given an electric shock upon certain behavior and given a food reward upon other behavior will adapt accordingly. The more subtle form of the technique is well suited to the interrogation setting. As long as the suspect resists, he will be subjected to negative stimuli. When he answers a question or otherwise behaves in a desired manner, the inquisitor will reward him with favorable words or treatment. Over time, the suspect is *conditioned.*

Another conditioning effect is sometimes called the "yes" mode. It involves asking a series of questions the answer to which must be "yes," followed by a question or questions that will incriminate the suspect. The repeated use of a word by the interrogator followed by a "yes" by the suspect creates a rhythm that can have a subconscious conditioning effect:

"You like to work out, right?"
  "Yes."
"You work out at a gym, right?"
  "Yes."
"You train hard, right?"
  "Yes."
"You want to get big, right?"
  "Yes."
"Steroids get you big, right?"
  "Yes."
"You've tried them, right?"
  "*..Yes.*"

Gradually, step by step, the skilled inquisitor leads the suspect further down the path. For example, having finally obtained an admission of a first-time Internet order, the interrogator may then confront the suspect with conflicting evidence. "You know, Joe, as I now look through this file from Customs, I see you've had packages seized from you before. They had steroids in them, Joe. You know, Joe, I really wanted to help you. I still want to help you, Joe. But if you're going to lie to me, I can't do that." Confronted with lying to his "friend," the suspect may be unable to resist admitting everything.

Putting Yourself in the Shoes

It is easy for the casual reader to underestimate the effectiveness of the art of a skilled inquisitor. It's difficult to fully imagine the subjective experience of undergoing a police interrogation, regardless of guilt or innocence. Think about it. Try to visualize yourself accused of a crime, being taken to an interrogation room in handcuffs. Your mind is spinning. You picture the faces of your loved ones, your friends, your employers and co-workers. What will they think of you now? You rehash every past act that may have brought you here. Your future becomes a great, gaping unknown, your mind swirling in a vortex of images of courtrooms and prison cells. What will become of you? How will this affect your future, your family and your job? Your sense of vulnerability will never be as high as at this moment. It is within this emotional maelstrom that the interrogator inserts his subtle manipulations.

As you can now see, the typical suspect – confused, vulnerable, nauseous and hopelessly searching for reassurance – is no match for modern interrogation tactics. The superb 1995 film "The Usual Suspects" details the grueling inquisition of a crippled suspect by a U.S. Customs agent. Students of interrogation techniques will enjoy the movie immensely, as the agent bears down on his suspect with relentless perseverance. "Verbal" Kint, played by actor Kevin Spacey, ultimately talks his way out of police custody by weaving a rich tapestry of information detailing every aspect of the crime. Spacey's character is a con man of unparalleled talent; besides, the film is fiction. Anyone who believes that he can talk his way out of trouble in the way this film portrays is self-deluded. In fact, even experienced interrogators have fallen victim to their own techniques. It's easy for a lawyer to blithely advise, "Keep your mouth shut." But the Supreme Court in *Miranda* expressly recognized the way interrogation techniques undermine such advice (these aren't *my* words, *but those of Chief Justice Warren*):

It's easy for a lawyer to blithely advise, "Keep your mouth shut." But the Supreme Court in *Miranda* expressly recognized the way interrogation techniques undermine such advice ...

> "The manuals also contain instructions for police on how to handle the individual who refuses to discuss the matter entirely, or who asks for an attorney or relatives. The examiner is to concede him the right to remain silent. "This usually has a very undermining effect. First of all, he is disappointed in his expectation of an unfavorable reaction on the part of the interrogator. Secondly, a concession of this right to remain silent impresses the subject with the apparent fairness of his interrogator." After this psychological conditioning, however, the officer is told to point out the incriminating significance of the suspect's refusal to talk:
>
> 'Joe, you have a right to remain silent. That's your privilege and I'm the last person in the world who'll try to take it away from you. If that's the way you want to leave this, O. K. But let me ask you this. Suppose you were in my shoes and I were in yours and you called me in to ask me about this and I told you, *I don't want to answer any of your questions*. You'd think I had something to hide, and you'd probably be right in thinking that. That's exactly what I'll have to think about you, and so will everybody else. So let's sit here and talk this whole thing over.'" [*Miranda, supra,* 453 (citations omitted)]

If the suspect asks if he should have an attorney, there are classic police responses, such as, "Why would you need one?" The goal is to make the suspect think that invoking his right to counsel will make him *more* of a suspect than he is already. Some suspects will answer questions just to show they "have nothing to hide." But most suspects *do* have something to hide. If you're in custody and being questioned by the police, the police have concluded that you're guilty. Invoking your Fifth Amendment privileges will not, I repeat, *not* make you any guiltier in their eyes. Obviously, if a suspect invokes his right to counsel, questioning should stop. In the real world, however, this doesn't always happen. Sometimes the police will sidestep the issue, and keep questioning. One police response to a request for an attorney is to imply that the delay to get a lawyer will result in a "missed opportunity." The pitch might be, "If you want to wait around until we can find one, fine. But I can only help you right now." Of course, the one who could really help the suspect is a criminal defense lawyer. Period.

"Yes or No" Technique

When normal procedures are slow to produce the needed result, the police may resort to more aggressive practices. One is the so-called "Yes or No" technique. The interrogator will lead up to it by using a variety of tactics to rattle the suspect and throw him off balance. Then he will present a "last chance" to confess: "My time is valuable, but I'm going to give you one last chance to save yourself. All I want to hear out of you is a yes or a no. Got it? All I want out of you is a yes or a no. Don't interrupt me. Yes or no. Nothing else, or I'll walk out that door and you're dead, dead, dead. Yes or no." The question that follows generally won't be the ultimate, "Did you do it?", but will rather be a slightly more palatable one that mildly incriminates the suspect. "Now we're getting somewhere," the interrogator will say as he follows up with progressively more damaging questions.

Good Cop/Bad Cop

Another time-tested and well-known approach is the classic "Good Cop/Bad Cop" routine. If the suspect persists in his refusal to talk, another law enforcement agent appears. His belligerent attitude is intended to bring the suspect's sense of guilt and discomfort up to near unbearable levels. He will gradually ratchet up the intensity of his accusations, citing the overwhelming proof of guilt in the case. He will attempt to demoralize and demean, e.g., "You're a very inept liar." He may promise that refusing to talk is a fatal mistake that will have a hefty price, such as by "turning a small case into a big one." Many suspects will finally begin talking under this sort of relentless assault. If the suspect is not receptive to this approach, however, the "bad cop" may profess delight that the suspect isn't talking, because then he can make nasty notes for the prosecutor to give to the judge at the bond hearing that the suspect was uncooperative.

> ... the bad cop will storm out of the room, leaving only the suspect and the "friend." Released from the terrible pressure of the bad cop, the suspect will find it a great relief to talk to the "friend" ...

Dealing with the bad cop is extremely stressful. His assertions are intended to make the suspect rethink his interests. But the bad cop is often just a hiatus from the true inquisitor. It is the good cop or "friend" who is always the greatest danger – the most lethal weapon in the arsenal of law enforcement.

At some point, the bad cop will storm out of the room, leaving only the suspect and the "friend." Released from the terrible pressure of the bad cop, the suspect will find it a great relief to talk to the "friend," who will continue his soft-spoken and concerned efforts to seemingly help the suspect before the bad cop returns. At this point, most suspects are unable to resist. Once Joe finally confesses, the "friend" will thank him for doing so and assure him that he has done the right thing.

Police Trickery

If all else fails, the interrogator may resort to various forms of trickery to fool the suspect out of exercising his constitutional rights. The leading interrogation manual (Inbau & Reid, *supra*) vigorously espouses the merits of deceptive interrogation tactics. These techniques include misleading the suspect into thinking he's a witness when he's a suspect. Another is exaggerating the evidence, such as the quantity of steroids involved, or claiming to have evidence of other criminal conduct, such as the delivery of prior steroid packages to the suspect's home. This form of lying may be called "bluffing" among law enforcers. When bluffing, however, the interrogator takes a big chance if he claims to know something that the suspect is *certain* cannot be true, because it may cause the suspect to disbelieve all the interrogator's statements.

Another tactic is to imply that the interrogator has the power to cut a deal for the suspect, when in reality only the *prosecutor* is empowered to do so. Some unscrupulous interrogators will flat-out lie and tell a suspect he'll go home if he confesses, then later deny in court the promise was made. Where two suspects are arrested together, an old favorite is to play one against the other. Separated, each will be falsely told that the other has confessed and implicated him.

Another tactic is to imply that the interrogator has the power to cut a deal for the suspect, when in reality only the *prosecutor* is empowered to do so.

While there are some limits on the duplicity that law enforcers may employ, trickery is a well-established element of interrogation methodology. Police trickery is but one factor to consider in determining the voluntariness of a confession. For an analysis of the policy concerns and legal standards applicable to police deceit, and a suggestion for a per se standard in forbidding police trickery in inducing confessions, *see* D. Sasaki, "Guarding the Guardians: Police Trickery and Confessions," 40 *Stan. L. Rev.* 1593 [1988]. For a philosophical discussion of which police lies should be deemed acceptable, *see* C. Slobogin, "Deceit, Pretext, and Trickery: Investigative Lies by the Police," 76 *Or. L. Rev.* 775 [Winter, 1997].

Some authors have concluded that police lying undermines the integrity of the criminal justice system, and breeds distrust of police. Some even contend that the police should be held to a higher standard of ethics than the criminals they interrogate, and that lying in the station house leads naturally to lying elsewhere, such as in the courtroom. These issues are explored by D. Young in "Unnecessary Evil: Police Lying in Interrogations," 28 *Conn. L. Rev.* 425 [Winter, 1996].

Police interrogation has been responsible for solving many heinous crimes. Lying is considered a necessary evil for effective law enforcers, who must overcome the natural tendency of criminals to protect themselves from arrest. It is unlikely that restraints will be placed upon the existing parameters of proper interrogation. Those who find themselves in the unfortunate situation of being interrogated, however, should recognize that their own personal interests might diverge sharply from the societal interests of law enforcement. The United States Constitution, as interpreted through *Miranda,* is the rock upon which a suspect has every entitlement to stand.

Summing It All Up

While it may well be that nothing can truly prepare someone – innocent or otherwise – for the experience of interrogation, careful study of the points raised in this chapter should be of great assistance. It should also be pointed out that some of the techniques described are not limited to the interrogation room. Pre-employment screening examiners use lie detection techniques all the time. Applicants for jobs in law enforcement, in particular, should be mindful that interviewers are trained to detect deception and will sometimes employ minimization, self-disclosure, or other techniques to persuade the applicant to reveal unfavorable background information.

So, what's a suspect to do if he wishes to invoke his Constitutional protections? He can't sit there like a "wooden Indian" because the process requires some verbal interaction. But how does he cut off the conversation before his Constitutional rights just evaporate? There are two things a suspect must do:

> *First,* the suspect must consciously refuse to respond to any questions, statements or stimuli beyond the basic pedigree information, always keeping in mind that the interrogator's primary goal is to extract an incriminating statement.
>
> *Second,* he must immediately and repeatedly invoke his Fifth Amendment privilege and Sixth Amendment right to counsel by requesting a lawyer and stating that he does not wish to be questioned. It isn't easy, but it's the only way to safeguard the rights guaranteed under the Constitution. In this scenario, only the strong survive.

As a review of the lessons of this chapter and the last, the following short test is offered.

If you are asked whether you prefer to be called Joe, Joey, or Joseph, you should:

a) Admit your Aunt Sadie called you "Sugar Pants";
b) Say you'd like to talk a bit more before using first names;
c) Immediately say, "I don't want to talk and I want my lawyer," then say nothing else.

While the answers in both a) or b) are not incriminating in themselves, they open the door to continued discussion. That's bad if you're seeking to invoke your rights. Continued discussion will invariably lead to temptations to waive them. Only answer c) provides a firm and unequivocal refusal to continue the interview.

If you are asked about your maximum bench press or how you built your fabulous biceps peak, you should:

a) Demonstrate your favorite variation of preacher curls;
b) Pull off your shirt, smile, and hit your front double biceps shot for all it's worth;
c) Immediately say, "I don't want to talk and I want my lawyer," then say nothing else.

If you answered anything other than c), you're on a slippery slope. You are well on your way to confessing *everything* you've ever done wrong. Forgive me for beating you over the head with my point here, but I need to be sure that you fully understand this.

If you are told that there is a videotape of you committing the crime, you should:

a) Admit it, because they've got you cold, bro;
b) Deny it, and call their bluff by asking to see the tape right now;
c) Politely but immediately say, "I don't want to talk and I want my lawyer," then say nothing else.

If you picked answer a), start this chapter over. If you picked answer b), you're still not getting it. The goal is to politely *shut down communication,* not to engage in conversation. Don't admit, and don't deny. Admitting is a confession, and denying is a lie. You don't have to do either! You can look them squarely in the eye, ask for a lawyer immediately, and say nothing else. You can do this over and over and over for as long as it takes.

If you are asked if you have ever used steroids before, you should:

a) Proudly display your favorite injection sites;
b) Admit using a "a long time ago" but firmly deny involvement in this crime;
c) Again, politely but immediately say, "I don't want to talk and I want my lawyer," then say nothing else.

Did you say c)? I think you're getting it!

If they throw a bag of steroid tablets on the desk in front of you and say, "What are these?" you should:

a) Pop a handful in your mouth and ask for a glass of water;
b) Deny, deny, deny;
c) Again, politely but immediately say, "I don't want to talk and I want my lawyer," then say nothing else.

Any questions? Examination concluded.

Chapter 23

YOUR TAX DOLLARS AT WORK

"The government solution to a problem is usually
as bad as the problem."
– Milton Friedman (b. 1912)

I like Mike. He's got a friendly, selfless way about him, the kind of guy who'd do anything for a buddy. "Mike" is his real name, by the way; he insisted that I use it. That's just like him. Mike lives in Maryland with his wife and family. He's about the same age as me, and we share a seasoned knowledge of all aspects of physical culture, from exercise performance techniques to diet and nutrition, as well as a love of bodybuilding since we were teenagers. We're both reaching the age where those minor training injuries take a bit longer to heal, and we laughingly compare complaints from time to time. Like me, Mike works hard and then trains in the evenings. We both enjoy our time at the gym, bookending just a little social chitchat around an "all-business" workout. I met Mike after he was arrested. This is the true story of what they did to Mike.

I like Mike. He's got a friendly, selfless way about him, the kind of guy who'd do anything for a buddy.

About a year ago, John Romano, the Senior Editor of *Muscular Development* magazine, contacted me about a project he was thinking about. He wanted to write an article about a real life steroid bust, and he wanted to feature one of my cases. John is a talented and entertaining writer, and I was excited to work with him. The case I suggested was Mike's. Together, John, Mike, and I put together and published the true story of what happened. Here it is, updated and in John's own brash, colorful, inimitable language.

BUSTED!
A True Story
By John Romano

Steroid use flies in the face of the medical establishment because we who use them do so not to treat disease, but to enhance our looks or our performance, selfishly, for our own ego satisfaction or personal gain. You can bet that a solid chunk of the AMA is pretty much in agreement that it would be unethical to prescribe powerful hormones and medications to people who are not sick, and most doctors pretty much don't. Except, of course, for a teenage girl with nasty thoughts on her mind and a notion to do something about them; she can ask her doctor for birth control pills so she can shag her way through college and not get pregnant.

Her doctor can thus legally prescribe steroids so she can go have recreational sex. If, by the time she has graduated college and had enough bad sex to come to the conclusion there really is a man trapped in her body, she can go through a sex change procedure, which includes a lifetime of legally prescribed steroids to support her folly. However, bodybuilders can't get a script to help themselves become better at what they do. *They* have to break the law. In some corners of the world there are the odd medical professionals who will oblige us, and those fortunate enough to be availed to such a convenience will get a "*You go, boy!*" from me every time. At least there's a handful of us cheating death the right way.

Keep the Feds Busy

Our government decided for us that since all major national, and practically every international, sports federation has rules forbidding the use of performance enhancing drugs, the manufacturing, sale, distribution, and importation of such drugs would be deemed illegal by persons not licensed to do so. This ultimately led up to someone in the Bush administration having his/her arm so twisted by the do-gooders, that anabolic steroids were included in the Controlled Substances Act in 1990. This added steroids to Schedule III of the DEA's list of controlled substances, the only drugs on the list devoid of euphoric or consciousness-altering properties.

A tiny minority of alarmist members of the medical community proclaimed that they didn't want athletes to use steroids because steroids are supposedly dangerous to their health; you have to be in bad health first, then you can use them. So, they join the sports lobby and manage to get the Feds to agree, and they do, and why not? More civil servants have become agents; they need to be on task forces and special drug units so they can *do* something. The cops need something to do so they can justify letting the crackheads keep multiplying while asking the taxpayers for more money.

Then they get to go out and try to rub something as innocuous as steroids off the map by throwing everyone who buys and sells them into prison! Yeah, that makes sense – let guys work out all day and have the government pay for it. They don't want athletes to use steroids so they use taxpayer money to investigate, arrest, and prosecute the offenders with the intent of locking them up in a joint with a huge weight pile so the taxpayers can support the convicts while they train without drugs. Not even in a cavalier sense could this be considered purposeful government spending. The greatest risk there ever is to a bodybuilder is not his health; it's his freedom.

As much as this screams to be fixed, this is the usual course every so-called "battle" in the war on drugs takes. It's so retarded. The federal government has proven time and time again to fail, and fail miserably, fighting this war that it can't possibly win. It costs the taxpayers gazillions in the process, the government keeps losing, but it still keeps "fighting" in its tired, old, ineffective way. The Feds never accomplish anything but throw thousands of people in jail to suck on the tax rolls. All you have to do is reminisce about the touted scourges of the street throughout the 60s, 70s, 80s, and 90s to see the wreckage.

Has the use of heroin, cocaine, marijuana, amphetamines, and PCP declined significantly over the years? Not significantly; those drugs are certainly still around. Yet each of them, and others, have enjoyed the DEA's spotlight while it champions a reason to increase its budget. Look at all the attention Ecstasy has been getting. Far more people suffer health risks due to over-the-counter drugs, but, dog-gone-it, those rave parties are just not wholesome and by golly they've a mind to do something about it. Unfortunately, these are the very people who should be on Ecstasy. Eventually the news will ebb, the Feds will claim victory and they'll be off looking for another party to stop while the old one keeps rolling. They'll never get people to stop using Ecstasy, just like people still use the other drugs the government fought to get rid of.

The reality is, the Feds are not fighting anything; they are just feeding the machine that keeps the wheels turning. If steroids disappeared off the black market and everyone could get them as legitimately as aspirin, what would all those special agents and task forces and special drug units be going after? They're civil servants; they always have a job. And therein lies the rub. If a federal agency fails to spend all of its budget one year, it won't get what it wants the next. You never hear of a DEA agent getting laid off because there's not enough work. They'll find something for which to bust you, I promise.

However, while much of the media focus is on steroid testing in sports lately, they are as illegal as they ever were to buy, sell, transport, distribute, import, conceal, carry, etc. It's not illegal to use them though. I always thought that was kind of funny – yeah, okay, I can use them, but how the hell am I supposed to get them into my bathroom? Well, my friends, *that's* where you take the chance. And in doing so, you may end up just another casualty of the war on drugs.

Valid Medical Use? Not!

I'll bet you never think of that when you're getting ready to gear up. Too busy with those blood test results, and who's got what, and is it fake? And if it is a fake, is it a good fake? Will the guy over the Internet really send me my shit after I send him the money orders? And where are all those syringes supposed to come from? Am I going to strangle my girlfriend when the test kicks in? These are but many of the concerns drifting through a would-be steroid user's brain prior to fixing his cycle.

Most guys don't think the bad guys are ever going to get them for buying just a few measly bottles of this or that, and they shop for their gear pretty much like they would shop for a Mother's Day present. In fact, many Internet sites that are still working sell real live steroids delivered to your "address" just as conveniently and as efficiently as FlowersDirect.com will deliver that killer spring bouquet to your mom. That's where the similarities end, though. No matter what, your mom will get the flowers and she'll just love them. The same can't be said about you and your alleged delivery from FarmaciaJuarez.mx.com. Some packages make it, some don't; the ones that do aren't always a hit. That's the chance you take.

But what of the shipments that don't make it? They pile up somewhere and, if the pile gets big enough, it can eventually lead the way to your door. Since it can, I think it's only fitting that you guys understand what you're in for when you order something and instead receive a note from Uncle Sam telling you *they* have it. Your problems are not over if you just crumple it up and throw it away like you're supposed to. If you keep ordering, eventually a DEA agent dressed as the mailman will come knocking with your alleged package under his arm. He's not working a second job for the post office; he wants to arrest you.

According to renowned New York steroid defense lawyer Rick Collins, "The U.S. Customs Mail Division searches packages that arrive at international airports. Packages from 'hot' areas like Thailand, Eastern Europe and Mexico are reportedly often targeted. Suspicious packages can be opened and examined. When controlled substances are discovered, Customs will seize the package and exercise one of two options. The first is to send a "seizure letter" on "Department of the Treasury, U.S. Customs Service" letterhead. A seizure letter is a notice from Customs notifying the designated recipient that his package has been detained for investigation. In the case of anabolic steroids, this would occur because the importation of controlled substances is a federal offense.

"The letter offers the opportunity to contest the seizure by providing proof of a legitimate medical basis for the importation. Since using steroids for building muscle is not a valid medical basis, steroid seizures are almost never contested. If the designated recipient doesn't respond, there will generally be no follow-up (although the addresses of origin and destination and designated recipient's name will be entered into the Customs computerized data system to help "flag" future packages). A bunch of prior seizure notices will make future packages more likely to be inspected, and will make the second option, a controlled delivery, more probable."

A Normal Kind of Guy

The "controlled delivery" option (when a DEA agent gets to drive the FedEx truck) was the option exercised on one of Mr. Collins' clients – well, sort of. Let's call him Mike. His experience is truly a testament to why those on the "other side" dislike the cops. With all the brouhaha associated with the deleterious health consequences of steroid use, we never seem to hear mention of the deleterious effect getting busted can have on you, your wife and kids, not to mention your health and well-being. How odd is that? Far more steroid users are in jail or awaiting trial than in the hospital or the graveyard, yet you never hear about the legal end. Now, I know "using" steroids isn't, in fact, illegal. However getting them in the U.S. without a prescription, even for free, is. Mike got such a prescription for his first two cycles, yet found that the allotted amount – 200 milligrams of Deca twice a month for two months total – wasn't going to cut it, and he couldn't get a script for more. Mike had the next best thing though: access to the Internet.

As with most things in bodybuilding, everything works, but nothing works all the time. His story is certainly one you should be aware of the next time you order your gear electronically because it goes way beyond the scope of what you might be in for just scoring out of some guy's gym bag. His wife – a prominent member of the community who never had so much as a parking ticket on her record and who had absolutely nothing to do with his steroid use – was busted and charged along with him. Their children were home alone when 15 cops served the search warrant, and they were first rate dickheads. As insane an account as this may sound, the reality is that it not only happened, but it could also happen to you.

I met Mike and his wife, Kim. He's a pretty normal kind of guy; a 42- year-old computer analyst with a stable job. He owns his home with his wife of three years that they share with her three children from a previous marriage. Kim, 39, is a licensed funeral director and mortician, who was previously a registered nurse. Mike began bodybuilding at age 16 as a way to positively focus his energies while he ditched his recreational drug use. While he permanently gave up recreational drugs at 21, his weight training efforts continued, and he still trains today.

He trained naturally until his mid 20s, then became convinced by virtue of the popular bodybuilding publications he regularly read, that anabolic steroids could greatly enhance his training. He started by using 500 milligrams a week of testosterone with 20-30 milligrams a day of D-Bol and he gained 50 pounds in two years. He also experimented with Finajet, Bolasterone and Deca, partially on the advice of late steroid guru Dan Duchaine. He then quit steroids for approximately 10 years and continued to train naturally.

At 37, he decided to try steroids again to enhance his training. At Mike's age, natural hormones are in a state of decline and hard, dedicated training and proper diet and nutrition come with little reward for someone with more youthful aspirations. Of course, this can be terribly frustrating and certainly the impetus for using performance enhancing drugs, just as much as it would be for a 20-year-old Olympian. Although the argument could be made that the Olympian has better reason to use performance enhancing drugs, that argument could be bested easily by the dude in the mirror, as long as he believes: *To thine own self be true*. Mike's only regret was waiting so long.

ATTORNEY'S NOTE:

"Mike is pretty typical of guys arrested for juice. Without doubt, some teenagers do try steroids. We should target our societal efforts toward stopping them. But the overwhelming majority of my steroid clients are otherwise law-abiding guys in their late 20s to mid 40s with stable jobs and no criminal records. What happened to Mike in this case can happen to anyone ordering steroids through the mail. The extent of the indignities and the unusual coincidences in Mike's case were exceptional, though. So was the degree of combined ineptitude and zeal by the police involved and the degree of negligence by the court." — RC

The Thailand Connection

Mike established a rapport with overseas sources using the Internet and was able to order steroids for himself without restraint. What led to Mike's arrest was the D-Bol he was getting from Thailand. He'd order in 1,000-tablet amounts (the minimum order), typically sent in 10 separate envelopes, a hundred in each. At first, these were received with ease. But soon after, seizure notices were arriving instead of the steroids — a sign that Customs had become more aware of these particular shipments from Thailand.

It was a similar shipment from Thailand for 10 envelopes of 100 tabs each that caused Customs to alert the local authorities. And thus, a case that really should have had federal jurisdiction was handed over to a bunch of inexperienced redneck local cops. Obviously, the Feds couldn't be bothered with such a spindly little case, but to the county cops of this little suburban community just outside Baltimore, it was like Pablo Escobar had just hit town. They proceeded to obtain a warrant and conduct a search of Mike's home and cars, despite the fact that the destination of the order was a P.O. box and no controlled delivery was ever conducted. There really was no link between the drug intended to go to the P.O. Box, and Mike's home and cars, other than speculation that Mike was a big drug dealer. Well, big for Mike and Kim's sleepy little town.

ATTORNEY'S NOTE:

"The handling of the investigation – of Mike's entire prosecution, in fact – showed the total inexperience of the authorities involved. While Customs agents reportedly made nearly 9,000 steroid seizures last year, juice remains an area of confusion for most agents, prosecutors, judges and defense lawyers. A controlled delivery of the package is step one in mail importation busts. An agent posing as a courier or letter carrier attempts delivery supported by a hidden backup team often including postal investigators and local law enforcement. Once the package is accepted, the agents move in to arrest the suspect, question him and ransack his home.

"In situations where a mail drop or post office box is the destination, agents will usually invent some ruse to force the suspect to come out and personally claim the package. Or, if necessary, they'll stake out the scene to see who comes to pick it up. The controlled delivery is a way of getting the package into the suspect's hands, strengthening the case against him, and a way of justifying a warrant to raid the residence. In Mike's case, no delivery was done, yet a judge authorized a search of Mike's house. The validity of a search with little nexus, or connection, between a post office box and the box owner's residence like this is debatable, with courts in different states deciding cases differently." — RC

So, one day, Mike arrived home from the gym, opened the door and was accosted by three armed county cops. He was quickly handcuffed, read his rights and led to his kitchen to wait while more than a dozen other uniformed and plainclothes cops searched his house and car. The cops had been there for hours, entering the home while Mike's three daughters, ages 11, 13 and 17, were home alone. Soon thereafter, Kim arrived. The ladies were made to sit on the couch for five hours and were not even permitted to use the rest room.

As luck would have it, during the search, the children's biological father pulled up. He happened to have been visiting the children at their basketball game that evening. Kim told the officers executing the search that her ex-husband was a Delaware State trooper with a violent temper against whom she once had a restraining order. In deference to the problems her ex-husband could cause if he found out his daughters were home while the house was being searched for Mike's steroids, Kim asked the cops not to make the situation apparent. As soon as the words left her lips, several uniformed officers began hanging around the front of the home for no apparent reason other than to tip the children's father off. He, of course, flashed his badge and inquired as to the nature of the activity, and they explained that a search for anabolic steroids was underway. Let's just say that didn't go over too well and it was totally unnecessary.

Comedy of Errors

The cops concluded their search and made off with 1,000 D-Bol, 1,000 A-bombs, 25 bottles of test, some Primo and nonscheduled items – IGF-1 and insulin. They also took a bottle of Pamprin, the dog's heartworm medication, a blood pressure kit, all Mike's bodybuilding magazines, steroid books, and an old Dan Duchaine price list from the '80s that Mike was keeping as a remembrance of the guru. They got Mike's computer, too. The search warrant expressly stated that no cash was to be seized from the home, yet, $3,660 cash, which could be verified as wedding gifts, was seized and lost to forfeiture.

> ATTORNEY'S NOTE:
> *"While Mike hired local civil counsel to deal with the forfeiture issue, the illegal seizure of the wedding money was just the beginning of the bungling by law enforcement in this case. But, while most people who watch TV know police mishandling can be used to get a case tossed out or even sue a municipality, few realize that in the real world it's a stacked deck. Some non-malicious varieties of police or clerical screw-ups are deemed 'harmless error' by the courts and simply hurt the accused. Police mistakes can cut either way. I've seen hundreds of steroid cases with various legal infirmities, but Mike's case was an unprecedented 'comedy of errors.'"*
>
> – RC

The cops uncuffed Mike and left with their stash to go assemble their case against him. Mike then hired Rick Collins. Rick communicated with the authorities and found out that Mike *and* Kim were being charged with "intent to distribute anabolic steroids," at that point in the case a misdemeanor, and that they had to surrender themselves to the authorities. They were jailed for the day and eventually transferred to appear before the commissioner who released them on their own recognizance.

Charging Kim was absolutely ludicrous. She obviously wasn't a steroid user or involved with either the trafficking or the possession of such drugs. The county officer in charge of the case said that if this was repeated he would deny it, but Kim's arrest was only for leverage to insure a conviction of Mike in the case. If he pleaded guilty, Kim's charges would be dropped. Including Kim in Mike's case is just one of the dirty little tricks the cops can get away with. In Kim's case, a conviction would mean losing her mortician's license and putting her out of business, not to mention the extra legal fees for another lawyer.

ATTORNEY'S NOTE:

"Mike contacted me for help. In cases where two people get busted for the same crime, and especially where one is involved and the other has nothing to do with it, a conflict of interest arises. That means it's potentially unethical for one lawyer to represent both. My firm technically represented Kim, with another lawyer representing Mike. But, hey, my personal concern was for both Mike and Kim. A big portion of my work on the case involved supervising and consulting on issues specific to Mike's defense. A key issue in the case against Mike was whether the sheer quantities of anabolics involved were indicative of an 'intent to distribute.'

"While the list of various pharmaceuticals and the amounts recovered from Mike's house were substantial indeed, they were not necessarily inconsistent with personal use for a heavy, hardcore user. Of course, the prosecutors were used to dealing with street drugs like cocaine and heroin, where only 20 or 30 individual product units might prove intent to sell. They were totally convinced from the outset that they had a high-level dealer. In fact, they believed the 1,000 tablets of methandienone alone that came to the P.O. box proved an intent to sell (a totally ludicrous position given that 1,000 was the typical minimum order from the overseas supplier). They were out for blood, absolutely convinced of their position.

"In fact, we actually had a roundtable meeting at the courthouse in which I went head-to-head with the police department's 'steroid expert' on the issue of whether or not the quantity recovered was consistent with one man's personal use."

–RC

Misdemeanor to Felony

Months went by, and finally it seemed they had worked out a deal for a plea agreement that Mike and Kim would accept in court, in lieu of going through the trial. This would typically be a deal in which the defendant would plead guilty to lesser charges in exchange for saving the government the expense and effort, and sometimes embarrassment, of putting their show on at trial.

At 4 pm the day before the trial date, however, Rick found out that in both cases the misdemeanor charges were going to be dropped and that new felony charges had been filed. The deal was off, which meant Mike and Kim would now have to go through the indignities of being arrested for a felony. This usually includes getting fingerprinted, strip searched and locked up for hours, if not days, in a filthy cell and then formally brought before a judge, magistrate, commissioner, etc., to be charged and hear their plea.

ATTORNEY'S NOTE:

"The police in Mike's case originally charged misdemeanor violations related to prescription drugs, not felony 'controlled dangerous substances' charges. Why? Because they were confused about what the substances were and about what their legal status was. To coin a phrase, many cops don't know an Anavar from an aspirin."

– RC

Mike and Kim were promised that both Rick and Mike's local lawyer would be informed of their surrender date so they could surrender themselves by summonses directly to the court rather than go through the entire process of executing warrants and going to jail, etc., all over again. But that didn't happen. In a sad coincidence, the day the cops decided to execute Mike's warrant happened to be the day Mike's mother passed away. Four hours after her death, Mike arrived home from the hospice and found a county cop waiting for him. Mike assumed he would be served with a summons to appear in court. However, it was a warrant for his arrest. Apparently a "clerical error" caused the foul-up and Mike's warrant had not been changed to a summons as promised. He spent most of the day his mother died waiting to get bailed out of jail.

Kim, knowing she would likely be the victim of a similar "clerical error," surrendered herself to the county police department four days later. Rick made arrangements with the police to have her processed swiftly and requested that her transfer to the commissioner be immediate. That didn't happen either. Kim was made to wait for five hours in a filthy cell, strewn with human waste, where there was only a small patch of ground for her to stand where she felt least likely to contract hepatitis. She was finally transferred, in handcuffs and shackles, to the commissioner's office. In the process, she was led past crowded areas where she encountered many people she knew or with whom she had done business.

Kim and Mike's lawyers filed "notices of appearance," a routine procedure in criminal cases. Once filed, neither the lawyer nor the accused needs to make an initial appearance just to answer the charges. However, the paperwork on Kim's case, though properly filed, was lost by the court clerks in a backlog of papers to be filed. The judge, not in possession of the "notice of appearance" and not seeing Kim in court, issued *another* warrant for her arrest. The county police went to pick up Kim that evening and arrived while she was bathing. Her 12 year-old daughter answered the door and said that her mother was not there. The poor kid was totally badgered by the cops before they left, threatening to return to take her mother away. The lawyers straightened it out the next day, but not before Mike, Kim, and their kids spent a sleepless night waiting for the cops to return; they never did.

The First Degree

Some time after that incident, another county cop arrived at the house inquiring as to Mike's whereabouts. The same 12-year-old answered the door and was again badgered by the officer. She told the cop Mike would be home shortly, so he left, only to not return again.

Ultimately, several trial dates were postponed because, after a full year, the detective in charge was still busy reviewing all 1,300 pages of e-mail from Mike's computer. The cops needed to provide some evidence that warranted the felony charge of distribution. One sentence, of the 1,300 pages, stating to a supplier that Mike needed "to satisfy some people over here" was exhibited as evidence that he was a steroid dealer.

Switching the blame of urgency to fictitious, impatient associates is a common tactic to coerce a slow moving supplier to begin to send a delayed order. Obviously, if Mike were a big Internet steroid dealer, there would be more than just this one partial sentence out of 1,300 pages of e-mail. Even so, the state insisted on pressing for the felony regardless of the lack of evidence. Their determination to convict was unexplainable, especially in a case of such a victimless crime. One day, Mike was in court with a man who sodomized and raped a 14-year-old; an armed bank robber who had robbed four banks in a year; and an armed robber involved in an assault. What did Mike do to be in such company? According to Rick, sarcastically, it was *BODYBUILDING IN THE FIRST DEGREE*!

Finally, 15 months after the search warrant was served, a determination on Kim and Mike's case was made in the Circuit Court. Rick had tried to get the state to agree to "Probation Before Judgment" (PBJ) and to dispose of the case since it started, but the prosecution wouldn't hear of it. Ultimately, the prosecutor backed down and Mike received a PBJ with two years' probation and no criminal conviction on his record; Kim's case was dismissed outright.

The money seized has still not been returned. Nor have Mike's computer, or his steroid books and other items not relevant to the case. Mike and Kim also had to pay legal fees and deal with an extraordinary amount of stress and family strife throughout their ordeal with the cops and prosecutors. The good news is that Mike didn't go to jail. You can bet that's because he had Rick Collins and his law firm behind him. Rick is passionately committed to the cause, and has traveled across the country defending steroid cases himself or assisting other lawyers to do so.

So, what did this little skirmish on the drug war battlefield accomplish? Not a damn thing. I'm not an advocate for breaking the law, although I've certainly done my share of it and I've paid the price. However, you will never get me, nor many bodybuilders, to stop using anabolic steroids drugs simply because the government says we can't. First of all, the government doesn't know a damn thing about steroid use and its potential dangers relative to bodybuilding, other than the hype the equally ignorant medical community feeds it.

Any hardcore gym in America has more knowledgeable steroid experts as members than the AMA. The medical community and the government's efforts in eradicating steroid use are clearly a case of the blind leading the blind. So long as cigarettes and alcohol, responsible for tens of thousands of deaths each year, are legal to purchase and pay taxes on in the process, the illegality of steroid use by bodybuilders will always be looked upon as a ludicrous waste of government spending. Clearly, the steroid laws need to be changed to accommodate the mature bodybuilder; bodybuilding is not a crime, and bodybuilders should be free to bodybuild, to whatever degree they choose. We don't need to be protected from ourselves, we need to be protected from our government, and that sucks.

* * *

Well, that's Mike's story, in John Romano's vivid prose. I'll never forget Mike being dragged to jail on the day his mother died, for no other reason than bureaucratic bungling. The prosecutor subsequently apologized for it, but it was a little late at that point. Maybe his embarrassment is why he didn't try to freeze Mike's bank accounts or initiate forfeiture proceedings on the family residence. Mike's civil lawyers took the state to court to try to get back his money, but it was ultimately cheaper to compromise with them than drag it out. So Mike lost some of his wedding money, and by the time they returned his computer he'd already bought another.

The taxpayers lost, too. The government man-hours devoted to spying on Mike, drafting affidavits and warrants, conducting surveillance, executing the delivery and raid, drafting reams of court papers, arresting Mike's innocent wife, repeatedly arresting Mike by mistake, combing through 1,300 e-mails, bouncing in and out of court for various appearances, and taking space on the docket, were all financed by the unwitting populace. In an era of limited resources, all those precious hours devoted to the relentless pursuit of stopping Mike from juicing seems unspeakably wasteful. Mike's as peaceful as a lamb. Mike's not hurting anybody, perhaps not even himself. And here's the scariest part: there are a lot of guys like Mike. What happened to him is being planned for them. You can bet that tomorrow, agents somewhere will be spying on some new poor soul's packages, then bringing an affidavit before a judge. Once again, thousands of dollars will be spent and man-hours squandered in the misguided crusade to save a soul from himself. Another Mike will be put through the ringer.

But before we start bashing the police, though, let's not forget that we're paying them to enforce the laws on the books – not to pick and choose which ones to enforce. Once we allow our politicians to enact laws empowering authorities to act, we foist upon those authorities the *responsibility* to act. Looking the other way, even if it seems appropriate under all the circumstances at the moment, could later be viewed as dereliction of duty or arbitrary enforcement. You can't give law enforcement the direction to go after something and expect them to pull their punches. In fact, you should expect that many authorities will enforce the law to the highest *limit* of their authority. And why not? The system is designed to reward that. Next year's budgets will be based on this year's investigation and arrest numbers. In some cases there'll be abuse. You can't make an omelet without breaking a few eggs, as they say. There's a price to protecting society.

From an institutional standpoint, the days of common sense and enforcement discretion are pretty much gone in many jurisdictions, among both police and prosecutors. Their hands are tied. I recently spoke at length about anabolic steroid cases with a former high-ranking Assistant United States Attorney (AUSA) for the Middle District of Georgia. He served before the imposition of the sentencing guidelines, and commented on the policy differences that have emerged since he left the office:

> "Our philosophy was that every technical violation of federal law did not have to be enforced to its utmost without any input of common sense. In particular where a defendant was clearly a menace and danger to society, we did everything legal and ethical, and with great vigor, to put him (or her) away as long as possible. I understand we were known in the legal community as being basically fair but also very "hard nosed." It's just simple reality that some violations of the law are much more serious and require much more stringent enforcement than others.
>
> "From talking with AUSA's currently serving in an active capacity and former AUSA's from the more recent era, it seems that things have changed considerably, and in my opinion not for the better. I understand that now they basically "keep score" – the more convictions an AUSA gets and the more *time* the AUSA's defendants get to serve, the better the AUSA will appear on his or her next performance evaluation. It literally seems to be somewhat similar to the old joke about the police officer who has a traffic ticket quota to cover each month, but with far more serious consequences. They no longer are encouraged or even allowed to exercise any judgment or discretion as to how vigorously cases should be prosecuted, and against whom – they simply pursue each and every case with a view toward getting as many convictions as possible, and the harshest sentences possible, absolutely without any regard to the facts involved in each individual case.
>
> "Quite frankly, I am glad I served as a federal prosecutor prior to the demonization of steroids and the passage of the current steroid laws, because if one of those cases had come before me I would have some serious difficulty dealing with it with a clear conscience, given what I know about anabolic steroids. I have no philosophical problem with certain medications being by prescription only, and certainly believe that drugs like heroin and cocaine are very dangerous, and without question have severe addiction potential. However, it is totally incomprehensible to me that anabolic steroids came to be classified the same as morphine, for example, and treated as if they were addicting drugs that are as dangerous as street

> drugs such as crack or heroin. The process by which this occurred simply suited the ends of the media, sports, political and law enforcement communities. The average citizen has no idea how out of whack it is to apply the 'war on drugs' to anabolic steroids."

This ex-prosecutor's position is consistent with those of many enlightened members of the justice community, including many active police officers with whom I have spoken. These are definite law and order types, who favor an aggressive approach to narcotics interdiction. But with anabolics, they say that they find themselves enforcing laws they plainly disagree with. As for the rest of us, is this the way we want our tax dollars to be spent?

As for the rest of us, is this the way we want our tax dollars to be spent?

Anyway, long after the case was finished, I saw Mike at the Arnold Classic bodybuilding expo in Columbus. We hung around and had a few laughs. It's so rare for lawyers, especially criminal lawyers, to actually like their clients. How much can criminal lawyers have in common with the rapists, robbers, burglars, prostitutes, crackheads, murderers, and thieves so many of us represent on a regular basis? I'm thankful every day that I'm doing something that makes me feel passionate and righteous. I'm grateful that I have so many clients with whom I have much in common and whose company and conversations I enjoy. I like fighting for worthy principles, and for decent people. I like Mike. I think you would, too.

Chapter 24

THE LAW THAT FAILED

"Prohibition will work great injury to the cause of temperance. It is a species of intemperance within itself, for it goes beyond the bounds of reason in that it attempts to control man's appetite by legislation, and makes a crime out of things that are not crimes. A Prohibition law strikes a blow at the very principles upon which our government was founded."

– Abraham Lincoln (1809–1865)

Well, here we are, folks. It's been well over a decade since Congress "controlled" the steroid problem. Anabolics are federally criminalized for everybody, young and old, responsible or irresponsible, athletes and non-athletes, when used for cosmetic purposes. Consider this true steroid story:

Randy, 31, was a factory worker near Little Rock. He'd been working out for fifteen years, going from a scrawny 130 pounds to 227. Randy had never done any recreational drugs in his life. He lived, slept and ate bodybuilding, and was naturally athletic. He had begun making inroads into the professional wrestling circuit, starting with some local matches, but he needed a bit more size. At the age of 30, when he felt he had fully tapped his natural potential, Randy tried anabolic steroids for the first time. After three short cycles of roughly a gram of testosterone per week, his weight had gone up to 245, his maximum bench press had gone from 330 to 430 pounds, and his arms had gone from 17" to 19" around.

This past summer the factory hired a new guy, in his 30's, who later turned out to be an undercover narc. Apparently, there had been reports that somebody at the factory had been dealing narcotics. But when the guy got a look at Randy's arms one day, he saw the opportunity for a steroid bust, too. He asked Randy's friend Mitch if he could introduce him to Randy. Mitch did, and from then on the narc asked Randy every day to hook him up with some steroids. Randy looked at the guy, who had no physique to speak of, and gave him numerous exercise and diet strategies. The narc continued begging for anabolics. Randy repeatedly told him to stay away from anabolics until he had developed to his natural potential. The narc then started pressuring Mitch to convince Randy to sell him some steroids. Randy told Mitch that the guy shouldn't be using anabolics, but the guy kept badgering Mitch so Mitch kept asking Randy.

After several weeks of this, Randy told him that if he wanted steroids he should talk to his doctor. The guy said he did, and his doctor said they'd be fine for him, but that he couldn't prescribe them. To get rid of the guy, Randy said anyone could find steroids on the Internet. Making that suggestion was a big mistake for Randy. The narc then begged Randy to get the anabolics for him, but Randy explained to him where to look on the Internet to find them for himself. He also continued to advise against using them at his stage. The guy asked how much it would cost to get started, and Randy gave him an estimate. The guy asked if he could give the money to Randy to order it for him. It had now been well over a month of this nonsense, and Randy finally said he'd order it for the guy this once if he'd leave him alone. Randy ordered a bottle of testosterone and a bottle of boldenone online with his own money and gave it to the guy, who reimbursed him for his out-of-pocket costs. Randy made not a single penny on the deal, but was glad to get the guy off his back.

A few weeks went by, and then five local police officers showed up at the factory looking for Randy. In front of all the assembled workers, Randy was handcuffed and driven away in a patrol car. He was held on a $10,000 bond. When his family managed to post the money, he went to the factory to learn he had lost his job. His case is pending...

To enforce the law, we've targeted, spied on, lied to, tricked, and arrested thousands of hapless adult Americans for steroid use. We've fined them ridiculous amounts or even thrown them in jail. We've branded people felons and destroyed their future prospects of productive livelihoods. We've broken up families, thrown people out of the military and various other jobs. We've seized people's property, including the belongings of innocent third parties. In many cases, we've taken the property away forever. But at least we can say that we accomplished what we set out to do. We've solved the problem of anabolic steroids in America! Right?

But at least we can say that we accomplished what we set out to do. We've solved the problem of anabolic steroids in America! Right?

Let's take a look at that. Today, proponents of criminalization in the sports bodies and law enforcement authorities claim that the Control Act and similar state laws have worked. They say that the laws: (1) deter trafficking, (2) protect the public, (3) send the right message to young people, and (4) preserve fair competition in sports. After all, those were the original intended goals of the legislation. Have they been fulfilled? If they have, then maybe there's some argument, however shaky, that all the suffering we've caused in enforcing these laws was justified. But what if the law has failed? We've given the approach over ten years to work. What has the past decade really shown?

Deterring Steroid Trafficking

Sure, penalties can be stiff, especially in state courts. But proponents of criminalization contend that stiff penalties help deter trafficking, and that the strict controls associated with controlled substance status prevent pharmaceutical companies from manufacturing more product than could be legitimately used for FDA-approved purposes. In fact, this "diversion" problem was one reason why Congress scheduled anabolics even *against* the advice of most authorities including the AMA and the DEA (see Chapter 1). In the congressional hearings, Charles Yesalis, Sc.D., testified as an expert witness that pharmaceutical companies refused to cooperate with investigations to determine the level of diversion. The Control Act addresses the diversion problem by requiring a triplicate "paper trail," and every person who manufactures, distributes, or dispenses a controlled substance has to register annually with the Attorney General. So, if the manufacturers, distributors, and dispensers are forced to account for where all the products go, how can they fall into the hands of teens or athletes?

Well, the criminal penalties attached to steroids *have* had an effect on domestic production. A *big* effect: they pretty much stopped it. Maybe it was too much of a hassle to meet the requirements, or maybe Big Pharmacy really had been making a chunk of extra product to quietly divert to the non-medical market. That's all over now. The pharmaceutical companies have moved on to other ways of making profits, off drugs like Prozac®, Zoloft® and Viagra®. There's always plenty of money to be made from selling drugs to the public.

But a funny thing happened in the last decade. Back in the 1980s, it was estimated that about a third of the steroid black market consisted of foreign products unlawfully smuggled into the States. Now that Big Pharmacy was withdrawing from the picture, Big La Farmacia saw an opportunity to make a bundle. For foreign anabolic manufacturers, the Control Act was a dream come true. It's taken a few years, but now they can't make juice fast enough to fill the void. And not just Mexican companies, but manufacturers in Thailand, China, Eastern Europe, Australia and elsewhere. The Control Act has effectively become a foreign aid policy, helping other nations supplement their export revenues by shipping products to America that we're not allowed to make. Oh, we catch some of these smuggled shipments, mostly small packages mail-ordered by poor schnooks for personal use, but the vast majority gets through without a hitch.

The Control Act has effectively become a foreign aid policy, helping other nations supplement their export revenues by shipping products to America that we're not allowed to make.

At the time of the congressional hearings, it was estimated that about a third of the black market was comprised of foreign products. Today, the black market is comprised of almost exclusively *foreign* products. Not just foreign products, but foreign *veterinary* products. It's easier to manufacture and traffic the stuff if it's not for human consumption. So, AAS labs all over the world are putting pictures of horses and dogs on the labels of their products, even as they churn out volumes that would be too much to juice up every horse, cow, goat, pig, dog, and house cat in America. What Department of Justice officials estimated in 1990 to be a $300 million black market has grown tremendously, to colossal proportions about which we can only speculate. In January 2001, federal law enforcement officials announced that they seized more than 3.25 million anabolic steroid tablets in the single largest steroid seizure in U.S. history.

If deterring steroid trafficking was the goal, we've failed. There's more trafficking now than ever before. But surely, we've succeeded as to the other goals. Surely, we've protected the public from harm, particularly our young people, haven't we?

Protecting the Public

Protecting the citizenry, particularly our children and teenagers, is a worthy goal of any legislation. Who could argue with that? Although our friends on Capitol Hill seemed most concerned about preventing another Ben Johnson scandal, they threw in enough rhetoric about saving the children to rile up public support for their legislative bills. Now here we are, looking back. Did we save the children? No, unfortunately. A primary effect of the Control Act's restrictions has been to put the children at *greater* risk. Let's talk about why.

Because the Control Act and similar laws have failed miserably in deterring trafficking, teens are still using steroids. Except now the products they're using are even more dangerous. Without the supervision of the FDA or similar government regulatory agencies, foreign pharmaceutical makers can invent their own safety and quality control standards. Some may be good; others might be downright scary. How much quality control effort goes into a product made for a horse? Some are reportedly made under unsupervised and quite unsanitary conditions. [*See*

M.G. Di Pasquale, "Black Market Drugs," *Anabolic Research Review* 1, no.1 (1995)] Many AAS users have reported occasional infections as a result of dirty anabolics, particularly certain Mexican brands. One physician familiar with the issue said, "My colleagues at Mount Sinai Hospital in New York tell me they are treating many more athletes for side effects of counterfeit and bogus steroids than they did when reliable pharmacy-purchased steroids were available." [Quoting Dr. Robert Price in B. Allen, "Steroid-using Athletes and Liver Function," *MuscleMag International* 191, (May 1998) 129, 224] At one time it was estimated that up to 90% of black-market anabolic steroids were either tainted or contained ingredients that were not listed on the label. While the quality of some products has reportedly improved, others may be contaminated by bacteria or other impurities or may contain steroids other than what are represented on the label.

Some products may not even be made by the purported manufacturer at all. Steroid counterfeiters can make products that mimic the real ones. These counterfeited products may contain who-knows-what. One law reviewer who assessed the situation back in 1994 condemned the Control Act for this reason, quoting a 1993 article. He concluded that it seemed quite evident that "continued enforcement of steroid legislation will worsen health risks associated with steroid use. An investigation by The Atlanta Journal and Constitution concluded that 'tougher laws and heightened enforcement...have fueled thriving counterfeit operations that pose even more severe health risks.'" [John Burge, "Legalize and Regulate: A Prescription for Reforming Anabolic Steroid Legislation," 15 *Loy. L.A. Ent. L. J.* 33 (1994) 54-55, citing Mike Fish, "Steroids Riskier Than Ever, Drugs Easy to Buy South of the Border," *Atlanta J. & Const.*, Sept. 28, 1993, D1.]

Perhaps an even bigger backfire to the criminalization approach has been to discourage users, especially teens, from admitting their steroid usage to physicians. Since some of the greatest dangers inherent in self-administered steroid use involve the failure to be monitored by a doctor, the Control Act has succeeded in greatly escalating this danger and has created an even wider gap between the muscle world and the medical community. Because the self-administration of anabolics is a federal crime, few anabolic takers are willing to 'fess up to their physicians. And because both state and federal enforcement efforts have targeted physicians, few doctors want anything to do with healthy people taking anabolics. Doctors caught distributing steroids to athletes have been criminally prosecuted. [*See* Chapter 12] "By forbidding trained physicians from administering steroids in a controlled manner, the Legislature has forced athletes to either buy steroids off the black market or seek out unethical and possibly incompetent physicians to supply them steroids.... [I]t appears that Congress's attempt at preventing steroid prescription has at best been futile and at worst harmful." [Jeffrey Black, "The Anabolic Steroids Control Act of 1990: A Need for Change," 97 *Dick. L. Rev.* 131 (1992), at 140 (citations omitted)]

> Since some of the greatest dangers inherent in self-administered steroid use involve the failure to be monitored by a doctor, the Control Act has succeeded in greatly escalating this danger ...

The end result is that the athletes using steroids rarely get regular blood pressure checks, cholesterol readings, prostate exams, and liver enzyme tests, making steroid use far more hazardous than it would otherwise be. Because of criminalization, the distribution of anabolic steroids has been driven further underground, resulting in a thriving black market of counterfeit drugs. Furthermore, users are now more reluctant to seek, or are sometimes refused, medical supervision. And the criminalization of anabolics combined with the unavailability of hypodermic instruments in some regressive jurisdictions has created the potential for HIV-infected needle sharing among juicers (although only one case is reported in the medical literature among the millions of non-medical steroid users). Thus, the risks involving the use of anabolics have increased well beyond those of the drugs themselves.

Here's another way the Control Act has harmed the public: it has helped smother legitimate therapeutic applications. Anabolic steroids can be wonderful, *health-restoring* medicines. It seems almost scandalous or irresponsible to say it, so relentless has the Ministry of Truth's propaganda been these last few years. Many patients who might have benefited enormously from medical AAS therapy have gone without because their physicians were too frightened by the stigma attached to steroids to explore the therapeutic possibilities. Take the elderly, for example. The restoration of strength, muscle mass, and libido in such patients greatly benefits society. But the sweeping stroke with which the Control Act is applied has scared off many practitioners. One legal reviewer has observed that when "physicians prescribe steroids for other than approved illnesses, they open themselves up to a presumption of illegality based upon the reading of the Anabolic Steroid Control Act." He further noted that:

Many patients who might have benefited enormously from medical AAS therapy have gone without because their physicians were too frightened by the stigma ...

> "By respecting the federal law, physicians may not prescribe steroids to advance the physical strength and condition of the elderly. By subverting a doctor's determination concerning the best interests of a patient, elders are penalized as well - not for violating the law, but by submitting to it.... Many illnesses requiring managed care possibly could be eliminated with hormone treatments. This would not only trigger a social benefit but a financial benefit as well. Congress has created a barrier for the revitalizing effects of steroids for the elderly." [Jeffrey Hedges, "The Anabolic Steroids Act: Bad Medicine for the Elderly," 5 *Elder L. J.* 293 (Fall 1997).]

Today, a growing number of practitioners have begun exploring the parameters of using anabolics and growth hormone in anti-aging medicine. However, they must be careful about their practices or face investigation by state medical licensing boards. [*See* Chapter 12] AIDS researcher and author Michael Mooney has said that the criminalization of anabolic steroids has inadvertently had a tragic, often deadly effect on people with critical medical conditions who can benefit from the therapeutic use of anabolic steroids, such as those who suffer from HIV/AIDS. Mooney observes that:

> "Because of this law and the misinformation that was used to rally public support to pass it, early in the AIDS crisis a majority of medical doctors either thought that anabolic steroids were too dangerous for medical use or feared crimination if they prescribed anabolic steroids. This is especially unfortunate when we consider that anabolic steroids have subsequently been proven to address what was described in 1995 by the World Health Organization as the second leading cause of death in AIDS patients, the loss

of lean body mass called AIDS-related wasting. The exaggerated negative bias that was commonplace in this country resulted in the stifling of much needed research into medical uses for anabolic steroids and their appropriate prescription for many years.

"From the time AIDS was first reported in 1982 to the present, I have personally witnessed the deaths of dozens of friends who died from AIDS-related wasting. Many of them wasted to as little as half their normal body weight before dying as skin and bones. Thousands of others have suffered the same fate.

"Studies have shown that a decline in testosterone in people with HIV/AIDS is directly associated with the loss of lean body mass, and a decline in T-cell counts in HIV+ males. Studies also confirm that testosterone replacement and the use of other anabolic steroids for people with HIV/AIDS can provide multiple benefits, including improved lean body mass and quality of life, and improved mental outlook with reduced depression scores. Studies and reports have also indicated that anabolic steroid therapy can improve critically important barometers of immune competence, such as CD8 T-cell counts, which have been shown to be directly associated with better long-term survival in AIDS.

"This is why in spite of the tremendous early bias against their use, doctors' perception of testosterone and anabolic steroids has risen to allow steroids to attain a near standard of care status as prescribed medications in all major metropolitan areas in the United States. We must not forget, though, that thousands of people have died needlessly because of the bias against their medical use, and some doctors still do not understand their potential as life saving medications, and so their patients suffer or die needlessly. This is why the Anabolic Steroid Control Act and public opinion need to be changed. Americans should be informed that testosterone or anabolic steroids may be valuable therapeutic agents, not only for HIV/AIDS, but for osteoporosis, multiple sclerosis, diabetes, rheumatoid arthritis, lupus, and other pathologies." [Personal correspondence, October 2002]

Lastly, when we talk about protecting the public, shouldn't we be comparing the harms we cause with the harms we prevent? The Control Act has criminalized a generation of our citizens, old and young. The individual caught with steroids may be forever a felon. While anti-AAS crusaders try to minimize the real life effects of crim-inalization, I've seen it firsthand over and over. For those unfortunate enough to be caught, the effects of prosecution can be devastating. This is especially true since most adult steroid users lead otherwise responsible, law-abiding lives. An East Coast former long-term user was quoted as follows:

For those unfortunate enough to be caught, the effects of prosecution can be devastating.

"Unfortunately our society has been educated to believe that if you use steroids, you're no different from the guy with crack cocaine, and there is a big difference. In the '80s, I saw so many individuals who used steroids and in some cases abused them, and these individuals went on to become doctors, lawyers, DEA agents, and various other types of law-enforcement personnel at the state and federal levels - prominent citizens for this country ... And we're not talking about 10 or 20. We're talking about hundreds of people

> I've seen over the years ... I'd say at least 90, maybe 95 percent, of the steroid users I saw became productive citizens – just because the guys who did it in the '80s were trying to be the best they could be. They had that characteristic of trying to be the best, and they kept that same characteristic and applied it to other areas of their lives." [B. Allen, "Steroids and the Law," *MuscleMag International* 180, (June 1997): 48, at 56 (quoting an anonymous athlete)]

Can't the same be said of marijuana users, or even some cocaine users? No way. With steroid users, whether or not you agree with their choice, the forces behind these individuals' AAS use were ambition and perfectionism, not an attempt to escape from reality or anesthetize themselves.

This book is filled with the stories of the victims of the Control Act. Surely, the extreme, abusive practices by some people who take steroids have caused them harm. But despite all the propaganda from the Ministry of Truth, the terrible, irreparable harms caused by the Control Act and similar laws would seem to vastly outweigh the generally mild health risks associated with steroid use by most mature adults. [*See* Chapter 3] Our laws have caused more harm than they've prevented.

Sending the Right Message to Young People

Surely, discouraging teen steroid use is important. The enactment of the Control Act was supposed to send the message that cheating sports stars would be punished for steroid use. But virtually none of them have. Quite a message, eh? Further, the message that anabolic steroids are a cheater's approach to competitive sports misses the real mark, anyway. The misguided focus, probably based on the sports community's over-inflated view of its own significance, assumes that most teens are using steroids to become sports stars. That's completely contrary to my observations, and those of the many authorities with whom I've corresponded. While some of them may play football or run high school track, they're using anabolics primarily to look bigger in clothes and harder on the beach. They're trying to impress their peers and any girls who might be looking. Just like the adults who use steroids, the teens are also cosmetic users.

The whole steroids-and-sports connection has been overblown, and legislation, policies, and journalists that harp on it don't have relevance to the majority of AAS users of all ages. Granted, many teens harbor dreams of becoming professional bodybuilders someday. (Elite caliber physiques are largely the result of dedication to training and diet, and perhaps mostly the result of superior genetics.) Of course, AAS use does play a role. That's not a secret. It's silly to think that the Control Act is convincing *anybody* that anabolic steroids aren't a part of professional bodybuilding.

The whole steroids-and-sports connection has been overblown, and legislation, policies, and journalists that harp on it don't have relevance to the majority of AAS users of all ages.

A law that doesn't do much but ensnare people for whom it wasn't intended isn't the way to discourage teen steroid use. Nor are scare tactics. (See Chapter 11 for a fuller discussion of how we've failed to effectively discourage teen use.)

Preserving Fair Competition in Sports

Well, this is what it all comes down to, doesn't it? Ironically, this is where it all started. Whatever claims may be made to the contrary, issues of cheating, "hollow victories," "winning at any cost," etc., were the true ideological foundation for criminalizing juice. While the controversial hypothesis of "addictive" potential provided the necessary legal criterion and the purported health risks provided a "hot" sell for the media, the real "steroid problem" was always about purity in sporting games. The special interests of the sports establishments were what the Control Act was all about. As pointed out by international steroid expert Mauro Di Pasquale, M.D.:

> "Contrary to what most people believe (the media's irresponsible sensationalism has resulted in the widely held mistaken view that the use by athletes of anabolic steroids and other performance-enhancing drugs is a problem on par with heroin and cocaine abuse), the use of drugs, such as anabolic steroids, by athletes is a problem, not because of the addictive and dangerous side effects of these compounds, but because these drugs offer an unfair advantage to the athletes who use them." [M.G. Di Pasquale, Editorial: "Why Athletes Use Drugs," *Drugs in Sports* 1, no.1 (February 1992): 2.]

Another Ben Johnson scandal apparently would have ended civilization as we know it. The Control Act was supposed to help exorcise anabolics from competitive sports. Twelve years later, are steroids gone from sports? Only a fool would say they are. In fact, many would agree that there are more steroids in sports today than ever before. Open the papers. Look at major league baseball. And even in sports where testing is conducted, do you really think anabolics have been eradicated?

The problem is that many athletic establishments were never really interested in working too hard to catch doping athletes. Those that have tried valiantly have generally bungled it through administrative or procedural mistakes. It was their laziness and ineptitude that helped create the Control Act. It was easier for them to cry to Congress and have a law passed to "control" the whole country than take the challenging responsibility of cleaning their own mess, and Congress clearly didn't trust them to be capable of doing it. But after all the arrests and prosecutions of non-athletes for a dozen years, their mess is no better.

When was the last time you heard of an elite athlete being prosecuted under the Control Act?

Random high-technology testing within sports, not an overbroad Control Act, is the effective deterrent to elite level use. When was the last time you heard of an elite athlete being prosecuted under the Control Act? Sports stars obtain their steroid supplies through sophisticated channels that avoid detection by law enforcement. When an Olympic athlete, professional athlete, or other popular sports figure gets caught using steroids, it is almost invariably by failing a drug test. Whatever consequences may ensue, criminal prosecution is not one of them. The Control Act is completely *irrelevant* for deterring the population for which it was primarily intended. It's done absolutely nothing to keep "purity" in sports. Quite a piece of legislation it's turned out to be, huh?

Looking Back at a Big Mistake

At one point in the congressional subcommittee hearings that preceded the Control Act, Rep. Levine made an offhand remark that "prosecutors are going to have to exercise judgment" about simple possession cases. He said, "I certainly do not intend ... to go after kids who have additional steroids and who are making them available to their friends, I would hope that that would be pursued as a possession offense, if it is going to be pursued." His comment suggests that Congress really didn't intend to enforce the law against personal users who share steroids with their gym buddies.

Well, such cases *have* been pursued. Thousands of otherwise law-abiding Americans – and not kids, but mature adult males – have been arrested, handcuffed, searched, arraigned, prosecuted, convicted, and sentenced for the personal use or low-level sharing of anabolic steroids with their friends. Virtually *none* of them have been Olympic athletes or NFL players. They have been computer technicians, health care workers, factory assemblers, mechanics, police officers, and many other men – your friends and neighbors. They're not cheating in sports; they're not even *playing* sports. Yet they are being vacuumed up into the criminal justice system by a law that was never enacted to address them. Hundreds of congressional transcript pages were devoted to promoting fair play at the elite and collegiate levels. Nobody ever mentioned the idea that the 35-year-old guy who's paving the roads by day, feeding his family, and using a moderate amount of juice to enhance the effects of his training, would be arrested and prosecuted. No teens are looking up to him. He is cheating no other athletes. He's not bothering anybody. In the zeal of Congress to solve the problem of athletic cheating, steroids were forcibly inserted, like a square peg into a round hole, into the Controlled Substances Act. Overnight, the typical mature adult male steroid user was turned into a criminal desperado – and remains so today – by a law that was passed with barely a thought to the issue.

In the zeal of Congress to solve the problem of athletic cheating, steroids were forcibly inserted, like a square peg into a round hole, into the Controlled Substances Act.

Which makes me wonder about the legislative process in general. If Congress made such a mess with anabolic steroids, how can we be sure that *other* laws haven't been passed to cater to special interests at the expense of and contrary to the interests of the rest of us? Can we really rely on what Congress tells us is good for us? Should we be paying closer attention to the integrity of the process, to what's going on in those smoky, paneled conference rooms we imagined at the beginning of this book?

Chapter 25

A New Prescription

"Even when laws have been written down, they ought not always to remain unaltered."
– *Aristotle*

There's only one inescapable and irrefutable conclusion to be drawn – steroid criminalization has been an unmitigated failure in almost every way. There is mounting evidence that the actual health dangers associated with anabolic steroids for mature adults are significantly *less* than were suggested to Congress or are commonly perceived by the public. [See Chapter 3] There is evidence that the tight regulations have stifled research, undermined beneficial applications, and effectively severed any connection between physicians and most steroid users. Further, there are strong arguments that the legislation has failed to solve the very problems for which it was enacted; rather, it has exacerbated the situation in many other areas. The only ones in favor of the criminalization approach are the captains and soldiers in our "War on Drugs," the sports anti-doping lobby, their doctorate-toadies, the sports journalism machine, and the hapless public they have collectively misled.

There is mounting evidence that the actual health dangers associated with anabolic steroids for mature adults are significantly *less* than were suggested to Congress ...

More of the Same

Of course, some steroid prohibitionists will keep trying to meet any challenges to the status quo with resistance. They will continue to peddle the myth that steroid use is primarily athletic rather than cosmetic. In *The Steroids Game* (see Chapter 3 references), co-author Virginia Cowart is quoted on the issue of legalization:

> "However imperfect our present systems might be, it would be a terrible mistake to consider legalizing performance-enhancing drugs ... We cannot depend on athletes making judicious use of steroids during their athletic careers. From the earliest times, the pattern has always been one of excess. Alcohol regulation does not entirely prevent alcohol abuse by youngsters, but it serves as a check that is in the best interests of society."

Brilliant. Professor Cowart's argument invites two responses. First, her observation about athletes' irresponsibility to self-administer anabolics supports the contrary position. Reforming the law to again allow doctors to be involved in the dosage regulation, administration, and health monitoring of cosmetic users would vastly reduce the patterns of "excess." Second, her analogy to alcohol makes *my* point. Prohibition failed. Instead, we changed our approach from prohibition to *restriction*, permitting use by mature adults but banning sales to minors. The same goes for cigarettes. I can't fathom an argument that alcohol or cigarettes are more worthy of availability to mature responsible adults than a far less dangerous substance like anabolics. Some anti-AAS crusaders would place even *further* restrictions on the general public in the interests of purifying sports and sending an anti-doping message to young athletes. Back in 1998, the U.S. Olympic Committee reported a nutrition web site to the FBI, demanding that it be investigated for selling androstenedione online (*USA Today* ran the headline, "FBI asked to probe steroid Web site", 08/03/98). Gary I. Wadler, M.D., an anti-anabolics media darling and anti-doping advisor, offered this statement in October 1999 to a Senate subcommittee investigating "The Use of Performance Enhancing Drugs in Olympic Competition":

I can't fathom an argument that alcohol or cigarettes are more worthy of availability to mature responsible adults than a far less dangerous substance like anabolics.

> "We cannot allow performance-enhancing drugs to undermine the Olympic Movement. We cannot allow another generation of young people to approach adulthood with a pervading sense of cynicism, and a belief in the power of chemical manipulation rather than the power of character ... When a celebrated athlete like Mark McGwire admits using androstenedione – and make no mistake, androstenedione is a steroid – and millions of kids witness the presumed power of these drugs, we are clearly on a slippery slope to disaster ... Congress must revisit the DSHEA Act of 1994. Substances like androstenedione were never contemplated by this legislation, and if it requires the reclassification of steroid supplements as prescriptive drugs, then let the process begin."

A "slippery slope," indeed. When the so-called experts start talking like that, putting mature non-athlete adults in *jail* for using currently over-the-counter prohormones like androstenedione is not far behind. Sound far-fetched? Think again. The government has been salivating over the idea of doing just that. It started when Barry McCaffrey, President Clinton's anti-drug chief, announced in July 1999 that he was trying to finance a study that could lead to the specific regulation of androstenedione as a *controlled substance* for which mature adults could be arrested. He said, "I'd like to expedite the examination of androstenedione and determine whether it can be classified an anabolic steroid under the Anabolic Steroid Control Act." He told Congress that same year, "Andro, currently classed as a food supplement, is believed by many to improve performance. The DEA is engaged in a scientific process to determine if Andro actually produces muscle growth – and, in turn, whether it should be classed as a steroid." Improving performance. Growing muscle. These are the terrible harms to be addressed. Not one word about adverse health risks, mind you!

Aren't there any defenders of public choice, particularly for mature adults? What about Dr. Charles Yesalis, who tried to discourage Congress from enacting what became the Anabolic Steroid Control Act? A decade later, the battle for the public's perception has been lost. It's so politically incorrect to say anything good about anabolic steroids that very few academicians will. Much better to toe the line and spout the approved rhetoric. In recent statements by Dr. Yesalis on AAS use by young people, he called for an immediate ban on androstenedione and attacked over-the-counter prohormone products. When it comes to the issue of individual freedom and steroid use by mature informed adults, he says precious little, except to mention "liver damage" and "increased risk of stroke." That's particularly unsettling given that most of the unbiased research and reviews on anabolic steroid health risks in the years since the Control Act went into effect have been *positive*, not negative. Alas, I suppose that there's little reward in swimming against the stream. Maybe we should simply add another name to the roster of the Ministry of Truth.

The whole sorry process we witnessed with the Anabolic Steroid Control Act is starting all over again with over-the-counter prohormones. Two Republican congressmen have introduced a bill (H.R. 5564) in Washington. The new bill would reclassify androstenedione and other steroid precursors as controlled substances, subjecting every American to arrest and prosecution for merely possessing these supplements. Who's pushing the bill? Take a guess. Here's what ESPN had to say: "The bill has the support of the U.S. Antidoping Agency, the group charged with ferreting out drug cheats in Olympic sports. On hand at Wednesday's news conference in Washington was Frank Shorter, the USADA chairman, as well as U.S. Olympic Committee Chairman Lloyd Ward and Olympic speedskating gold medallist Christine Witty. The NCAA and NFL have also expressed support for the bill." [www.msn.espn.go.com/gen/news/2002/1009/1443414.html] Once again, the special interests of the sports lobby are dictating what the rest of America can and can't do. It's a classic case of the tail wagging the dog. How many more Americans will be arrested and convicted as drug felons – for what are now dietary supplements – if this bill sees the light of day?

The new bill would reclassify androstenedione and other steroid precursors as controlled substances, subjecting every American to arrest and prosecution for merely possessing [them] ...

Well, we can listen to these characters and get more of the same overbroad, oppressive laws we're already suffering from. We can further and further restrict our freedoms, painting ourselves into a smaller and smaller corner. Steroids in 1990, prohormones today, and who knows what tomorrow? Is that what we want for ourselves? Is that what the Founding Fathers envisioned for us over two hundred years ago? Where did our freedoms go? How can we get them back?

The Acceptance of Cosmetic AAS Use

Changing the laws is not enough. We need to change some minds. It's time for the medical community to embrace the legitimacy of prescribing anabolics for the cosmetic purposes of reducing fat, building muscle, and improving self-esteem. Are there inherent risks involved in cosmetic AAS use? Absolutely. But we allow lots of other surgical or cosmetic procedures to be performed by doctors, despite the risks. In fact, they're becoming more and more popular. For actors and models, whose physical appearance is important to their work, it's often accepted as a necessity. For the rest of society, it speaks to our preoccupation with looking younger and better.

Physicians are now permitted to inject muscle-paralyzing toxins into patients' foreheads purely for the sake of vanity. Hey, the manufacturer of Botox® made $310 million in sales last year, with numbers rising dramatically. We're a nation obsessed with appearance, and all these nip-and-tucks are not without risk. Think about this: under the current views and laws of our society, it's criminal for a physician to administer anabolics to a healthy adult for purposes of cosmetic physical enhancement. However, it's perfectly acceptable and enormously lucrative to perform the much more radical, invasive, and dangerous procedure of surgically implanting foreign prosthetics into virtually all parts of the human anatomy for the same purpose. Well, that's different, some might say. Really, how? Both cosmetic anabolics and cosmetic surgery are intended to make us look better, and sometimes younger and fitter. Neither is medically necessary and both have risks. One might say that both suggest an inordinate preoccupation with appearance or, in some cases, outright narcissism. Maybe I'll grant you that. But why would one be legal and the other subject to devastating criminal consequences? How can that make sense? And what does that say about the American Medical Association and most state medical boards? They too have been brainwashed by years of demonizing propaganda, largely by their own sports medicine sector, to further the all-important anti-doping agenda.

> ... cosmetic anabolics and cosmetic surgery are intended to make us look better ... Neither is medically necessary and both have risks ... why would one be legal and [not] the other?

With all due respect to the "High Counsel" of old white heads that think this way, there are professionals in both the medical and legal communities who disagree. And with good reason, too. The health risks are far more speculative and transitory than we've been led to believe. The substantial benefits, at least to mature adult men, would seem to be *under*estimated. What makes the non-medical use of anabolics *abuse* in all cases? Why can't a mature adult patient make an educated and responsible decision to improve his appearance with the tools that modern science has to offer? Well, the High Counsel may counter, because there's a *risk* involved! It's unethical for a doctor to put his patient at risk! Oh, really? That's quite simply a crock.

Not only do physicians subject their patients to substantial and life-threatening risks all the time, they actually make them fully acknowledge them in written *Informed Consent* forms. Well, the High Counsel argues, those are medically necessary risks! You're kidding, right? Since when is full-body liposuction medically necessary? How necessary is it to put implants the size of beach balls into a stripper's chest? Not to even mention gender reassignment surgery! A few years ago, a perfectly healthy young man in New York wanted to increase the size of his calves. Of course, no physician could prescribe anabolics for that purpose – too risky! So he had prosthetic implants surgically inserted, which is perfectly acceptable to the medical establishment. A massive infection developed, necessitating amputation of both legs above the knees.

Look, nobody is saying anabolic steroids can't be abused. As a former competitive bodybuilder and personal trainer, I've seen it firsthand in people I've known. But one of the greatest dangers inherent in the cosmetic, non-medical use of anabolics is the *lack* of involvement on the part of the medical establishment. The rigid and myopic perspective of some members of the medical community is exemplified by the woefully misguided comments of a reviewer for a state medical licensing board: "If it needs to be said, the dangers of taking anabolic-androgenic steroids that are not medically indicated, are the same dangers whether the drugs are bought illegally on the black market or prescribed legally." The utterance of such nonsense defies belief. It is incomprehensible that anyone with a medical degree would compare physician-supervised androgen administration to taking non-FDA-approved, potentially tainted black-market drugs, often not intended for human use, in the absence of any examination for contraindications, without any advice or guidance as to dosages, and without any supervision or monitoring as to adverse effects. Sadly, though, this is the current state of thinking among many in the medical establishment, and progressive physicians need to be aware of it.

It's time to reevaluate. Comparing the risks of steroids to liposuction, for example, is startling. According to the FDA, liposuction, a relatively new procedure, may have been responsible for up to 140 deaths nationwide – some caused by post-operative problems like infections and blood clotting. Patients have died or been permanently disfigured by everything from nose jobs to face-lifts. As much as 7% of all breast enlargements get infected, and implants can cause a lifetime of complications. Cosmetic surgery can kill and has killed, with no justified medical necessity whatsoever. The point here is not to demonize cosmetic surgery, which in the vast majority of cases can make people look better and feel better about themselves. Rather, it is to demonstrate the arbitrary and illogical bias against anabolics.

The "Absence of Evidence"

How strong is the "case" against anabolics? Steroid authorities have long stated that there is an absence of evidence of long-term health risks of anabolic steroids for healthy mature adult males. This has been used to support the current policies. Even Dr. Yesalis once said, "Don't mistake the 'absence of evidence' with the 'evidence of absence'" with regard to long-term health risks. I wholeheartedly agree. If there was irrefutable evidence confirming the absence of any health risks from anabolics, and proving that their only effect was to make you bigger, stronger, and leaner, why wouldn't almost everyone be taking them as mature, healthy, non-competing active adults, along with our vitamins?

> Mature healthy adults are being convicted and imprisoned on an "absence of evidence" that what they're doing is significantly harmful to them ...

Of course, that's not the case. There's an *absence* of proof about what may happen in the long run. We just don't know. Which brings me to my point. I'm a lawyer. I go to court and fight cases. If the prosecutor's case is built on an absence of evidence, he loses. He *should* lose. Nobody should ever be convicted on an absence of evidence. Agreed? But that's *exactly* what we're doing to Americans who are arrested and prosecuted for anabolic steroids every day. Mature healthy adults are being convicted and imprisoned on an "absence of evidence" that what they're doing is significantly harmful to them or to anybody else.

Now, I can hear the anti-steroid crusaders shrieking, "We may not have proof, but we've got theories and hypotheses from which we can draw inferences and speculations! We've got suspicions that there could be long-term risks." *Suspicions?* If a prosecutor said that to a jury, they'd send him packing, and well they should. You need a lot more than that to convict somebody in America. What we've been doing to most steroid defendants over the last decade is the real crime. Causing what we know to be a harm in the present in order to protect against a speculative future harm is a shameful policy. I've seen its consequences, and they aren't pretty.

Informed Choice Versus Paternalism

Look, if we really want to eradicate *all* risk, we'd outlaw *everything*. There's inherent risk in all things and activities. The law doesn't prevent individuals from skiing, scuba diving, or even hang gliding, although all are extremely dangerous activities. As one reviewer noted:

> "People in this country can choose to have tummy tucks, breast implants, nose jobs, smoke cigarettes, drink alcohol excessively, or watch strippers as long as they don't hurt

> other people. Actually, smokers are allowed free rein to harm others with secondhand smoke in most places in the country except California, so why aren't people allowed to exert their freedom of choice in regards to use of things like marijuana and anabolic steroids, either of which can be credibly argued to be less dangerous or no more dangerous than cigarettes and alcohol." [Michael Mooney, *Decriminalizing Anabolic Steroids*, May 28, 2001 [www.decriminalizesteroids.com/michael.html]

Smokers are not subject to arrest and criminal prosecution, even though many more deaths result from tobacco *annually* than in all fifty years of non-medical steroid use. According to the U.S. Centers for Disease Control, from 1990 through 1994 there was an average of 430,700 deaths annually attributed to smoking. [*See*, www.drugwarfacts.org/causes.htm, citing "Smoking – Attributable Mortality and Years of Potential Life Lost", *Morbidity and Mortality Weekly Report* (Atlanta, GA: Centers for Disease Control, 1997), May 23, 1997, Vol. 46, No. 20: 449.]

But despite over fifty years of AAS use by bodybuilders, "there is little evidence to show that their use will cause long-term detriment; furthermore, the use of moderate doses of androgens results in side effects that are largely benign and reversible." [Street et al., see references in Chapter 3] Although the inherent risks of dangerous sports and cosmetic surgery are unnecessary, and may well outweigh the benefits, we do not prohibit these activities. Is it appropriate, then, to prevent mature, informed adults from choosing cosmetic enhancement through physician-administered hormones?

But aren't anabolics addictive? No, and yes. There's no good evidence that they're addictive in the way that narcotics are. They are, however, clearly addictive in the way that anything you do that makes you feel or look better is going to make you want to keep doing it. Going to the gym is addictive, if you ask me. Are some folks likely to abuse anabolics because of their own immaturity, irresponsibility, or stupidity? Of course, just like they might abuse alcohol. That's why we prohibit the use of alcohol by minors. But we let adults make up their own minds. Of course, we once tried locking people up for alcohol, and that didn't work any better than the Anabolic Steroid Control Act.

... we prohibit the use of alcohol by minors. But we let adults make up their own minds.

Well, then some might ask, why not legalize all drugs? A growing consensus from across the political spectrum, from liberal to conservative, is becoming highly critical of America's approach to the drug problem (you can read more at web sites like www.drugpolicy.org and www.csdp.org). Many think the current approach has downright *failed*, and that a new strategy is needed that's both more effective *and* more *cost*-effective. However, that's an issue for another writer to take on. My concern isn't with psychoactive drugs taken to escape reality; it's with hormones used for productive physical improvement. How totally insane it seems that we're open to talking about as radical an idea as legalizing mind-altering recreational drugs when anabolics are illegal because we don't like them in sports. Obviously, physique enthusiasts have traditionally had some really lousy lobbyists.

Let's Keep Steroids Out of Sports

The public almost exclusively associates steroids with cheating in sports. And why not? That's virtually the only context in which we hear about them. The big public steroid scandals, from

Ben Johnson's Olympic disgrace to José Canseco's baseball revelations, have all been about juice in competitive athletics and the concerns about the unfair playing field that results. Salacious coverage in *Sports Illustrated* helped to whip not only the public, but also our members of Congress, into a frenzy. When the press prints sensationalistic news bites about the supposed evils of anabolic steroids, the typical sources are physicians with ties to organized sports. How candid or objective are physicians who are wrapped up with anti-doping committees or professional team management? Moreover, you'll notice that the health-related aspects are always inextricably bound to the athletic cheating concerns.

Is using steroids "cheating"? Breaking the rules is cheating. If using steroids breaks the rules, then it's cheating. To analogize, let's say you're a powerlifter and it's against the rules to wear more than one lift-improving bench shirt in a particular meet. You find a way to sneak an extra bench shirt on underneath, so that you're wearing two and won't get caught. Are you cheating? Sure you are. It's not that there's anything inherently ethically wrong about wearing more than one bench shirt. Rather, what's wrong is that you've taken an unfair and unethical advantage over your competitors. It's the same with anabolics. If the rules of the game are that anabolics are disallowed, whether or not you get caught, you're a cheater.

Most competitive sports have banned anabolic steroids. Some athletes may disagree with the rules, and say steroids *should* be allowed. After all, if everyone were allowed to use them, nobody would have an unfair advantage. The playing field would be quite level, wouldn't it? They argue that the judicious use of anabolics is a training tool like any other, and that banning them is really somewhat capricious. Why not ban vitamins and protein supplements and psychological performance improvement techniques? Why not ban practicing? All of these training tools may provide an advantage to those who use them over those who don't.

The answer is, simply, that we have to draw the line *somewhere*. Choosing where to draw it is inherently somewhat arbitrary and subjective. Perhaps anabolics provide just too *great* an advantage for users, or maybe it's the public distaste for the injectable method of administration. Perhaps anabolics seem like a short cut around hard work and discipline, even though most juice users train as hard or, due to the steroids, even *harder* than non-juicers. Maybe anabolics, whether by injection or tablet, just seem more like *chemicals* to the public than vitamins or minerals. Clearly, AAS use by some is unfair to an athlete who can't use them because of a preexisting health condition. For any or all of these reasons, most sports establishments long ago decided that anabolics demean the purity, integrity and values of athletics. Whether or not you agree, "dem's da rules." If you don't like the rules, don't play the game.

What About the Rest of Us?

But what about people who *don't* compete in athletics? They're not taking juice to run faster or jump farther. Are they cheating if they use anabolics? Let's take the 42-year-old dockworker who does an annual pre-summer cycle of juice to feel stronger in the gym and to look better on the beach? Whether or not you approve of his choice, who's he cheating? Let's say he uses responsible dosages and visits his doctor regularly throughout the cycle. Let's say he's fully aware of the speculative long-range risks, and is willing to accept them. Let's say that, overall, the observable effects on his health are positive. Where's the problem?

Well, the fat cats from the sports bodies might argue, condoning the cosmetic use of anabolics for mature adults undermines our anti-doping agenda. That's nonsense, of course. There are lots of substances that are banned in competition but acceptable for the rest of us to consume. Too much caffeine, for example, can get an Olympic athlete disqualified. Does my freedom to drink coffee undermine that policy? Or should their competition policy override my freedom to have ten damned cups of java if I so please? Would the fat cats like to limit my visits to Starbuck's, or maintain surveillance of me so that if I go for a second cup I'll be subject to an arrest? That's ridiculous, isn't it? But that's exactly what's happening to mature non-competing adults who use anabolics. Again, it's the tail wagging the dog. The concerns of a tiny but vocal minority have dictated policies for the overwhelming majority. Cheating athletes should be punished; cosmetic non-athletic users should not be their scapegoats. Most anabolic users probably don't watch the Olympics, much less compete in them.

I can hear the Olympic fat cats, blood boiling, enraged at my voicing these heretical thoughts. They'd say that the fellow is cheating *himself*. Really? Says who, them? He's a mature adult, making an informed decision. How about if he opted for liposuction instead, or calf implants? What if he wore a toupee, or got hair transplants like some legislators have, or used diet drugs? What if he had a face lift or got Botox® injections – is that cheating? Even if it is, with all due respect, why is it *their* business? He's not playing their games.

A Plan for the Future

It's time for a new prescription to treat society's AAS issues. Criminalizing productive Americans is *not* a solution. Returning anabolic steroids to simple prescription drug status would end the many evils caused by the Control Act. Heavy penalties for illegal trafficking could and should continue, especially for those who distribute to teens. The anti-trafficking law that existed before the Control Act was more than adequate to investigate and prosecute illegal AAS distribution.

What about cheating athletes? Punish them. Abolishing the national and state criminalization approach to steroids would *not* require sports bodies to soften their stance. On the contrary, they would be completely free to maintain or toughen their policies on ergogenic substances like steroids, in order to promote fair athletic competition. Improved drug testing technologies and more frequent random testing procedures could be employed to help ensure that adult athletes wishing to compete in such events would need to refrain from using such substances. While testing for steroids may never be perfect, it does remove identified steroid users from sports and is the only effective deterrent. Serious athletes devote huge amounts of time, energy and resources into training for an event. The effect of drug testing – preventing steroid-using athletes from competing – is both a more effective and more appropriate deterrent. Where will the money for tougher testing come from? Let's take all the money we're putting into spying on non-athletic cosmetic AAS users and put it into teen education and athletic testing. Any bored postal inspector who gets the bright idea to do a controlled delivery of fifteen stanozolol tablets to some 40-year old gym rat should be hung out to dry. There are far better uses of our tax dollars.

Abolishing the national and state criminalization approach to steroids would *not* require sports bodies to soften their stance.

What about the diversion issue? The sad joke of it all is that we never even needed controlled substance status to create a paper trail. It could have been done simply by making special rules for anabolics to establish records of sales, orders, and prescriptions, all without changing their prescription drug status. We could have kept track of everything without arresting anyone for personal use.

Regardless of the scheduling status, however, it's time to return the AAS issue for non-competing mature adults to where it belongs: the physician's office. Just like the decision of whether or not to have liposuction or breast augmentation, the decision of whether or not to use hormonal therapies for cosmetic enhancement should be one that takes place after careful discussion with a qualified doctor. It's a matter that should be between physician and patient. You may not like cosmetic AAS use. You may not like liposuction either. But nobody ought to be arrested for either one. It's time to let paternalism give way to the freedom for mature adults to make their own informed health decisions in the confines of their doctor's offices. To accomplish this, two things must take place:

- *First,* the state and federal laws must be changed to give discretion back to physicians.
- *Second,* the rigid and archaic views of the AMA and state medical licensing boards regarding AAS use must be jettisoned.

What would happen? Physicians would no longer fear being arrested for dispensing moderate amounts of anabolics. Mature adults seeking anabolics for cosmetic enhancement would no longer be driven to contaminated black-market products, discouraged from health monitoring, and faced with arrest and imprisonment. Those suffering from AIDS or age-related infirmities would have greater access to needed medications. Funding for anabolic steroid research would increase. The foreign black market would be decimated. Of course, anabolic steroids would be restricted to adults, and non-physicians caught trafficking in steroids, or anyone dispensing or selling anabolics to minors, would be subjected to stiff criminal sanctions.

You may agree with my position, but think, well, what can I do? Make some noise. Lend a copy of this book to your physician, tell him to read it, and tell him to talk to his colleagues about it. Sneak a copy onto the doorstep of your local police department. If you're the member of a police organization, discuss it with your colleagues – if nothing else, your agency will have something in black and white that might have a chilling effect on claims that a hundred tablets of D-bol necessarily indicates distribution intent. If you're an attorney, spread the word among your professional community. Whatever you may do for a living, call up your legislators and ask them how they feel about the issue. If you don't like what you hear, tell them you'll let them know it loud and clear on Election Day. Then get off your butt and vote. The law won't change overnight; change is a long and painful process often met with great resistance. But it's long overdue.

There's nothing wrong with waving our flag. But it should be waved as a genuine expression of the spirit of freedom we all feel as Americans, not as a cheap way to manipulate popular support for the special interests of an influential minority. There's also nothing wrong with criticizing bad laws and policies. This nation was born out of a revolution against unjust laws, and founded on principles of individual liberty and tolerance. The dream of freedom from government oppression is what united America in the first place. Our love of liberty should always be what sets us apart from other places in this world. Sometimes, all these years later, we forget that. When it comes to anabolics, we have lost our way. Together, we need to find our way back.

Appendix I

State AAS Laws

What are the AAS laws in *your* state? Since most steroid prosecutions are brought under state laws, this is absolutely *vital* information for juicers, law enforcers, prosecutors and criminal defense lawyers, most all of whom are surprisingly uncertain on the topic. Here you'll find the crucial specifics for every state, with references to the applicable statutes or codes, including:

How are anabolic steroids defined?
What is their scheduling status?
What conduct is prohibited?
What is the potential jail or prison exposure for simple possession?
How is possessing with intent to sell treated?
How are more substantial quantities dealt with?
What are the maximum prison penalties for distribution or trafficking?
How are first offenses typically handled in practice?
What are previous offenders facing, or those who sell near schools or to minors?
What sorts of diversionary programs exist, such as Drug Courts, Pre-Trial Intervention, Probation Before Judgment, Interim Probation, Suspended Imposition of Sentence, etc.?

Since most AAS defendants are first offenders, the status and the maximum jail or prison penalties for first offenders charged with simple possession or sale are bolded for easy reference. Also bolded are certain unusual provisions, such as maximum misdemeanor jail exposure of less than a year, offense levels based upon weight, or explicit restrictions on physicians.

Also provided within this Appendix is a convenient, state-by-state First-Time Personal Use Possession Chart. It also includes the scheduling status of HCG and hGH in each state.

***

ALABAMA

Title 20, Chapter 2 of the Code of Alabama deals with controlled substances. Take a look through the five lists of controlled substances (Code of Ala. §§ 20-2-23, -25, -27, -29, and -31). You won't see any mention of anabolic steroids! That's because § 20-2-32 directs the State Board of Health to revise and republish the schedules annually, obviating the need to update or revise the Code itself.

So, for information about the scheduling status of anabolic steroids, you need to go to the Rules of the State Board of Health, Chapter 420-7-2 (available online at www.adph.org/administration/controlled.pdf). The revised and republished Alabama Controlled Substances List appears there as an Appendix to the chapter. The list as of this writing, effective October 1, 2001, classifies anabolic steroids under subsection (f) of Schedule III, and explicitly exempts "[a]ny anabolic steroid products exempted by the Federal Drug Enforcement Administration."

Unfortunately, what constitutes an anabolic steroid under Alabama law cannot be explicitly gleaned from this subsection of the Appendix, which circuitously defines "anabolic steroids" to include "any material, compound, mixture or preparation containing any quantity of ... Anabolic Steroids". Unlike the federal law and regulations, the Alabama definition makes no references to testosterone or to the promoting of muscle growth, and provides no list of specific substances. While it specifically includes "salts, isomers and salts of isomers" (although there are no AAS salts), it fails to specifically include *esters* - a puzzling omission. The Rules acknowledge that Alabama originally scheduled anabolic steroids in 1986 as Schedule V drugs, and that when federal scheduling took place in 1991, steroids were transferred into Schedule III (effective March 29, 1991) to comport with the federal law. While officials at the Alabama State Board of Health claim that the Alabama definition of anabolic steroids is identical to the federal definition, there appears to be nothing explicitly saying so. Accordingly, there might be some basis for an argument that the law is impermissibly vague. Of course, that doesn't mean that people can't be convicted based on the existing definition. They have been. For example, in *R.W. v. State* [808 So. 2d 122, 82001 Ala. Crim. App. LEXIS 8], a young man was convicted of possession of testosterone cypionate (although the conviction was overturned based upon unrelated evidentiary weaknesses).

The Code of Alabama's drug offense laws are set forth in Title 13A, Criminal Code; Chapter 12, Offenses Against Public Health and Morals; Article 5, Drug Offenses. Anabolic steroids fall under the criminal laws because the annual controlled substance schedules of the State Board of Health are applicable to criminal prosecutions under § 13A-12-216.

Simple unlawful *possession* or receipt of an anabolic steroid – *in any amount* – is a Class C *felony*. The law (§ 13A-12-212) states:

(a) A person commits the crime of unlawful possession of controlled substance if:
  (1) Except as otherwise authorized, he possesses a controlled substance enumerated in Schedules I through V.
  (2) He obtains by fraud, deceit, misrepresentation or subterfuge or by the alteration of a prescription or written order or by the concealment of a material fact or by the use of a false name or giving a false address, a controlled substance enumerated in Schedules I through V.
(b) Unlawful possession of a controlled substance is a Class C felony.

It is noteworthy that **there is no separate law regarding "possession with intent to distribute."** Nor is there an aggravated offense based on quantity. The same § 13A-12-212 covers *all* possession cases, no matter how much or how little is possessed or for what reason, and it's a Class C felony.

Unlawful *distribution* of anabolic steroids is a Class B felony, covered by § 13A-12-211:

(a) A person commits the crime of unlawful distribution of controlled substances if, except as otherwise authorized, he sells, furnishes, gives away, manufactures, delivers or distributes a controlled substance enumerated in Schedules I through V.
(b) Unlawful distribution of controlled substances is a Class B felony.

Selling, furnishing or giving anabolic steroids to a minor is a Class A felony under § 13A-12-215:

> If the offender is over the age of 18 and the offense consists of selling, furnishing or giving such controlled substances as enumerated in [Schedule III] to a person who has not attained the age of 18 years the offender shall be guilty of a Class A felony. The imposition or execution of sentence shall not be suspended and probation shall not be granted.

A *five-year prison sentence* without the possibility for probation is mandated if the sale takes place on or near a school campus (§ 13A-12-250) or within three miles of a public housing project (§ 13A-12-270). Although a separate Class A felony of "trafficking" in large quantities of controlled substances exists in Alabama (§ 13A-12-231), it does *not* apply to anabolic steroids.

In Alabama, there is *no* misdemeanor drug charge (other than for certain first-time marijuana offenders). So, the bad news is that if a guilty plea in a steroid case is going to be entered, it is generally as a plea to a *felony*. The good news, however, is that there is enough flexibility in many Alabama counties for persuasive plea negotiating to make a difference. Like most states, Alabama has begun to institute drug courts and diversion programs, particularly in larger counties with better-funded justice systems. In these counties, a plea to a felony may be entered but the sentence *postponed* for a lengthy period of time, during which the offender may be required to participate in a program of therapy, drug testing, probationary supervision and/or other negotiated conditions. If the offender succeeds in the program, the felony plea will be *vacated* and the case *dismissed*. Of course, these sorts of diversion programs are mostly targeted toward first offenders, however at least one county in Alabama allows repeat offenders admission to drug court.

If a drug diversion program can't be negotiated, the case may proceed to sentencing on a felony. Under § 13A-5-6, the sentencing ranges for potential imprisonment on the three classes of Alabama felonies are wide:

(a) Sentences for felonies shall be for a definite term of imprisonment, which imprisonment includes hard labor, within the following limitations:
   (1) For a Class A felony, for life or not more than 99 years or less than 10 years.
   (2) **For a Class B felony, not more than 20 years or less than 2 years.**
   (3) **For a Class C felony, not more than 10 years or less than 1 year and 1 day.**

Under § 15-22-50, the court, upon a conviction, may *suspend* execution of sentence (if not more than fifteen years) and place the defendant on probation, or may impose a fine within the limits fixed by law and also place the defendant on probation. The current maximum term of probation was recently increased to seven (7) years.

Note that upon conviction or adjudication of, or finding of delinquency based on, any of the steroid possession or sale offenses described above, § 13A-12-290 requires a *suspension of the offender's driver's license* for a period of six months.

ALASKA

The Alaska Statutes deal with controlled substances under Title 11, Criminal Law; Chapter 11.71. You'll find Schedules IA through VIA in Alaska Stat. §§ 11.71.040 through 11.71.090. Look carefully, particularly in Schedule IIIA (§ 11.71.060). You will find not a single mention of anabolic steroids! That's because **anabolic steroids are not controlled substances under Alaska state law!** Hard to believe? Yes, indeed, but true.

Does this mean Alaska is the unrestricted juice capital of America? Not quite. There is federal jurisdiction over most drug crimes (plus, most of Alaska is, in fact, federal land). Since anabolic steroids are scheduled federally, importing (by mail order or otherwise) would violate federal law, as would situations of distributing or possessing with intent to distribute. Don't expect agents from U.S. Customs, D.E.A., or the Postal Inspector to look the other way!

What would state or local law enforcement do if confronted with a situation of unlawful possession? Representatives from Alaska law enforcement have indicated that in situations of significant quantity or where other factors suggest distribution, the case would typically be handed over to the state Attorney General and the federal authorities for assessment. But what about, for example, a small amount of anabolic steroids recovered in a car? It is unclear what authority (e.g., possession of a prescription drug without a prescription?) might provide for the prosecution of a simple personal use possession situation, and no lawyer we contacted in Alaska has ever seen the prosecution of a personal use steroid possession case.

ARIZONA

Arizona's laws define and list anabolic steroids not once, but twice! Anabolic steroids are defined and listed as "controlled substances" under the Public Health and Safety law and also, defined slightly differently, as "dangerous drugs" under the Criminal Code.

The Arizona Revised Statutes puts steroids in Schedule III under Title 36, Public Health and Safety; Chapter 27, Uniform Controlled Substances Act; Article 2, Schedules (A.R.S. § 36-2514):

A. The following controlled substances are, unless specifically excepted, included in schedule III:
...5. Any material, compound, mixture or preparation containing any of the following anabolic steroids but not including United States food and drug administration approved over-the-counter preparations, labeled for animal use or those prescription-only anabolic steroid preparations in combination with a therapeutic amount of a non-anabolic steroid and intended for human use:
(a) Boldenone. (b) Chlorotestosterone. (c) Clostebol. (d) Dehydrochlormethyltestosterone. (e) Dihydrotestosterone. (f) Drostanolone. (g) Ethylestrenol. (h) Fluoxymesterone. (i) Formebulone. (j) Mesterolone. (k) Methandienone. (l) Methandranone. (m) Methandriol. (n) Methandrostenolone. (o) Methenolone. (p) Methyltestosterone. (q) Mibolerone. (r) Nandrolone. (s) Nore-

thandrolone. (t) Oxandrolone. (u) Oxymesterone. (v) Oxymetholone. (w) Stanolone. (x) Stanozolol. (y) Testolactone. (z) Testosterone. (aa) Trenbolone. (bb) Any salt, ester or isomer of a drug or substance described or listed in this paragraph, if that salt, ester or isomer promotes muscle growth.

B. The board may except by rule any compound, mixture or preparation containing any substance listed in this section from the application of all or any part of this chapter if the compound, mixture or preparation contains one or more active medicinal ingredients and if the admixtures are included therein in combinations, quantity, proportion or concentration that vitiates the potential for abuse.

C. For the purposes of this section, "anabolic steroid" means a growth promoting drug or hormonal substance that promotes growth and that is chemically or pharmacologically related to testosterone, other than estrogens, progestins and corticosteroids.

The scheduling of anabolic steroids under the Public Health and Safety law is intended to address the state regulation of the manufacture, distribution and dispensation of controlled substances, and is primarily applicable to drug manufacturers, physicians, pharmacists, and the like. It specifically **prohibits (as a class 4 felony) knowingly dispensing or delivering "anabolic steroids without a written prescription or for a nontherapeutic use"** (A.R.S. § 36-2531). The "nontherapeutic use" language is presumably intended to authorize prosecution of a physician who writes a steroid prescription for a healthy athlete.

Arizona also defines anabolic steroids as a "dangerous drug." It is under the Criminal Code's "dangerous drug" status that Arizona authorities initiate the majority of criminal prosecutions of drug offenses. The definition of "dangerous drug" is located in Title 13, Criminal Code; Chapter 34, Drug Offenses. A.R.S. § 13-3401(6)(d) refers to anabolic steroids:

(d) Any material, compound, mixture or preparation which contains any quantity of the following anabolic steroids and their salts, isomers or esters: (i) Boldenone; (ii) Clostebol (4-Chlorotestosterone); (iii) Dehydrochloromethyltestosterone; (iv) Drostanolone; (v) Ethylestrenol; (vi) Fluoxymesterone; (vii) Formebulone (Formebolone); (viii) Mesterolone; (ix) Methandriol; (x) Methandrostenolone (Methandienone); (xi) Methenolone; (xii) Methyltestosterone; (xiii) Mibolerone; (xiv) Nandrolone; (xv) Norethandrolon; (xvi) Oxandrolone; (xvii) Oxymesterone; (xviii) Oxymetholone; (xix) Stanolone (4-Dihydrotestosterone); (xx) Stanozolol; (xxi) Testolactone; (xxii) Testosterone; (xxiii) Trenbolone.

Significantly and in contrast to the federal law, the Criminal Code definition lacks a "catch-all" provision enabling the prosecution of muscle-promoting anabolic steroid formulations that are not salts, esters or isomers of the specifically listed compounds. There are far more anabolic androgens than could be practically listed in any definition, and the lack of a catch-all provision fails to cover the prosecution of non-listed or even newly-discovered anabolic steroids. Further, if there are salts, isomers or esters of the listed compounds that do not promote muscle growth, they would fall within the statute (possible overbreadth argument?)

The knowing possession, use, administration, acquisition, sale, manufacture or transportation of dangerous drugs are all covered by the same section of Arizona law: A.R.S. § 13-3407. The same section also sets forth the applicable penalties.

The *simple possession or use* of "dangerous drugs" such as anabolic steroids is considered a "class 4 felony" in Arizona. However, the judge, on motion of the state, considering the nature and circumstances of the offense, may reduce the case to a "class 1 misdemeanor" for many persons who have no previous drug or felony convictions. A misdemeanor conviction may be entered, or the person may be placed on probation without designating the offense as a felony or misdemeanor until the probation is successfully terminated, in which case this "open-ended" offense shall be treated as a felony for all purposes until the court enters an order designating the offense a misdemeanor.

Arizona's "Proposition 200" (A.R.S. § 13-901.01), provides for mandatory probation with drug treatment in lieu of prison sentences for certain offenders. The law is new and its scope is still being defined by the courts. For example, the Supreme Court of Arizona recently held that Prop 200 (as it's commonly called) applies not only to substantive drug possession charges but (despite the plain language of the statute) also to associated drug paraphernalia charges, as long as the paraphernalia is related solely to the personal use or possession of the drugs. *State v. Estrada*, 34 P.3d 356, 361 Ariz. Adv. Rep. 20 (2001). Expect further litigation to define the parameters of Prop 200.

One alternative that is available for possession cases, depending on the county, is referral to Drug Court. Drug Court is available only to first time drug offenders who do not have a violent criminal history and have no more that 2 prior felonies on their record. Prop 200 divides Drug Court into two tracks:

> Track One– Offenses that fall within this classification will receive jail time. These are Prop 200 second offenses and non Prop 200 offenses. The defendants are sentenced but if they successfully complete their drug court program the jail time will be wiped away.
>
> Track Two– Offenses that fall within this classification will not receive jail time. These are Prop 200 first offenses. This is a reward-based program, featuring four levels, that offers incentives such as tickets, ice cream, etc., when a participant is promoted or successfully completes the program.

Knowingly manufacturing a dangerous drug, administering a dangerous drug to another person, possessing a dangerous drug for sale, or selling or offering to sell a dangerous drug is each considered a "class 2 felony" under A.R.S. § 13-3407(B).

Imprisonment for first felony offenders is set forth in A.R.S. § 13-701(C). **For a class 2 felony, it's five years; for a class 4 felony, it's two and one-half years.** The law provides alternative sentencing for exceptional circumstances, aggravation and mitigation (A.R.S. § 13-702 and § 13-702.01), and specifically addresses the use of minors in drug offenses § 13-3409. Note that Arizona doesn't provide for "suspended sentences."

Another interesting section involves using "threshold amounts" as an aggravating factor that prevents probation in multiple drug offense cases (A.R.S. § 13-3419). Under A.R.S. § 13-3401(36), the threshold amount of most common drugs is based on weight. But under subparagraph (j), **for unlisted drugs like anabolic steroids, the threshold amount is defined as a quantity that has a value of at least one thousand dollars.** This could spell major trouble because law enforcement agents have been notoriously inaccurate in assessing steroid prices [see Chapter 14]. There is no mandatory drivers' license suspension or revocation.

ARKANSAS

The Arkansas Code addresses anabolic steroids and other controlled substances under Title 5, Criminal Offenses; Subtitle 6, Offenses Against Public Health, Safety or Welfare; Chapter 64, Controlled Substances. Anabolic steroids are defined in the Arkansas Controlled Substances Act, A.C.A. § 5-64-101 (unlike the federal law, Arkansas provides no list of specific compounds):

> (x) The term "anabolic steroid" means any drug or hormonal substance, chemically and pharmacologically related to testosterone, other than estrogens, progestin, and corticosteroid, that promotes muscle growth. Except that such term does not include an anabolic steroid which is expressly intended for administration through implants to cattle or other nonhuman species and which has been approved by the Director of the Department of Health for such administration. If any person prescribes, dispenses, or distributes such steroid for human use, such person shall be considered to have prescribed, dispensed, or distributed an anabolic steroid within the meaning of this subdivision.

In Arkansas, there are not five but *six* schedules of controlled substances. While the criteria for each schedule are published in the Arkansas Code, the schedules themselves are not codified. Rather, they are governed by administrative regulation and are revised and republished annually by the Director of the Arkansas Department of Health or his authorized agent. For a copy of the most recent rescheduling of controlled substances, you can contact the Department of Health. The most recent rescheduling places anabolic steroids in Schedule III:

A personal use possession conviction for anabolic steroids is a misdemeanor for first timers, but subsequent convictions are felonies under A.C.A. § 5-64-401(c):

> (c) It is unlawful for any person to possess a controlled substance ... unless the substance was obtained directly from, or pursuant to, a valid prescription or order of a practitioner while acting in the course of his professional practice, or except as otherwise authorized by this chapter. Any person convicted of a first offense for violation of this subsection is guilty of a Class A misdemeanor. Provided any person who is convicted of a second offense for a violation of this subsection is guilty of a Class D felony. Provided, any person who is convicted of a third or subsequent offense for violation of this subsection shall be guilty of a Class C felony...

A typical first time possession charge is often dealt with in a manner that avoids a lasting criminal record. One mechanism by which this is accomplished is found in A.C.A. § 5-64-407, which provides for "Probation – Discharge and dismissal." A plea to a misdemeanor is entered, but the conviction may be vacated and the charge dismissed upon successful completion of a probationary period. Another popular mechanism of avoiding a conviction in Arkansas is under "Act 346," which is found in A.C.A. § 16-90-901, and permits a criminal record to be expunged and sealed. This *can* apply to both sale and possession cases.

The manufacture, delivery, or possession with intent to manufacture or deliver an anabolic steroid falls within A.C.A. § 5-64-401(a). It is a Class B felony regardless of the quantity involved, but the statute is referenced to the *aggregate weight* of the drug for *sentencing* purposes. The pertinent parts state:

> (1) Any person who violates this subsection with respect to..
>
> ...(ii) Any other controlled substance classified in Schedules I, II, or III which by aggregate weight, including adulterants or diluents, is less than twenty-eight grams (28 g.), is guilty of a felony and shall be imprisoned for not less than five (5) years nor more than twenty (20) years and shall be fined an amount not to exceed fifteen thousand dollars ($15,000). For all purposes, other than disposition, this offense is a Class B felony.
>
> Any other controlled substance classified in Schedules I, II, or III which by aggregate weight, including adulterants or diluents, is twenty-eight grams (28 g.) or more but less than four hundred grams (400 g.), is guilty of a felony and shall be imprisoned for not less than ten (10) years nor more than forty (40) years, or life, and shall be fined an amount not to exceed fifty thousand dollars ($50,000). For all purposes other than disposition, this offense is a Class B felony.
>
> Any other controlled substance classified in Schedules I, II, or III which by aggregate weight, including adulterants or diluents, is four hundred grams (400 g.) or more, is guilty of a felony and shall be imprisoned for not less than fifteen (15) years nor more than forty (40) years, or life, and shall be fined an amount not exceeding one hundred thousand dollars ($100,000). For all purposes other than disposition, this offense is a Class B felony.

The statute measures aggregate weight in grams. Using such a standard is easy with most drugs, especially powdered substances. This is an appropriated standard of measure for powders, such as cocaine and heroin, as they are both bought and sold in these quantities. Anabolic steroids are not bought, sold or used in these quantities and therefore "grams" is an inappropriate way of measuring them. Additionally, if you were to attempt this type of quantification, one would assume that the aggregate weight of a gram of injectable steroid should refer to the steroid itself, minus the oil. Again, there is the problem of ignoring the potency issue, with regard to both tablets and injectables. The potency of the particular type and brand of steroid has much to do with the amount of steroid actually contained in the tablet or vial. [*See* Case Notes, *Wall v. Texas*, for a disturbing example of how aggregate weight can be interpreted to include the oil in injectables and the fillers and binders in steroid tablets.]

Note that a separate subsection (d) of A.C.A. § 5-64-401 creates a *presumption* of possession with intent to deliver if a controlled substance quantity exceeds certain specified amounts. There is a list of various controlled substances and their quantity limits to trigger this presumption (which is rebuttable), but anabolic steroids are *not* included on the list. The prosecution, unable to enjoy the benefit of this presumption in a steroid case, would have to rely on other evidence and arguments to prove that a quantity of steroids was not possessed for personal use.

The imprisonment ranges for crimes in Arkansas are set forth in A.C.A. § 5-4-401:

a) A defendant convicted of a felony shall receive a determinate sentence according to the following limitations:
 ...(3) **For a Class B** felony, the sentence **shall be not less than five (5)** years **nor more than twenty (20)** years;
 (4) For a Class C felony, the sentence shall be not less than three (3) years nor more than ten (10) years;
 (5) For a Class D felony, the sentence shall not exceed six (6) years;
(b) A defendant convicted of a misdemeanor may be sentenced according to the following limitations:
 (1) For a Class A misdemeanor, the sentence shall not exceed one (1) year;

Under A.C.A. § 5-64-408, persons with previous drug convictions are may be imprisoned for up to *twice* the term otherwise authorized, and fines may be doubled. A separate statute addresses distribution to minors (A.C.A. § 5-64-406) by doubling potential imprisonment terms from those indicated above. Note that aggressive or creative prosecutors could try to use various other aggravating statutory provisions to up the ante on the potential sentence. For example, the continuing criminal enterprise crime of A.C.A. § 5-64-414 could be applied to a steroid distribution ring engaged in a continuing series of felonies if the offender was in a management position derived substantial income or resources from the enterprise, etc.

Arkansas currently provides for a mandatory six-month driver's license suspension for conviction of a controlled substances offense under A.C.A. § 27-16-915.

CALIFORNIA

California law contains 29 codes covering various subject areas. Anabolic steroids have been controlled substances in California since 1986. They are both defined and classified as a Schedule III controlled substance in the California Health and Safety Code; Division 10, Uniform Controlled Substances Act; Chapter 2, Standards and Schedules. Cal Health & Saf Code § 11056:

Schedule III list of controlled substances...
(f) Anabolic steroids and chorionic gonadotropin. Any material, compound, mixture, or preparation containing chorionic gonadotropin or an anabolic steroid (excluding anabolic steroid products listed in the "Table of Exempt Anabolic Steroid Products" (Section 1308.34 of Title 21 of the Code of Federal Regulations), as exempt from the federal Controlled Substances Act (Section 801 and following of Title 21 of the United States Code)), including, but not limited to, the following: (1) Androisoxazole. (2) Androstenediol. (3) Bolandiol. (4) Bolasterone. (5) Boldenone. (6) Chlormethandienone. (7) Clostebol. (8) Dihydromesterone. (9) Ethylestrenol. (10) Fluoxymesterone. (11) Formyldienolone. (12) 4-Hydroxy-19-nortestosterone. (13) Mesterolone. (14) Methandriol. (15) Methandrostenolone. (16) Methenolone. (17) 17-Methyltestosterone. (18) Methyltrienolone. (19) Nandrolone. (20) Norbolethone. (21) Norethandrolone. (22) Normethandrolone. (23) Oxandrolone. (24) Oxymestrone. (25) Oxymetholone. (26) Quinbolone. (27) Stanolone. (28) Stanozolol. (29) Stenbolone. (30) Testosterone. (31) Trenbolone. (32) Chorionic Gonadotropin (HGC).

Although it fails to mention salts, isomers or esters, the California law provides a list of anabolic steroid preparations and excludes the products exempted by federal regulations. But it also throws in *chorionic gonadotropin* (which it spells out correctly - unlike the New York law - but then misspells the abbreviation as "HGC" instead of HCG) with anabolic steroids despite the fact that HCG doesn't fit any legal definition of "anabolic steroid," nor is it a controlled substance under federal law. As in New York, it seems to have been bootstrapped into the statute because some steroid users administer HCG to boost their own endogenous testosterone production during or after a cycle of steroids. Also, note the inclusion of androstenediol, a prohormone.

The *simple possession* of anabolic steroids and HCG without a valid prescription is a misdemeanor under Cal Health & Saf Code § 11377:

> (a) Except as authorized by law ... every person who possesses any controlled substance which is (1) classified in Schedule III ... unless upon the prescription of a physician, dentist, podiatrist, or veterinarian, licensed to practice in this state, shall be punished by imprisonment in a county jail for a period of not more than one year or in the state prison.
>
> (b)(1) Any person who violates subdivision (a) by unlawfully possessing a controlled substance specified in subdivision (f) of Section 11056, and who has not previously been convicted of such a violation involving a controlled substance specified in subdivision (f) of Section 11056, is guilty of a misdemeanor.

The California law, therefore, makes a special provision for anabolic steroids. Unlike the possessors of other non-narcotic Schedule III drugs who are punishable by imprisonment either in a county jail for up to a year or in state prison, first-time steroid possessors are *misdemeanor* violators and don't face state prison. Second convictions may be punished by jail or state prison.

"Proposition 36" has been codified under Cal Pen Code § 1210.1. It is a new drug program providing probation and treatment for eligible individuals charged with possession for personal use. They enter a guilty plea for the charge, are sentenced immediately, and are referred to the probation department, which provides them with a list of programs that are acceptable to provide counseling. The program directors determine the level of counseling. Initially the offenders don't serve any time and they are allowed three chances; but if they fail in the drug program they can serve the maximum. If a person fails to comply, their probation will be revoked and they will be sentenced for a second time. A successful completion can result in dismissal as if it never happened. Section 1210.1 states:

> (a) Notwithstanding any other provision of law, and except as provided in subdivision (b), any person convicted of a nonviolent drug possession offense shall receive probation. As a condition of probation the court shall require participation in and completion of an appropriate drug treatment program. The court may also impose, as a condition of probation, participation in vocational training, family counseling, and literacy training and/or community service. A court may not impose incarceration as an additional condition of probation. Aside from the limitations imposed in this subdivision, the trial court is not otherwise limited in the type of probation conditions it may impose. Probation shall be imposed by suspending the imposition of sentence.

Possession of steroids or HCG for sale is a felony covered by Cal Health & Saf Code § 11378, and is punishable under Cal Pen Code § 18 by imprisonment in any of the **state prisons for 16 months, or two or three years.**

Sale, distribution and transportation of anabolic steroids and HCG is covered by Cal Health & Saf Code § 11379:

> (a) Except as otherwise provided ... every person who transports, imports into this state, sells, furnishes, administers, or gives away, or offers to transport, import into this state, sell, furnish, administer, or give away, or attempts to import into this state or transport any controlled substance which is
> (1) classified in Schedule III ... unless upon the prescription of a physician, dentist, podiatrist, or veterinarian, licensed to practice in this state, **shall be punished by imprisonment in the state prison for a period of two, three, or four years.**
>
> (b) Notwithstanding the penalty provisions of subdivision (a), any person who transports for sale any

controlled substances specified in subdivision (a) within this state from one county to another noncontiguous county shall be punished by imprisonment in the state prison for three, six, or nine years.

Drug Court is an option available for drug users who don't have much of a record but are considered addicts and heavy drug users. The program is intensively supervised by the Drug Court judge and successful completion can earn you a dismissal. Sale or intent to sell cases are generally not eligible for any of the above "diversionary" programs, however, in some cases when the quantity is a small amount, a judge might grant long term treatment as an option.

Determinate Sentencing in California can be found within the definition of the crime itself or under Cal Pen Code § 1170, Determinate Sentencing. Section (a)(3) states that, "In any case in which the punishment prescribed by statute for a person convicted of a public offense is a term of imprisonment in the state prison of any specification of three time periods, the court shall sentence the defendant to one of the terms of imprisonment specified unless the convicted person is given any other disposition provided by law, including a fine, jail, probation, or the suspension of imposition or execution of sentence..." The judge starts with the middle term and the sentence can be mitigated down or aggravated up.

License revocation is discretionary for the DMV; based on registration as narcotic offenders.

COLORADO

Anabolic steroids are covered by the Uniform Controlled Substances Act of 1992, located in Title 18 of the Colorado Criminal Code. The definition is found in C.R.S. §18-18-102:

(3) (a) "Anabolic steroid" means any material, drug, hormonal compound, salt, isomer or salts of isomers of testosterone, or synthetic or natural derivatives of testosterone having pronounced anabolic properties which is used primarily to promote growth of muscle tissue, which includes, but is not limited to, any of the following: (I) Boldenone; (II) Chlorotestosterone; (III) Clostebol; (IV) Dehydrochlormethyltestosterone; (V) Dihydrotestosterone; (VI) Drostanolone; (VII) Ethylestrenol; (VIII) Fluoxymesterone; (IX) Formebulone; (X) Human chorionic gonadotropin; (XI) Human growth hormone; (XII) Mesterolone; (XIII) Methandienone; (XIV) Methandranone; (XV) Methandriol; (XVI) Methandrestenolone; (XVII) Methenolone; (XVIII) Methyltestosterone; (XIX) Mibolerone; (XX) Nandrolone; (XXI) Norethandrolone; (XXII) Oxandrolone; (XXIII) Oxymesterone; (XXIV) Oxymetholone; (XXV) Stanolone; (XXVI) Stanozolol; (XXVII) Testolactone; (XXVIII) Testosterone; (XXIX) Trenbolone; (XXX) Any salt, ester, or isomer of a drug or substance described or listed in this paragraph (a) if that salt, ester, or isomer promotes muscle growth.

(b) (I) Except as provided in subparagraph (II) of this paragraph (b), such term does not include an anabolic steroid which is expressly intended for administration through implants to cattle or other nonhuman species and which has been approved by the secretary of health and human services for such administration.

(II) If any person prescribes, dispenses, or distributes a steroid described in subparagraph (I) of this paragraph (b) for human use, such person shall be considered to have prescribed, dispensed, or distributed an anabolic steroid within the meaning of paragraph (a) of this subsection (3).

Anabolic steroids are classified as schedule III controlled substances under C.R.S. §18-18-205:

(2) Unless specifically excepted by Colorado or federal law, or Colorado or federal regulation, or more specifically included in another schedule, the following controlled substances are listed in schedule III:

...(e) Anabolic steroids

***Using* anabolic steroids or HCG or hGH is a misdemeanor** under C.R.S. §18-18-404. The statute specifically talks about "use," not "possession," of controlled substances, and subsection (1) applies to steroids (as a schedule III substance) in pertinent part:

> ... [A]ny person who uses any controlled substance, except when it is dispensed by or under the direction of a person licensed or authorized by law to prescribe, administer, or dispense such controlled substance for bona fide medical needs, commits:
> ...(b) A class 1 misdemeanor, if the controlled substance is listed in schedule III....

Subsections (2) and (3) of C.R.S. §18-18-404 demonstrate Colorado's interest in promoting drug treatment as an alternative to traditional sentencing concepts for persons in need of treatment.

Now here's the kicker! **While using steroids or HCG or hGH is a misdemeanor, *possessing* them is a class 4 *felony*.** One law (C.R.S. 18-18-405) covers both personal possession and possession to distribute:

> (1) (a) Except as authorized ... , it is unlawful for any person knowingly to manufacture, dispense, sell, distribute, possess, or to possess with intent to manufacture, dispense, sell, or distribute a controlled substance; or induce, attempt to induce, or conspire with one or more other persons, to manufacture, dispense, sell, distribute, possess, or possess with intent to manufacture, dispense, sell, or distribute a controlled substance...
> (2) Except as is otherwise provided for ... offenses involving minors in section 18-18-407 (1) (g), any person who violates any of the provisions of subsection (1) of this section: ...
> (b) In the case of a controlled substance listed in schedule III ... commits:
> (I) A class 4 felony; or
> (II) A class 3 felony, if the violation is committed subsequent to any prior conviction [under this section for schedule I, II, or III drugs]...

Clearly, distinguishing between personal *use* of drugs and *possession for* personal use of drugs seems a bit specious. It's difficult to imagine a real world factual scenario where a person could use a drug without possessing it, so to make one charge a misdemeanor and another a felony seems ludicrous. The Colorado courts have acknowledged the absurdity: While an individual may unlawfully possess a controlled substance without voluntarily using it, it is simply not feasible for an individual to voluntarily use a controlled substance without also possessing it. [*People v. Villapando, 984 P.2d 51 (Colo. 1999)*] However, courts have held that ... Equal protection is not violated when a defendant is charged for the same conduct under both this section and § 18-18-404(1)(a) because unlawful use and unlawful possession are distinct offenses that each require proof of at least one fact that the other does not. [*People v. District of Ct. of 11th Jud. Dist., 964 P. 2d 498 (Colo. 1998)*]

In Colorado, a criminal offense falls into one of eleven classes. There are six classes of felonies, distinguished by their presumptive ranges of penalties, as defined in §18-1-105; three classes of misdemeanors as defined in § 18-1-106; and two classes of petty offenses as defined in § 18-1-107.

The presumptive sentence ranges (post-1993) are set forth under C.R.S. §18-1-105(1)(a)(V)(A). **For a Class 4 felony, the presumptive range of imprisonment is a minimum sentence of two years to six years,** with a mandatory period of post-incarceration parole of three years. For a Class 3 felony, the range is four years to twelve years, with a mandatory period of post-incarceration parole of five years. Under subparagraph (VI), offenders must generally be punished by the imposition of a definite sentence within the presumptive ranges, in consideration of the nature and elements of the offense, the character and record of the offender, and all aggravating or mitigating circumstances surrounding the offense and the offender (although some provisions permit the court to depart upwardly or downwardly based upon extraordinary aggravating or mitigating circumstances).

However, under C.R.S. §18-1-105(1)(a)(III)(E), a person who's been twice convicted of any federal or state felony prior to the conviction for which he or she is being sentenced is not be eligible to receive a fine in lieu of any sentence to imprisonment, community corrections, or work release, but must be sentenced to at least the minimum sentence and may receive a fine in addition to said sentence.

Further, §18-1-105(10) permits suspended sentences in meet the ends of justice and the best interest of the public, as well as the defendant. The courts have the power to suspend the imposition or execution of a sentence for such period and upon such terms and conditions as it may deem best; except that in no instance shall the court have the power to suspend a sentence to a term of incarceration when the defendant is sentenced pursuant to a mandatory sentencing provision. Where the defendant has two prior felony convictions, the district attorney must recommend and the court must approve any suspended sentence arrangement.

Misdemeanors carry the following potential punishments under §18-1-106(1):

> Class 1 misdemeanors: minimum of six months jail or $500 fine or both to a maximum of 18 months jail or $5,000 fine, or both;
> Class 2 misdemeanors: minimum of three months jail or $250 fine or both to a maximum of 12 months jail or $1,000 fine, or both;
> Class 3 misdemeanors: minimum of $50 fine or a maximum of 6 months jail or $750 fine, or both.

First time offenders are usually granted probation. Possession cases are eligible for deferred judgment or probation, depending on the history of the offender. Intent to sell cases may be eligible, depending on the quantity involved.

License revocation is mandated for drug convictions, but some judges still may not order it.

CONNECTICUT

Connecticut addresses controlled substances in Title 21a, Consumer Protection; Chapter 420b, Dependency-Producing Drugs. Its controlled substance schedules are not found in its statutes. Rather, Conn. Gen. Stat. § 21a-243 (2001) authorizes the Commissioner of Consumer Protection to adopt *regulations* for the efficient enforcement of the statutes, either by adopting the existing federal regulations or by scheduling specific substances upon the advice of the Commission of Pharmacy.

Accordingly, Connecticut regulations, Sec. 21a-243-9, lists the controlled substances in schedule III:

> The controlled substances listed in this regulation are included by whatever official, common, usual, chemical, or trade name des-ignation in Schedule III:
> ...(e) Unless expressly intended for administration through im-plants to nonhuman species and approved for such use by the Fed-eral Food and Drug Administration, any anabolic steroid including but not limited to, any of the following, or any isomer, ester, salt or derivative of the following that acts in the same manner on the human body:
> (1) Boldenone; (2) Chlorotestosterone; (3) Clostebol; (4) Dehydrochlormethyltestosterone; (5) Dihydrotesterone; (6) Drostanolone; (7) Ethylestrenol; (8) Fluoxymesterone; (9) Formebulone; (10) Mesterolone; (11) Methandienone; (12) Methandranone; (13) Methandriol; (14) Methandrostenolone; (15) Methenolone; (16) Methyltesterone; (17) Mibolerone; (18) Nandrolone; (19) Norethandrolone; (20) Oxandrolone; (21) Oxymesterone; (22) Oxymetholone; (23) Stanolone; (24) Stanozolol; (25) Testolactone; (26) Testosterone; (27) Trenbolone. (f) Chorionic gonadotropin.

Note the absence of the typical federal "catch-all" provision about any growth-producing substances chemically or pharmacologically related to testosterone. Note also that Connecticut schedules chorionic gonadotropin as a controlled substance. It does this under a separate subparagraph, unlike New York, which erroneously puts it under the anabolic steroids heading.

Where a conflict arises between the federal schedules and Connecticut's schedules, Conn. Gen. Stat. § 21a-243 applies:

> (f) In the event of any inconsistency between the contents of schedules I, II, III, IV and V of the controlled substance scheduling regulations and schedules I, II, III, IV and V of the federal Controlled

> Substances Act, as amended, the provisions of the federal act shall prevail, except when the provisions of the Connecticut controlled substance scheduling regulations place a controlled substance in a schedule with a higher numerical designation, schedule I being the highest designation.

In Connecticut, **simple first-time unlawful possession of steroids or HCG is a misdemeanor (subsequent offenses are felonies)**, and the penalties are right in the offense statute rather than in general sentencing laws. Conn. Gen. Stat. § 21a-279:

> ...(c)Any person who possesses or has under his control any quantity of any controlled substance other than a narcotic substance ... except as authorized in this chapter, for a first offense, may be fined not more than one thousand dollars or be imprisoned not more than one year, or be both fined and imprisoned; and for a subsequent offense, may be fined not more than three thousand dollars or be imprisoned not more than five years, or be both fined and imprisoned.

There is also a provision in subparagraph (d) adding 2 years of consecutive imprisonment if the violation occurs within one thousand five hundred feet of a school or licensed day care center.

Situations of selling anabolic steroids or HCG or possessing steroids or HCG with the intent to sell them are proscribed under Conn. Gen. Stat. § 21a-277:

> ...(b) Any person who manufactures, distributes, sells, prescribes, dispenses, compounds, transports with intent to sell or dispense, possesses with intent to sell or dispense, offers, gives or administers to another person any controlled substance, except a narcotic substance, or a hallucinogenic substance other than marijuana, except as authorized in this chapter, **may, for the first offense, be fined not more than twenty-five thousand dollars or be imprisoned not more than seven years or be both fined and imprisoned**; and, for each subsequent offense, may be fined not more than one hundred thousand dollars or be imprisoned not more than fifteen years, or be both fined and imprisoned.
>
> ...(d) As an alternative to the sentences specified in subsections (a) and (b) of this section, the court may sentence the person to the custody of the Commissioner of Correction for an indeterminate term not to exceed three years or the maximum term specified for the offense, whichever is the lesser, and, at any time within such indeterminate term and without regard to any other provision of law regarding minimum term of confinement, the Commissioner of Correction may release the convicted person so sentenced subject to such conditions as he may impose including, but not limited to, supervision by suitable authority. At any time during such indeterminate term, the Commissioner of Correction may revoke any such conditional release in his discretion for violation of the conditions imposed and return the convicted person to a correctional institution.

Under Conn. Gen. Stat. § 21a-278a, selling to minors is punishable by an added two years of prison time, without suspension of sentence.

An option available to most first time drug offenders is accelerated rehabilitation, which generally entails probation and dismissal upon successful completion. Other alternatives that first time offenders may receive are drug education programs or community service. A first time sale offender may be offered a "cap." He would enter a guilty plea and there would be a pre-sentence investigation. An alternative to incarceration plan is developed, and the case may continue for 10 weeks during probation. Other options are suspended sentence with probation (sentences can be suspended, in whole or in part, under Conn. Gen. Stat. § 53a-28) or serve time or take on the alternative sentence. Drug Court may be an option for repeat offenders who would otherwise be serving time. Those charged with a sale case are ineligible. It's a long-term, intensive treatment, mostly outpatient but with strict guidelines.

Driver's license revocations are only for DWI and driving related drug offenses.

DELAWARE

The Delaware Code addresses controlled substances in its Title 16, Health and Safety; Part IV, Food and Drugs; Chapter 47, Uniform Controlled Substances Act. There is a basic definition in the general definitions section and a more detailed one in the scheduling section. The more basic definition is under 16 Del. C. § 4701:

> ...(5)The term "anabolic steroid" means any drug or hormonal substance, chemically and pharmacologically related to testosterone (other than estrogens, progestins, and corticosteroids) that promotes muscle growth. Except such terms does not include an anabolic steroid which is expressly intended for administration through implants to cattle or other nonhuman species and which has been approved by the Secretary of Health and Human Services for such administration.

Note that this section also provides the following:

> ...(18)"Human growth hormone" is synonymous with the term "human chorionic gonadotropin."

Wrong! Human growth hormone is most assuredly *not* human chorionic gonadotropin. In effect, the statute defines an apple as an orange, and it's arguably anybody's guess as to what is meant! Of course, neither substance is included in the section prohibiting anabolic steroids, and officials at the Board of Pharmacy seemed totally confused when we asked them what substances were actually controlled.

Now, like many states, Delaware has a separate definition for anabolic steroids within its schedule of controlled substances. Pursuant to 16 Del. C. § 4718, anabolic steroids are a Schedule III controlled substance (although a exemption exists for combination hormones for hormone-deficient women):

> Schedule III:
>
> ...(f) Anabolic steroids and combinations:
>
> (1) Boldenone; (2) Chlorotestosterone (4-dihydrotestosterone); (3) Clostebol; (4) Dehydrochlormethyltestosterone; (5) Dihydrotestosterone (4-dihydrotestosterone); (6) Drostanolone; (7) Ethylestrenol; (8) Fluoxymesterone; (9) Formebulone (formebulone); (10) Mesterolone; (11) Methandienone; (12) Methandranone; (13) Methandriol; (14) Methandrostenolone; (15) Methenolone; (16) Methyltestosterone; (17) Mibolerone; (18) Nandrolone; (19) Norethandrolone; (20) Oxandrolone; (21) Oxymesterone; (22) Oxymetholone; (23) Stanolone; (24) Stanozolol; (25) Testolactone; (26) Testosterone; (27) Trenbolone; and (28) Any salt, ester, or isomer of a drug or substance described or listed in this paragraph, if that salt, ester, or isomer promotes muscle growth.
>
> ...(m) Any anabolic steroid, as listed in subsection (f), which is a combination of estrogen and anabolic steroid and which is expressly intended for administration to hormone-deficient women, shall be exempt from the provisions of this chapter. If any person prescribes, dispenses or distributes an anabolic steroid which is a combination of estrogen and anabolic steroid for use by persons who are not hormone-deficient women, such person shall be considered to have prescribed, dispensed or distributed an anabolic steroid within the meaning of this chapter.

Simple unlawful possession (or use or consumption) of anabolic steroids without a valid prescription is considered a class B misdemeanor under 16 Del. C. § 4754:
(a) It is unlawful for any person knowingly or intentionally to possess, use or consume any controlled substance [in Schedule III] unless the substance was obtained directly from, or pursuant to, a valid prescription or order of a practitioner while acting in the course of the practitioner's professional practice, or except as otherwise authorized by this chapter. Any person who violates this subsection shall be guilty of a class B misdemeanor.

Class B misdemeanors are punishable by up to 6 months in jail under 11 Del. C. § 4206:

> (b) The sentence for a class B misdemeanor may include up to 6 months incarceration at Level V and such fine up to $1,150, restitution or other conditions as the court deems appropriate.

Delivery or possession with the intent to deliver steroids is a class E felony punishable by up to 5 years in prison under 16 Del. C. § 4752, Prohibited acts B; penalties:

(a) Except as authorized by this chapter, any person who manufactures, delivers or possesses with intent to manufacture or deliver a controlled substance [in Schedule III] is guilty of a class E felony and upon conviction shall be fined not less than $1,000 nor more than $10,000 and imprisoned not more than 5 years.

The punishments are consistent with 11 Del. C. § 4205(b)(5), the general Delaware section on sentences for class E felonies. But the interesting thing about 16 Del. C. § 4752 is the inclusion of the two subsections that follow:

(b) Any person who distributes, sells, offers to sell, dispenses, administers, or prescribes any anabolic steroid or any counterfeit substance purporting to be an anabolic steroid for the purposes of human body building or enhancement of human athletic performance is guilty of a class E felony. For purposes of this section, **it is not a valid medical practice to distribute, sell, offer to sell, dispense, administer or prescribe any anabolic steroid for purposes of human body building or enhancement of human athletic performance.**
(c) For purposes of this section, the words "body building" shall mean the increasing of muscle weight. For purposes of this section, the words "athletic enhancement" shall mean the improvement of performance in any form of exercise, sport or game.

These subsections are targeted at physicians. Delaware has gone out of its way to explicitly declare bodybuilding to be an invalid medical application for steroids right in their section for all non-narcotic drugs! A critic might say, sarcastically, that Delaware has ensured that steroid use will be kept out of doctors' offices and remain instead on the black market where it belongs.

Now, other provisions impose various enhanced punishments in the presence of aggravating factors. These include distribution, delivery or possession of a controlled substance within 1,000 feet of a school (16 Del. C. § 4767) and in or within 300 feet of a park, recreation area, church, synagogue or other place of worship (16 Del. C. § 4768). Certain affirmative defenses do apply.

The available options include a newly instated drug court; however, there is no Probation Before Judgment for drug cases. A first time sale case is likely to entail a 2 -3 year probation sentence and up to 15 months is recommended under the guidelines for an E felony. Delaware has a tiered sentencing system, with levels ranging from Level 5, which is jail, to level 1, which is unsupervised release.

A driver's license may be suspended for 2 years on any misdemeanor drug offense and 3 years on felonies. Up until recently, restricted licenses for work were not granted.

DISTRICT OF COLUMBIA

The District of Columbia Official Code defines and schedules anabolic steroids in Title 48, Foods and Drugs; Subtitle III, Illegal Drugs; Chapter 9, Controlled Substances, § 48-902.08:

(a) The controlled substances listed in this section are included in Schedule III, unless and until removed therefrom pursuant to § 48-902.01:
...(5)Unless specifically excepted or unless listed in another schedule, any material, compound, mixture, or preparation containing any quantity of the following substances, drug, or hormonal substance, chemically and pharmacologically related to testosterone (other than estrogens, progesterons, and corticorsteroids) that promotes muscle growth and includes: (A) Boldenone; (B) Chlortestosterone (4-chlortestosterone); (C) Clostebol; (D) Dehydrochlormethyltestosterone; (E) Dihydrotestosterone (4-dihydrotestosterone); (F) Drostanolone; (G) Ethylestrenol; (H) Fluoxymestorone; (I) Formebulone (formebolone); (J) Mesterolone; (K) Meth-

andienone; (L) Methandranone; (M) Methandriol; (N) Methandrostenolone; (O) Methenolone; (P) Methyltestosterone; (Q) Mibolerone; (R) Nandrolone; (S) Norethandrolone; (T) Oxandrolone; (U) Oxymesterone; (V) Oxymetholone; (W) Stanolone; (X) Stanozolol; (Y) Testolactone; (Z) Testosterone; (AA) Trenbolone; and (BB) Any salt, ester or isomer of a drug or substance described or listed in this paragraph, if that salt, ester, or isomer promotes muscle growth. Except such term does not include an anabolic steroid which is expressly intended for administration through implants to cattle or other nonhuman species and which has been approved by Secretary of Health and Human Services for such administration. If any person prescribes, dispenses or distributes such steroid for human use such person shall be considered to have prescribed, dispensed or distributed an anabolic steroid within the meaning of this paragraph;

Penalties for the basic anabolic steroid offenses are all set forth under D.C. Code § 48-904.01. **Simple unlawful possession is a misdemeanor punishable by up to 180 days in jail** under subsection (d):

(d) It is unlawful for any person knowingly or intentionally to possess a controlled substance unless the substance was obtained directly from, or pursuant to, a valid prescription or order of a practitioner while acting in the course of his or her professional practice, or except as otherwise authorized by this chapter. Any person who violates this subsection is guilty of a misdemeanor and upon conviction may be imprisoned for not more than 180 days, fined not more than $1,000, or both.

Distributing steroids or possessing them with the intent to distribute is punishable by up to 5 years in prison under D.C. Code § 48-904.01 (a):

(a) (1) Except as authorized by this chapter, it is unlawful for any person knowingly or intentionally to manufacture, distribute, or possess, with intent to manufacture or distribute, a controlled substance.
(2) Any person who violates this subsection with respect to:
...(B) Any other controlled substance classified in [Schedule III] is guilty of a crime and upon conviction may be imprisoned for not more than 5 years, fined not more than $50,000, or both..

However, subsection (f) permits the prosecutor to charge an offender only with a misdemeanor under subsection (d) "if the interests of justice so dictate." Also, subsection (e)(1) provides a mechanism by which first-time offenders convicted of the misdemeanor possession charge under subsection (d) may be placed on probation, for up to one year, without an adjudication of guilt. Upon successful completion of the probationary terms, the case is dismissed, and records of the matter can be expunged under subsection (e)(2) as if the case never happened.

Other provisions escalate punishments when there are aggravating factors. Second or subsequent offenders face stiffer treatment under D.C. Code § 48-904.08. Under D.C. Code § 48-904.06, the potential imprisonment for selling steroids to minors is escalated to up to twice that otherwise authorized. Punishments are also escalated for those who enlist minors to distribute steroids under D.C. Code § 48-904.07, or who distribute steroids within 1,000 feet of a day care center, school, public library, public swimming pool, playground, video arcade, youth center, or public housing (so-called "drug free zones") under D.C. Code § 48-904.07a.

Drug Court may be an option for both misdemeanor possession cases as well as felony sale cases, resulting in dismissal upon successful completion. Diversion options are generally not provided in drug cases.

Currently there is no mandatory driver's license suspension for drug crimes.

FLORIDA

Florida addresses anabolic steroids under Florida Statutes Title XLVI, Crimes; Chapter 893, Drug Abuse Prevention and Control. Anabolic steroids are defined and classified as Schedule III controlled substances pursuant to the schedules and standards section, Fla. Stat. § 893.03(3): Schedule III:

> (d) Anabolic steroids.
>
> 1. The term "anabolic steroid" means any drug or hormonal substance, chemically and pharmacologically related to testosterone, other than estrogens, progestins, and corticosteroids, that promotes muscle growth and includes: a. Androsterone. b. Androsterone acetate. c. Boldenone. d. Boldenone acetate. e. Boldenone benzoate. f. Boldenone undecylenate. g. Chlorotestosterone (4-chlortestosterone). h. Clostebol. i. Dehydrochlormethyltestosterone. j. Dihydrotestosterone (4-dihydrotestosterone). k. Drostanolone. l. Ethylestrenol. m. Fluoxymesterone. n. Formebulone (formebolone). o. Mesterolone. p. Methandienone. q. Methandranone. r. Methandriol. s. Methandrostenolone. t. Methenolone. u. Methyltestosterone. v. Mibolerone. w. Nandrolone. x. Norethandrolone. y. Nortestosterone. z. Nortestosterone decanoate. aa. Nortestosterone phenylpropionate. bb. Nortestosterone propionate. cc. Oxandrolone. dd. Oxymesterone. ee. Oxymetholone. ff. Stanolone. gg. Stanozolol. hh. Testolactone. ii. Testosterone. jj. Testosterone acetate. kk. Testosterone benzoate. ll. Testosterone cypionate. mm.Testosterone decanoate. nn. Testosterone enanthate. oo. Testosterone isocaproate. pp. Testosterone oleate. qq. Testosterone phenylpropionate. rr. Testosterone propionate. ss. Testosterone undecanoate. tt.Trenbolone. vv. Any salt, ester, or isomer of a drug or substance described or listed in this subparagraph if that salt, ester, or isomer promotes muscle growth.
> 2. The term does not include an anabolic steroid that is expressly intended for administration through implants to cattle or other nonhuman species and that has been approved by the United States Secretary of Health and Human Services for such administration. However, any person who prescribes, dispenses, or distributes such a steroid for human use is considered to have prescribed, dispensed, or distributed an anabolic steroid within the meaning of this paragraph.

The statute also specifically exempts the cattle implants listed under 21 C.F.R. § 1308.34. As can be seen, Florida's list of anabolic steroids is more extensive than the federal definition, and actually recites a number of boldenone and testosterone esters (as well as the typical redundancies).

Penalties for the basic anabolic steroid offenses are all set forth under Fla. Stat. § 893.13, Prohibited acts; penalties. **Simple unlawful possession is considered a third degree felony** under subsection (6):

> (6) (a) It is unlawful for any person to be in actual or constructive possession of a controlled substance unless such controlled substance was lawfully obtained from a practitioner or pursuant to a valid prescription or order of a practitioner while acting in the course of his or her professional practice or to be in actual or constructive possession of a controlled substance except as otherwise authorized by this chapter. Any person who violates this provision commits a felony of the third degree....

Under subsection (2)(a)(2), **unlawfully purchasing an anabolic steroid, or possessing it "with intent to purchase" (an odd factual anomaly), is also a felony in the third degree.** So is bringing a Schedule III drug into the state unlawfully, under subsection (5)(b).

Distributing steroids or possessing them with the intent to distribute is also a felony in the third degree under subsection (1)(a) of Fla. Stat. § 893.13:

> (1)(a) Except as authorized ..., it is unlawful for any person to sell, manufacture, or deliver, or possess with intent to sell, manufacture, or deliver, a controlled substance. Any person who violates this provision with respect to...:
>
> 2. A controlled substance [in Schedule III] commits a felony of the third degree....

Under § 893.13(1), various aggravating circumstances escalate selling anabolic steroids or possessing them with intent to sell from a felony in the third degree to a felony in the second degree. They include doing so within 1,000 feet of a school or child care facility (under subparagraph (c)(2)), within 200 feet of a college, university or public park (under subparagraph (d)(2)), within 1,000 feet of a church or convenience business (under subparagraph (e)(2)), and within 200 feet of a public housing facility (subparagraph (f)(2)). Delivering to a minor or using or hiring a minor to deliver Schedule III drugs is a felony in the second degree under Fla. Stat. § 893.13(4)(b), and the offender is ineligible for probation or a suspended or deferred sentence.

Felony charges are punishable by imprisonment under Fla. Stat. § 775.082:

> (3) A person who has been convicted ... may be punished as follows...:
> (c) For a felony of the second degree, by a term of imprisonment not exceeding 15 years.
> (d) For a felony of the third degree, by a term of imprisonment not exceeding 5 years.

Fines are set forth under Fla. Stat. § 775.083(1), and permit imposition of up to $10,000 on felonies in the second degree and up to $5,000 on felonies in the third degree.

Enhanced sentencing applies to "habitual felony offenders" under Fla. Stat. § 775.084. Offenders with prior state or federal drug sale or trafficking convictions are also subject to additional penalties pursuant to Fla. Stat. § 775.16.

When we look at the practical application of these laws, there are a number of plea bargains available. For a simple possession case, a first time offender may make an application for drug court. Some counties that have a drug court will require that the defendant have no prior convictions. As is the case in most every state that offers a drug court, the program allows for dismissal of the charges contingent upon successful completion and satisfaction of the requirements. Alternatively, distribution or sale cases are not eligible for drug court and are likely to receive a much stiffer penalty.

If there is adjudication on the merits leading to a conviction, a drivers' license can be revoked for two years.

GEORGIA

Anabolic steroids are dealt with under the Georgia Code, Title 16, Crimes and Offenses; Chapter 13, Controlled Substances. O.C.G.A. § 16-13-27 states:

> Schedule III:
> ...(6)Any anabolic steroid or any salt, ester, or isomer of a drug or substance described or listed in this paragraph, if that salt, ester, or isomer promotes muscle growth. Such term does not include an anabolic steroid which is expressly intended for administration through implants to cattle or other nonhuman species and which has been approved by the secretary of health and human services for such administration: (A) Boldenone; (B) Chlorotestosterone; (C) Clostebol; (D) Dehydrochlormethyltestosterone; (E) Dihydrotestosterone; (F) Drostanolone; (G) Ethylestrenol; (H) Fluoxymesterone; (I) Formebolone; (J) Mesterolone; (K) Methandienone; (L) Methandranone; (M) Methandriol; (N) Methandrostenolone; (O) Methenolone; (P) Methyltestosterone; (Q) Mibolerone; (R) Nandrolone; (S) Norethandrolone; (T) Oxandrolone; (U) Oxymesterone; (V) Oxymetholone; (W) Stanolone; (X) Stanozolol; (Y) Testolactone; (Z) Testosterone; (AA) Trenbolone.

Georgia also lists anabolic steroids that are exempt from federal Schedule III by DEA by name of the steroid and its manufacturer under O.C.G.A. § 16-13-27.1:

> The following anabolic steroid containing compounds, mixtures, or preparations have been exempted as Schedule III Controlled Substances by the United States Drug Enforcement Administration, as listed in 21 C.F.R. 1308.34, and are therefore exempted from paragraph (6) of Code Section 16-13-27... [the list contains a variety of combination androgen/estrogen products].

All steroid crimes are under one section. **First offense for unlawful possession or purchase is a felony, with one to five years in prison. Trafficking crimes are punishable with one to ten years in prison**. Under O.C.G.A. § 16-13-30:

(a) Except as authorized by this article, it is unlawful for any person to purchase, possess, or have under his control any controlled substance.
(b) Except as authorized by this article, it is unlawful for any person to manufacture, deliver, distribute, dispense, administer, sell, or possess with intent to distribute any controlled substance.
...(g) Any person who violates subsection (a) of this Code section with respect to a controlled substance in Schedule III ... shall be guilty of a felony and, upon conviction thereof, shall be punished by imprisonment for not less than one year nor more than five years. Upon conviction of a second or subsequent offense, he shall be imprisoned for not less than one year nor more than ten years.
(h) Any person who violates subsection (b) of this Code section with respect to a controlled substance in Schedule III ... shall be guilty of a felony and, upon conviction thereof, shall be punished by imprisonment for not less than one year nor more than ten years.

Subsection (k) makes it a felony, with escalated punishments, to hire, solicit, engage or use an individual under the age of 17 years to manufacture, distribute or dispense controlled substances. A person who manufactures, distributes, dispenses, or possesses with intent to distribute a controlled substance within 1,000 feet of a school (O.C.G.A. § 16-13-32.4), within 1,000 feet of a park, playground, recreation center or public housing project (O.C.G.A. § 16-13-32.5), or in a designated "drug-free commercial zone" (O.C.G.A. § 16-13-32.6) faces significantly enhanced sentencing.

The simple possession case in Georgia, for the first time offender, will most likely result in straight probation with no jail time. Probation will likely be for a period of approximately one year and will require drug counseling and random drug testing as conditions of probation. For repeat offenders, boot camp programs vary by county, with some setting age limits as low as age 25. The boot camp may be at a local jail and the type of program would be up to the discretion of the sheriff. Some programs may have the defendant working on a GED if he does not have a high school diploma. The boot camp will last from 90 to 120 days, with the balance of the time being done on probation. If probation is satisfactorily completed and the defendant is a first time offender, the file will indicate merely a "first offender" conviction. Mere possession alone will not result in a mandatory suspension of motor vehicle driving privileges.

The case of a drug sale is a different story, and will depend upon the county. However, for the most part, according to one Georgia criminal defense practitioner, "if you do the sale, you go to jail." While it will depend upon the county; the district attorney will probably seek jail time in all sale cases. Most often, the undercover police will make several controlled buys from the defendant, up to as many as five to six, thereby solidifying the state's case. However, depending upon the circumstances, the judge may grant a first offender conviction status in a drug sale case.

HAWAII

Chapter 329 of the Hawaii Revised Statutes is the Uniform Controlled Substances Act, defining and classifying anabolic steroids. HRS § 329-18:

(a) The controlled substances listed in this section are included in schedule III.
...(g) Any anabolic steroid. The term "anabolic steroid" means any drug or hormonal substance chemically and pharmacologically related to testosterone (other than estrogens, progestins, and corticosteroids) that promotes muscle growth, and includes: (1) Boldenone; (2) Clostebol (4-Chlorotestosterone); (3) Dehydrochlormethyltestosterone; (4) Dihydrotestosterone (4-dihydrotestosterone); (5) Drostanolone; (6) Ethylestrenol; (7) Fluoxymesterone; (8) Formebolone (Formyldienolone); (9) Mesterolone; (10) Methandranone; (11) Methandriol; (12) Methandrostenolone (Methandienone); (13) Methenolone; (14) Methyltestosterone; (15) Mibolerone; (16) Nandrolone; (17) Norethandrolone; (18) Oxandrolone; (19) Oxymesterone; (20) Oxymetholone; (21) Stanolone (Dihydrotestoster-

> one); (22) Stanozolol; (23) Testolactone; (24) Testosterone; (25) Trenbolone; and (26) Any salt, ester, or isomer of a drug or substance described or listed in this subsection, if that salt, ester, or isomer promotes muscle growth, except the term "anabolic steroid" does not include an anabolic steroid which is expressly intended for administration through implants to cattle or other nonhuman species and which has been approved by the Secretary of Health and Human Services for nonhuman administration. If any person prescribes, dispenses, or distributes an anabolic steroid intended for administration to nonhuman species for human use, the person shall be considered to have prescribed, dispensed, or distributed an anabolic steroid within the meaning of this paragraph.

Hawaii seems to have consulted with qualified chemists prior to drafting its laws. Unlike the statutes passed by our Congress and most state lawmakers, the Hawaii legislature acknowledges that methandrostenolone and methandienone, and stanolone and dihydrotestosterone (a.k.a. DHT), are the same. Even so, they still couldn't avoid the mistake of listing DHT twice – as (4) and (21), or in referring to a mysterious AAS "salt."

Drug offenses are covered under Hawaii Revised Statutes Chapter 712, Offenses Against Public Health and Morals, Part IV, Offenses Related to Drugs and Intoxicating Compounds. The definitions section, under HRS § 712-1240, distinguishes "dangerous drugs" (Schedule I or II), "detrimental drugs" (Schedule V) and "harmful drugs (Schedule III, such as anabolic steroids, and Schedule IV).

Hawaii has a hierarchy of drug offenses, primarily focusing on the "promoting" of drugs. Starting at the most serious level, we have the crime of promoting a harmful drug in the first degree, under HRS § 712-1244:

> (1) A person commits the offense of promoting a harmful drug in the first degree if the person knowingly:
> (a) **Possesses one hundred or more capsules or tablets or dosage units** containing one or more of the harmful drugs ...or
> (b) **Possesses one or more preparations, compounds, mixtures, or substances, of an aggregate weight of one ounce** or more containing one or more of the harmful drugs ... or
> (c) **Distributes twenty-five or more capsules or tablets or dosage units** containing one or more of the harmful drugs ... or
> (d) **Distributes one or more preparations, compounds, mixtures, or substances, of an aggregate weight of one-eighth ounce or more**, containing one or more of the harmful drugs ... or
> (e) **Distributes any harmful drug ... in any amount to a minor**.
> (2) Promoting a harmful drug in the first degree **is a class A felony**.

Next comes promoting a harmful drug in the second degree, under HRS § 712-1245:

> (1) A person commits the offense of promoting a harmful drug in the second degree if the person knowingly:
> (a) **Possesses fifty or more capsules or tablets or dosage units** containing one or more of the harmful drugs ... or
> (b) **Possesses one or more preparations, compounds, mixtures, or substances, of an aggregate weight of one-eighth ounce or more**, containing one or more of the harmful drugs ... or
> (c) **Distributes** any harmful drug ... in any amount.
> (2) Promoting a harmful drug in the second degree **is a class B felony**.

Then we have promoting a harmful drug in the third degree, under HRS § 712-1246:

> (1) A person commits the offense of **promoting a harmful drug in the third degree if the person knowingly possesses twenty-five or more capsules or tablets or dosage units containing one or more of the harmful drugs....**
> (2) Promoting a harmful drug in the third degree **is a class C felony**.

Least serious is the misdemeanor of promoting a harmful drug in the fourth degree, under HRS § 712-1246.5:

(1) A person commits the offense of **promoting a harmful drug in the fourth degree if the person knowingly possesses any harmful drug in any amount**.
(2) Promoting a harmful drug in the fourth degree **is a misdemeanor.**

The maximum sentence for a misdemeanor is a definite sentence of one year under HRS § 706-663.

Regarding drug felonies, under HRS § 706-610 there are three classes. A person convicted of a class A drug felony must get the maximum twenty-year sentence under HRS § 706-659. Under HRS § 706-660, a person convicted of a class B felony must get the maximum ten years, and a person convicted of a class C felony must get the maximum five years. In all cases, the minimum length of imprisonment is determined by the paroling authority in accordance with HRS § 706-669.

Offenders may be eligible for alternative programs in lieu of incarceration (.i.e., drug court programs, house arrest, electronic monitoring, etc.) under HRS § 706-605.1. A separate section, HRS § 706-605.5, authorizes courts to order offenders to complete a rigorous offender program based on "regimental discipline." Under HRS § 706-605(3), the court may sentence a person convicted of a misdemeanor to a suspended sentence. A provision also exists for "conditional discharge" under HRS § 712-1255, wherein the court may, without entering a judgment of guilt, defer further proceedings and place many first offenders on probation. Upon fulfillment of the probationary terms and conditions, the court discharges the person and dismisses the proceedings. Under HRS § 712-1256, the court records may then be expunged, but only if the offender was not over twenty years of age.

Aggravating factors can escalate the severity of the charges. Distributing or possessing with the intent to distribute any controlled substance on or within 750 feet of school property or on or near a school bus is a class C felony under HRS § 712-1249.6. Certain offenders face escalated sentencing under HRS § 706-606.5 as repeat offenders, or pursuant to HRS § 706-661 and § 706-662 as "persistent," "dangerous" or "professional" criminals.

Hawaii's controlled substance **laws are based on quantity rather than intent, so there is no "possession with intent" offense.** Consequently, the charges in a personal use possession case can vary disturbingly. Many steroid users, for example, will purchase a tub of a thousand methandrostenolone tablets for personal use, often consuming five to ten of these 5 mg tablets each day. A person caught with a hundred of these tablets in his gym bag faces a class A felony with a twenty-year maximum, but a person with twenty-four tablets faces a misdemeanor with a maximum of only a year!

Under HRS § 853-1, a defendant may receive a Deferred Acceptance of a guilty plea. This requires a nolo contendre (no contest) or guilty plea and results in discharge, dismissal and expungement of the record. With a deferred acceptance the case does not appear in drug court and does not require that the defendant participate in the drug court program, which is quite stringent. The drug court program requires that the defendant report before the judge on a weekly basis, among other things. As such, the drug court program has a high success rate.

There is no mandatory suspension of driving privileges for drug offenses.

IDAHO

The Idaho Statutes schedule drugs and substances under Title 37 of the General Laws, which represents the Food, Drugs, and Oil section. The Uniform Controlled Substances Act is Chapter 27 of Title 37. Idaho classifies anabolic steroids as Schedule III substances, similar to the federal law, except that Idaho has snuck "human growth hormones" into the mix. Although clearly not belonging here from a chemical perspective, Idaho has done what Congress chose not to do: make human growth hormone a controlled substance. Schedule III of Idaho Code §37-2709 includes:

f) Anabolic steroids and human growth hormones. Any drug or hormonal substance, chemically and pharmacologically related to testosterone (other than estrogens, progestins and corticosteroids) that promotes muscle growth including any salt, ester or isomer of a drug or substance listed in this paragraph, if that salt, ester or isomer promotes muscle growth. (1) Boldenone; (2) Chlorotestosterone (4-chlortestosterone); (3) Chorionic gonadotropin; (4) Clostebol; (5) Dehydrochlormethyltestosterone; (6) Dihydrotestosterone (4-dihydrotestosterone); (7) Drostanolone; (8) Ethylestrenol; (9) Fluoxymesterone; (10) Formebulone; (11) Human growth hormones; (12) Mesterolone; (13) Methandienone; (14) Methandranone; (15) Methandriol; (16) Methandrostenolone; (17) Methenolone; (18) Methyltestosterone; (19) Mibolerone; (20) Nandrolone; (21) Norethandrolone; (22) Oxandrolone; (23) Oxymesterone; (24) Oxymetholone; (25) Stanolone; (26) Stanozolol; (27) Testolactone; (28) Testosterone; (29) Testosterone cypionate; (30) Testosterone enanthate; (31) Testosterone propionate; (32) Trenbolone.

The section goes on to exempt bovine implants:

> Anabolic steroids that are expressly intended for administration through implants to cattle or other nonhuman species, and that are approved by the federal Food and Drug Administration for such use, shall not be classified as controlled substances under this act and shall not be governed by its provisions.

Further, the section specifically criminalizes (as a felony) conduct that promotes anabolic steroids or growth hormone for muscle building:

> In addition to the penalties prescribed in article IV of the Uniform Controlled Substances Act, any person shall be guilty of a felony who prescribes, dispenses, supplies, sells, delivers, manufactures or possesses with the intent to prescribe, dispense, supply, sell, deliver or manufacture **anabolic steroids or any other human growth hormone for purposes of enhancing performance in an exercise, sport or game or hormonal manipulation intended to increase muscle mass**, strength or weight without a medical necessity as determined by a physician.

Idaho's Uniform Controlled Substances Act provides for penalties related to the possession of anabolic steroids in the state. The prohibited acts are set forth in Idaho Code § 37-2732, Prohibited acts A - Penalties. **Possession of steroids or growth hormone, without a prescription, is punishable as a misdemeanor:**

c) It is unlawful for any person to possess a controlled substance unless the substance was obtained directly from, or pursuant to, a valid prescription or order of a practitioner while acting in the course of his professional practice, or except as otherwise authorized by this chapter.
...(3) Any person who violates this subsection and has in his possession a controlled substance which is a [schedule III controlled substance] is guilty of a misdemeanor and upon conviction thereof may be imprisoned for not more than one (1) year, or fined not more than one thousand dollars ($1,000), or both.

Note too that Idaho makes presence at a drug location a misdemeanor. Idaho Code § 37-2732:

(d) It shall be unlawful for any person to be present at or on premises of any place where he knows illegal controlled substances are being manufactured or cultivated, or are being held for distribution, transportation, delivery, administration, use, or to be given away. A violation of this section shall deem those persons guilty of a misdemeanor and upon conviction shall be punished by a fine of not more than three hundred dollars ($300) and not more than ninety (90) days in the county jail, or both.

Subsection (a) of § 37-2732 covers **delivery and possession with intent of steroids or growth hormone, which may be punished by up to five years in prison**:

> (a) Except as authorized by this chapter, it is unlawful for any person to manufacture or deliver, or possess with intent to manufacture or deliver, a controlled substance.
> (1) Any person who violates this subsection with respect to:
> ...(B) [a schedule III substance] is guilty of a felony and upon conviction may be imprisoned for not more than five (5) years, fined not more than fifteen thousand dollars ($15,000), or both;

Under § 37-2737, distribution to persons under age 18 calls for enhanced punishments. Other aggravating factors are set forth in § 37-2739A (mandatory minimum penalties) and § 37-2739B (fixed minimum sentences in drug cases).

If you have been found guilty of possession, manufacture or delivery of a Schedule III controlled substance, including steroids or growth hormone, then under Idaho Code §37-2738 you must attend a substance abuse evaluation directed by the state. Failure to make good faith efforts to comply with this provision are aggravating factors for sentence. Note that while a "withheld judgment" is an available option for many first-time offenders, there are strings attached. Under § 37-2738, the accused must have "satisfactorily cooperated with law enforcement authorities in the prosecution of drug related crimes of which the defendant has previously had involvement" and must complete a period of not less than one hundred (100) hours of community service work.

Idaho provides for wide discretion to suspend sentences and withhold judgments, placing the accused on probation, under Idaho Code § 19-2601. Idaho has also set up a Drug Court Act, authorized by Title 19, Criminal Procedure, Chapter 56.

There is no mandatory driver's license suspension for conviction of drug crimes.

ILLINOIS

In the Illinois Complied Statutes, anabolic steroids are dealt with in Chapter 720, Criminal Offenses; 570, Illinois Controlled Substances Act. Anabolic steroids are defined under § 720 ILCS 570/102:

> (c-1)"Anabolic Steroids" means any drug or hormonal substance, chemically and pharmacologically related to testosterone (other than estrogens, progestins, and corticosteroids) that promotes muscle growth, and includes: (i) boldenone, (ii) chlorotestosterone, (iii) chostebol, (iv) dehydrochlormethyltestosterone, (v) dihydrotestosterone, (vi) drostanolone, (vii) ethylestrenol, (viii) fluoxymesterone, (ix) formebulone, (x) mesterolone, (xi) methandienone, (xii) methandranone, (xiii) methandriol, (xiv) methandrostenolone, (xv) methenolone, (xvi) methyltestosterone, (xvii) mibolerone, (xviii) nandrolone, (xix) norethandrolone, (xx) oxandrolone, (xxi) oxymesterone, (xxii) oxymetholone, (xxiii) stanolone, (xxiv) stanozolol, (xxv) testolactone, (xxvi) testosterone, (xxvii) trenbolone, and (xxviii) any salt, ester, or isomer of a drug or substance described or listed in this paragraph, if that salt, ester, or isomer promotes muscle growth. Any person who is otherwise lawfully in possession of an anabolic steroid, or who otherwise lawfully manufactures, distributes, dispenses, delivers, or possesses with intent to deliver an anabolic steroid, which anabolic steroid is expressly intended for and lawfully allowed to be administered through implants to livestock or other nonhuman species, and which is approved by the Secretary of Health and Human Services for such administration, and which the person intends to administer or have administered through such implants, shall not be considered to be in unauthorized possession or to unlawfully manufacture, distribute, dispense, deliver, or possess with intent to deliver such anabolic steroid for purposes of this Act.

> (kk)"Practitioner" means a physician licensed to practice medicine in all its branches, dentist, podiatrist, veterinarian, scientific investigator, pharmacist, physician assistant, advanced practice nurse,

licensed practical nurse, registered nurse, hospital, laboratory, or pharmacy, or other person licensed, registered, or otherwise lawfully permitted by the United States or this State to distribute, dispense, conduct research with respect to, administer or use in teaching or chemical analysis, a controlled substance in the course of professional practice or research.

[The above subsection seems to say that practitioner is defined differently than in other states]

A separate section, § 720 ILCS 570/208, classifies steroids under Schedule III, with certain exemptions for mixed androgen/estrogen preparations:

> (a) The controlled substances listed in this Section are included in Schedule III.
> ...(f) Anabolic steroids, except the following anabolic steroids that are exempt: (1) Androgyn L.A.; (2) Andro-Estro 90-4; (3) depANDROGYN; (4) DEPO-T.E.; (5) depTESTROGEN; (6) Duomone; (7) DURATESTRIN; (8) DUO-SPAN II; (9) Estratest; (10) Estratest H.S.; (11) PAN ESTRA TEST; (12) Premarin with Methyltestosterone; (13) TEST-ESTRO Cypionates; (14) Testosterone Cyp 50 Estradiol Cyp 2; (15) Testosterone Cypionate-Estradiol Cypionate injection; and (16) Testosterone Enanthate-Estradiol Valerate injection.

A further exemption is set forth in § 720 ILCS 570/214:

> Excluded Substances.
> (a) Products containing an anabolic steroid, that are expressly intended for administration through implants to cattle or other nonhuman species and that have been approved by the Secretary of Health and Human Services for that administration, and that are excluded from all schedules under [the federal CSA] are also excluded from ... this Act.

And another exemption is in § 720 ILCS 570/217:

> Exempt anabolic steroid products.
> Compounds, mixtures, or preparations that contain an anabolic steroid that have been exempted by the Administrator of the federal Drug Enforcement Administration from application ... of the federal Controlled Substances Act are also exempt from ... this Act.

Unless otherwise set forth, Illinois has a catch-all provision that makes simple unlawful possession of any amount of a controlled substance a Class 4 felony, with a fine of up to $25,000. However, Illinois has carved out a special subsection just for anabolic steroids. **Steroids are the only drugs in the state that are punishable only as a (Class B) misdemeanor for simple possession. Even subsequent violations are only misdemeanors.** Simple unlawful possession of steroids is covered by § 720 ILCS 570/402:

> Except as otherwise authorized by this Act, it is unlawful for any person knowingly to possess a controlled or counterfeit substance. A violation of this Act with respect to each of the controlled substances listed herein constitutes a single and separate violation of this Act.
> ...(d) Any person who violates this Section with regard to any amount of anabolic steroid is guilty of a Class C misdemeanor for the first offense and a Class B misdemeanor for a subsequent offense committed within 2 years of a prior conviction.

Simple possession cases are eligible for § 720 ILCS 570/410 probation, under which a defendant pleads guilty or is found guilty of possession of a controlled substance and the court, without entering a judgment, may sentence him to probation. Upon successful completion, the defendant may receive dismissal but upon violation of a condition of probation, the original judgment may be entered against him. Two years later, the defendant may petition for the case to be expunged.

Making, delivering, or possessing with intent is covered under § 720 ILCS 570/401:

Except as authorized by this Act, it is unlawful for any person knowingly to: (i)manufacture or deliver, orpossess with intent to manufacture or deliver [a controlled substance]...

...(f) Any person who violates this Section with regard to any other amount of a controlled or counterfeit substance classified in Schedule III **is guilty of a Class 3 felony**. The fine for violation of this subsection (f) shall not be more than $125,000.

Note too that **practitioners in Illinois are specifically prevented from administering steroids for "improving physical appearance"** under § 720 ILCS 570/312, Requirements for dispensing controlled substances:

...(j) No person shall manufacture, dispense, deliver, possess with intent to deliver, prescribe, or administer or cause to be administered under his direction any anabolic steroid, for any use in humans other than the treatment of disease in accordance with the order of a physician licensed to practice medicine in all its branches for a valid medical purpose in the course of professional practice. The use of anabolic steroids for the purpose of hormonal manipulation that is intended to increase muscle mass, strength or weight without a medical necessity to do so, or for the intended purpose of improving physical appearance or performance in any form of exercise, sport, or game, is not a valid medical purpose or in the course of professional practice.

Illinois also criminalizes the non-medical distribution of human growth hormone in § 410 ILCS 620/3.22, Illinois Food, Drug and Cosmetic Act, Chapter 410, Public Health:

> Whoever knowingly distributes, or possesses with intent to distribute, human growth hormone for any use in humans other than the treatment of a disease or other recognized medical condition, where the use has been authorized by the Secretary of Health and Human Services and under the order of a physician, is guilty of a Class 3 felony, and may be fined an amount not to exceed $50,000. Whoever commits any offense set forth in this Section and the offense involves an individual under 18 years of age is punishable by not more than 10 years imprisonment, and twice the fine authorized above. Any conviction for a violation of this Section shall be considered a violation of the Illinois Controlled Substances Act for the purposes of forfeiture.... As used in this Section the term "human growth hormone" means somatrem, somatropin, or an analogue of either of them. The Department of State Police and Department of Professional Regulation are authorized to investigate offenses punishable by this Section.

Criminal sentencing in Illinois is covered by Chapter 730, Corrections. The classifications of offenses are set forth under § 730 ILCS 5/5-5-1. For misdemeanors, § 730 ILCS 5/5-8-3(a) sets forth the applicable determinate terms:

(1) for a Class A misdemeanor, for any term less than one year;
(2) for a **Class B misdemeanor, for not more than 6 months**;
(3) for a Class C misdemeanor, for not more than 30 days.

Sentences of imprisonment for felonies are covered by § 730 ILCS 5/5-8-1:

(a) Except as otherwise provided in the statute defining the offense, a sentence of imprisonment for a felony shall be a determinate sentence set by the court under this Section, according to the following limitations:
...(6) for a **Class 3 felony, the sentence shall be not less than 2 years and not more than 5 years**;
(7) for a Class 4 felony, the sentence shall be not less than 1 year and not more than 3 years.

Enhanced sentencing for aggravating factors can bump up the sentencing to a more "extended term" under § 730 ILCS 5/5-8-2 (for a Class 3 felony, not less than 5 years and not more than 10 years, and for a Class 4 felony, not less than 3 years and not more than 6 years).

Illinois has a Drug Court Treatment Act, § 730 ILCS 166, in its Chapter 730, Corrections.

Now, here's something really interesting. Illinois has a statute, § 720 ILCS 570/411, setting forth the conduct in drug offenses warranting the most severe punishments. While any of these could apply in a steroid case, take particular note of subsection (8):

> In determining the appropriate sentence for any conviction under this Act, the sentencing court may consider the following as indicative of the type of offenses which the legislature deems most damaging to the peace and welfare of the citizens of Illinois and which warrants the most severe penalties:
> ...(2) offenses involving unusually large quantities of controlled substances, as measured by their wholesale value at the time of the offense;
> (3) the unlawful delivery of controlled substances by a non-user to a user of controlled substances;
> (4) non-possessory offenses by persons who have no other visible means of support;
> (5) offenses involving the large-scale manufacture of controlled substances;
> (6) offenses which indicate any immediate involvement whatsoever with organized crime in terms of the controlled substance's manufacture, importation, or volume distribution;
> (7) the manufacture for, or the delivery of controlled substances to persons 3 years or more junior to the person(s) convicted under this Act;
> (8) **the unlawful delivery of anabolic steroids by an athletic trainer, coach, or health club personnel.**

Illinois has statutory provisions for "steroid abuse education." These include:

> § 105 ILCS 5/27-23.3 (2001):
> Education in steroid abuse prevention. School districts shall provide instruction in relation to the prevention of abuse of anabolic steroids in grades 7 through 12 and shall include such instruction in science, health, drug abuse, physical education or other appropriate courses of study. Such instruction shall emphasize that the use of anabolic steroids presents a serious health hazard to persons who use steroids to enhance athletic performance or physical development. The State Board of Education may assist in the development of instructional materials and teacher training in relation to steroid abuse prevention.

> § 20 ILCS 301/20-15 (2001):
> Steroid education program. The Department may develop and implement a statewide steroid education program to alert the public, and particularly Illinois physicians, other health care professionals, educators, student athletes, health club personnel, persons engaged in the coaching and supervision of high school and college athletics, and other groups determined by the Department to be likely to come into contact with anabolic steroid abusers to the dangers and adverse effects of abusing anabolic steroids, and to train these individuals to recognize the symptoms and side effects of anabolic steroid abuse. Such education and training may also include information regarding the education and appropriate referral of persons identified as probable or actual anabolic steroid abusers. The advice of the Illinois Advisory Council ... shall be sought in the development of any program established under this Section.

There's no mandatory driver's license revocation for conviction of drug crimes in Illinois.

INDIANA

The Indiana Code explicitly deals with anabolic steroids under two distinct Titles. It deals with them as "controlled substances" under Title 35, Criminal Law and Procedure; Article 48, Controlled Substances. It also deals with them as "legend drugs" under Title 16, Health; Article 42, Regulation of Food, Drugs and Cosmetics; Chapter 19, Drugs: Indiana Legend Drug Act. Curiously, the definitions are not identical.

Let's first look at the more typical concept of anabolics as controlled substances. They are defined as controlled substances under the section that classifies Schedule III drugs, Ind. Code § 35-48-2-8:

> (a) The controlled substances listed in this section are included in schedule III.
> ...(f) Anabolic steroid (as defined in 21 U.S.C. 802(41)(A) and 21 U.S.C. 802(41)(B)).

Simple unlawful possession of Schedule III controlled substances is a Class D felony under Ind. Code § 35-48-4-7(a):

> A person who, without a valid prescription or order of a practitioner acting in the course of his professional practice, knowingly or intentionally possesses a controlled substance (pure or adulterated) classified in schedule [III], except marijuana or hashish, commits possession of a controlled substance, a Class D felony. However, the offense is a Class C felony if the person in possession of the controlled substance possesses the controlled substance:
> (1) on a school bus; or
> (2) in, on, or within one thousand (1,000) feet of:
> (A) school property;
> (B) a public park;
> (C) a family housing complex; or
> (D) a youth program center.

Distribution of Schedule III controlled substances is a Class B felony covered by Ind. Code § 35-48-4-2:

> (a) A person who:
> (1) knowingly or intentionally:
> (A) manufactures;
> (B) finances the manufacture of;
> (C) delivers; or
> (D) finances the delivery of; a [Schedule III] controlled substance ... or
> (2) possesses, with intent to:
> (A) manufacture;
> (B) finance the manufacture of;
> (C) deliver; or
> (D) finance the delivery of; a [Schedule III] controlled substance ... commits ... a Class B felony, except as provided in subsection (b).
> (b) The offense is a Class A felony if:
> (1) the person:
> (A) delivered; or
> (B) financed the delivery of; the substance to a person under eighteen (18) years of age at least three (3) years junior to the person; or
> (2) the person delivered or financed the delivery of the substance:
> (A) on a school bus; or
> (B) in, on, or within one thousand (1,000) feet of:
> (i) school property;
> (ii) a public park;
> (iii) a family housing complex; or
> (iv) a youth program center.

Interestingly, selling hashish is treated *much* more leniently than selling steroids (see Ind. Code § 35-48-4-10)!

Now let's look at anabolic steroids under the Indiana Legend Drug Act, which primarily focuses on the conduct of medical practitioners in the context of the physician-patient relationship. The applicable definitions are in a different article of Title 16: Article 18, General Provisions and Definitions; Chapter 2, Definitions. There, anabolic steroids are defined under Ind. Code § 16-18-2-15:

> "Anabolic steroid" [for purposes of the Indiana Legend Drug Act], means a material, compound, mixture, or preparation that contains an anabolic steroid that includes any of the following: Chorionic gonadotropin; Clostebol; Dehydrochlormethyltestosterone; Ethylestrenol; Fluoxymesterone; Mesterolone; Metenolone; Methandienone; Methandro stenolone; Methyltestosterone; Nandrolone decanoate; Nandrolone phenpropionate; Norethandrolone; Oxandrolone; Oxymesterone; Oxymetholone; Stanozolol; Testosterone propionate; Testosterone-like related compounds.

Note that this definition differs from the federal definition adopted by the Indiana article on controlled substances. For some reason, the Indiana Legend Drug Act definition explicitly lists testosterone propionate as an anabolic steroid, but fails to mention several equally popular esters including cypionate and enanthate. It misspells methenolone, and makes methandrostenolone two words. The term "testosterone-like related compounds" is unnecessarily broad enough to include many compounds, including products available in health food stores, which do not promote muscle growth. **Note also that Indiana includes human "chorionic gonadotropin" as an anabolic steroid for application of its Legend Drug Act, but not for application of its Controlled Substances Act.**

Under the Indiana Legend Drugs Act, simple unlawful possession is covered under Ind. Code § 16-42-19-19:

> Except as provided ..., a person may not possess or use an anabolic steroid without a valid prescription or drug order issued by a practitioner acting in the usual course of the practitioner's professional practice.

Under the Legend Drugs Act, situations of unlawful distribution or possession with intent are set out under Ind. Code § 16-42-19-25. That **section forbids practitioners to be involved with steroids to build muscle** in subsection (a), and addresses everyone else in subsection (b):

> (a) A practitioner may not prescribe, order, distribute, supply, or sell an anabolic steroid for any of the following:
> (1) Enhancing performance in an exercise, sport, or game.
> (2) Hormonal manipulation intended to increase muscle mass, strength, or weight without a medical necessity.
> (b) Except as provided, ... a person who is not a practitioner or lawful manufacturer of anabolic steroids may not do any of the following:
> (1) Knowingly or intentionally manufacture or deliver an anabolic steroid, pure or adulterated.
> (2) Possess, with intent to manufacture or deliver, an anabolic steroid.

The applicable offense levels under the Legend Drug Act are set out in Ind. Code § 16-42-19-27. Under subsection (a), simple unlawful possession of anabolic steroids and non-medical administration of steroids by a practitioner are Class D felonies (the offense is a Class C felony if the person has a prior drug conviction). For non-practitioners dealing in steroids, the offense is more serious:

> (c) A person who violates section 25(b) [IC 16-42-19-25(b)] of this chapter commits dealing in an anabolic steroid, a Class C felony. However, the offense is a Class B felony if the person delivered the anabolic steroid to a person who is:

(1) Less than eighteen (18) years of age; and
(2) At least three (3) years younger than the delivering person.

There appears to be an offense level conflict between the Indiana Controlled Substances Act and the Legend Drug Act. Manufacturing or delivering anabolic steroids to an adult is prosecuted as a Class B felony under the Controlled Substances Act, but as a Class C felony under the Legend Drug Act.

The applicable penalties for steroid offenses are found in Title 35, Article 50, Sentences, and are as follows:

Ind. Code § 35-50-2-5:
A person who commits a **Class B felony shall be imprisoned for a fixed term of ten (10) years**, with not more than ten (10) years added for aggravating circumstances or not more than four (4) years subtracted for mitigating circumstances; in addition, he may be fined not more than ten thousand dollars ($10,000).

Ind. Code § 35-50-2-6:
(a) A person who commits a Class C felony shall be imprisoned for a fixed term of four (4) years, with not more than four (4) years added for aggravating circumstances or not more than two (2) years subtracted for mitigating circumstances. In addition, he may be fined not more than ten thousand dollars ($10,000).

Ind. Code § 35-50-2-7:
(a) A person who commits a **Class D felony shall be imprisoned for a fixed term of one and one-half (1½) years,** with not more than one and one-half (1½) years added for aggravating circumstances or not more than one (1) year subtracted for mitigating circumstances. In addition, he may be fined not more than ten thousand dollars ($10,000).
(b) Notwithstanding subsection (a), if a person has committed a Class D felony, the court may enter judgment of conviction of a Class A misdemeanor and sentence accordingly. However, the court shall enter a judgment of conviction of a Class D felony if:
 (1) the court finds that:
  (A) the person has committed a prior, unrelated felony for which judgment was entered as a conviction of a Class A misdemeanor; and
  (B) the prior felony was committed less than three (3) years before the second felony was committed....

Ind. Code § 35-50-3-2:
A person who commits a Class A misdemeanor shall be imprisoned for a fixed term of not more than one (1) year; in addition, he may be fined not more than five thousand dollars ($5,000).

Suspended sentences are authorized and regulated under Ind. Code § 35-50-2-2. Persons with prior felony convictions can be sentenced as "habitual offenders" under Ind. Code § 35-50-2-8.

While Indiana still imposes stiff penalties in both the Schedule III simple possession and drug sale cases, there has been some softening. In the larger counties, a simple possession case may be handled by a special drug court. Nonetheless, all drug possession cases are suspendable and a treatment program in lieu of jail is available if the defendant is accepted. If treatment is offered in lieu of prosecution, the case may ultimately be dismissed or the defendant may be placed on probation. The simple possession case carries with it a mandatory suspension of the privilege to drive. A traffic infraction need not even be involved for driving privileges to be suspended. In fact, the defendant need not even be in or near their motor vehicle; the defendant may be merely walking down the street.

Boot camp-type programs are available for juvenile offenders. Cases involving juveniles will be adjudicated in the juvenile division of the court unless such juvenile status is waived. In such case, the juvenile would be subject to the adult criminal justice system.

In the drug sale cases there has recently been a change in the law, which makes the penalties not as harsh. Whereas in the past there was mandatory jail time, the suspendability statute allows the court to suspend part of the sentence where there are no prior felonies and where the case does not come within one of the exclusions. Cases which come within the exclusion include a sale of Schedule III controlled substances with possession of a firearm, or sale to an individual under the age of 18. Suspendability allows for more discretion by the judge, depending upon the facts and circumstances of the case, and can result in a sentence of work release or home detention.

IOWA

Scheduling of anabolic steroids in Iowa is under the Iowa Code, Title IV, Public Health; Subtitle 1, Alcoholic Beverages and Controlled Substances. Chapter 124, Controlled Substances, defines anabolic steroids and classifies them as Schedule III controlled substances. Iowa Code § 124.208, Schedule III - substances included:

6. *Anabolic steroids.* Anabolic steroids, except any anabolic steroid which is expressly intended for administration through implants to cattle or other nonhuman species unless such steroid is prescribed, dispensed, or distributed for human use. Anabolic steroids include any salt, ester, or isomer of the following drugs or substances if that salt, ester, or isomer promotes muscle growth: *a.* Boldenone. *b.* Chlorotestosterone (4-chlortestosterone). *c.* Clostebol. *d.* Dehydrochlormethyltestosterone. *e.* Dihydrotestosterone (4-dihydrotestosterone). *f.* Drostanolone. *g.* Ethylestrenol. *h.* Fluoxymesterone. *i.* Formebulone (formebolone). *j.* Mesterolone. *k.* Methandienone. *l.* Methandranone. *m.* Methandriol. *n.* Methandrostenolone. *o.* Methenolone. *p.* Methyltestosterone. *q.* Mibolerone. *r.* Nandrolone. *s.* Norethandrolone. *t.* Oxandrolone. *u.* Oxymesterone. *v.* Oxymetholone. *w.* Stanolone. *x.* Stanozolol. *y.* Testolactone. *z.* Testosterone. *aa.* Trenbolone.

Prohibited acts involving anabolic steroids are covered under Iowa Code § 124.401 in Chapter 124, Division IV, Offenses and Penalties. **First time simple unlawful possession is a "serious misdemeanor"** under subsection (5):

5. It is unlawful for any person knowingly or intentionally to possess a controlled substance unless such substance was obtained directly from, or pursuant to, a valid prescription or order of a practitioner while acting in the course of the practitioner's professional practice, or except as otherwise authorized by this chapter. Any person who violates this subsection is guilty of a serious misdemeanor for a first offense. A person who commits a violation of this subsection and who has previously been convicted of violating this chapter or [various drug-related offenses] is guilty of an aggravated misdemeanor. A person who commits a violation of this subsection and has previously been convicted two or more times of violating this chapter or [various drug-related offenses] is guilty of a class "D" felony.
   ...All or any part of a sentence imposed pursuant to this subsection may be suspended and the person placed upon probation upon such terms and conditions as the court may impose including the active participation by such person in a drug treatment, rehabilitation or education program approved by the court.

Under Iowa Code § 124.409, first offenders convicted of simple unlawful possession are eligible for interim probation without judgment, and discharge and dismissal upon successful completion. Note that under Iowa Code § 124.401B, if the possession occurs within one thousand feet of the real property comprising a public or private elementary or secondary school, public park, public swimming pool, public recreation center, or on a marked school bus, the offender may be sentenced to one hundred hours of community service work for a public agency or a nonprofit charitable organization.

Under subsection (1) of § 124.401, **distribution situations are a class C felony**:

1. Except as authorized by this chapter, it is unlawful for any person to manufacture, deliver, or possess with the intent to manufacture or deliver, a controlled substance ... or to act with, enter into a common scheme or design with, or conspire with one or more other persons to manufacture, deliver, or possess with the intent to manufacture or deliver a controlled substance...
   c. Violation of this subsection with respect to the following controlled substances ... is a class "C" felony, and in addition to [prison] shall be punished by a fine of not less than one thousand dollars nor more than fifty thousand dollars:
   ...(8) Any other controlled substance ... classified in schedule ... III.

Under (Iowa Code § 124.413), an offender convicted of a distribution charge must serve one-third the maximum indeterminate sentence before being eligible for parole. Further, enhanced penalties apply to second or subsequent offenders (Iowa Code § 124.411) and in situations of distribution to minors (Iowa Code § 124.406), use of minors in the drug trade (Iowa Code § 124.406A), and for distribution within one thousand feet of the real property comprising a public or private elementary or secondary school, public park, public swimming pool, public recreation center, or on a marked school bus (Iowa Code § 124.401A).

It should be noted that under a separate chapter on Drugs, Devices, and Cosmetics within the Public Health title, anabolic steroids are defined and regulated. Iowa Code § 126.2 defines anabolic steroids:

2. *"Anabolic steroid"* means any anabolic steroid, including, but not limited to oxymetholone, oxandrolone, ethylestrenol, methandrostenolone, stanozolol, nandrolone phenpropionate, nandrolone decanoate, and any other substance designated by the board as an anabolic steroid through the adoption of rules pursuant to chapter 17A.

Iowa Code § 126.3 makes it unlawful to tender steroids to teens unless to treat disease:

Prohibited acts. The following acts and the causing of the acts within this state are unlawful:
...23. Selling, dispensing, or distributing; causing to be sold, dispensed, or distributed; or possessing with intent to sell, dispense, or distribute, an anabolic steroid to a person under eighteen years of age, with knowledge that the anabolic steroid is not necessary for the legitimate treatment of disease pursuant to an order of a physician.

Violation of this section is an "aggravated misdemeanor" under Iowa Code § 126.5(4). Under Iowa Code § 903.1(2), the punishment is imprisonment not to exceed two years.

Iowa Code Title XVI, Criminal Law and Procedure; Subtitle 3, Criminal Corrections deals with sentencing. Chapter 902, Felonies, sets out the maximum sentence for anabolic steroid felonies in 902.9:

4. **A class "C" felon**, not an habitual offender, **shall be confined for no more than ten years**...
5. A class "D" felon, not an habitual offender, shall be confined for no more than five years...

"Habitual offenders" are subject to heightened minimum sentencing under Iowa Code § 902.8.

Chapter 903, Misdemeanors, provides that **"serious misdemeanors" such as unlawful possession of anabolic steroids carry up to a year in prison** and a fine of up to $1500. Iowa Code § 903.1:

1. If a person eighteen years of age or older is convicted of a simple or serious misdemeanor and a specific penalty is not provided for or if a person under eighteen years of age has been waived to adult court pursuant to section 232.45 on a felony charge and is subsequently convicted of a simple, serious, or aggravated misdemeanor, the court shall determine the sentence, and shall fix the period of confinement or the amount of fine, which fine shall not be suspended by the court, within the following limits:
   a. For a simple misdemeanor, there shall be a fine of at least fifty dollars but not to exceed five hundred dollars. The court may order imprisonment not to exceed thirty days in lieu of a fine

or in addition to a fine.

b. For a serious misdemeanor, there shall be a fine of at least two hundred fifty dollars but not to exceed one thousand five hundred dollars. In addition, the court may also order imprisonment not to exceed one year.

Provisions for leniency also exist within the Criminal Corrections subtitle. Chapter 907 provides for deferred judgments, deferred sentences, suspended sentences and probation for eligible offenders.

Possession cases may be eligible for probation, deferred judgment, or Drug Court. Deferred judgment can lead to expungement or no conviction, though your record may indicate that there was a deferred judgment. Drug Court is available only for possession cases.

Sale or delivery cases can be pleaded down but there are mandatory minimums.

There is an automatic 180-day driver's license suspension for drug convictions; however, two deferred judgments can also lead to a license suspension.

KANSAS

The Kansas Statutes address anabolic steroids in Chapter 65, Public Health; Article 41, Controlled Substances. K.S.A. § 65-4109 includes the following substances in Schedule III:

(f) Anabolic steroids...

"Anabolic steroid" means any drug or hormonal substance, chemically and pharmacologically related to testosterone (other than estrogens, progestins, and corticosteroids) that promotes muscle growth, and includes: (1) boldenone; (2) chlorotestosterone (4-chlortestosterone); (3) clostebol; (4) dehydrochlormethyltestosterone; (5) dihydrotestosterone (4-dihydrotestosterone); (6) drostanolone; (7) ethylestrenol; (8) fluoxymesterone; (9) formebulone (formebolone); (10) mesterolone; (11) methandienone; (12) methandranone; (13) methandriol; (14) methandrostenolone; (15) methenolone; (16) methyltestosterone; (17) mibolerone' (18) nandrolone; (19) norethandrolone; (20) oxandrolone; (21) oxymesterone; (22) Oxymetholone; (23) stanolone; (24) stanozolol; (25) testolactone; (26) testosterone; (27) trenbolone; (28) any salt, ester, or isomer of a drug or substance described or listed in this paragraph, if that salt, ester, or isomer promotes muscle growth.

(A) Except as provided in (B), such term does not include an anabolic steroid which is expressly intended for administration through implants to cattle or other nonhuman species and which has been approved by the United States' secretary of health and human services for such administration.

(B) If any person prescribes, dispenses or distributes such steroid for human use, such person shall be considered to have prescribed, dispensed or distributed an anabolic steroid within the meaning of this subsection (f).

Simple first-time unlawful possession is a misdemeanor under K.S.A. § 65-4162:

(a) Except as authorized by the uniform controlled substances act, it shall be unlawful for any person to possess or have under such person's control:

...(5) any anabolic steroids as defined in subsection (f) of K.S.A. 65-4109, and amendments thereto. Except as otherwise provided, any person who violates this subsection shall be guilty of a class A nonperson misdemeanor. If any person has a prior conviction under this section, a conviction for a substantially similar offense from another jurisdiction or a conviction of a violation of an ordinance of any city or resolution of any county for a substantially similar offense if the substance involved was marijuana or tetrahydrocannabinol as designated in subsection (d) of K.S.A. 65-4105 and amendments thereto, then such person shall be guilty of a drug severity level 4 felony.

Distribution situations are generally a drug severity level 3 felony under K.S.A. § 65-4163:

(a) Except as authorized by the uniform controlled substances act, it shall be unlawful for any person to sell, offer for sale or have in such person's possession with the intent to sell, deliver or distribute; cultivate; prescribe; administer; deliver; distribute; dispense or compound:

...(5) any anabolic steroids as defined in subsection (f) of K.S.A. § 65-4109, and amendments thereto. Except as provided in subsection (b), any person who violates this subsection shall be guilty of a drug severity level 3 felony.

(b) Notwithstanding any other provision of law, upon conviction of any person pursuant to subsection (a) for an offense in which the substances involved were possessed with intent to sell, sold or offered for sale in or on, or within 1,000 feet of any school property upon which is located a structure used by a unified school district or an accredited nonpublic school for student instruction or attendance or extracurricular activities of pupils enrolled in kindergarten or any of the grades one through 12 and such person is 18 or more years of age, such person shall be guilty of a drug severity level 2 felony.

In Kansas, sentencing guidelines are set forth in Chapter 21, Crimes and Punishment; Article 47, Sentencing Guidelines. **Kansas has created a "grid" of guidelines by which to determine the sentence in a given case.** A grid block is formed by the intersection of the crime severity ranking of a current crime of conviction and an offender's criminal history classification. The grid for drug felonies is provided and explained in K.S.A. § 21-4705.

21-4705. Sentencing guidelines; grid for drug crimes applied in felony cases under uniform controlled substances act; authority and responsibility of sentencing court; presumptive disposition.

(a) For the purpose of sentencing, the following sentencing guidelines grid for drug crimes shall be applied in felony cases under the uniform controlled substances act for crimes committed on or after July 1, 1993:

(b) The provisions of subsection (a) will apply for the purpose of sentencing violations of the uniform controlled substances act except as otherwise provided by law. Sentences expressed in the sentencing guidelines grid for drug crimes in subsection (a) represent months of imprisonment.

(c) (1) The sentencing court has discretion to sentence at any place within the sentencing range. The sentencing judge shall select the center of the range in the usual case and reserve the upper and lower limits for aggravating and mitigating factors insufficient to warrant a departure. The sentencing court shall not distinguish between the controlled substances cocaine base (9041L000) and cocaine hydrochloride (9041L005) when sentencing within the sentencing range of the grid block.

(2) In presumptive imprisonment cases, the sentencing court shall pronounce the complete sentence which shall include the prison sentence, the maximum potential reduction to such sentence as a result of good time and the period of postrelease supervision at the sentencing hearing. Failure to pronounce the period of postrelease supervision shall not negate the existence of such period of postrelease supervision.

(3) In presumptive nonprison cases, the sentencing court shall pronounce the prison sentence as well as the duration of the nonprison sanction at the sentencing hearing.

(d) Each grid block states the presumptive sentencing range for an offender whose crime of conviction and criminal history place such offender in that grid block. If an offense is classified in a grid block below the dispositional line, the presumptive disposition shall be nonimprisonment. If an offense is classified in a grid block above the dispositional line, the presumptive disposition shall be imprisonment. If an offense is classified in grid blocks 3-E, 3-F, 3-G, 3-H, 3-I, 4-E or 4-F, the court may impose an optional nonprison sentence upon making the following findings on the record:

(1) An appropriate treatment program exists which is likely to be more effective than the presumptive prison term in reducing the risk of offender recidivism; and

(2) the recommended treatment program is available and the offender can be admitted to such program within a reasonable period of time; or

(3) the nonprison sanction will serve community safety interests by promoting offender reformation.

Any decision made by the court regarding the imposition of an optional nonprison sentence if the offense is classified in grid blocks 3-E, 3-F, 3-G, 3-H, 3-I, 4-E or 4-F shall not be considered a departure and shall not be subject to appeal.

(e) The sentence for a second or subsequent conviction of K.S.A. 65-4159 and amendments thereto, manufacture of any controlled substance or controlled substance analog shall be a presumptive term of imprisonment of two times the maximum duration of the presumptive term of imprisonment. The court may impose an optional reduction in such sentence of not to exceed 50% of the mandatory increase provided by this subsection upon making a finding on the record that one or more of the mitigating factors as specified in K.S.A. 21-4716 and amendments thereto justify such a reduction in sentence. Any decision made by the court regarding the reduction in such sentence shall not be considered a departure and shall not be subject to appeal.

21-4708. Sentencing; crime severity scale for drug offenses, application; sentencing rules for certain crimes; plea bargain agreements.

(a) The crime severity scale contained in the sentencing guidelines grid for drug offenses as provided in K.S.A. 21-4705 and amendments thereto consists of 4 levels of crimes. Crimes listed within each level are considered to be relatively equal in severity. Level 1 crimes are the most severe crimes and level 4 crimes are the least severe crimes.

(b) The provisions of this section shall also be applicable to the presumptive sentences for anticipatory crimes committed on or after July 1, 1993, contained in the sentencing guidelines grid for drug crimes as provided in K.S.A. 21-4705 and amendments thereto:

(1) The sentencing rule for a conviction of an attempt to commit a drug offense shall be as provided in K.S.A. 21-3301 and amendments thereto. The sentencing rule for a conviction of a conspiracy to commit a drug offense shall be as provided in K.S.A. 21-3302 and amendments thereto. The sentencing rule for conviction of a solicitation to commit a drug offense shall be as provided in K.S.A. 21-3303 and amendments thereto.

(2) No plea bargaining agreement may be entered into whereby the prosecutor agrees to decline to use a prior drug conviction of the defendant to elevate or enhance the severity level of a drug crime as provided in K.S.A. 65-4127a, 65-4127b and 65-4159 or K.S.A. 1995 Supp. 65-4160 through 65-4164 and amendments thereto, or agrees to exclude any prior conviction from the defendant's criminal history.

21-4709. Criminal history categories in criminal history scale. The criminal history scale is represented in abbreviated form on the horizontal axis of the sentencing guidelines grid for nondrug crimes and the sentencing guidelines grid for drug crimes. The relative severity of each criminal history category decreases from left to right on such grids. Criminal history category A is the most serious classification. Criminal history category I is the least serious classification. The criminal history categories in the criminal history scale are:

Descriptive Criminal History

A The offender's criminal history includes three or more adult convictions or juvenile adjudications, in any combination, for person felonies.

B The offender's criminal history includes two adult convictions or juvenile adjudications, in any combination, for person felonies.

C The offender's criminal history includes one adult conviction or juvenile adjudication for a person felony, and one or more adult conviction or juvenile adjudication for a nonperson felony.

D The offender's criminal history includes one adult conviction or juvenile adjudication for a person felony, but no adult conviction or juvenile adjudications for a nonperson felony.

E The offender's criminal history includes three or more adult convictions or juvenile adjudications for nonperson felonies, but no adult conviction or juvenile adjudication for a person felony.

F The offender's criminal history includes two adult convictions or juvenile adjudications for nonperson felonies, but no adult conviction or juvenile adjudication for a person felony.

G The offender's criminal history includes one adult conviction or juvenile adjudication for a nonperson felony, but no adult conviction or juvenile adjudication for a person felony.
H The offender's criminal history includes two or more adult convictions or juvenile adjudications for nonperson and/or select misdemeanors, and no more than two adult convictions or juvenile adjudications for person misdemeanors, but no adult conviction or juvenile adjudication for either a person or nonperson felony.
I The offender's criminal history includes no prior record; or, one adult conviction or juvenile adjudication for a person, nonperson, or select misdemeanor, but no adult conviction or juvenile adjudication for either a person or nonperson felony.

KSA § 21-4717 sets forth various aggravating factors the presence of which can provide substantial and compelling reasons to "depart" upward in the guidelines. These include, for example, under subsection (1), evidence of participation in a major organized drug operation, or under subsection (2), possession of drugs with intent to sell to minors or in their presence.

Sentencing options are set forth in KSA § 21-4603(d). The option of "house arrest" is authorized under KSA § 21-4603(b).

Sentencing options in Kansas are set forth in Chapter 21, Crimes and Punishment, Article 46, Sentencing (§ 21-4603d. Authorized dispositions, crimes committed on or after July 1, 1993).

21-4502. Classification of misdemeanors and terms of confinement; possible disposition.
(1) For the purpose of sentencing, the following classes of misdemeanors and the punishment and the terms of confinement authorized for each class are established:
(a) Class A, the sentence for which shall be a definite term of confinement in the county jail which shall be fixed by the court and shall not exceed one year.
(b) Class B, the sentence for which shall be a definite term of confinement in the county jail which shall be fixed by the court and shall not exceed six months.
(c) Class C, the sentence for which shall be a definite term of confinement in the county jail which shall be fixed by the court and shall not exceed one month.
(d) Unclassified misdemeanors, which shall include all crimes declared to be misdemeanors without specification as to class, the sentence for which shall be in accordance with the sentence specified in the statute that defines the crime; if no penalty is provided in such law, the sentence shall be the same penalty as provided herein for a class C misdemeanor.

There is still a lot of leeway within the grid system for plea-bargaining. There are many grounds for downward departure. For example, meth lab cases are typically closer to 3-4 year sentences than the suggested 11 years. However, there are some pleas that are disallowed statutorily because, for example, the defendant has prior offenses on his record. These cannot be ignored. When choosing a sentence that provides a range within the box, they will generally choose the middle number in the box.

The plea agreement rules are subject to K.S.A. § 21-4708(b)(2) and K.S.A. § 21-4713. The parties may move to dismiss any charge or counts pursuant to a plea bargain. The parties may stipulate to a particular sentence within the grid block classification appropriate for an offender given his or her crime of conviction and complete criminal history score. The parties may agree to recommend a sentence outside the presumptive range on the gird when departure factors exist. These factors must be stated on the record. The State may agree to file or not to file specific charges or counts. A plea agreement involving the deliberate deletion of an offender's prior convictions from criminal history or an agreement by the prosecution to disregard any prior convictions of the offender which will elevate the severity level of the offense or count in the offender's criminal history is impermissible.

The sentencing court is free to accept or reject any plea agreement entered into by the parties. Before accepting any plea of guilty or nolo contendre, the court must inform the offender of the specific severity level of the crime and the range of penalties associated with that severity level. [*See* K.S.A. 2001 Supp. § 22-3210]

Diversion agreements cannot be entered into for a class A or B felony, or for crimes committed on or after July 1, 1993 for off-grid crimes, nondrug severity level 1, 2 and 3 felonies, and drug severity level 1 and 2 felonies. [*See* K.S.A. 22-2908]

Obviously, there is a lot of room to improve upon the grid system. Currently, there is a panel reviewing the grid for revisions, so we can expect changes in the future. Some counties have instituted a drug court as a pilot program.

There is no mandatory driver's license revocation for conviction of drug offenses.

KENTUCKY

The Kentucky Revised Statutes address anabolic steroids in Title XVIII, Public Health, Chapter 218A, Controlled Substances. The definitions for the Controlled Substances chapter are found in KRS § 218A.010: As used in this chapter... (2) "Anabolic steroid" means any drug or hormonal substance chemically or pharmacologically related to testosterone that promotes muscle growth and includes those substances listed in KRS 218A.090(5) but does not include estrogens, progestins, and anticosteroids.

Anabolic steroids are more specifically defined in the section that classifies them as controlled substances, which is KRS § 218A.090:

> Unless otherwise rescheduled by regulation of the Cabinet for Health Services, the controlled substances listed in this section are included in Schedule III:
>
> ...(5)Any material, compound, mixture, or preparation containing any quantity of any of the following anabolic steroid substances, or any isomer, ester, salt, or derivative thereof:
> (a) Boldenone; (b) Clostebol; (c) Dehydrochlormethyltestosterone; (d) Drostanolone; (e) Ethylestrenol; (f) Fluoxymesterone; (g) Formebulone; (h) Mesterolone; (i) Methandienone; (j) Methandriol; (k) Methenolone; (l) Methyltestosterone; (m) Mibolerone; (n) Nandrolone; (o) Norethandrolone; (p) Oxandrolone; (q) Oxymesterone; (r) Oxymetholone; (s) Stanolone; (t) Stanozolol; (u) Testolactone; (v) Testosterone; and (w) Trenbolone.
>
> (6) This section shall not apply to any material, compound, mixture, or preparation containing any quantity of an anabolic steroid substance, or any isomer, ester, salt, or derivative thereof that is expressly intended for administration through implant to livestock or other nonhuman species, and that is approved by the United States Food and Drug Administration for such use.

One section proscribes all the related conduct. **First-time trafficking and dispensing is a Class D felony but simple possession for personal use is a misdemeanor on the first go-round**:

> KRS § 218A.1404: Prohibited activities relating to controlled substances – Penalties
>
> (1) No person shall traffic in any controlled substance except as authorized by law.
> (2) No person shall possess any controlled substance except as authorized by law.
> (3) No person shall dispense, prescribe, distribute, or administer any controlled substance except as authorized by law.
> (4) Unless another specific penalty is provided in this chapter, any person who violates the provisions of subsection (1) or (3) of this section shall be guilty of a Class D felony for the first offense and a Class C felony for subsequent offenses and any person who violates the provisions of subsection (2) of this section shall be guilty of a Class A misdemeanor for the first offense and a Class D felony for subsequent offenses.

Selling to a minor jacks up the offense by one level, thereby enhancing the sentence:

KRS § 218A.1401:

> (1) A person is guilty of selling controlled substances to a minor when he, being eighteen (18) years of age or older, knowingly and unlawfully sells or transfers any quantity of a controlled substance to any person under eighteen (18) years of age.

(2) Selling controlled substances to a minor is a Class C felony for a first offense, and a Class B felony for each subsequent offense, unless a more severe penalty for trafficking in controlled substances is applicable, in which case the higher penalty shall apply.

Possession of a firearm at the time of the commission of the offense enhances the seriousness of the crime pursuant to KRS § 218A.992.

Kentucky has specifically addressed the **conduct of physicians** in its statutes, although these sections essentially duplicate the penalties set forth in the controlled substances section KRS § 218A.1404:

KRS § 218A.1413:
(1) A person is guilty of trafficking in a controlled substance in the second degree when:
(a) He knowingly and unlawfully traffics in ... a controlled substance classified in Schedule III; but not lysergic acid diethylamide, phencyclidine, or marijuana; or
(b) He knowingly and unlawfully prescribes, orders, distributes, supplies, or sells an anabolic steroid for:
1. **Enhancing performance in an exercise, sport, or game**; or
2. **Hormonal manipulation intended to increase muscle mass**, strength, or weight in the human species without a medical necessity.
(2) Any person who violates the provisions of subsection (1) of this section shall:
(a) For the first offense be guilty of a Class D felony.
(b) For a second or subsequent offense be guilty of a Class C felony.

KRS § 218A.1416:
(1) A person is guilty of possession of a controlled substance in the second degree when he knowingly and unlawfully possesses: ... a controlled substance classified in Schedule III; but not lysergic acid diethylamide, phencyclidine, or marijuana.
(2) Possession of a controlled substance in the second degree is:
(a) For a first offense a Class A misdemeanor.
(b) For a second or subsequent offense a Class D felony.

Trying to get steroids by fraud is a felony:

KRS § 218A.140:
(1) (a) No person shall obtain or attempt to obtain a prescription for a controlled substance by knowingly misrepresenting to, or knowingly withholding information from, a practitioner.
(b) No person shall procure or attempt to procure the administration of a controlled substance by knowingly misrepresenting to, or withholding information from, a practitioner.
(c) No person shall obtain or attempt to obtain a controlled substance or procure or attempt to procure the administration of a controlled substance by the use of a false name or the giving of a false address.
(d) No person shall knowingly make a false statement regarding any prescription, order, report, or record required by this chapter.
(e) No person shall, for the purpose of obtaining a controlled substance, falsely assume the title of or represent himself to be a manufacturer, wholesaler, distributor, repacker, pharmacist, practitioner, or other authorized person.
(f) In order to obtain a controlled substance, no person shall present a prescription for a controlled substance that was obtained in violation of this chapter.
(g) No person shall affix any false or forged label to a package or receptacle containing any controlled substance.
(2) No person shall possess, manufacture, sell, dispense, prescribe, distribute, or administer any counterfeit substance.
(3) Any person who violates any subsection of this section shall be guilty of a Class D felony for a first offense and a Class C felony for subsequent offenses.

Further, under KRS § 218A.280, information communicated to a physician or other practitioner in an effort to unlawfully procure a controlled substance is not deemed a privileged communication.

The sentences for offenses under Kentucky law are set forth as follows:

KRS § 532.060:
(2) The authorized maximum terms of imprisonment for felonies are:
- (a) For a Class A felony, not less than twenty (20) years nor more than fifty (50) years, or life imprisonment;
- (b) For a Class B felony, not less than ten (10) years nor more than twenty (20) years;
- (c) For a Class C felony, not less than five (5) years nor more than ten (10) years; and
- (d) **For a Class D felony, not less than one (1) year nor more than five (5) years.**

KRS § 532.090:
A sentence of imprisonment for a misdemeanor shall be a definite term and shall be fixed within the following maximum limitations:
(1) For a Class A misdemeanor, the term shall not exceed twelve (12) months; and
(2) For a Class B misdemeanor, the term shall not exceed ninety (90) days.

Pretrial diversion of certain offenders charged with anabolic steroid cases, including Class D felonies, is available with the consent of the Commonwealth's Attorney under KRS § 533.250, and a variety of less severe sentencing options are available under KRS § 533.010, including probation, probation with an alternative sentencing plan, and conditional discharge.

Kentucky does have some other diversion programs available, but the prosecutor has a lot of discretion in determining which cases are eligible. Drug Court is another possible alternative.

Driver's license suspension is only for a DUI case or another driving related violation.

LOUISIANA

The Louisiana Revised Statutes address anabolic steroids in Title 40, Public Health and Safety, which deals with "controlled dangerous substances." La. R.S. 40:964:

Schedule III:

E. Anabolic steroids and muscle building substances. Unless specifically excepted or unless listed in another schedule, any material compound, mixture, or preparation, which contains any quantity of anabolic steroids including but not limited to the following substances, or material which contains any of their salts, esters, isomers, or salts of isomers whenever the existence of such salts, esters, isomers, or salts of isomers is possible within the specific chemical designation. The term anabolic steroid means any drug or hormonal substance, chemically and pharmacologically related to testosterone other than estrogens, progestins, and corticosteroids that promote muscle growth and include the following: (1) Boldenone (2) Clostebol (Chlorotestosterone) (3) Dehydrochlormethyltestosterone (4) Drostanolone (5) Ethylestrenol (6) Fluoxymesterone (7) Formebolone (8) Mesterolone (9) Methandienone (Methandrostenolone) (10) Methandriol (11) Methenolone (12) Methlytestosterone (13) Mibolerone (14) Nandrolone (15) Norethandrolone (16) Oxandrolone (17) Oxymesterone (18) Oxymetholone (19) Stanolone (Dihydrotestosterone) (20) Stanozolol (21) Testolactone (22) Testosterone (23) Trenbolone

F. (1) Except as provided in Paragraph (2) of this Subsection, the term anabolic steroid does not include a substance listed in Subsection E above but which is expressly intended for administration to livestock or other nonhuman species and which has been approved by the secretary of health and hospitals for such an administration.

(2) If any person prescribes, dispenses, or distributes such steroid for human use, such person shall be considered to have prescribed, dispensed, or distributed an anabolic steroid within the mean-

ing of Subsection E above.

(3) A physician, dentist, or veterinarian shall not prescribe, dispense, deliver, or administer an anabolic steroid for human use or cause an anabolic steroid to be administered under his direction or supervision for human use except for a valid medical purpose and when required by demonstrable generally accepted medical indications. Bodybuilding, muscle enhancement, or increasing muscle bulk or strength through the use of an anabolic steroid by a person who is in good health is hereby declared not a valid medical purpose.

Note that subsection (F)(3) declares that **bodybuilding is not a valid reason for prescribing or dispensing anabolic steroids by a physician.**

Louisiana law permits the exemption of anabolic steroids that are deemed not to have an abuse potential in La. R.S. 40:965:

§ 965 Secretary of health and hospitals; authority to except

...B. The secretary of health and hospitals, may, by regulation, exempt any compound, mixture, or preparation containing any anabolic steroids substances listed in Schedule III(E) of R.S. 40:964 from the application of all or any part of this Part if, because of its concentration, preparation, mixture, or delivery system, it has no significant potential for abuse.

Now, as far as penalties for steroid crimes are concerned, how about five years of hard labor for first-time personal juice use? Welcome to Louisiana! Here it is: La. R.S. 40:968:

A. **Manufacture; distribution**. Except as authorized by this part, it shall be unlawful for any person knowingly or intentionally:

(1) To produce, manufacture, distribute or dispense or possess with intent to produce, manufacture, distribute, or dispense, a controlled dangerous substance classified in Schedule III; ...

...B. Penalties for violation of Subsection A. Any person who violates Subsection A with respect to any controlled dangerous substance classified in Schedule III **shall be sentenced to a term of imprisonment at hard labor for not more than ten years**; and, in addition, may be sentenced to pay a fine of not more than fifteen thousand dollars.

C. **Possession**. It is unlawful for any person knowingly or intentionally to possess a controlled dangerous substance classified in Schedule III unless such substance was obtained directly or pursuant to a valid prescription or order from a practitioner, or as provided in R.S. 40:978 or R.S. 40:1239, while acting in the course of his professional practice or except as otherwise authorized by this Part. Any person who violates this Subsection **shall be imprisoned with or without hard labor for not more than five years** and, in addition, may be required to pay a fine of not more than five thousand dollars.

First offenses usually receive probation and drug treatment, though the sentence can range from 0-5 years. Second or subsequent offenses merit double the prison time under R.S. 40:982:

A. Any person convicted of any offense under this part, if the offense is a second or subsequent offense, shall be sentenced to a term of imprisonment that is twice that otherwise authorized or to payment of a fine that is twice that otherwise authorized, or both. If the conviction is for an offense punishable under [R.S. 40:968(B)], and if it is the offender's second or subsequent offense, the court may impose in addition to any term of imprisonment and fine, twice the special parole term otherwise authorized.

B. For purposes of this section, an offense shall be considered a second or subsequent offense, if, prior to the commission of such offense, the offender had at any time been convicted of any violation of this state, the United States, any other state of or any foreign country, relating to the unlawful use, possession, production, manufacturing, distribution, or dispensation of any narcotic drug, marijuana, depressant, stimulant, or hallucinogenic drugs.

Stiffer penalties apply for distribution to persons under age eighteen under R.S. 40:981:

> ...C. Any person who is at least eighteen years of age who violates [R.S. 40:968] by distributing [any] controlled dangerous substance listed in [Schedule III], to a person under eighteen years of age who is at least three years his junior, shall, upon conviction, be punished by a term of imprisonment up to one and one-half times the longest term of imprisonment authorized by R.S. 40:966 through R.S. 40:970 or by payment of not more than twice the fine authorized by R.S. 40:966 through R.S. 40:970, or both.

Double prison time also applies for distributing to students (this crime is dependent on distributing to an enrolled student, not on the proximity to the school facility, which is addressed in R.S. 40:981.3). La. R.S. 40:981.1:

> Any person who violates any provision of [R.S. 40:968] by distributing any controlled dangerous substance listed in [Schedule III] to any student enrolled in any public or private elementary, secondary, vocational-technical training, special, or postsecondary school or institution in Louisiana shall, upon conviction, be punished by a term of imprisonment of not more than twice that authorized ... or by payment of not more than twice the fine authorized ... or both.

A separate crime criminalizes soliciting minors to distribute controlled dangerous substances. R.S. 40:981.2:

> A. No person eighteen years of age or older shall solicit, procure, or counsel any person under eighteen years of age to distribute or attempt to distribute [any Schedule III controlled dangerous substance]....
> B. ...[A]ny person who violates the provisions of this Section [for a Schedule III controlled dangerous substance] shall upon conviction be punished by a term of imprisonment of not more than one and one-half times the longest term of imprisonment authorized by the applicable provisions ... or by a fine of not more than twice that authorized by such applicable provisions, or both.

Distributing on or near school grounds or school busses is covered under La. R.S. 40:981.3:

> A. (1) Any person who violates a felony provision of R.S. 40:966 through R.S. 40:970 of the Uniform Controlled Dangerous Substances Law while on any property used for school purposes by any school, within one thousand feet of any such property, or while on a school bus, shall, upon conviction, be punished in accordance with Subsection E.
> (2) Any person who violates a felony provision of R.S. 40:966(A), 967(A), 968(A), 969(A), or 970(A) while on property used as a drug treatment facility or within one thousand feet of any such property, when included within an area marked as a drug free zone pursuant to R.S. 40:1058.10 shall, upon conviction, be punished in accordance with Subsection E.
> (3)(a) Any person who violates a felony provision of R.S. 40:966 through R.S. 40:970 of the Uniform Controlled Dangerous Substances Law while on any religious building property, public housing authority property, or within one thousand feet of any such property, if the area is posted as a drug-free zone, shall, upon conviction, be punished in accordance with Subsection E of this Section...
> ...E.(1) On a first conviction, whoever violates a provision of this Section shall be punished by the imposition of the maximum fine and not less than one-half nor more than the maximum term of imprisonment authorized by the applicable provisions of R.S. 40:966 through R.S. 40:970, with the minimum mandatory term of imprisonment being served without benefit of parole, probation, or suspension of sentence, provided in no case shall the term of imprisonment be less than the minimum term provided in R.S. 40:966 through R.S.40:970.
> (2) On a second or subsequent conviction, whoever violates a provision of this Section shall be punished by the imposition of the maximum fine and maximum term of imprisonment authorized by

> the applicable provisions of R.S. 40:966 through R.S. 40:970, without benefit of parole, probation, or suspension of sentence. An offense shall be considered a second or subsequent offense, if, prior to the commission of such offense, the offender had at any time been convicted of any felony violation of this state, the United States, any other state, or any foreign country, relating to an act prohibited by the Uniform Controlled Dangerous Substances Law.

Now, **physicians are covered under a separate section, and a different schedule is written up. This one includes HCG**, the other doesn't!!! La. R.S. 40:1239:

§ 1239 Uses authorized; regulation; penalties

A. The provisions of this Section and of the Uniform Controlled Dangerous Substances Law [FN1] do not apply to anabolic steroids that are expressly intended for administration to livestock or other nonhuman species, that are approved by the federal Food and Drug Administration for such use.

B. "Anabolic steroid" as used herein means any anabolic steroid or synthetic derivative of testosterone, including but not limited to the following: (1) Bodenone; (2) Chlorotestosterone; (3) Clostebol; (4) Chorionic gonadotropin; (5) Dehydrochlormethyltestosterone; (6) Dihydrotestosterone; (7) Drostanolone; (8) Ethylestrenol; (9) Fluoxymesterone; (10) Mesterolone; (11) Methandienone; (12) Methandranone; (13) Methandriol; (14) Methandrostenolone; (15) Methyltestosterone; (16) Mibolerone; (17) Nandrolone; (18) Norethandrolone; (19) Oxandrolone; (20) Oxymesterone; (21) Oxymetholone; (22) Stanolone; (23) Stanozolol; (24) Testolactone; (25) Testosterone; (26) Trenbolone.

C. (1) A physician, dentist, or veterinarian shall not prescribe, dispense, deliver, or administer an anabolic steroid for human use or cause an anabolic steroid to be administered under his direction or supervision for human use except for a valid medical purpose and when required by demonstrable generally accepted medical indications. Bodybuilding, muscle enhancement, or increasing muscle bulk or strength through the use of an anabolic steroid by a person who is in good health is not a valid medical purpose.
(2) Whoever violates the provisions of this Subsection shall be subject to suspension or revocation of his license to practice medicine, dentistry, or veterinary medicine by his governing board.
(3) Whoever violates the provisions of this Subsection shall also be fined not more than five thousand dollars or imprisoned with or without hard labor for not more than five years, or both

There is no mandatory driver's license suspension for drug crimes.

* * *

MAINE

In the Maine Revised Statutes, scheduled drugs are dealt with in Title 17-A: Maine Criminal Code; Part 2, Substantive Offenses; Chapter 45, Drugs. The Maine Legislature has amended many sections of Chapter 45 with changes that will become effective as of January 31, 2003. Although the amendments are minor as applied to anabolic steroids, both the currently effective laws and the new laws that will become effective as of January 31, 2003 are recited here.

Maine has only four drug schedules, and they are designated not by numerals but by letters: Schedules W, X, Y and Z. The schedules are set out in 17-A M.R.S. § 1102. Anabolic steroids are *not* listed in schedules W, X, or Y (nor are they defined in the definitions section, 17-A M.R.S. § 1101). Accordingly, as prescription drugs they fall into the catch-all provision of schedule Z, under § 1102(4)(A): "All prescription drugs other than those included in schedules W, X or Y."

The Maine Statutes don't talk about felonies and misdemeanors. Instead, Maine has a hierarchy of offenses ranging from Class A crimes down to Class E crimes. Class D and E crimes have maximum terms of imprisonment less than one year, and so would be tantamount to misdemeanors.

Simple unlawful possession of a schedule Z drug like steroids is a Class E crime. As of this writing and until January 31, 2003, simple unlawful possession is covered under 17-A M.R.S. § 1107. Unless expressly authorized:

1. A person is guilty of unlawful possession of a scheduled drug if that person intentionally or knowingly possesses what that person knows or believes to be a scheduled drug, and which is, in fact, a scheduled drug...
2. Violation of this section is:
   ...C. A Class E crime if the drug is a schedule Y or Z drug;

As of January 31, 2003, the new section is 17-A M.R.S. § 1107-A.

1. Except [if expressly authorized], a person is guilty of unlawful possession of a scheduled drug if that person intentionally or knowingly possesses what that person knows or believes to be a scheduled drug, which is in fact a scheduled drug, and the drug is:
   ... F. A schedule Z drug. Violation of this paragraph is a Class E crime.

"Trafficking" in scheduled drugs like anabolic steroids includes to make, create, manufacture, sell, barter, trade, exchange or otherwise furnish for consideration, or to possess with the intent to do any of the above. 17-A M.R.S. § 1101(17). Under 17-A M.R.S. § 1103, **trafficking in schedule Z drugs like anabolic steroids is a Class D crime**. Until January 31, 2003, the section provides:

1. A person is guilty of unlawful trafficking in a scheduled drug if the person intentionally or knowingly trafficks in what the person knows or believes to be a scheduled drug and that is in fact a scheduled drug, unless the conduct that constitutes such trafficking is [expressly authorized]:
2. Violation of this section is:
   ...C. A Class D crime if the drug is a schedule Y or schedule Z drug.

As of January 31, 2003, the section provides:

1-A. Except [as expressly authorized], a person is guilty of unlawful trafficking in a scheduled drug if the person intentionally or knowingly trafficks in what the person knows or believes to be a scheduled drug, which is in fact a scheduled drug, and the drug is:
   ...H. A schedule Z drug. Violation of this paragraph is a Class D crime.

Note that under subsection (6) of § 1103, *a person who uses a motor vehicle to facilitate trafficking of a scheduled drug risks suspension of his or her driver's license, permit, privilege to operate a motor vehicle or right to apply for or obtain a license for a period not to exceed 5 years*. In fact, the vehicle can be forfeited when involved in drug trafficking violations.

Several sections provide for enhanced penalties for "aggravated trafficking." Section 1105 covers "Aggravated trafficking, furnishing or cultivation of scheduled drugs." Under the old law § 110S:

> A person is guilty of aggravated trafficking, furnishing or cultivating of scheduled drugs if: Trafficking or furnishing to minors, having a prior certain convictions for drugs or other felonies, uses or carries a firearm, is within 1000 feet of a school or on a school bus, solicits the aid of a child
>
> 2. Aggravated trafficking, furnishing or cultivation of scheduled drugs is a crime one class more serious than such trafficking, furnishing or cultivation would otherwise be.

The new law, § 1105-A, shortens the heading to "Aggravated trafficking of scheduled drugs" and spells out explicitly that the various conducts that constitute aggravated trafficking in a schedule Z drug is a Class C crime.

There's also § 1118, which prohibits the unauthorized and illegal importation of scheduled drugs into Maine from either outside the U.S. or from another state. For schedule Z drugs, it's a Class D crime.

The punishments under Maine law are found in 17-A: Maine Criminal Code, Part 3; Chapter 51: Sentences of Imprisonment. Imprisonment for crimes other than murder are found in § 1252:

> 2. The court shall set the term of imprisonment as follows:...
>
> C. In the case of a Class C crime, the court shall set a definite period not to exceed 5 years;
>
> D. **In the case of a Class D crime, the court shall set a definite period of less than one year**; or
>
> E. **In the case of a Class E crime, the court shall set a definite period not to exceed 6 months.**

Maine has a provision (§ 1252(5-A)) that sets out minimum sentences of imprisonment that may not be suspended in drug trafficking cases under § 1105 or the new § 1105-A. Under the law both before and after January 31, 2003, the minimum term of imprisonment which may not be suspended in a Class C crime is one year. However, the provision sets forth standards by which a court can extend leniency and impose a lesser sentence, although the minimum term of imprisonment then becomes 3 months in a Class C crime.

Chapter 49 covers Probation and Unconditional Discharge. Eligibility for a sentence that includes a period of probation is set forth in § 1201. The court may, under § 1203-C, suspend the entire term of imprisonment in a case and sentence the offender to probation. Authorized sentences and alternatives under § 1152 include unconditional discharge, split sentence of imprisonment with probation, a fine, suspended in whole or in part, with probation, a suspended term of imprisonment with probation, a split sentence of imprisonment with one part served and followed by probation, a county jail reimbursement fee, and community service. Drug Court is another available option for some non-violent drug offenders who will receive intensive treatment.

MARYLAND

In the Maryland Code, drugs are covered under Article 27, Crimes and Punishments, Controlled Dangerous Substances. Every scheduled drug is called a "controlled dangerous substance," not simply a controlled substance. The definition of anabolic steroids is under the definition subsection Md. Ann. Code art. 27, § 277. It then goes on to classify anabolic steroids as a schedule III controlled substance under the schedule provision of Crimes and Punishments. Md. Ann. Code art. 27, § 277:

> (c)(1) "Anabolic steroid" means any material, compound, or preparation (other than estrogens, progestins, and corticosteroids) that includes any of the following, or any isomer, ester, salt, or

derivative of the following: (i) Boldenone; (ii) Chlorotestosterone; (iii) Clostebol; (iv) Dehydrochlormethyltestosterone; (v) Dihydrotestosterone; (vi) Drostanolone; (vii) Ethylestroenol; (viii) Fluoxymesterone; (ix) Formobulone; (x) Mesterolone; (xi) Methandienone; (xii) Methandranone; (xiii) Methandriol; (xiv) Methandrostenolone; (xv) Methenolone; (xvi) Methystestosterone; (xvii) Mibolerone; (xviii) Nandrolone; (xix) Norethandrolone; (xx) Oxandrolone; (xxi) Oxymesterone; (xxii) Oxymetholone; (xxiii) Stanolone; (xxiv) Stanozolol; (xxv) Testolactone; (xxvi) Testosterone; and (xxvii) Trenbolone.

(2) "Anabolic steroid" does not include a substance described in paragraph (1) of this subsection which is expressly intended for administration through implants to cattle or other nonhuman species and which has been approved for such use by the Food and Drug Administration.

Md. Ann. Code art. 27, § 279: Schedule III:
(g.) Anabolic steroid.

Unlawful possession of a controlled substance without a prescription in Maryland may be found guilty of a "misdemeanor" with a possible jail sentence of up to 4 years and fines up to $25,000. These provisions are also listed under Code of Maryland, Crimes and Punishments.

Md. Ann. Code art. 27, § 287:
Except as authorized by this subheading, it is unlawful for any person:

(a) To possess or administer to another any controlled dangerous substance, unless such substance was obtained directly, or pursuant to a valid prescription or order from a practitioner, while acting in the course of his professional practice.

(b) To obtain or attempt to obtain a controlled dangerous substance or controlled paraphernalia or to procure or attempt to procure the administration of any controlled dangerous substance by (1) fraud, deceit, misrepresentation or subterfuge, or (2) by the forgery or alteration of a prescription or a written order, or (3) by the concealment of any material fact or by the use of false name or address, or (4) by falsely assuming the title of or representing himself to be a manufacturer, distributor or practitioner, or (5) by making or uttering any false or forged prescription or written order.

...(e) Any person who violates this section shall, upon conviction, be deemed guilty of a misdemeanor and be sentenced to a term of imprisonment for not more than four (4) years, a fine of not more than twenty-five thousand dollars ($25,000), or both; provided, however, that any such person convicted of a violation of this section involving the use or possession of marihuana shall be punished by a period of imprisonment not to exceed one (1) year or by a fine not to exceed $1,000.00, or both.

Distributing is a felony with up to 5 years in prison under Md. Ann. Code art. 27, § 286:

(a) Except as authorized by this subheading, it is unlawful for any person:
  (1) To manufacture, distribute, or dispense, or to possess a controlled dangerous substance in sufficient quantity to reasonably indicate under all circumstances an intent to manufacture, distribute, or dispense, a controlled dangerous substance;

...(b) Any person who violates any of the provisions of subsection (a) of this section with respect to:
  ...(3) Any other controlled dangerous substance classified in [Schedule III] shall, upon conviction, be deemed guilty of a felony and sentenced to a term of imprisonment for not more than 5 years or a fine of not more than $15,000, or both. Any person who has previously been convicted under this paragraph shall be sentenced to imprisonment for not less than 2 years. The prison sentence of a person sentenced under this paragraph as a repeat offender may not be suspended to less than 2 years, and the person may be paroled during that period only in accordance with § 4-305 of the Correctional Services Article.

Several provisions enhance the crime as aggravating factors, such as selling to minors or involving them in controlled dangerous substances:

Md. Ann. Code art. 27, § 286C.

(a) A person may not hire, solicit, engage, or use a minor, in any manner, for the purpose of manufacturing, distributing, or delivering, on behalf of that person, any controlled dangerous substance in sufficient quantity to reasonably indicate under all the circumstances an intent to distribute, unless the manufacturing, delivery, or distribution has a lawful purpose.

(b) Any person who violates this section is guilty of a felony and, upon conviction, shall be sentenced to imprisonment for up to 20 years, or fined up to $20,000, or both.

Also, the manufacture, distribution, etc., of controlled dangerous substances in, on, or within 1,000 feet of schools or on school vehicles sets higher penalties.

Md. Ann. Code art. 27, § 286D.

(b) Penalty. –

(1) A person who violates the provisions of this section, on conviction, shall be subject to the following penalties:

(i) For a first offense, imprisonment for not more than 20 years or a fine of not more than $20,000 or both; or

(ii) For a second or subsequent offense, imprisonment for not less than 5 or more than 40 years or a fine of not more than $40,000 or both. It is mandatory for the court to impose a minimum sentence of 5 years, which may not be suspended, and a person is not eligible for parole during that period, except in accordance with § 4-305 of the Correctional Services Article.

(2) A sentence imposed under this subsection shall be served consecutively to any other sentence imposed.

Simple possession cases may be eligible for a number of diversionary programs and first offenders are not likely to serve any prison time. Probation Before Judgment (PBJ) is another option where the imposition of sentence is stayed for three years, after which the defendant will receive expungement of their record, assuming successful completion of the probationary period. Baltimore, Maryland has the largest Drug Court in the country. Maryland Drug Courts are seeking the habitual, non-violent drug offenders.

The court cannot attach driver's license revocation to drug convictions.

MASSACHUSETTS

Drugs are covered in the General Laws of Massachusetts Title XV, Regulation of Trade; Chapter 94C, Controlled Substances Act.

The definition of anabolic steroids is not found under Mass. Ann. Laws Chapter 94C, § 1, nor in the section that classifies controlled substances (Mass. Ann. Laws ch. 94C, § 31). Accordingly, as in Maine, **steroids fall into the controlled substances schedule merely by virtue of their status as prescription drugs**:

§ 31. Classification of Controlled Substances for Purpose of Establishing Penalties.

For the purposes of establishing criminal penalties for violation of, a provision of this chapter, there are established the following five classes of controlled substances:

...CLASS E

...(b)Prescription drugs other than those included in Classes A, B, C, D, and subsection (a) of this Class.

Simple possession is a misdemeanor punishable by up to six months under Mass. Ann. Laws ch. 94C, § 34:

§ 34. Unauthorized Possession; Penalties; Dismissal and Sealing of Record in Certain Cases of First Offense.

No person knowingly or intentionally shall possess a controlled substance unless such substance was obtained directly, or pursuant to a valid prescription or order, from a practitioner while acting in the course of his professional practice, or except as otherwise authorized by the provisions of this chapter.... Any person who violates this section by possession of ... a controlled substance in Class E of section thirty-one shall be punished by imprisonment in a house of correction for not more than six months or a fine of five hundred dollars, or both...

If any person who is charged with a violation of this section has not previously been convicted of a violation of any provision of this chapter or other provision of prior law relative to narcotic drugs or harmful drugs as defined in said prior law, or of a felony under the laws of any state or of the United States relating to such drugs, has had his case continued without a finding to a certain date, or has been convicted and placed on probation, and if, during the period of said continuance or of said probation, such person does not violate any of the conditions of said continuance or said probation, then upon the expiration of such period the court may dismiss the proceedings against him, and may order sealed all official records relating to his arrest, indictment, conviction, probation, continuance or discharge pursuant to this section; provided, however, that departmental records which are not public records, maintained by police and other law enforcement agencies, shall not be sealed; and provided further, that such a record shall be maintained in a separate file by the department of probation solely for the purpose of use by the courts in determining whether or not in subsequent proceedings such person qualifies under this section. The record maintained by the department of probation shall contain only identifying information concerning the person and a statement that he has had his record sealed pursuant to the provisions of this section. Any conviction, the record of which has been sealed under this section, shall not be deemed a conviction for purposes of any disqualification or for any other purpose. No person as to whom such sealing has been ordered shall be held thereafter under any provision of any law to be guilty of perjury or otherwise giving a false statement by reason of his failure to recite or acknowledge such arrest, indictment, conviction, dismissal, continuance, sealing, or any other related court proceeding, in response to any inquiry made of him for any purpose.

Notwithstanding any other penalty provision of this section, any person who is convicted for the first time under this section for the possession of ... a controlled substance in Class E and who has not previously been convicted of any offense pursuant to the provisions of this chapter, or any provision of prior law relating to narcotic drugs or harmful drugs as defined in said prior law shall be placed on probation unless such person does not consent thereto, or unless the court files a written memorandum stating the reasons for not so doing. Upon successful completion of said probation, the case shall be dismissed and records shall be sealed.

The unlawful manufacture, distribution, dispensing, or possession with intent to manufacture, etc., of Class E controlled substances like anabolic steroids is covered under Chapter 94C, Section 32D. **First-time offenders face nine months jail, while repeat offenders face one and a half years.**

Section 32D. (a) Any person who knowingly or intentionally manufactures, distributes,dispenses, or possesses with intent to manufacture, distribute, or dispense a controlled substance in Class E of section thirty-one shall be imprisoned in a jail or house of correction for not more than nine months, or by a fine of not less than two hundred and fifty nor more than two thousand and five hundred dollars, or both such fine and imprisonment.

(b) Any person convicted of violating this section after one or more prior convictions of manufacturing, distributing, dispensing or possessing with the intent to manufacture, distribute or dispense a controlled substance as defined by section thirty-one under this or any prior law of this jurisdiction or of any offense of any other jurisdiction, federal, state, or territorial which is the same as or necessarily includes the elements of said offense shall be punished by a term of imprison-

> ment in a jail or house of correction for not more than one and one-half years, or by a fine of not less than five hundred nor more than five thousand dollars, or both such fine and imprisonment.

Under Section 32J, controlled substances violations in, on, or within 1,000 feet of a school (lack of knowledge of school boundaries is no defense) or within 100 feet of a public park or playground are punishable by state prison for not less than two and one-half nor more than fifteen years or by imprisonment in a jail or house of correction for not less than two nor more than two and one-half years, with no less than a mandatory minimum of two years imprisonment.

Under Section 32K, inducing or abetting a minor to distribute or sell controlled substances is punishable by state prison for not less than five years nor more than fifteen years, with no less than a mandatory minimum of five years imprisonment.

If the defendant is charged with selling near a school or to a minor, plea bargaining policies in some counties may not allow the complaint to be amended to drop this charge. Mandatory sentencing will usually lead to sentencing especially if the crime involves sale or distribution. Where there is no mandatory sentence promulgated, there is a vast amount of discretion with regard to sentencing. There is no fixed sentencing grid.

Chapter 279, Judgment and Execution; Section 1, provides for suspension of execution, payment of fine, probation; revocation of suspension; exceptions, ...

> Section 1. When a person convicted before a court is sentenced to imprisonment, the court may direct that the execution of the sentence, or any part thereof, be suspended and that he be placed on probation for such time and on such terms and conditions as it shall fix. When a person so convicted is sentenced to pay a fine and to stand committed until it is paid, the court may direct that the execution of the sentence, or any part thereof, be suspended for such time as it shall fix and in its discretion that he be placed on probation on condition that he pay the fine within such time. If the fine does not exceed two hundred dollars and the court finds that the defendant is unable to pay it when imposed, the execution of the sentence shall be suspended and he may in its discretion be placed on probation, unless the court shall find that he will probably default, or that such suspension will be detrimental to the interests of the public...
>
> ...When a person is sentenced by a court upon conviction of any crime, he shall be informed by the probation department on a form providejd by the criminal history systems board that he will have a criminal record that may be accessible to the public under certain conditions, and of his rights pertaining thereto, as provided in sections one hundred and sixty-seven through one hundred and seventy-eight of chapter six.

A driver's license may be revoked on a drug conviction.

MICHIGAN

Michigan does not schedule anabolic steroids as a typical controlled substance. They are covered under their own separate statutes. "Androgenic anabolic steroids" and "counterfeit androgenic anabolic steroids" are defined, listed and regulated under the Michigan Public Health Code Article 15, Part 177 Pharmacy Practice and Drug Control. The legislature did an awful job of defining and listing the substances, duplicating references to some and *completely* overlooking others. In light of the absence of the inclusion of a catch-all provision, prosecutions involving steroids not specifically referenced ought to be vigorously challenged. MCLS § 333.17766a:

(10) As used in this section:

(a) Except as provided in subdivision (b), "androgenic anabolic steroid" includes any of the following or any isomer, ester, salt, or derivative of the following that acts in the same manner on the human body: (i) Dehydrochlormethyltestosterone. (ii) Ethylestrenol. (iii) Fluoxymesterone. (iv) Mesterolone. (v) Methandienone. (vi) Methandrostenolone. (vii) Methenolone. (viii) Methyltestosterone. (ix) Nandrolone. (x) Nandrolone deconoate. (xi) Norethandrolone. (xii) Oxandrolone. (xiii) Oxymesterone. (xiv) Oxymetholone. (xv) Stanozolol. (xvi) Testosterone. (xvii) Testosterone enanthate. (xviii) Testosterone propionate. (xix) Testosterone cypionate.

(b) "Androgenic anabolic steroid" does not include any anabolic steroids which are expressly intended for administration through implants to livestock or other nonhuman species and which are approved by the federal food and drug administration for such use.

(c) "Counterfeit androgenic anabolic steroid" means 1 or more of the following:

(i) An androgenic anabolic steroid that, without authorization, bears a trade name, identifying mark, imprint, or number of a person other than the manufacturer, distributor, or dispenser of that androgenic anabolic steroid.

(ii) An androgenic anabolic steroid that, without authorization, is packaged in a container that bears a trade name, identifying mark, imprint, or number of a person other than the manufacturer, distributor, or dispenser of that androgenic anabolic steroid.

(iii) A substance other than an androgenic anabolic steroid that bears a trade name, identifying mark, imprint, or number that misrepresents the substance as an androgenic anabolic steroid.

(iv) A substance other than an androgenic anabolic steroid that is packaged in a container that bears a trade name, identifying mark, imprint, or number that misrepresents the substance as an androgenic anabolic steroid.

(d) "Deliver" means the actual, constructive, or attempted transfer of an androgenic anabolic steroid or counterfeit androgenic anabolic steroid from 1 person to another, whether or not there is an agency relationship.

Personal use or first-time simple possession are each a misdemeanor punishable by up to 90 days jail. Delivery is a felony, punishable by up to 7 years imprisonment. MCLS § 333.17766a:

(1) A person shall not knowingly use an androgenic anabolic steroid except as provided in this act. A person who violates this subsection is guilty of a misdemeanor, punishable by imprisonment for not more than 90 days or by a fine of not more than $100.00, or both.

(2) A person shall not knowingly possess an androgenic anabolic steroid except pursuant to the lawful prescription of a practitioner. A person who violates this subsection is guilty of a misdemeanor, punishable by imprisonment for not more than 90 days or by a fine of not more than $100.00, or both. A person who commits a second or subsequent violation of this subsection is guilty of a felony, punishable by imprisonment for not more than 4 years or by a fine of not more than $2,000.00, or both.

(3) A person shall not knowingly deliver an androgenic anabolic steroid to another person except as provided in this act or knowingly possess an androgenic anabolic steroid with the intent to deliver that androgenic anabolic steroid to another person except as provided in this act. A person who violates this subsection is guilty of a felony, punishable by imprisonment for not more than 7 years or by a fine of not more than $5,000.00, or both.

(4) A person shall not knowingly deliver a counterfeit androgenic anabolic steroid to another person or knowingly possess a counterfeit androgenic anabolic steroid with the intent to deliver that counterfeit androgenic anabolic steroid to another person. A person who violates this subsection is guilty of a felony, punishable by imprisonment for not more than 7 years or by a fine of not more than $5,000.00, or both. This subsection does not apply to a person who knowingly delivers a counterfeit androgenic anabolic steroid to another person or knowingly possesses a counterfeit androgenic anabolic steroid with the intent to deliver that androgenic anabolic steroid to another person for legitimate and professionally recognized therapeutic or scientific purposes.

(5) It is not necessary for this state to negate any exemption or exception in a complaint, information, indictment, or other pleading or in a trial, hearing, or other proceeding pursuant to this section.

The burden of proof of an exemption or exception is upon the person claiming that exemption or exception.

(6) In the absence of proof that a person is the authorized holder of an appropriate license or order form, the person is presumed not to be the holder of the license or order form. The burden of proof is upon the person to rebut the presumption.

(7) A liability is not imposed by this section upon an authorized state, county, or local officer, engaged in the lawful performance of his or her duties.

(8) Property is subject to forfeiture for a violation of this section as provided under sections 7521 to 7524.

(9) A person who violates this section is subject to licensing sanctions under section 7408a.

Simple possession cases are eligible for MCL § 333.7411, which is a plea that allows for interim probation and sentencing. The plea is not technically accepted, but this allows the offender to avoid serving time. Otherwise, felony cases may serve time if convicted though first offenses may receive only one year. Another option is a rehabilitation program, which may or may not be available for AAS cases depending on the circumstances. The program requires a plea to offense charged and then rehab which can lead to dismissal. Drug Court may be another option available in some jurisdictions.

There is no driver's license suspension unless convicted.

MINNESOTA

While federal law makes anabolic steroids Schedule III controlled substances, Minnesota lists "anabolic substances" as **Schedule IV** controlled substances under the Minnesota Statutes Health Code, Chapter 152, Drugs, controlled substances: Minn. Stat. § 152.02:

Subd. 5. Schedule IV. (a) The following items are listed in Schedule IV: Anabolic substances;

...(b)For purposes of this subdivision, "anabolic substances" means the naturally occurring androgens or derivatives of androstane (androsterone and testosterone); testosterone and its esters, including, but not limited to, testosterone propionate, and its derivatives, including, but not limited to, methyltestosterone and growth hormones, except that anabolic substances are not included if they are: (1) expressly intended for administration through implants to cattle or other nonhuman species; and (2) approved by the United States Food and Drug Administration for that use.

What does it all mean? Why is "naturally occurring" used when anabolic steroids are typically defined as *synthetic* analogues of testosterone? What are "growth hormones"? Are methyltestosterone and "growth hormones" supposedly derivatives of testosterone propionate? Note that there's no reference to any muscle-promoting characteristics anywhere. And what about "androstane" - would prohormones be included? Can the law be struck down as void for vagueness? The only sure thing is that cattle implants are excepted. But what if they are diverted for human administration? Clearly, a bit of a mess.

Both sale and possession of anabolic substances are considered crimes in the fifth degree. The statute is constructed with the sale, possession and penalty stuff all in one:

Minn. Stat. § 152.025:

Subdivision 1. Sale crimes. A person is guilty of controlled substance crime in the fifth degree if:

(2) the person unlawfully sells one or more mixtures containing a controlled substance classified in schedule IV.

Subd. 2. Possession and other crimes. A person is guilty of controlled substance crime in the fifth degree if:

(1) the person unlawfully possesses one or more mixtures containing a controlled substance classified in [schedule IV];

For fifth degree crimes, the penalty for first offenses is five years. Under Subd. 3 of Minn. Stat. § 152.025:

Subd. 3. Penalty.
(a) A person convicted under subdivision 1 or 2 may be sentenced to imprisonment for not more than five years or to payment of a fine of not more than $ 10,000, or both.
(b) If the conviction is a subsequent controlled substance conviction, a person convicted under subdivision 1 or 2 shall be committed to the commissioner of corrections or to a local correctional authority for not less than six months nor more than ten years and, in addition, may be sentenced to payment of a fine of not more than $ 20,000.

Therefore, the possession of even a tiny bit of anabolic substances is a felony subject to five years on a first offense!

Selling anabolic substances can escalate to a fourth degree crime when minors are involved.

Minn. Stat. § 152.024:
Subdivision 1. Sale crimes. A person is guilty of controlled substance crime in the fourth degree if:
...(2) the person unlawfully sells one or more mixtures containing [schedule IV controlled substance] to a person under the age of 18;
(3) the person conspires with or employs a person under the age of 18 to unlawfully sell a [schedule IV controlled substance];

For fourth degree crimes:

Minn. Stat. § 152.024:
Subd. 3. Penalty.
(a) A person convicted under subdivision 1 or 2 may be sentenced to imprisonment for not more than 15 years or to payment of a fine of not more than $ 100,000, or both.
(b) If the conviction is a subsequent controlled substance conviction, a person convicted under subdivision 1 or 2 shall be committed to the commissioner of corrections or to a local correctional authority for not less than one year nor more than 30 years and, in addition, may be sentenced to payment of a fine of not more than $ 100,000.

First time drug offenders may be eligible for deferred prosecution under Minn. Stat. § 152.18(1). The court may, without an adjudication of guilt, defer further proceedings and place the offender on probation. If during the period of probation the person does not violate any of the conditions of the probation, then upon expiration of the period the court shall discharge the person and dismiss the proceedings against that person, leaving only a "not public" record.

Drug Court may be another available option as virtually all drug cases are sent to Drug Court in Minnesota. The Drug Court program requires that the case stay open for one year during which time the offender will receive treatment, court appearances and review, reports and drug testing.

Under Minn. Stat. § 152.0271, the sentencing court in a drug case determines *if the sale or possession of the controlled substance occurred while the offender was driving a motor vehicle. If so, a 30 day license revocation results.*

MISSISSIPPI

The Mississippi Uniform Controlled Substances Law, Title 41 Public Health; Chapter 29 Article 3, defines and classifies anabolic steroids as a Schedule III controlled substance.

Miss. Code Ann. § 41-29-117:
(A) The controlled substances listed in this section are included in Schedule III.
...(f) Any material, compound, mixture or preparation containing any quantity of any of the fol-

lowing anabolic steroids, which means any drug or hormonal substance chemically and pharmacologically related to testosterone (other than estrogens, progestins and corticosteroids) that promotes muscle growth, unless listed in another schedule or excepted: (1) Boldenone (dehydrotestosterone); (2) Chlorotestosterone (clostebol, 4-chlorotestosterone, 4-chlortestosterone); (3) Dehydrochlormethyltestosterone; (4) Dihydrotestosterone (stanolone, 4-dihydrotestosterone); (5) Drostanolone; (6) Ethylestrenol; (7) Fluoxymesterone; (8) Formebulone (formebolone); (9) Mesterolone; (10) Methandienone (methandrostenolone); (11) Methandriol; (12) Methenolone; (13) Methyltestosterone; (14) Mibolerone; (15) Nandrolone; (16) Norethandrolone; (17) Oxandrolone; (18) Oxymesterone; (19) Oxymetholone; (20) Stanozolol; (21) Testolactone; (22) Testosterone; (23) Trenbolone; (24) Any salt, ester, or isomer of a drug or substance described or listed in this paragraph, if that salt, ester, or isomer promotes muscle growth;

...(B) Any material, compound, mixture or preparation which contains any quantity of a Schedule III controlled substance and is listed as an exempt substance in 21 C.F.R., Section 1308.22, 1308.24, 1308.26, 1308.32 or 1308.34, shall be exempted from the provisions of the Uniform Controlled Substances Law.

Admirably, the Mississippi legislators did some homework before defining anabolic substances, avoiding the redundancies of the federal statute (but still those mysterious AAS "salts"?). As will be seen, however, they failed to follow the United States Sentencing Guidelines as to defining steroid *dosage units*, resulting in quantity calculations that are *up to fifty times* as harsh as under federal guidelines!

Penalties under Mississippi law for possession of controlled substances without a valid prescription are listed under the Mississippi Uniform Controlled Substances Law.

Miss. Code Ann. § 41-29-139:

(c) It is unlawful for any person knowingly or intentionally to possess any controlled substance unless the substance was obtained directly from, or pursuant to, a valid prescription or order of a practitioner while acting in the course of his professional practice, or except as otherwise authorized by this article. The penalties for any violation of this subsection (c) with respect to a controlled substance classified in [Schedules III], shall be based on dosage unit as defined herein or the weight of the controlled substance as set forth herein as appropriate: **"Dosage unit (d.u.)" means a tablet or capsule, or in the case of a liquid solution, one (1) milliliter.** In the case of lysergic acid diethylamide (LSD) the term, "dosage unit" means a stamp, square, dot, microdot, tablet or capsule of a controlled substance. For any controlled substance that does not fall within the definition of the term "dosage unit," the penalties shall be based upon the weight of the controlled substance. The weight set forth refers to the entire weight of any mixture or substance containing a detectable amount of the controlled substance. If a mixture or substance contains more than one (1) controlled substance, the weight of the mixture or substance is assigned to the controlled substance that results in the greater punishment.

Note the disparity between the federal definition of "dosage unit" and that of Mississippi. In federal courts, 500 tablets of oral steroids would be 10 dosage units; in Mississippi's courts, the same amount would be 500 units. Ten bottles each containing 10 cc's of injectable steroids would be 10 dosage units in federal court, but 100 units in Mississippi's courts. [At least it makes more sense than in Texas, where injectable steroids are weighed in grams, *including the oil!*]

Maximum imprisonment sentences for unlawful possession of Schedule III controlled substances are based on weight, and may range from one year to twenty-four years! Miss. Code Ann. § 41-29-139(c):

...(3) A controlled substance classified in [Schedule III]...may be punished as follows:

(A) Less than fifty (50) grams or less than one hundred (100) dosage units is a misdemeanor and punishable by not more than one (1) year and a fine of not more than One Thousand Dollars ($1,000.00).

(B) Fifty (50) grams but less than one hundred fifty (150) grams or one hundred (100) dosage units but less than five hundred (500) dosage units, by imprisonment for not less than one (1) year nor more than four (4) years and a fine of not more than Ten Thousand Dollars ($10,000.00).
(C) One hundred fifty (150) grams but less than three hundred (300) grams or five hundred (500) dosage units but less than one thousand (1,000) dosage units, by imprisonment for not less than two (2) years nor more than eight (8) years and a fine of not more than Fifty Thousand Dollars ($50,000.00).
(D) Three hundred (300) grams but less than five hundred (500) grams or one thousand (1,000) dosage units but less than two thousand five hundred (2,500) dosage units, by imprisonment for not less than four (4) years nor more than sixteen (16) years and a fine of not more than Two Hundred Fifty Thousand Dollars ($250,000.00).
(E) Five hundred (500) grams or more or two thousand five hundred (2,500) dosage units or more, by imprisonment for not less than six (6) years nor more than twenty-four (24) years and a fine of not more than Five Hundred Thousand Dollars ($500,000.00).

Ouch! A tub of one thousand tablets of Thai Anabol can garner a sentence of between four and sixteen years in prison - even if personal use is conceded!!!

Under Miss. Code Ann. § 41-29-139(a), **it is unlawful for any person knowingly or intentionally to sell, barter, transfer, manufacture, distribute, dispense, or to possess with intent to do the same, and violators face up o twenty years in prison**:

(4) In the case of [Schedule III controlled substances], such person may, upon conviction, be imprisoned for not more than twenty (20) years and shall be fined not less than One Thousand Dollars ($1,000.00) nor more than Two Hundred Fifty Thousand Dollars ($250,000.00), or both;

Now, Miss. Code Ann. § 41-29-149 may provide relief by permitting suspended sentences:

(a) Regardless of the penalties provided heretofore for the violation of any section or portion of this article, the judge of the court of jurisdiction of any defendant may, in his discretion, suspend such penalty, penalties, or portions thereof, for any person charged with a first offense.

Under § 41-29-142, doubled terms of imprisonment apply for selling, etc., within 1,500 feet of a building or outbuilding which is all or part of a school, church, public park, ballpark, public gymnasium, youth center or movie theatre, or within 1,000 feet of the real property comprising a school, church, public park, ballpark, public gymnasium, youth center or movie theatre. Subsequent convictions under this section may be punished by mandatory imprisonment of not less than three years and up to life in prison or by, in the discretion of the court, tripled terms of imprisonment.

Distributing controlled substances to persons under age 21, under § 41-29-145, subject the offender to doubled terms of imprisonment or sentencing pursuant to the section authorizing doubled or tripled imprisonment for violations near schools (§ 41-29-142), and § 41-29-152 authorizes doubled imprisonment for controlled substance violations committed while in possession of a firearm.

"Trafficking" is defined and punished under § 41-29-139(g). Under subd. (2):

Trafficking in controlled substances" as used herein means to engage in three (3) or more component offenses within any twelve (12) consecutive month period where at least two (2) of the component offenses occurred in different counties. A component offense is any act which would constitute a violation of subsection (a) of this section. Prior convictions shall not be used as component offenses to establish the charge of trafficking in controlled substances.

Under subd. (1), a person convicted of trafficking gets imprisonment for a term of thirty (30) years and the sentence can't be reduced or suspended nor shall such person be eligible for probation or parole.

The options available for simple possession cases and some low level sale cases include Drug Court, and diversionary programs. The diversionary programs can result in expungement upon successful completion of the program, for first offenders. This option is not available for repeat offenders.

Driver's license suspension is for minors under the age of 21 that have a drug related charge involving a vehicle.

MISSOURI

Missouri's drug regulations collectively comprise the "Comprehensive Drug Control Act of 1989" under Missouri Revised Statutes, Title XII, Public Health and Welfare, Chapter 195, Drug Regulations.

The definition of anabolic steroids is found in § 195.017 R.S.Mo.:

> 6. The controlled substances listed in this subsection are included in Schedule III:
>
> ...(5)Anabolic steroids. Unless specially excepted or unless listed in another schedule, any material, compound, mixture or preparation containing any quantity of the following substances, including its salts, isomers and salts of isomers whenever the existence of such salts of isomers is possible within the specific chemical designation: (a) Boldenone; (b) Chlorotestosterone (4-Chlortestosterone); (c) Clostebol; (d) Dehydrochlormethyltestosterone; (e) Dihydrostestosterone (4-Dihydro-testosterone); (f) Drostanolone; (g) Ethylestrenol; (h) Fluoxymesterone; (i) Formebulone (Formebolone); (j) Mesterolone; (k) Methandienone; (l) Methandranone; (m) Methandriol; (n) Methandrostenolone; (o) Methenolone; (p) Methyltestosterone; (q) Mibolerone; (r) Nandrolone; (s) Norethandrolone; (t) Oxandrolone; (u) Oxymesterone; (v) Oxymetholone; (w) Stanolone; (x) Stanozolol; (y) Testolactone; (z) Testosterone; (aa) Trenbolone; (bb) Any salt, ester, or isomer of a drug or substance described or listed in this subdivision, if that salt, ester or isomer promotes muscle growth except an anabolic steroid which is expressly intended for administration through implants to cattle or other nonhuman species and which has been approved by the secretary of health and human services for that administration.

Simple AAS "possession or control" is a class C felony under in § 195.202 R.S.Mo.:

1. Except as authorized ..., it is unlawful for any person to possess or have under his control a controlled substance.
2. Any person who violates this section with respect to any controlled substance except thirty-five grams or less of marijuana is guilty of a class C felony.

Distribution crimes are class B felonies under § 195.211 R.S.Mo.:

1. Except as authorized by sections 195.005 to 195.425 and except as provided in section 195.222, it is unlawful for any person to distribute, deliver, manufacture, produce or attempt to distribute, deliver, manufacture or produce a controlled substance or to possess with intent to distribute, deliver, manufacture, or produce a controlled substance.
2. Any person who violates or attempts to violate this section with respect to any controlled substance except five grams or less of marijuana is guilty of a class B felony.

Distribution to a minor is covered under § 195.212 R.S.Mo.:

1. A person commits the offense of unlawful distribution of a controlled substance to a minor if he violates section 195.211 by distributing or delivering any controlled substance to a person under seventeen years of age who is at least two years that person's junior.
2. Unlawful distribution of a controlled substance to a minor is a class B felony.

3. It is not a defense to a violation of this section that the defendant did not know the age of the person to whom he was distributing or delivering.

Under § 195.213 R.S.Mo., knowingly permitting a minor child to purchase or transport illegally obtained controlled substances is a class B felony.

Under § 195.214 R.S.Mo., unlawfully distributing or delivering any controlled substance to a person in or on, or within 2,000 feet of, the real property comprising a school or college, or on any school bus, is a class A felony.

Under § 195.218 R.S.Mo., unlawfully distributing or delivering any controlled substance to a person in or on, or within 1,000 feet of the real property comprising public housing or other governmental assisted housing is a class A felony.

The penalties for the various felonies are set forth under § 558.011 R.S.Mo.:

1. The authorized terms of imprisonment, including both prison and conditional release terms, are:
   (1) For a class A felony, a term of years not less than ten years and not to exceed thirty years, or life imprisonment;
   (2) **For a class B felony, a term of years not less than five years and not to exceed fifteen years;**
   (3) **For a class C felony, a term of years not to exceed seven years;**
   (4) For a class D felony, a term of years not to exceed five years; ...
2. In cases of class C and D felonies, the court shall have discretion to imprison for a special term not to exceed one year in the county jail or other authorized penal institution, and the place of confinement shall be fixed by the court. If the court imposes a sentence of imprisonment for a term longer than one year upon a person convicted of a class C or D felony, it shall commit the person to the custody of the department of corrections for a term of years not less than two years and not exceeding the maximum authorized terms provided in subdivisions (3) and (4) of subsection 1 of this section.

In practice, most first-time drug offenses arising from personal use can be resolved with a suspended imposition of sentence ("suspended imp"). A suspended sentence may also be possible in low level sale situations. In higher level distribution situations, a three or four year sentence may be imposed but, pursuant to § 559.115 R.S.Mo., in-patient drug treatment through the Department of Corrections may be initiated. If the offender does well, he gets a "call back" to the sentencing court in 120 days and may then receive probation. Another option for first offenders is Drug Court, with criteria that vary by jurisdiction (small quantity sale cases may still be eligible).

Provisions provide escalation for prior offenders. Under § 195.285 R.S.Mo., persons convicted of simple possession or control [§ 195.202(2)] who are prior drug offenders face imprisonment for a class B felony. Persistent drug offenders can receive class A felony imprisonment. Under § 195.291 R.S.Mo., persons convicted of class B felony distribution [§ 195.211] who are prior drug offenders face imprisonment for a class A felony. Persistent drug offenders face class A felony imprisonment, but without the possibility of probation or parole.

Driver's license revocation only applies to driving offenses.

MONTANA

The Montana Code covers anabolic steroids in Title 45, Crimes; Chapter 9, Dangerous Drugs, and in Title 50, Health and Safety; Chapter 32, Controlled Substances.

Steroids are Schedule III controlled substances under Mont. Code Anno., § 50-32-226:

...(5)Anabolic steroids. The term "anabolic steroid" means any drug or hormonal substance, chemically and pharmacologically related to testosterone, other than estrogens, progestins, and corticosteroids, that promotes muscle growth. Unless specifically excepted or listed in another schedule, any

> material, compound, mixture, or preparation containing any quantity of the following substances is an anabolic steroid, including salts, isomers, and salts of isomers whenever the existence of those salts of isomers is possible within the specific chemical designation: (a) boldenone; (b) chlorotestosterone, also known as 4-chlortestosterone; (c) clostebol; (d) dihydrochlormethyltestosterone; (e) dihydrotestosterone, also known as 4-dihydrotestosterone; (f) drostanolone; (g) ethylestrenol; (h) fluoxymesterone; (i) formebulone, also known as formebolone; (j) mesterolone; (k) methandienone; (l) methandranone; (m) methandriol; (n) methandrostenolone; (o) methenolone; (p) methyltestosterone; (q) mibolerone; (r) nandrolone; (s) norethandrolone; (t) oxandrolone; (u) oxymestrone; (v) oxymetholone; (w) stanolone; (x) stanozolol; (y) testolactone; (z) testosterone; or (aa) trenbolone.

Various products are exempted under Mont. Code Anno., § 50-32-233:

> The following anabolic steroid-containing compounds, mixtures, or preparations are exempt from this chapter: (1) androgyn L.A.; (2) andro-estro 90-4; (3) depandrogyn; (4) DEPO-T.E.; (5) deptestrogen; (6) duomone; (7) duratestrin; (8) duo-span II; (9) estratest; (10) estratest HS; (11) pan estra test; (12) premarin with methyltestosterone; (13) synovex H pellets in process; (14) synovex H pellets in process granulation; (15) test-estro cypionates; (16) testagen; (17) testosterone cyp 50 estradiol cyp 2; (18) testosterone, cypionate-estradiol, cypionate injection; (19) testosterone, enanthate-estradiol, valerate injection; and (20) tilapia sex reversal feed (investigational).

Under Mont. Code Anno., § 50-32-101, the following definition applies:

> (6) "Dangerous drug" means a drug, substance, or immediate precursor in Schedules I through V set forth in part 2.

Montana makes a special provision for first-time personal use of anabolic steroids. While possession of other drugs (except marijuana) is a felony, with up to five years in prison time, anabolic steroids are treated more leniently. Under Mont. Code Anno., § 45-9-102, **criminal possession of steroids is a misdemeanor facing up to 6 months in jail**:

> ...(3)A person convicted of criminal possession of an anabolic steroid as listed in 50-32-226 is, for the first offense, guilty of a misdemeanor and shall be punished by a fine of not less than $ 100 or more than $ 500 or by imprisonment in the county jail for not more than 6 months, or both.

Possession with intent to distribute anabolics is punishable by up to 20 years in prison under Mont. Code Anno., § 45-9-103:

> (1) A person commits the offense of criminal possession with intent to distribute if the person possesses with intent to distribute any dangerous drug as defined in 50-32-101.
> ...(3) A person convicted of criminal possession with intent to distribute [drugs like steroids] shall be imprisoned in the state prison for a term of not more than 20 years or be fined an amount not to exceed $ 50,000, or both.

Criminal distribution of anabolics is punishable by between one year in prison and life in prison under Mont. Code Anno., § 45-9-101:

> (1) A person commits the offense of criminal distribution of dangerous drugs if the person sells, barters, exchanges, gives away, or offers to sell, barter, exchange, or give away any dangerous drug...
> (4) A person convicted of criminal distribution of dangerous drugs [like anabolic steroids] shall be imprisoned in the state prison for a term of not less than 1 year or more than life or be fined

an amount of not more than $50,000, or both.

(5) A person who was an adult at the time of distribution and who is convicted of criminal distribution of dangerous drugs to a minor shall be sentenced as follows:

...(d) If convicted pursuant to subsection (4), the person shall be imprisoned in the state prison for not less than 2 years or more than life and may be fined not more than $50,000, except as provided in 46-18-222.

(6) Practitioners and agents under their supervision acting in the course of a professional practice, as defined by 50-32-101, are exempt from this section.

Under Mont. Code Anno., § 45-9-109, distributing drugs in, on, or within 1,000 feet of the real property of a school is punishable Except as provided in 46-18-222, by imprisonment in the state prison for a term of not less than 3 years or more than life.

In Montana, for some unknown reason, carrying dangerous drugs on a train is a designated offense under Mont. Code Anno., § 45-9-127.

Mont. Code Anno., § 45-9-202 provides alternative sentencing authority:

(1) A person convicted of a dangerous drug felony offense under this chapter may, in lieu of imprisonment, be sentenced according to the alternatives provided in subsection (2).

(2) If the court determines, either from the face of the record or from a presentence investigation and report, that incarceration of the defendant is not appropriate, the court may, as a condition of a suspended or deferred sentence, impose one or more of the following alternatives:

(a) imposition of a fine not to exceed the maximum amount provided by statute for those offenses that specify a fine as part of the penalty or $1,000 for those offenses that do not specify a fine;

(b) commitment to a residential drug treatment facility licensed and approved by the state for rehabilitative treatment for not less than the minimum recommended time determined necessary by the facility and not more than 1 year;

(c) mandatory service of not more than 2,000 hours in a community-based drug treatment or drug education program with compliance to be monitored by the probation and parole bureau of the department of corrections based upon information provided by the treatment or education program;

(d) if recommended by the probation and parole bureau, placement in a program of intensive probation that requires, at a minimum, that the defendant comply with all of the following conditions:

(i) maintain employment or full-time student status at an approved school, making progress satisfactory to the probation officer, or be involved in supervised job searches and community service work designated by the probation officer;

(ii) pay probation supervision fees through the clerk of the district court of not less than $50 per month to be deposited in an account in the state special revenue fund to the credit of the department of corrections;

(iii) find a place to reside approved by the probation officer that may not be changed without the officer's approval;

(iv) remain at the residence at all times except to go to work, to attend school, or to perform community service or as otherwise specifically allowed by the probation officer;

(v) remain drug free and submit to drug and alcohol tests administered randomly not less than once each month by or under supervision of the probation officer;

(vi) perform not less than 10 hours of community service each month as approved by the pro bation officer, except that full-time students may be exempted or required to perform fewer hours of community service;

(vii) enroll or make satisfactory effort to seek enrollment in an approved drug rehabilitation program; and

(viii) comply with any other conditions imposed by the court to meet the needs of the community and the defendant;

(e) suspension or revocation of the defendant's driver's license issued under Title 61, chapter 5, subject to the following terms and conditions:

(i) upon the first conviction of an offense under this chapter, the driver's license must be suspended for 6 months;

(ii) upon the second conviction, the driver's license must be revoked for 1 year;

(iii) upon a third or subsequent conviction, the driver's license must be revoked for 3 years.

Most first time offenders receive a deferred imposition of sentence. Upon a successful term of probation, the guilty plea is withdrawn and the case dismissed. Only some counties have drug courts.

NEBRASKA

The Nebraska Statutes address controlled substances in the Criminal Code. Anabolic steroids are defined in R.R.S. Neb § 28-401:

...(31) Anabolic steroid shall mean any drug or hormonal substance, chemically and pharmacologically related to testosterone (other than estrogens, progestins, and corticosteroids), that promotes muscle growth and includes any controlled substance in Schedule III(d) of section 28-405. Anabolic steroid shall not include any anabolic steroid which is expressly intended for administration through implants to cattle or other nonhuman species and has been approved by the Secretary of Health and Human Services for such administration, but if any person prescribes, dispenses, or distributes such a steroid for human use, such person shall be considered to have prescribed, dispensed, or distributed an anabolic steroid within the meaning of this subdivision ...

Nebraska lists anabolic steroids as a Schedule III controlled substance under its Criminal Code. Statutes of Nebraska Annotated Chapter 28 Crimes and Punishments, Article 4 Drugs and Narcotics lists the contents of Schedule III. R.R.S. Neb. § 28-405:

Schedule III:

(d) Any anabolic steroid, which shall include any material, compound, mixture, or preparation containing any quantity of the following substances, including its salts, isomers, and salts of isomers whenever the existence of such salts of isomers is possible within the specific chemical designation: (1) Boldenone; (2) chlorotestosterone (4-chlortestosterone); (3) clostebol; (4) dehydrochlormethyltestosterone; (5) dihydrotestosterone (4-dihydrotestosterone); (6) drostanolone; (7) ethylestrenol; (8) fluoxymesterone; (9) formebulone (formebolone); (10) mesterolone; (11) methandienone; (12) methandranone; (13) methandriol; (14) methandrostenolone; (15) methenolone; (16) methyltestosterone; (17) mibolerone; (18) nandrolone; (19) norethandrolone; (20) oxandrolone; (21) oxymesterone; (22) oxymetholone; (23) stanolone; (24) stanozolol; (25) testolactone; (26) testosterone; (27) trenbolone; and (28) any salt, ester, or isomer of a drug or substance described or listed in this subdivision if the salt, ester, or isomer promotes muscle growth.

All of the prohibited acts concerning anabolic steroids are covered by one section, as are the aggravating factors.

Simple possession of anabolic steroids without a valid prescription is a Class IV felony under subsection (3) of R.R.S. Neb. § 28-416:

(3) A person knowingly or intentionally possessing a controlled substance, except marijuana, unless such substance was obtained directly or pursuant to a valid prescription or order from a practitioner while acting in the course of his or her professional practice, or except as otherwise authorized by the act, shall be guilty of a Class IV felony.

Trafficking AAS crimes are considered Class III felonies under subsections (1) and (2):

(1) Except as authorized by the Uniform Controlled Substances Act, it shall be unlawful for any person knowingly or intentionally: (a) To manufacture, distribute, deliver, dispense, or possess with intent to manufacture, distribute, deliver, or dispense a controlled substance; or (b) to create, distribute, or possess with intent to distribute a counterfeit controlled substance.
(2) Except as [otherwise] provided ..., any person who violates subsection (1) of this section with respect to: ...(b) any [Schedule III substance] shall be guilty of a Class III felony;

Under subsection (4), there are heavier penalties for aggravating factors in trafficking crimes:

(4) (a) Except as authorized by the Uniform Controlled Substances Act, any person eighteen years of age or older who knowingly or intentionally manufactures, distributes, delivers, dispenses, or possesses with intent to manufacture, distribute, deliver, or dispense a controlled substance or a counterfeit controlled substance (i) to a person under the age of eighteen years, (ii) in, on, or within one thousand feet of the real property comprising a public or private elementary, vocational, or secondary school, a community college, a public or private college, junior college, or university, or a playground, or (iii) within one hundred feet of a public or private youth center, public swimming pool, or video arcade facility shall be punished by the next higher penalty classification than the penalty prescribed in subsection (2), (7), (8), (9), or (10) of this section, depending upon the controlled substance involved, for the first violation and for a second or subsequent violation shall be punished by the next higher penalty classification than that prescribed for a first violation of this subsection, but in no event shall such person be punished by a penalty greater than a Class IB felony.

Nebraska has nine classes of felonies and seven classes of misdemeanors! Under R.R.S. Neb. § 28-105:

Class IB felony - Maximum- life imprisonment
Minimum — twenty years imprisonment
Class II felony - Maximum- fifty years imprisonment
Minimum — one year imprisonment
Class III felony - Maximum- Twenty years imprisonment, or twenty-five thousand dollars fine, or both.
Minimum-one year imprisonment
Class IV felony - Maximum- Five years imprisonment, or ten thousand dollars fine, or both.
Minimum-none

Nebraska has both pretrial diversion programs and drug courts. *There's no mandatory driver's license revocation provision for drug convictions.*

NEVADA

The Nevada Revised Statutes don't contain the schedules of controlled substances or the definition of anabolic steroids (although Nev. Rev. Stat. Ann. § 453.137 provides that "'Steroid' means any of the compounds that contain a hydrogenated cyclopentophenanthrene-ring system, and includes the sterols"). The controlled substance schedules are found in the Nevada Administrative Code. Schedule III drugs are listed in NAC § 453.530:

9. Except as otherwise provided in subsections 10 and 11, or specifically excepted or listed in another schedule, any material, compound, mixture or preparation containing any quantity of anabolic steroids, including their salts, isomers, esters and salts of isomers, whenever the existence of such salts of isomers is possible within the specific chemical designation, is hereby enumerated on schedule III: (a) Androisoxazole; (b) Androstenediol; (c) Bolandiol; (d) Bolasterone; (e) Boldenone; (f)

Chlormethandienone; (g) Clostebol; (h) Chorionic gonadotropin (HGC); (i) Dihydrochlormethyltestosterone; (j) Dihydromesterone; (k) Drostanolone; (l) Ethylestrenol; (m) Fluoxymesterone; (n) Formebolone; (o) Formyldienolone; (p) 4-Hydroxy-19-nortestosterone; (q) Mesterolone; (r) Methandrenone; (s) Methandriol; (t) Methandrostenolone; (u) Methenolone; (v) 17-Methyltestosterone; (w) Methyltrienolone; (x) Mibolerone; (y) Nandrolone; (z) Norbolethone; (aa) Norethandrolone; (bb) Normethandrolone; (cc) Oxandrolone; (dd) Oxymesterone; (ee) Oxymetholone; (ff) Quinbolone; (gg) Stanolone; (hh) Stanozolol; (ii) Stenbolone; (jj) Testolactone; (kk) Testosterone; or (ll) Trenbolone.

10. Any anabolic steroid described in subsection 9 which is used solely for implantation in cattle or any other nonhuman species and is approved by the Food and Drug Administration for that use is not a controlled substance.
11. The following classifications are not controlled substances for the purposes of this section:
    (a) Oral combinations containing therapeutic doses of estrogen and androgen;
    (b) Parenteral preparations containing therapeutic doses of estrogen and androgen;
    (c) Topical preparations containing androgens or combinations of androgen and estrogen; and
    (d) Vaginal preparations.

Note that at least one prohormone as well as HCG (misspelled HGC) are "anabolic steroids" in Nevada.

Controlled substance violations are governed under the Nevada Revised Statutes, Title 40, Public Health and Safety; Chapter 453, Controlled Substances. **First or second offenses for simple unlawful possession of steroids or HCG is a category E felony** under Nev. Rev. Stat. Ann. § 453.336:

1. A person shall not knowingly or intentionally possess a controlled substance, unless the substance was obtained directly from, or pursuant to, a prescription or order of a physician, physician's assistant, dentist, podiatric physician, optometrist or veterinarian while acting in the course of his professional practice, or [except as otherwise authorized].
2. Except as otherwise provided [by the discharge and dismissal provisions of NRS 453.3363], and [for possession of a controlled substance in a prison], ... a person who violates this section shall be punished:
    (a) For the first or second offense, if the controlled substance is listed in [schedule III], for a category E felony....
    (b) For a third or subsequent offense, if the controlled substance is listed in [schedule III], or if the offender has previously been convicted two or more times in the aggregate of any violation of the law of the United States or of any state, territory or district relating to a controlled substance, for a category D felony....

Under NRS 453.391 and 453.421, it's a category C felony in Nevada if a person who is being treated or prescribed any controlled substance from one practitioner, knowingly obtains any controlled substance or a prescription for a controlled substance from another practitioner without disclosing this fact to the second practitioner.

Unlawful possession for sale of anabolics or HCG is a category D felony for first and second offenders under NRS 453.338:

1. Except as authorized..., it is unlawful for a person to possess for the purpose of sale any controlled substance classified in schedule III...
2. A person who violates this section shall be punished:
    (a) For the first and second offense, for a category D felony...
    (b) For a third or subsequent offense, or if the offender has been previously convicted two or more times of a felony under the Uniform Controlled Substances Act or of any offense under the laws of the United States or any state, territory or district which, if committed in this state, would amount to a felony under the Uniform Controlled Substances Act, for a category C felony..

3. The court shall not grant probation to or suspend the sentence of a person convicted of violating this section and punishable under paragraph (b) of subsection 2.

Distribution of steroids or HCG is a category C felony for first offenders, prohibited under NRS 453.321:

1. Except as authorized ... it is unlawful for a person to:
   (a) Import, transport, sell, exchange, barter, supply, prescribe, dispense, give away or administer a controlled ... substance [or]...
   (c) Offer or attempt to do [the same]...
4. Unless a greater penalty is provided ... if a person violates [with a schedule III substance] he shall be punished:
   (a) For the first offense, for a category C felony...
   (b) For a second offense, or if, in the case of a first conviction of violating this subsection, the offender has previously been convicted of violating this section or of any offense under the laws of the United States or any state, territory or district which, if committed in this state, would amount to a violation of this section, for a category B felony by imprisonment in the state prison for a minimum term of not less than 2 years and a maximum term of not more than 10 years, and may be further punished by a fine of not more than $15,000.
   (c) For a third or subsequent offense, or if the offender has previously been convicted two or more times of violating this section or of any offense under the laws of the United States or any state, territory or district which, if committed in this state, would amount to a violation of this section, for a category B felony by imprisonment in the state prison for a minimum term of not less than 3 years and a maximum term of not more than 15 years, and may be further punished by a fine of not more than $20,000 for each offense.
5. The court shall not grant probation to or suspend the sentence of a person convicted under subsection 4 and punishable pursuant to paragraph (b) or (c) of subsection 4.

Under NRS 453.334, escalated penalties apply for second or subsequent offenses of sale of a controlled substance to a minor. Under NRS 453.3345, additional, consecutive penalties apply for violations at or within 1,000 feet of schools, school bus stops (during school days), youth recreational facilities or public parks.

The terms of imprisonment for felonies are set forth under NRS 193.130:

1. Except when a person is convicted of a category A felony, and except as otherwise provided by specific statute, a person convicted of a felony shall be sentenced to a minimum term and a maximum term of imprisonment which must be within the limits prescribed by the applicable statute, unless the statute in force at the time of commission of the felony prescribed a different penalty. The minimum term of imprisonment that may be imposed must not exceed 40 percent of the maximum term imposed.
2. Except as otherwise provided by specific statute, for each felony committed on or after July 1, 1995:
   (a) A category A felony is a felony for which a sentence of death or imprisonment in the state prison for life with or without the possibility of parole may be imposed, as provided by specific statute.
   (b) A category B felony is a felony for which the minimum term of imprisonment in the state prison that may be imposed is not less than 1 year and the maximum term of imprisonment that may be imposed is not more than 20 years, as provided by specific statute.
   (c) **A category C felony is a felony for which a court shall sentence a convicted person to imprisonment in the state prison for a minimum term of not less than 1 year and a maximum term of not more than 5 years**. In addition to any other penalty, the court may impose a fine of not more than $10,000, unless a greater fine is authorized or required by statute.
   (d) **A category D felony is a felony for which a court shall sentence a convicted person to imprisonment in the state prison for a minimum term of not less than 1 year and a maximum**

term of not more than 4 years. In addition to any other penalty, the court may impose a fine of not more than $5,000, unless a greater fine is authorized or required by statute.

(e) **A category E felony is a felony for which a court shall sentence a convicted person to imprisonment in the state prison for a minimum term of not less than 1 year and a maximum term of not more than 4 years.** Except as otherwise provided ..., **upon sentencing a person who is found guilty of a category E felony, the court shall suspend the execution of the sentence and grant probation to the person** upon such conditions as the court deems appropriate. Such conditions of probation may include, but are not limited to, requiring the person to serve a term of confinement of not more than 1 year in the county jail. In addition to any other penalty, the court may impose a fine of not more than $5,000, unless a greater penalty is authorized or required by statute.

Under NRS 453.3363, suspension of the proceedings and placement on probation is available for certain first-time drug offenders. After the successful completion of an educational program or a program of drug treatment, the court discharges the accused and dismisses the proceedings without adjudication of guilt. A nonpublic record of the dismissal must be retained solely for the use of the courts in determining whether, in later proceedings, the person qualifies under this section. However, a professional licensing board may consider a proceeding under this section in determining suitability for a license or liability to discipline for misconduct. Such a board is entitled to a truthful answer from the applicant or licensee concerning any such proceeding. If the accused does well for three years after discharge from probation, NRS 453.3365 provides for sealing of a variety of court and agency documents.

Title 14, Procedure in Criminal Cases: Chapter 176A, deals with probation and suspension of sentence. NRS 176A.100 gives courts the authority and discretion to suspend sentence and grant probation in many cases:

1. Except as otherwise provided ..., if a person is found guilty in a district court upon verdict or plea of:
   (b) A category E felony, except as otherwise provided in this paragraph, the court shall suspend the execution of the sentence imposed and grant probation to the person. The court may, as it deems advisable, decide not to suspend the execution of the sentence imposed and grant probation to the person if, at the time the crime was committed, the person:
      (1) Was serving a term of probation, whether in this state or elsewhere, for a felony conviction;
      (2) Had previously had his probation revoked, whether in this state or elsewhere, for a felony conviction; or
      (3) Had previously been two times convicted, whether in this state or elsewhere, of a crime that under the laws of the situs of the crime or of this state would amount to a felony....
   (c) Another felony, a gross misdemeanor or a misdemeanor, the court may suspend the execution of the sentence imposed and grant probation as the court deems advisable....

Drug Court is also an option, and can result in a plea less than a felony or even in an outright dismissal and expungement. *No mandatory driver's license revocation; however, it may be revoked for driving/drug related offenses.*

NEW HAMPSHIRE

In New Hampshire's Revised Statutes, the Controlled Drug Act, Chapter 318-B, is found in Title XXX, Occupations and Professions. Section 318-B:1 defines the term "anabolic steroid" as follows:

II-a. "Anabolic steroid" includes any of the following or any isomer, ester, salt, or derivative of the following that acts in the same manner on the human body: (a) Clostebol; (b) Dehydrochlormethyltestosterone; (c) Ethylestrenol; (d) Fluoxymesterone; (e) Mesterolone; (f) Methandienone; (g) Methandrostenolone; (h) Methenolone; (i) Methyltestosterone; (j) Nandrolone; (k) Norethandrolone; (l)

Oxandrolone; (m) Oxymesterone; (n) Oxymetholone; (o) Stanozolol; and (p) Testosterone

Standing alone, this definition would seem to exclude various compounds, including trenbolone and stanolone. But Section 318-B:1-a authorizes the Commissioner to schedule in conformity with federal laws. New Hampshire follows the federal definition, and states that what substances are listed federally shall be listed in the New Hampshire Controlled Drug Act. Therefore, although there appears to be some confusion with respect to some substances, for purposes of scheduling, steroids are classified as Schedule III controlled substances.

The New Hampshire Controlled Drug Act Section 318-B:2 proscribes a variety of conduct regarding controlled substances:

> I. It shall be unlawful for any person to manufacture, possess, have under his control, sell, purchase, prescribe, administer, or transport or possess with intent to sell, dispense, or compound any controlled drug, or controlled drug analog, or any preparation containing a controlled drug, except as authorized in this chapter.

A distinction is made between personal use situations and situations involving sale or possessing to sell. **First-time simple possession of anabolics is a class B felony** pursuant to Section 318-B:26(II):

> Any person who knowingly or purposely obtains, purchases, transports, or possesses actually or constructively, or has under his control, [any controlled drug or any preparation containing a controlled drug] except as authorized in this chapter, shall be sentenced as follows...:
>
> (a) In the case of a [schedule III controlled drug], the person shall be guilty of a class B felony [and] a fine of not more than $25,000 may be imposed. If any person commits such a violation after one or more prior [controlled drug offenses], such person shall be guilty of a class A felony [and] a fine of up to $50,000 may be imposed;

Selling steroids and possessing them for sale are punishable by up to seven years in prison for a first offense under 318-B:26(I), which states:

> Any person who manufactures, sells, prescribes, administers, or transports or possesses with intent to sell, dispense, or compound any controlled drug, controlled drug analog or any preparation containing a controlled drug ... shall be sentenced as follows, except as otherwise provided in this section...:
>
> (c) In the case of a violation involving [a schedule III controlled drug], a person may be sentenced to a maximum term of imprisonment of not more than 7 years, a fine of not more than $100,000, or both. If any person commits such a violation after one or more prior [controlled drug offenses], such person may be sentenced to a maximum term of imprisonment of not more than 15 years, a fine of not more than $200,000, or both:

The two classes of felonies in New Hampshire are Class A and B felonies, distinguished as follows under RSA 625:9(III)(a):

> (1) Class A felonies are crimes so designated by statute within or outside this code and any crime defined by statute outside of this code for which the maximum penalty, exclusive of fine, is imprisonment in excess of 7 years.
>
> (2) Class B felonies are crimes so designated by statute within or outside this code and any crime defined outside of this code for which the maximum penalty, exclusive of fine, is imprisonment in excess of one year but not in excess of 7 years.

So, simple possession of steroids as a Class B felony faces seven years — the same maximum prison punishment as the first offense of selling them.

Sentencing for Class A and B felonies is determined by the New Hampshire Criminal Code, Title LXII, Section 651:2. The section covers all aspects of sentencing, including terms of imprisonment, probation, community service, home electronic home detention, fines, etc. While there are reportedly no formal diversion programs or drug courts, treatment may be mandated.

Driver's license revocation is automatic for those under age 18. But for adults, revocation only applies in vehicular transporting cases.

NEW JERSEY

Title 2C is the New Jersey Code of Criminal Justice. Sections 2C:35-1. et seq. are collectively known as and may be cited as the "Comprehensive Drug Reform Act of 1987." New Jersey uses the term "controlled dangerous substances," defined in 2C:35-2, to refer to drugs in Schedules I through V:

> "Controlled dangerous substance" means a drug, substance, or immediate precursor in Schedules I through V, any substance the distribution of which is specifically prohibited ... and any drug or substance which, when ingested, is metabolized or otherwise becomes a controlled dangerous substance in the human body. When any statute refers to controlled dangerous substances, or to a specific controlled dangerous substance, it shall also be deemed to refer to any drug or substance which, when ingested, is metabolized or otherwise becomes a controlled dangerous substance or the specific controlled dangerous substance, and to any substance that is an immediate precursor of a controlled dangerous substance or the specific controlled dangerous substance. The term shall not include distilled spirits, wine, malt beverages, ... or tobacco and tobacco products. The term, wherever it appears in any law or administrative regulation of this State, shall include controlled substance analogs.

Under N.J. Stat. § 24:21-7, Schedule III, anabolic steroids are not listed as controlled dangerous substances. However, under the Administrative Code [N.J.A.C. § 8:65-10.3(b)(4)] they are listed under Schedule III:

> 4. Anabolic steroids (CDS Code 4000), with the exception of those anabolic steroid products specified in (b)5 below, as follows: i. Boldenone; ii. Chlorotestosterone (4-chlorotestosterone); iii. Clostebol; iv. Dehydrochlormethyltestosterone; v. Dihydrotestosterone (4-dihydrotesterone); vi. Drostanolone; vii. Ethylestrenol; viii. Fluoxymesterone; ix. Formebulone (formebolone); x. Mesterolone; xi. Methandienone; xii. Methandranone; xiii. Methandriol; xiv. Methandrostenolone; xv. Methenolone; xvi. Methyltestosterone; xvii. Mibolerone; xviii. Nandrolone; xix. Norethandrolone; xx. Oxandrolone; xxi. Oxymesterone; xxii. Oxymetholone; xxiii. Stanolone; xxiv. Stanozolol; xxv. Testolactone; xxvi. Testosterone; xxvii. Trenbolone; and xxviii. Any salt, ester, or isomer of a drug or substance described or listed above, if that salt, ester, or isomer promotes muscle growth.

Subd. 5 provides an extensive list of excluded products, such as mixed androgen/estrogens and cattle implants.

Simple AAS possession is a crime of the third degree (felony) under N.J. Stat. § 2C:35-10:

> a. It is unlawful for any person, knowingly or purposely, to obtain, or to possess, actually or constructively, a controlled dangerous substance or controlled substance analog, unless the substance was obtained directly, or pursuant to a valid prescription or order form from a practitioner, while acting in the course of his professional practice, or except as otherwise authorized .... Any person who violates this section with respect to:
> (1) A controlled dangerous substance, or its analog, classified in [Schedule III] is guilty of a crime of the third degree except that, notwithstanding the provisions of subsection b. of N.J.S.2C:43-3, a fine of up to $35,000.00 may be imposed;

Under N.J. Stat. § 2C:35-5, **unlawful distribution, manufacturing or dispensing of anabolic steroids is also a crime of the third degree**:

a. Except as authorized ... it shall be unlawful for any person knowingly or purposely:
   (1) To manufacture, distribute or dispense, or to possess or have under his control with intent to manufacture, distribute or dispense, a controlled dangerous substance or controlled substance analog ...

b. Any person who violates subsection a. with respect to:
   ...(13) Any other controlled dangerous substance classified in [Schedule III] is guilty of a crime of the third degree, except that, notwithstanding the provisions of subsection b. of N.J.S. 2C:43-3, a fine of up to $25,000.00 may be imposed;

Now, why would simple possession and possession to distribute be the same level, and the fine for simple possession have a higher cap?

Under N.J. Stat. § 2C:35-7, distribution offenses including possession with intent that occur within 1,000 feet of a school or school bus subject the offender to mandatory imprisonment. The term of imprisonment includes the imposition of a minimum term which shall be fixed at, or between, one-third and one-half of the sentence imposed, or three years, whichever is greater, during which the offender is ineligible for parole. A fine of up to $150,000.00 may also be imposed upon any conviction for a violation of this section. Not knowing that a school is within 1,000 feet is no defense, but an affirmative defense provision is set forth in the statute. Now, the range provided under the statute is wide enough for greatly disparate treatment. The case of *State v. Brimage,* 153 N.J. 1 (Supreme Court of N.J., 1998), addressed the lack of uniformity. The "Brimage guidelines" address situations of selling controlled substances within 1,000 feet of a school.

Under N.J. Stat. § 2C:35-7.1, distribution offenses including possession with intent that occur within 500 feet of a public housing facility or public park pr building is guilty of a crime in the second degree.

Under 2C:35-8, distribution to pregnant females or persons under age 18 provokes enhanced punishment, including twice the term of imprisonment, fine and penalty, including twice the term of parole ineligibility, if any, authorized or required to be imposed.

The degrees of crimes in New Jersey are set forth under D2C:43-1:

a. Crimes defined by this code are classified, for the purpose of sentence, into four degrees, as follows:
   (1) Crimes of the first degree;
   (2) Crimes of the second degree;
   (3) Crimes of the third degree; and
   (4) Crimes of the fourth degree.

   A crime is of the first, second, third or fourth degree when it is so designated by the code. An offense, declared to be a crime, without specification of degree, is of the fourth degree.

b. Notwithstanding any other provision of law, a crime defined by any statute of this State other than this code and designated as a high misdemeanor shall constitute for the purpose of sentence a crime of the third degree. Except as provided in sections 2C:1-4c. and 2C:1-5b. and notwithstanding any other provision of law, a crime defined by any statute of this State other than this code and designated as a misdemeanor shall constitute for the purpose of sentence a crime of the fourth degree.

Regarding sentences, fines and restitutions for the various degrees of crimes are set forth in 2C:43-3. Sentences of imprisonment are covered in N.J. Stat. § 2C:43-6;

a. Except as otherwise provided, a person who has been convicted of a crime may be sentenced to imprisonment, as follows:
   (1) In the case of a crime of the first degree, for a specific term of years which shall be fixed by the court and shall be between 10 years and 20 years;
   (2) In the case of a crime of the second degree, for a specific term of years which shall be fixed by the court and shall be between five years and 10 years;

(3) **In the case of a crime of the third degree, for a specific term of years which shall be fixed by the court and shall be between three years and five years;**

(4) In the case of a crime of the fourth degree, for a specific term which shall be fixed by the court and shall not exceed 18 months.

b. As part of a sentence for any crime, where the court is clearly convinced that the aggravating factors substantially outweigh the mitigating factors, as set forth in subsections a. and b. of 2C:44-1, the court may fix a minimum term not to exceed one-half of the term set pursuant to subsection a., or one-half of the term set pursuant to a maximum period of incarceration for a crime set forth in any statute other than this code, during which the defendant shall not be eligible for parole; provided that no defendant shall be eligible for parole at a date earlier than otherwise provided by the law governing parole.

..f. A person convicted of manufacturing, distributing, dispensing or possessing with intent to distribute any dangerous substance or controlled substance analog under N.J.S. 2C:35-5, of maintaining or operating a controlled dangerous substance production facility under N.J.S. 2C:35-4, of employing a juvenile in a drug distribution scheme under N.J.S. 2C:35-6, leader of a narcotics trafficking network under N.J.S. 2C:35-3, or of distributing, dispensing or possessing with intent to distribute on or near school property or buses under section 1 of P.L.1987, c.101 (C.2C:35-7), who has been previously convicted of manufacturing, distributing, dispensing or possessing with intent to distribute a controlled dangerous substance or controlled substance analog, shall upon application of the prosecuting attorney be sentenced by the court to an extended term as authorized by subsection c. of N.J.S. 2C:43-7, notwithstanding that extended terms are ordinarily discretionary with the court. The term of imprisonment shall, except as may be provided in N.J.S. 2C:35-12, include the imposition of a minimum term. The minimum term shall be fixed at, or between, one-third and one-half of the sentence imposed by the court or three years, whichever is greater, not less than seven years if the person is convicted of a violation of N.J.S. 2C:35-6, or 18 months in the case of a fourth degree crime, during which the defendant shall be ineligible for parole. The court shall not impose an extended term pursuant to this subsection unless the ground therefor has been established at a hearing. At the hearing, which may occur at the time of sentencing, the prosecutor shall establish the ground therefor by a preponderance of the evidence. In making its finding, the court shall take judicial notice of any evidence, testimony or information adduced at the trial, plea hearing, or other court proceedings and shall also consider the presentence report and any other relevant information.

The criteria for imposing or withholding sentences of imprisonment are set out under N.J.S.2C:44-1.

A statewide program of Pretrial Intervention exists to provide supervisory treatment to first offenders, set forth in sections 2C:43-12 through 2C:43-22. At any time prior to trial but after the filing of a criminal complaint, or the filing of an accusation or the return of an indictment, with the consent of the prosecutor and upon written recommendation of the program director, the assignment judge or a judge designated by him may postpone all further proceedings against an applicant and refer said applicant to a program of supervisory treatment approved by the Supreme Court. During a period of supervisory treatment the charge or charges on which the participant is undergoing supervisory treatment shall be held in an inactive status. Upon completion of supervisory treatment, and with the consent of the prosecutor, the complaint, indictment or accusation against the participant may be dismissed with prejudice.

Section 2C:35-12 provides for negotiated agreements between the defense and the prosecution to reduce or waive mandatory sentences or minimum terms of parole ineligibility. Section 2C:43-6.2 permits the prosecutor to move the court for leniency for certain first offenders facing mandatory minimum terms of imprisonment. Under 2C:35-14, rehabilitation programs for drug or alcohol dependent offenders and special probation for five years are authorized.

As an additional deterrent, New Jersey provides for civil actions against "drug dealers" under 2C:35B-2.

New Jersey has provisions targeted at teen steroid use. Under Title 18A, Education, Subtitle 6, School Conduct, Chapter 40A, Substance Abuse, provisions exist to institute instructional public school programs about anabolic steroids and other substances of abuse. N.J. Stat. § 18A:40A-1 sets forth the curriculum guidelines. Under N.J. Stat. § 18A:40A-12(b), **teaching staff members, school nurses and other educational school personnel who have reason to believe that a pupil has used or may be using** anabolic **steroids must report the matter as soon as possible to the school nurse, medical inspector or substance awareness coordinator and to the principal.**

Section 2C:35-16 provides for mandatory forfeiture or postponement of driving privileges for violations. Forfeiture of the privilege to operate a motor vehicle in New Jersey for a period set by the court (not less than six months or more than two years) begins on the day the sentence is imposed. A court may in its discretion suspend, revoke or postpone the driving privileges of a person admitted to supervisory treatment under N.J.S. 2C:36A-1 or N.J.S. 2C:43-12 without a plea of guilty or finding of guilt. Upon conviction or adjudication of, or finding of delinquency based on, any of the steroid possession or sale offenses described above, § 13A-12-290 requires a *suspension of the driver's license* of the offender for a period of six months.

In the simple possession case an adult, first-time offender would most likely receive a "conditional discharge." The defendant must make the application to the court for the conditional discharge and it would have to be approved by the district attorney and evaluated and approved by the probation department. In addition to the conditional discharge, fines will be imposed as well.

In the distribution case the conditional discharge will not be available. The defendant could be sentenced to probation; however, it is more likely that some time will have to be served.

NEW MEXICO

Although anabolic steroids are considered a "dangerous drug"(under N.M. Stat. Ann. § 26-1-2(F), any prescription drug under federal law) in the state, the statutory list of Schedule III substances, found in N.M. Stat. Ann. § 30-31-8, does not include them. New Mexico defines anabolic steroids by regulation in its Administrative Code, Title 16, Occupational and Professional Licensing; Chapter 19, Pharmacists; Part 20, Controlled Substances. Here, in the context of regulations for pharmacists, is a schedule of controlled substances. The section that sets forth Schedule III substances, 16 NMAC 19.20.28(2), states:

> 28(2).E ANABOLIC STEROIDS. The term "anabolic steroid" means any drug or hormonal substance, chemically and pharmacologically related to testosterone (other than estrogens, progestins, and corticosteroids) that promotes muscle growth. Unless specifically exempt or unless listed in another schedule, any material, compound, mixture or preparation which contains any quantity of the following substances listed in this section:
>
> **1.** boldenone
> **2.** chlorotestosterone
> **3.** clostebol
> **4.** dehydrochlormethyltestosterone
> **5.** dihydrotestosterone
> **6.** drostanolone
> **7.** ethylestrenol
> **8.** fluoxymesterone
> **9.** formebolone
> **10.** mesterolone
> **11.** methandienone
> **12.** methandranone
> **13.** methandriol
> **14.** methandrostenolone
> **15.** methenolone
> **16.** methyltestosterone
> **17.** mibolerone
> **18.** nandrolone
> **19.** norethandrolone
> **20.** oxandrolone
> **21.** oxymesterone
> **22.** oxymetholone
> **23.** stanolone
> **24.** stanozolol
> **25.** testolactone
> **26.** testosterone
> **27.** trenbolone; and
> **28.** any salt, ester, or isomer of a drug or substance described or listed in this paragraph, if that salt, ester, or isomer promotes muscle growth.

Under the New Mexico Annotated Statutes, Chapter 30, Criminal Offenses; Article 31, Controlled Substances, the state has criminalized unlawful conduct regarding steroids, with **simple possession being a misdemeanor and typical distribution crimes being a fourth degree felony**:

N.M. Stat. Ann. § 30-31-41 (Anabolic steroids; possession; distribution; penalties; notice):

A. Except as authorized by the New Mexico Drug, Device and Cosmetic Act, it is unlawful for any person to intentionally possess anabolic steroids. Any person who violates this subsection is guilty of a misdemeanor.

B. Except as authorized by the New Mexico Drug[, Device] and Cosmetic Act, it is unlawful for any person to intentionally distribute or possess with intent to distribute anabolic steroids. Any person who violates this subsection is guilty of a fourth degree felony...

C. Except as authorized by the New Mexico Drug[, Device] and Cosmetic Act, it is unlawful for any person eighteen years of age or older to intentionally distribute anabolic steroids to a person under eighteen years of age. Any person who violates this subsection is guilty of a third degree felony...

Misdemeanor sentencing is covered under N.M. Stat. Ann. § 31-19-1:

A. Where the defendant has been convicted of a crime constituting a misdemeanor, the judge shall sentence the person to be imprisoned in the county jail for a definite term less than one year or to the payment of a fine of not more than one thousand dollars ($1,000) or to both such imprisonment and fine in the discretion of the judge.

...C. When the court has deferred or suspended sentence, it shall order the defendant placed on supervised or unsupervised probation for all or some portion of the period of deferment or suspension.

Felony sentencing authority for imprisonment in noncapital cases is established under 31-18-15(A), and set forth as follows:

(1) for a first degree felony, eighteen years imprisonment;
(2) for a second degree felony resulting in the death of a human being, fifteen years imprisonment;
(3) for a second degree felony, nine years imprisonment;
(4) for a third degree felony resulting in the death of a human being, six years imprisonment;
(5) for a third degree felony, three years imprisonment; or
(6) **for a fourth degree felony, eighteen months imprisonment**

Section 31-18-17 provides for heightened sentences for offenders with prior felony convictions. Section 31-18-22 establishes a special incarceration alternative program.

Former Governor Gary E. Johnson was a vocal critic of the "war on drugs" throughout his tenure, and supported a number of drug policy reform initiatives. Governor Johnson believed that drug reform bills would head New Mexico in the right direction of helping to treat people with drug problems rather than locking them up in prison. "The current failed war on drugs is draining the nation and state of vital resources that could be spent more wisely and effectively. I believe New Mexicans are beginning to realize that the nation's drug war is not working and that treatment can be more effective and costs less than prison for drug offenders," the Governor said. "Now more than ever, we don't have money to waste on things that are not working."

Whether the new governor will share his progressive approach will remain to be seen. Currently, there are pending bills that would mandate "Treatment Instead of Incarceration" Sentencing Reform (Rep. Joe Thompson, R-Albuquerque) for first and second time drug possession offenders, and Civil Asset Forfeiture Reform (Senator Manny Aragon, D-Albuquerque) amending the current law allowing police officers to seize property used in certain crimes without a criminal conviction. Under the Forfeiture Reform bill, a person whose property is seized would be provided certain guarantees with regard to the forfeiture proceeding. Money obtained by the state from property seizures would go into the state's general fund, instead of directly into the funds of the law enforcement entity that accomplished the seizure.

In New Mexico, probation, and conditional discharge are available for simple possession cases. Misdemeanor offenses can receive probation and referrals to treatment. The Misdemeanor Court actually has a DWI and Drug Court. Additionally, there is a Drug Court for felony offenses. Sale cases may be eligible for this court depending on the quantity. N.M. Stat. Ann. § 30-31-28 provides for a Conditional discharge for possession as a first offense:

> A. If any person who has not previously been convicted of violating the laws of any state or any laws of the United States relating to narcotic drugs, marijuana, hallucinogenic or depressant or stimulant substances, is found guilty of a violation of Section 23 [30-31-23 NMSA 1978], after trial or upon a plea of guilty, the court may, without entering a judgment of guilty and with the consent of the person, defer further proceedings and place him on probation upon reasonable conditions and for a period, not to exceed one year, as the court may prescribe...

§ 30-31-29 provides for a Probationary period:

> Notwithstanding any other provision of law, the court may place on probation for a period not to exceed one year any person convicted of a violation of the Controlled Substances Act [30-31-1 NMSA 1978] where the maximum length of the term of imprisonment is one year or less if: A. the judge does not impose a prison sentence; or B. the judge suspends all of any prison sentence which he imposes.

Driver's license suspension is only for (alcohol / drug) driving related offenses.

NEW YORK

In New York, the controlled substance schedules are found in the Public Health Law, Article 33, Controlled Substances. Under federal law (and the laws of most states), anabolic steroids are classified as Schedule III controlled substances. In New York State, Public Health Law § 3306 classifies them as *Schedule II* controlled substances, defining them as follows:

> (h) Anabolic steroids. Unless specifically excepted or unless listed in another schedule, 'anabolic steroid' shall mean any drug or hormonal substance, chemically and pharmacologically related to testosterone (other than estrogens, progestins and corticosteroids) that promotes muscle growth, any drug or hormonal substance that stimulates the endogenous production of steroids in the human body which acts in the same manner, or any material, compound, mixture, or preparation which contains any amount of the following substances: (1) Boldenone. (2) Clostebol. (3) Dehydrochlormethyltestosterone. (4) Drostanolone. (5) Ethylestrenol. (6) Fluoxymesterone. (7) Formebulone (formebolone). (8) Mesterolene. (9) Methandriol. (10) Methandrostenolone. (11) Methenolone. (12) Methyltestosterone. (13) Mibolerone. (14)Nandrolone. (15) Norethandrolone. (16) Oxandrolone. (17) Oxymesterone. (18) Oxymetholone. (19) Stanolone. (20) Stanozolol. (21) Testosterone. (22) Trenbolone. (23) Any salt, ester or isomer of a drug or substance described or listed in this subdivision, if such salt, ester or isomer promotes muscle growth.
>
> (i) Subdivision (h) of this section shall not include any substance containing anabolic steroids expressly intended for administration through implants to cattle or other nonhuman species and that are approved by the federal food and drug administration solely for such use. Any individual who knowingly and willfully administers to himself or another person, prescribes, dispenses or distributes such substances for other than implantation to cattle or nonhuman species shall be subject to the same penalties as a practitioner who violates the provisions of this section or any other penalties prescribed by law.
>
> (j) Chorionic gonadotrophin. Unless specifically excepted or unless listed in another schedule any material, compound, mixture, or preparation which contains any amount of chorionic gonadotrophin.

Note that in subsection (j), the New York statute schedules human chorionic gonadotropin (commonly called HCG), which it misspells, as a Schedule II substance. It seems to have been bootstrapped into the statute because some steroid users administer HCG to boost their own endogenous testosterone production during or after a cycle of steroids. [Note that HCG is also scheduled in California, but in Schedule III.)

The New York State Penal Law, Title M, Offenses Against Public Health and Morals; Article 220, Controlled Substances Offenses, covers anabolic steroid crimes. New York has no specific statutes proscribing anabolic steroids beyond the Public Health Law definition and classification. Steroids are controlled substances, but they are not "narcotic drugs" as defined in New York.

The simple unlawful possession of a anabolic steroids or HCG is a class A misdemeanor under NYS Penal Law § 220.03, Criminal Possession of a Controlled Substance in the Seventh Degree:

> A person is guilty of criminal possession of a controlled substance in the seventh degree when he knowingly and unlawfully possesses a controlled substance. Criminal possession of a controlled substance in the seventh degree is a class A misdemeanor.

In many first-offender cases of personal use, the misdemeanor charge will be reduced to a non-criminal violation of the law unless there are aggravating circumstances. Typically, the reduced charge will be Disorderly Conduct, under NYS PL § 240.20(7). Violations are not punishable by terms of probation. Although up to fifteen days incarceration may be imposed, most first offenders receive fines or a "conditional discharge." Drug counseling may be required as a condition.

If the possession is with "intent to sell," the crime is a class D felony under § 220.06, Criminal possession of a controlled substance in the fifth degree.

> A person is guilty of criminal possession of a controlled substance in the fifth degree when he knowingly and unlawfully possesses: 1. a controlled substance with intent to sell it;

While New York does have escalating felony provisions based upon the weight of a controlled substance, these provisions do not apply to anabolic steroids. Accordingly, a class D felony is the top count in any possession case regardless of quantity.

Steroid or HCG sales are a class D felony in New York regardless of the quantity sold under § 220.31, Criminal Sale of a Controlled Substance in the Fifth Degree:

> A person is guilty of criminal sale of a controlled substance in the fifth degree when he knowingly and unlawfully sells a controlled substance. Criminal sale of a controlled substance in the fifth degree is a class D felony.

In New York, "sell" is defined under § 220.00(1) PL to mean "to sell, exchange, give or dispose of to another, or to offer or agree to do the same." If the sale takes place upon school grounds or at a known child day care or educational facility, the conduct violates § 220.34 of the New York State Penal Law, Criminal Sale of a Controlled Substance in the Fourth Degree. This is a class C felony.

Note that New York has certain statutory presumptions applicable to all drug cases. Found in § 220.25, they authorize presumptions of knowing possession in some situations involving automobiles and where the drugs are in open view in a room.

The NY Penal Law, Title E, Sentences; Article 70, Sentences of Imprisonment, sets forth the sentences of imprisonment authorized for various levels of offenses. Class A misdemeanors are punishable by up to one year in jail under Section 70.15:

> 1. Class A misdemeanor. A sentence of imprisonment for a class A misdemeanor shall be a definite sentence. When such a sentence is imposed the term shall be fixed by the court, and shall not exceed one year; ...

Sentences of imprisonment for felonies are set forth in Section 70.00 PL:

> [Except as provided], a sentence of imprisonment for a felony shall be an indeterminate sentence. When such a sentence is imposed, the court shall impose a maximum term in accordance with the provisions of subdivision two of this section and the minimum period of imprisonment shall be as provided in subdivision three of this section.
>
> 2. Maximum term of sentence. The maximum term of an indeterminate sentence shall be at least three years and the term shall be fixed as follows:
>   ...(c) For a class C felony, the term shall be fixed by the court, and shall not exceed fifteen years;
>   (d) **For a class D felony, the term shall be fixed by the court, and shall not exceed seven years**; and
>   (e) For a class E felony, the term shall be fixed by the court, and shall not exceed four years.
> 3. Minimum period of imprisonment. The minimum period of imprisonment under an indeterminate sentence shall be at least one year and shall be fixed as follows:
>   ...(b) ... Where the sentence is for [the felonies above] the minimum period shall be fixed by the court and specified in the sentence and shall be not less than one year nor more than one-third of the maximum term imposed.
> 4. Alternative definite sentence for class D, E, and certain class C felonies. When a person, other than a second or persistent felony offender, is sentenced for a class D or class E felony, or to a class C felony specified in article two hundred twenty ... and the court, having regard to the nature and circumstances of the crime and to the history and character of the defendant, is of the opinion that a sentence of imprisonment is necessary but that it would be unduly harsh to impose an indeterminate or determinate sentence, the court may impose a definite sentence of imprisonment and fix a term of one year or less.

Enhanced statutory penalties apply for those with prior felony convictions. Article 480 of the PL authorizes forfeiture of property in controlled substance cases.

Probationary sentences are authorized under Article 65 of the Penal Law. The applicable periods of probation are as follows: for felony convictions, five years; for "A" misdemeanors, three years.

A drug conviction requires the suspension of the offender's drivers' license.

NORTH CAROLINA

North Carolina defines anabolic steroids as schedule III controlled substances under the North Carolina Controlled Substances Act, General Statutes of North Carolina, Chapter 90, Article 5.

N.C. Gen. Stat. § 90-91:

> Schedule III:
>
> (k) Anabolic steroids. The term "anabolic steroid" means any drug or hormonal substance, chemically and pharmacologically related to testosterone (other than estrogens, progestins, and corticosteroids) that promotes muscle growth, including, but not limited to, the following: 1. Methandrostenolone, 2. Stanozolol, 3. Ethylestrenol, 4. Nandrolone phenpropionate, 5. Nandrolone deconoate, 6. Testosterone propionate, 7. Chorionic gonadotropin, 8. Boldenone, 9. Chlorotestosterone (4-chlorotestosterone), 10. Clostebol, 11. Dehydrochlormethyltestosterone, 12. Dibydrostestosterone (4-dihydrotestosterone), 13. Drostanolone, 14. Fluoxymesterone, 15. Formebulone (formebolone), 16. Mesterolene, 17. Methandienone, 18. Methandranone, 19. Methandriol, 20. Methenolene, 21. Methyltestosterone, 22. Mibolerone, 23. Nandrolene, 24. Norethandrolene, 25. Oxandrolone, 26. Oxymesterone, 27. Oxymetholone, 28. Stanolone, 29. Testolactone, 30. Testosterone, 31. Trenbolone, and 32. Any salt, ester, or isomer of a drug or substance described or listed in this subsection, if that salt, ester, or isomer promotes muscle growth. Except such term does not include an anabolic steroid which is expressly intended for administration through implants to cattle or other

> nonhuman species and which has been approved by the Secretary of Health and Human Services for such administration. If any person prescribes, dispenses, or distributes such steroid for human use, such person shall be considered to have prescribed, dispensed, or distributed an anabolic steroid within the meaning of this subsection.

Situations of sale and possession of controlled substances are all covered under N.C. Gen. Stat. § 90-95. Under subd. (d)(2), **first-time unlawful possession of steroids - including HCG - is a Class 1 misdemeanor unless it exceeds one hundred tablets or dosage units, in which case it becomes a Class I felony**:

> (d) Except as provided ... any person who violates G.S. 90-95(a)(3) with respect to:
> ...(2) A controlled substance classified in Schedule [III] shall be guilty of a Class 1misdemeanor. If the controlled substance exceeds ... one hundred tablets, capsules or other dosage units, or equivalent quantity, the violation shall be punishable as a Class I felony..

Under N.C. Gen. Stat. § 14-3, a Class 1 misdemeanor is one with a maximum punishment of more than six months imprisonment. North Carolina provides for, in § 90-96, conditional discharge and expunction of records for a first offense. A previous conviction escalates the misdemeanor to a class I felony under subsection (e)(3).

Distribution offenses involving steroids or HCG are Class I felonies except for an actual sale, which is a Class H felony. The wording of the statute is as follows:

> (a) Except as authorized by this Article, it is unlawful for any person:
> (1) To manufacture, sell or deliver, or possess with intent to manufacture, sell or deliver, a controlled substance;...
> (3) To possess a controlled substance.
> (b) Except as provided ..., any person who violates G.S. 90-95(a)(1) with respect to:
> ...(2) A controlled substance classified in [Schedule III] shall be punished as a Class I felon, except that the sale of a [Schedule III substance] shall be punished as a Class H felon...

Under subsection (e)(5), an adult who sells to a pregnant female or a teen between 14 and 16 is faces a Class D felony, and one who sells to a child 13 years old or younger faces a Class C felony. Under § 90-95.4, employing or intentionally using a minor to commit a drug law violation enhances the seriousness of the charges, as does promoting drug sales by a minor under § 90-95.6. Interestingly, North Carolina has a statutory mechanism to encourage teens to turn in their sources. Under § 90-96.1, teens without prior records can receive immunity from prosecution if they disclose the identity of the person or persons from whom they obtained the controlled substances for which they were accused.

North Carolina has an elaborate chart for sentencing, like the federal guidelines. Prior record level and offense category determine the months of imprisonment authorized. Under § 15A-1340.23, the punishment limits for each class of misdemeanor offense and prior conviction level are set forth. Under § 15A-1340.17, the same is set forth for felonies, including presumptive, mitigated and aggravated ranges for the various prior record levels and levels of offense.

Simple possession cases may receive deferred prosecution under the T.A.S.C. Program (Treatment Alternatives to Street Crimes). To be eligible for this program, you must not have a criminal history, and you must be charged with only a small amount with no evidence of sale and no weapons. Probation and drug treatment is another possibility for lower level felonies; however repeat offenders are still eligible. Drug Court is available if there is evidence that the offender is an addict and there is no evidence of sale or violence. Successful completion can result in dismissal. Sale cases can possibly receive probation or a split sentence (prison / probation) dependent upon the record of the offender.

There is no requirement of driver's license revocation, but reportedly no restriction against it.

NORTH DAKOTA

The North Dakota Century Code, Title 19, Foods, Drugs, Oils, and Compounds, contains the Uniform Controlled Substances Act in Chapter 19-03.1. N.D. Cent. Code §19-03.1-01(3) defines "anabolic steroids" as "any drug or hormonal substance, chemically and pharmacologically related to testosterone, other than estrogens, progestins, and corticosteroids." Anabolic steroids are classified as Schedule III controlled substances pursuant to §19-03.1-09(7):

> Anabolic steroids. Unless specifically excepted or unless listed in another schedule, any material, compound, mixture, or preparation that contains any of the following anabolic steroids: (a) Boldenone; (b) Chlorotestosterone; (c) Clostebol; (d) Dehydrochlormethyltestosterone; (e) Dihydrotestosterone; (f) Drostanolone; (g) Ethylestrenol; (h) Fluoxymesterone; (i) Formebulone; (j) Mesterolone; (k) Methandienone; (l) Methandranone; (m) Methandriol; (n) Methandrostenolone; (o) Methenolone; (p) Methyltestosterone; (q) Mibolerone; (r) Nandrolone; (s) Norethandrolone; (t) Oxandrolone; (u) Oxymesterone; (v) Oxymetholone; (w) Stanolone; (x) Stanozolol; (y) Testolactone; (z) Testosterone; (aa) Trenbolone; or any salt, ester, or isomer of a drug or substance described or listed in this subsection, if that salt, ester, or isomer promotes muscle growth. The term does not include an anabolic steroid that is expressly intended for administration through implants to cattle or other nonhuman species and which has been approved by the secretary of health and human services for administration unless any person prescribes, dispenses, possesses, delivers, or distributes for human use.

North Dakota does not differentiate between the schedules of controlled substances when it comes to penalties and sentencing. North Dakota has made it a felony to willfully possess all controlled substances without a prescription, anabolic steroids included. **Simple possession of an anabolic steroid is a class C felony** under N.D. Cent. Code §19-03.1-23(6):

> 6. It is unlawful for any person to willfully ... possess a controlled substance unless the substance was obtained directly from, or pursuant to, a valid prescription or order of a practitioner while acting in the course of the practitioner's professional practice. ... Except as provided in this subsection, any person who violates this subsection is guilty of a class C felony...

The crime is raised to a class B felony if the person is in or on, or within one thousand feet [300.48 meters] of the real property comprising a public or private elementary or secondary school or a public vocational school.

Note that North Dakota defines drug paraphernalia to include hypodermic instruments under § 19-03.4-01(11). The stringent North Dakota statutes make possession of syringes or needles used to inject schedule III substances such as steroids a class C felony (§ 19-03.4-03).

Manufacturing, delivering or possessing with intent to manufacture or deliver steroids is a class B felony under N.D. Cent. Code §19-03.1-23(1):

> 1. Except as authorized by this chapter, it is unlawful for any person to willfully ... manufacture, deliver, or possess with intent to manufacture or deliver, a controlled substance.... Any person who violates this subsection with respect to:
>
> ...b. Any [schedule III substance] is guilty of a class B felony ... [and] any person found guilty under this subdivision must be sentenced:
>
> (1) For a second offense, to imprisonment for at least three years.
>
> (2) For a third or subsequent offense, to imprisonment for ten years...

The sentencing for penalties of offenses is located in North Dakota Criminal Code, Chapter 12.1-32 covers Penalties and Sentencing. Under N.D. Cent. Code §12.1-32-01 in pertinent part:

> 3. **Class B felony, for which a maximum penalty of ten years' imprisonment**, a fine of ten thousand dollars, or both, may be imposed.

4. **Class C felony, for which a maximum penalty of five years' imprisonment**, a fine of five thousand dollars, or both, may be imposed.

N.D. Cent. Code § 12.1-32-02 provides flexibility in sentencing. Pursuant to N.D. Cent. Code § 12.1-32-02(1), offenders need not necessarily be sentenced to jail, but to one or more of several alternatives including imprisonment, probation, or payment of fines, court costs, or drug treatment costs. For first-time anabolic steroid offenders there is no mandated imprisonment, under N.D. Cent. Code § 12.1-32-02(8). However, aggravating factors, such as selling too minors or near a school, can escalate the punishment.

Controlled substance offenders must undergo a drug addiction evaluation by an appropriate licensed addiction treatment program. The evaluation must indicate the prospects for rehabilitation and whether addiction treatment is required. The evaluation must be submitted to the court for consideration when imposing punishment for a felony violation and may be submitted before or after the imposing of punishment for a misdemeanor violation. Whether a first offender gets imprisonment is within the discretion of the judge. The court may consider fourteen different factors in assessing the appropriate sentence pursuant to N.D. Cent. Code § 12.1-32-04 Now, a person who is convicted of a felony and sentenced to imprisonment of not more than one year is deemed to have been convicted of a misdemeanor. If the person violates probation and has probation revoked, then the conviction reverts to a felony. N.D. Cent. Code § 12.1-32-02 (9)

> The court may suspend the execution of all or part of a sentence imposed, if it places the offender on probation during the term of the suspension. N.D. Cent. Code § 12.1-32-02(3).

Drug Court may be an option for possession cases, depending on the jurisdiction. First offense possession cases are likely to receive a deferred imposition of sentence. Successful probation will receive expungement. Sale or distribution cases though charged as an A or B felony, can be pled down.

Driver's license revocation can only be attached in DUI or other driving related offenses.

OHIO

In Ohio, anabolic steroids are scheduled under Ohio Revised Code Title 37, Health, Safety and Morals, Chapter 3719 Controlled Substances. Steroids are listed the same as under Federal law, in Schedule III. ORC Ann. 3719.41(E):

Schedule III:

(E) Anabolic steroids Unless specifically excepted under federal drug abuse control laws or unless listed in another schedule, any material, compound, mixture, or preparation that contains any quantity of the following substances, including their salts, esters, isomers, and salts of esters and isomers, whenever the existence of these salts, esters, and isomers is possible within the specific chemical designation:

(1) Anabolic steroids. Except as otherwise provided in division (E)(1) of schedule III, "anabolic steroids" means any drug or hormonal substance that is chemically and pharmacologically related to testosterone (other than estrogens, progestins, and corticosteroids) and that promotes muscle growth. "Anabolic steroids" does not include an anabolic steroid that is expressly intended for administration through implants to cattle or other nonhuman species and that has been approved by the United States secretary of health and human services for that administration, unless a person prescribes, dispenses, or distributes this type of anabolic steroid for human use. "Anabolic steroid" includes, but is not limited to, the following: (1) Boldenone; (2) Chlorotestosterone (4-chlortestosterone); (3) Clostebol; (4) Dehydrochlormethyltestosterone; (5) Dihydrotestosterone (4-dihydrotestosterone); (6) Drostanolone; (7) Ethylestrenol; (8) Fluoxymesterone; (9) Formebulone (formebolone); (10) Mesterolone; (11) Methandienone; (12) Methandranone; (13) Methandriol; (14) Methandrostenolone; (15) Methenolone; (16) Methyltest-

osterone; (17) Mibolerone; (18) Nandrolone; (19) Norethandrolone; (20) Oxandrolone; (21) Oxymesterone; (22) Oxymetholone; (23) Stanolone; (24) Stanozolol; (25) Testolactone; (26) Testosterone; (27) Trenbolone; (28) Any salt, ester, isomer, or salt of an ester or isomer of a drug or hormonal substance described or listed in division (E)(1) of schedule III if the salt, ester, or isomer promotes muscle growth.

Penalties for possession of steroids in Ohio are located in Ohio Code Title 29, crimes and Procedure, Chapter 2529 Drug Offenses. **First-time illegal possession of steroids is a third degree misdemeanor** under ORC Ann. § 2925.11, Possession of drugs:

No person shall knowingly obtain, possess, or use a controlled substance.

...(C) Whoever violates division (A) of this section is guilty of one of the following:

...(2) If the drug involved in the violation is a compound, mixture, preparation, or substance included in schedule III ..., whoever violates division (A) of this section is guilty of possession of drugs. The penalty for the offense shall be determined as follows:

(a) Except as otherwise provided in division (C)(2)(b), (c), or (d) of this section, possession of drugs is a misdemeanor of the third degree or, if the offender previously has been convicted of a drug abuse offense, a misdemeanor of the second degree. If the drug involved in the violation is an anabolic steroid included in schedule III and if the offense is a misdemeanor of the third degree under this division, in lieu of sentencing the offender to a term of imprisonment in a detention facility, the court may place the offender on conditional probation pursuant to division (F) of section 2951.02 of the Revised Code.

(b) **If the amount of the drug involved equals or exceeds the bulk amount but is less than five times the bulk amount, possession of drugs is a felony of the fourth degree**, and division (C) of section 2929.13 of the Revised Code applies in determining whether to impose a prison term on the offender.

(c) **If the amount of the drug involved equals or exceeds five times the bulk amount but is less than fifty times the bulk amount, possession of drugs is a felony of the third degree**, and there is a presumption for a prison term for the offense.

(d) **If the amount of the drug involved equals or exceeds fifty times the bulk amount, possession of drugs is a felony of the second degree**, and the court shall impose upon the offender as a mandatory prison term one of the prison terms prescribed for a felony of the second degree.

The "bulk amount" for anabolic steroids is defined to be two hundred tablets or sixteen milliliters of substance. The statute reads:

§ 2925.01 Definitions.

As used in this chapter:

(E) "Bulk amount" of a controlled substance means any of the following:

...(11) An amount equal to or exceeding two hundred solid dosage units, sixteen grams, or sixteen milliliters of a compound, mixture, preparation, or substance that is or contains any amount of a schedule III anabolic steroid.

(F) "Unit dose" means an amount or unit of a compound, mixture, or preparation containing a controlled substance, such amount or unit being separately identifiable and in such form as to indicate that it is the amount or unit by which the controlled substance is separately administered to or taken by an individual.

So, possession of two hundred tablets is a felony in the fourth degree and a thousand is a felony of the third degree with a presumption of prison. Only two ten milliliter bottles of testosterone is a felony.

A separate section of the Code, ORC Ann. § 2925.06, specifically proscribes the illegal administration or distribution of anabolic steroids:

(A) No person shall knowingly administer to a human being, or prescribe or dispense for administration to a human being, any anabolic steroid not approved by the United States food and drug administration for administration to human beings.

(B) This section does not apply to any person listed in division (B)(1), (2), or (3) of section 2925.03 of the Revised Code to the extent and under the circumstances described in those divisions.

(C) Whoever violates division (A) of this section is guilty of illegal administration or distribution of anabolic steroids, a felony of the fourth degree, and division (C) of section 2929.13 of the Revised Code applies in determining whether to impose a prison term on the offender.

(D) In addition to any prison term authorized or required by division (C) of this section and sections 2929.13 and 2929.14 of the Revised Code and in addition to any other sanction imposed for the offense under this section or sections 2929.11 to 2929.18 of the Revised Code, the court that sentences an offender who is convicted of or pleads guilty to a violation of division (A) of this section shall do both of the following:

(1) The court shall revoke or suspend the offender's driver's or commercial driver's license or permit in accordance with division (G) of section 2925.03 of the Revised Code. If an offender's driver's or commercial driver's license or permit is revoked in accordance with that division, the offender may request termination of, and the court may terminate, the revocation in accordance with that division.

(2) If the offender is a professionally licensed person or a person who has been admitted to the bar by order of the supreme court in compliance with its prescribed and published rules, the court shall comply with section 2925.38 of the Revised Code.

(E) If a person commits any act that constitutes a violation of division (A) of this section and that also constitutes a violation of any other provision of the Revised Code, the prosecutor, as defined in section 2935.01 of the Revised Code, using customary prosecutorial discretion, may prosecute the person for a violation of the appropriate provision of the Revised Code.

Under § 2925.02, "Corrupting another with drugs" is a separate offense with escalated penalties. It is applicable in various situations, including to those who use force, threat, or deception to induce somebody to use a controlled substance, and to those who furnish drugs to juveniles or involve them in drug trafficking. In the case of anabolic steroids, the crime is a felony of the second degree, and the court must impose a sentence of actual incarceration of three years (five years for prior drug felony offenders). If the crime occurs on school premises, in a school building, or within one thousand feet of the boundaries of any school premises, it's a felony of the first degree, and the court must impose a sentence of actual incarceration of seven years (twelve years for prior drug felony offenders). The section also provides for license revocation or suspension of up to five years.

For the misdemeanor of possession of steroids, Ohio has set limits on its misdemeanor prison sentencing under Title 29 Criminal Procedure, Chapter 29 Sentencing. Under ORC Ann. § 2929.21(B)(3), **a jail sentence for a misdemeanor of the third degree is limited to not more than sixty days**.

For felonies, ORC Ann. § 2929.14 sets forth the basic prison terms.

(A) Except as [otherwise] provided ... the court shall impose a definite prison term that shall be one of the following:

(1) For a felony of the first degree, the prison term shall be three, four, five, six, seven, eight, nine, or ten years.

(2) **For a felony of the second degree, the prison term shall be two, three, four, five, six, seven, or eight years.**

(3) **For a felony of the third degree, the prison term shall be one, two, three, four, or five years.**

(4) **For a felony of the fourth degree, the prison term shall be six, seven, eight, nine, ten, eleven, twelve, thirteen, fourteen, fifteen, sixteen, seventeen, or eighteen months.**

(5) For a felony of the fifth degree, the prison term shall be six, seven, eight, nine, ten, eleven, or twelve months.

Trafficking in drugs is addressed under § 2925.03. This section proscribes most situations of distribution and possession of more substantial amounts. Subsection (A) sets forth the proscribed conduct and subsection (D) sets forth the applicable offense levels. For simplicity, subsection (A) is set forth with the applicable offense levels pursuant to subsection (D) indicated in brackets:

(A) No person shall knowingly do any of the following:

(1) Sell or offer to sell a controlled substance in an amount less than the minimum bulk amount [a felony of the fourth degree; however, it's a felony of the third degree if committed in, on or within 1,000 feet of a school, within one hundred feet of any juvenile or within the view of any juvenile, or where the offender previously has been convicted of a drug offense];

(2) Prepare for shipment, ship, transport, deliver, prepare for distribution, or distribute a controlled substance, when the offender knows or has reasonable cause to believe the controlled substance is intended for sale or resale by the offender or another [a felony of the fourth degree; but a felony of the third degree where the offender previously has been convicted of a drug offense];

(3) Cultivate, manufacture, or otherwise engage in any part of the production of a controlled substance [a felony of the third degree requiring a sentence of actual incarceration of one year; but a felony of the second degree requiring a sentence of actual incarceration of two years where the offender previously has been convicted of a drug offense];

(4) Possess a controlled substance in an amount equal to or exceeding the bulk amount, but in an amount less than three times that amount [a felony of the fourth degree requiring a sentence of actual incarceration of six months; but a felony of the third degree requiring a sentence of actual incarceration of eighteen months where the offender previously has been convicted of a drug offense];

(5) Sell or offer to sell a controlled substance in an amount equal to or exceeding the bulk amount, but in an amount less than three times that amount [a felony of the third degree requiring a sentence of actual incarceration of one year; however, it's a felony of the second degree requiring two years incarceration if committed in, on or within 1,000 feet of a school, within one hundred feet of any juvenile or within the view of any juvenile, or where the offender previously has been convicted of a drug offense];

(6) Possess a controlled substance in an amount equal to or exceeding three times the bulk amount, but in an amount less than one hundred times that amount [a felony of the third degree requiring a sentence of actual incarceration of eighteen months; but a felony of the second degree requiring a sentence of actual incarceration of three years where the offender previously has been convicted of a drug offense];

(7) Sell or offer to sell a controlled substance in an amount equal to or exceeding three times the bulk amount, but in an amount less than one hundred times that amount; [a felony of the second degree requiring a sentence of actual incarceration of two years; however, it's a felony of the first degree requiring four years incarceration if committed in, on or within 1,000 feet of a school, within one hundred feet of any juvenile or within the view of any juvenile, or where the offender previously has been convicted of a drug offense];

(8) Provide money or other items of value to another person with the purpose that the recipient of the money or items of value would use them to obtain controlled substances for the purpose of selling or offering to sell the controlled substances in amounts exceeding a bulk amount or for the purpose of violating division (A)(3) of this section [a felony of the first degree requiring a sentence of actual incarceration of five years; but requiring a sentence of actual incarceration of seven years where the offender previously has been convicted of a drug offense];

(9) Possess a controlled substance in an amount equal to or exceeding one hundred times the bulk amount [a felony of the third degree requiring a sentence of actual incarceration of eighteen months; but a felony of the second degree requiring a sentence of actual incarceration of three years where the offender previously has been convicted of a drug offense];

(10) Sell or offer to sell a controlled substance in an amount equal to or exceeding one hundred times the bulk amount; [a felony of the second degree requiring a sentence of actual incarceration of two years; however, it's a felony of the first degree requiring four years incarceration if committed in, on or within 1,000 feet of a school, within one hundred feet of any juvenile

or within the view of any juvenile, or where the offender previously has been convicted of a drug offense];

(11) Administer to a human being, or prescribe or dispense for administration to a human being, any anabolic steroid not approved by the United States food and drug administration for administration to human beings [a felony of the fourth degree; but a felony of the third degree where the offender previously has been convicted of a drug offense].

Under subsection (F), it's **an affirmative defense to a bulk amount possession charge that the substance was possessed solely for personal use**. *The section also provides for license revocation or suspension of up to five years.* Under subsection (N), a person violating division (A)(11) of this section for administering veterinary or unapproved steroids may be prosecuted for any other appropriate provision of the Revised Code.

Suspended sentence and probation with a fine, community service and drug treatment may be available for first time possession cases. Even a felony charge for possession of more than a bulk amount will likely be granted "community control," which entails a fine, community service and the possibility of some local jail time. License suspension, drug testing and treatment would also follow. Some trafficking offenses may receive community control, dependant upon circumstances such as the quantity involved. Ohio law provides a specific process for avoiding drug convictions in cases involving less serious offenses, which is known as "Intervention in Lieu of Conviction." To be eligible, the defendant must have no prior felony convictions or cases where intervention in lieu of conviction was granted and the charge must be either a misdemeanor or a fourth or fifth degree felony. The program requires the defendant plead guilty to the charge and agree to comply with all the terms and conditions the court imposes. Successful completion of the program will get the case closed without a finding of guilt and in some cases the case may be sealed all together. Drug court may be another available option depending on the jurisdiction.

There is mandatory driver's license suspension for not less than 6 months and up to three years for all drug offenses.

OKLAHOMA

The scheduling of steroids in Oklahoma is located in Oklahoma Statutes Title 63, Public Health and Safety, Chapter 2, Uniform Controlled Dangerous Substances Act. Steroids are defined and listed under 63 Okl. St. § 2-208(A) in Schedule III:

...19.Any material, compound, mixture, or preparation which contains any quantity of the following hormonal substances or steroids, including their salts, isomers, esters and salts of isomers and esters, when the existence of these salts, isomers, esters, and salts of isomers and esters is possible within the specific chemical designation: (a) Boldenone, (b) Chlorotestosterone, (c) Clostebol, (d) Dehydrochlormethyltestosterone, (e) Dihydrotestosterone, (f) Drostanolone, (g) Ethylestrenol, (h) Fluoxymesterone, (i) Formebolone, (j) Mesterolone, (k) Methandienone, (l) Methandranone, (m) Methandriol, (n) Methandrostenolone, (o) Methenolone, (p) Methyltestosterone, except as provided in subsection E of this section, (q) Mibolerone, (r) Nandrolone, (s) Norethandrolone, (t) Oxandrolone, (u) Oxymesterone, (v) Oxymetholone, (w) Stanolone, (x) Stanozolol, (y) Testolactone, (z) Testosterone, except as provided in subsection E of this section, and (aa) Trenbolone. Livestock implants as regulated by the Federal Food and Drug Administration shall be exempt.

Subsection (E) exempts androgen / estrogen combination hormonal substances or steroids from classification as Schedule III controlled dangerous substances:

In Oklahoma, **first time illegal possession of steroids is a misdemeanor** under 63 Okl. St. § 2-402:

A. 1. It shall be unlawful for any person knowingly or intentionally to possess a controlled dangerous substance unless such substance was obtained directly, or pursuant to a valid prescription or order from a practitioner, while acting in the course of his professional practice, or except as otherwise authorized by this act.

... B. Any person who violates this section with respect to:

...2. Any [Schedule III substance] is guilty of a misdemeanor punishable by confinement for not more than one (1) year. A second or subsequent violation of this section with respect to any [Schedule III substance] is a felony punishable by imprisonment for not less than two (2) years nor more than ten (10) years.

Leniency is extended to possession first offenders under § 2-410:

> Whenever any person who has not previously been convicted of any [drug] ... pleads guilty to or is found guilty of possession of a controlled dangerous substance under Section 63-2-402, the court may, without entering a judgment of guilt and with the consent of such person, defer further proceedings and place him on probation upon such reasonable terms and conditions as it may require including the requirement that such person cooperate in a treatment and rehabilitation program of a state-supported or state-approved facility, if available. Upon violation of a term or condition, the court may enter an adjudication of guilt and proceed as otherwise provided. Upon fulfillment of the terms and conditions, the court shall discharge such person and dismiss the proceedings against him. Discharge and dismissal under this section shall be without court adjudication of guilt and shall not be deemed a conviction for purposes of this section or for purposes of disqualifications or disabilities imposed by law upon conviction of a crime. Discharge and dismissal under this section may occur only once with respect to any person.
>
> Any expunged arrest or conviction shall not thereafter be regarded as an arrest or conviction for purposes of employment, civil rights, or any statute, regulation, license, questionnaire or any other public or private purpose; provided, that, any such plea of guilty or finding of guilt shall constitute a conviction of the offense for the purpose of this act or any other criminal statute under which the existence of a prior conviction is relevant.

Distribution crimes involving steroids are covered by § 2-401:

Prohibited acts A—Penalties

A. Except as authorized ... it shall be unlawful for any person:

1. To distribute, dispense, transport with intent to distribute or dispense, possess with intent to manufacture, distribute, or dispense, a controlled dangerous substance or to solicit the use of or use the services of a person less than eighteen (18) years of age to cultivate, distribute or dispense a controlled dangerous substance;

...B. Any person who violates the provisions of this section with respect to:

...2. Any [Schedule III substance], upon conviction, shall be guilty of a felony and **shall be sentenced to a term of imprisonment for not less than two (2) years nor more than life** and a fine of not more than Twenty Thousand Dollars ($ 20,000.00), which shall be in addition to other punishment provided by law and shall not be imposed in lieu of other punishment. Any sentence to the custody of the Department of Corrections shall not be subject to statutory provisions for suspended sentences, deferred sentences, or probation except when the conviction is for a first offense;

Second or subsequent violations face doubled terms of imprisonment under subsection (D), and subsection (F) establishes harsher penalties for offenses within 2,000 feet of schools, public parks and housing projects. Adults who use minors to distribute steroids or who distribute steroids to minors under subsection (E) also face doubled prison terms. [A separate section of law, 63 Okl. St. § 2-419.1, also provides for doubled imprisonment for involving minors in the drug trade, with even more serious punishments for subsequent offenses and for using minors under fifteen in drug transactions.]

In 1994, Oklahoma enacted a Drug Dealer Liability Act establishing civil liability under Sec 2-423 against certain persons who knowingly participate in the drug trade by certain aggrieved parties who are injured from use of illegal drugs. Section 2-424 sets out the persons eligible to bring actions for damages, including parents, guardians, employers, and medical and drug treatment programs that expended money on behalf of the individual drug user.

Oklahoma 63 Okl. St. § 2-312.1 focuses on anabolic steroids and health care practitioners:

> A. A licensed practitioner ... shall not prescribe, dispense, deliver, or administer an anabolic steroid or human growth hormone or cause an anabolic steroid or human growth hormone to be administered under the direction or supervision of the practitioner except for a valid medical purpose and in the course of a professional practice. A valid medical purpose for the use of anabolic steroids or human growth hormones shall not include bodybuilding, muscle enhancement or increasing muscle bulk or strength of a person who is in good health. This section shall not prohibit the use of anabolic steroids for the treatment of livestock or domestic animals in accordance with state or federal law.
>
> B. The prescribing, dispensing, delivering or administering of an anabolic steroid by a licensed practitioner in violation of the provisions of subsection A of this section shall be grounds for revocation or nonrenewal of the license of such licensed practitioner to practice in this state. In addition, any licensed practitioner prescribing, dispensing, delivering or administering an anabolic steroid in violation of the provisions of subsection A of this section, upon conviction thereof shall be guilty of a felony punishable by imprisonment in the State Penitentiary for a term of not more than three (3) years, or by a fine not to exceed Ten Thousand Dollars ($10,000.00), or by both such imprisonment and fine.

Note that **subsection (A) explicitly prevents physicians from administering either anabolic steroids or human growth hormone for bodybuilding. However, perhaps due to an oversight, the wording of subsection (B), the penalties provision, only refers to anabolic steroids and fails to include human growth hormone.**

Simple possession cases are eligible for deferred prosecution or deferred sentence, based on quantity. To be eligible for Drug Court, the defendant must have at least two prior felony drug charges. Possession with intent to distribute cases may be eligible for a suspended sentence. Distribution cases are likely to face jail time.

Driver's license revocation is mandatory based on adjudication on the merits.

OREGON

In the Oregon Revised Statutes, Chapter 475 covers Controlled Substances. The term "controlled substance" is defined in ORS § 475.005:

> (6) "Controlled substance" means a drug or its immediate precursor classified in Schedules I through V under the federal Controlled Substances Act, 21 U.S.C. 811 to 812, as modified [by the State Board of Pharmacy].

So, Oregon controlled substances are those listed federally, unless modified by the Oregon Board of Pharmacy, which has the responsibility for implementing and regulating the chapters of the Oregon Statutes dealing with controlled substances and pharmacists. Modifications are set forth in the Oregon Administrative Rules, Chapter 855, Division 080, Board of Pharmacy, which is available online as an Adobe Acrobat document at www.pharmacy.state.or.us/rules/div080.pdf. The Oregon Schedule III list under 855-080-0023 is not anabolic steroids, but a list of what are called "Anabolic Substances" in (5)(a) through (bb):

> Anabolic Substances. Any quantity of the following substances or its isomer, ester, salt or derivative except that anabolic substances in a dosage form approved by the Food and Drug Administration for administration through implants to cattle or other nonhuman species shall not be classified as con-

trolled substances: (a) Boldenone; (b) Chlorotestosterone (4-chlortestosterone); (c) Clostebol; (d) Dehydrochlormethyltestosterone; (e) Dihydrotestosterone (4-dihydrotestosterone); (f) Dostanolone; (g) Ethylestrenol; (h) Fluoxymesterone; (i) Formebulone (formebolone); (j) Human growth hormone; (k) Mesterolone; (l) Methandienone; (m) Methandranone; (n) Methandriol; (o) Methandrostenolone; (p) Methenolone; (q) Methyltestosterone; (r) Mibolerone; (s) Nandrolone; (t) Norethandrolone; (u) Oxandrolone; (v) Oxymesterone; (w) Oxymetholone; (x) Stanolone; (y) Stanozolol; (z) Testolactone; (aa) Testosterone; (bb) Trenbolone.

Note that "Human growth hormone" is a controlled substance in Oregon. Note that Oregon departs from the federal definition by omitting any general or catch-all phrase. If a substance is not listed and is not an isomer, ester, salt or derivative of a listed substance, by what authority is it then a controlled substance? Under ORS § 475.005, does the Oregon rule replace the federal schedule, or simply "modify" it?

Simple AAS of hGH possession is a Class A misdemeanor under subsection (4) of ORS 475.992:

> (4) It is unlawful for any person knowingly or intentionally to possess a controlled substance unless the substance was obtained directly from, or pursuant to, a valid prescription or order of a practitioner while acting in the course of professional practice, or except as otherwise authorized by ORS 475.005 to 475.285 and 475.940 to 475.999. Any person who violates this subsection with respect to:
> ...(c) A controlled substance in Schedule III, is guilty of a Class A misdemeanor.

In Oregon, "Deliver" or "Delivery" is defined in ORS § 475.005(8) to mean "the actual, constructive or attempted transfer, other than by administering or dispensing, from one person to another of a controlled substance, whether or not there is an agency relationship." (Administering and dispensing refer to "practitioners," which includes physicians, veterinarians and others but not pharmacists) **Manufacturing or delivering a controlled substance is a Class C felony** under ORS § 475.992:

> (1) Except as authorized ... it is unlawful for any person to manufacture or deliver a controlled substance. Any person who violates this subsection with respect to:
> ...(c) A controlled substance in Schedule III, is guilty of a Class C felony.

Penalties for delivery to minors is covered by ORS § 475.995:

> Except as authorized ... , it is unlawful for any person to deliver a controlled substance to a person under 18 years of age. Any person who violates this section with respect to:
> ...(2) A controlled substance in Schedule III, is guilty of a Class B felony.

Sentencing for controlled substance violations is governed by Chapter 161. ORS § 161.615 sets forth the prison terms for misdemeanors:

> Sentences for misdemeanors shall be for a definite term. The court shall fix the term of imprisonment within the following maximum limitations:
> (1) For a Class A misdemeanor, 1 year.
> (2) For a Class B misdemeanor, 6 months.
> (3) For a Class C misdemeanor, 30 days.

Under ORS § 161.605, the maximum prison terms for felonies are set forth:

> The maximum term of an indeterminate sentence of imprisonment for a felony is as follows:
> (1) For a Class A felony, 20 years.
> (2) For a Class B felony, 10 years.
> (3) **For a Class C felony, 5 years.**

Aggravating factors may enhance sentencing. Under § 475.996, certain conduct under ORS § 475.992 requires enhanced crime category classification as a "commercial drug offense." Section 475.999 makes it a Class A felony to manufacture or deliver a schedule III controlled substance within 1,000 feet of a school.

Various mechanisms for leniency exist. Section 475.245 provides for "Conditional discharge" in simple personal use cases. The section provides for probation without entering a judgment of guilt and deferment of the proceedings in cases of drug dependence. The district attorney must consent and this provision is available one time only. Also, under ORS § 137.533, the court may impose probation without entering judgment of guilt upon first offenders in misdemeanor cases. Additionally, Chapter 135, covering Arraignments and Pretrial Provisions, provides for "Diversion" – referral of the accused to a supervised performance program prior to adjudication.. Section 135.886 sets forth the factors to be considered by the district attorney before offering a diversion agreement to the accused. Under Section 135.901, if the accused fulfills the terms of the diversion agreement, the case is dismissed. Even where a sentence of imprisonment is imposed, ORS § 137.010 gives the judge the power to suspend the imposition or execution of any part of a sentence for any period of not more than five years. The court may also impose and execute a sentence of probation on the defendant for a definite or indefinite period of not more than five years. Upon a later finding that a defendant sentenced to probation for a felony has violated his probation, the court may, if it wishes to, order the period of both the suspended sentence and the sentence of probation extended until a date not more than six years from the date of original imposition of sentence.

Simple possession cases may be eligible for the STOP Program, which is the Oregon version of Drug Court. To be eligible for this program you must have no prior convictions and you must stipulate to the information in the police report. This is an intensive program with continuous monitoring and visits with a treatment provider up to five times per week for six weeks. Successful completion of the program will result in dismissal while unsuccessful completion might result in a conviction or removal into the new "clean court" program. This is a more intensive program and the rules and criteria are changing regularly. Sale or delivery cases may receive treatment, work release or community service, if the quantities are small and the offense is minor.

Driver's license suspension is discretionary rather than mandatory for drug crimes.

PENNSYLVANIA

The Pennsylvania Statutes address anabolic steroids in Title 35, Health and Safety. All "Drugs, Poisons and Dangerous Substances" are covered in the Controlled Substance, Drug, Device, and Cosmetic Act.

Anabolic steroids are defined under the Controlled Substance, Drug, Device, and Cosmetic Act, Pennsylvania Statutes Title 35, Chapter 6. They are classified as schedule III controlled substances. 35 P.S. § 780-104(3):

> (vii) Anabolic steroid includes any material, compound, mixture or preparation that includes any of the following or any isomer, ester, salt or derivative of any of the following that acts in the same manner on the human body: 1. Chorionic gonadotropin. 2. Clostebol. 3. Dehydrochlormethyltestosterone. 4. Ethylestrenol. 5. Fluoxymesterone. 6. Mesterolone. 7. Metenolone. 8. Methandienone. 9. Methandrostenolone. 10. Methyltestosterone. 11. Nandrolone decanoate. 12. Nandrolone phenpropionate. 13. Norethandrolone. 14. Oxandrolone. 15. Oxymesterone. 16. Oxymetholone. 17. Stanozolol. 18. Testosterone propionate. 19. Testosterone-like related compounds. Human Growth Hormone (HGH) shall not be included as an anabolic steroid under the provisions of this act. An anabolic steroid which is a combination of estrogen and anabolic steroid and which is expressly intended for administration to hormone-deficient women shall be exempt from the provisions of this act. A person who prescribes, dispenses or distributes an anabolic steroid which is a combination of estrogen and anabolic steroids and which is intended for administration to hormone-deficient women for use by persons who are not hormone-deficient women shall be considered to have prescribed, dispensed or distributed an anabolic steroid within the meaning of this subclause.

Pennsylvania departs from the federal law. The law apparently intends to cover substances that are not explicitly listed (like stanolone, for example) under the catch-all phrase "Testosterone-like related compounds." Note that there is no requirement that these unidentified compounds promote muscle growth. The inherent vagueness in this term leaves open the question of exactly what substances (including, for example, over-the-counter sports supplements) might be regarded as "like" or "related" to testosterone. Mixed androgen/estrogens are excluded in the statute, but cattle implants are not addressed. **Unlike most States, Pennsylvania has included human chorionic gonadotropin (HCG) as an anabolic steroid and has explicitly excluded human growth hormone (hGH).**

Prohibited conduct regarding controlled substances is set forth in subsection (a) of 35 P.S. § 780-113. **Typical situations of illegal personal use possession of steroids or HCG carry a misdemeanor charge, as does the intentional purchase or knowing receipt of steroids or HCG.** Subsection (b) sets forth the penalties. For simplicity, the applicable sentencing to each clause is set forth in brackets.

35 P.S. § 780-113:

(a) The following acts and the causing thereof within the Commonwealth are hereby prohibited:

...(16) Knowingly or intentionally possessing a controlled ... substance by a person not registered under this act, or a practitioner not registered or licensed by the appropriate State board, unless the substance was obtained directly from, or pursuant to, a valid prescription order or order of a practitioner, or except as otherwise authorized by this act [punishment is of up to one year imprisonment and/or up to a $ 5,000 fine]

...(19) The intentional purchase or knowing receipt in commerce by any person of any controlled substance, other drug or device from any person not authorized by law to sell, distribute, dispense or otherwise deal in such controlled substance, other drug or device [punishment is of up to three years imprisonment and/or up to a $ 5,000 fine].

...(37) The possession by any person, other than a registrant, of more than thirty doses labeled as a dispensed prescription or more than three trade packages of any anabolic steroids listed in section 4(3)(vii) [punishment is of up to one year imprisonment and/or up to a $ 5,000 fine].

Subsection (b) makes each of these acts a misdemeanor. **Aside from the problem of calling a crime with up to three years in jail a misdemeanor, it seems capricious if not bizarre to punish the act of obtaining steroids more seriously than the act of then having them!** Enhanced punishment applies to repeat offenders.

Regarding distribution, under 35 P.S. § 780-113(a)(30), the following acts are prohibited:

(30)Except as authorized by this act, the manufacture, delivery, or possession with intent to manufacture or deliver, a controlled substance by a person not registered under this act, or a practitioner not registered or licensed by the appropriate State board,...

The prison term for distribution acts can be as much as five years, under subsection (f):

(f) Any person who violates clause ... (30) of subsection (a) with respect to:

(2) Any other [Schedule III controlled substance], is guilty of a felony and upon conviction thereof shall be sentenced to imprisonment not exceeding five years, or to pay a fine not exceeding fifteen thousand dollars ($ 15,000), or both.

Under 35 P.S. § 780-114, distribution to persons under age eighteen can escalate punishment:

Any person who is at least twenty-one years of age and who is not himself a drug dependent person who violates this act by distributing a controlled substance listed in schedules I through V to a person under eighteen years of age who is at least four years his junior is punishable by a term of imprison-

> ment up to twice that otherwise authorized by subsection (f) of section 13 of this act, in addition to any fine authorized by this act.

Pennsylvania provides for, under § 780-117, probation without verdict for certain first-time "drug dependent" offenders. However, for the purposes of proving drug dependency, the person must present the testimony of a physician or psychologist trained in the field of drug abuse. Further, the statute, subsection (1)(vi), makes those charged under clauses (30) and (37) ineligible – so those with more than three trade packages of anabolic steroids are ineligible.

Another provision for one-time-only leniency is contained in § 780-118: Disposition In Lieu Of Trial Or Criminal Punishment. This section applies if a person charged with a nonviolent crime claims to be drug dependent or a drug abuser requests, prior to trial, appropriate treatment in lieu of criminal prosecution. A physician experienced or trained in the field of drug dependency or drug abuse is appointed by the court to examine, if necessary, and to review the accused's record and advise in writing if for the treatment and rehabilitation of the accused it would be preferable for the criminal charges to be held in abeyance or withdrawn in order to institute treatment for drug dependence, or for the criminal charges to be prosecuted. With the consent of the government and the court, the criminal charge may be held in abeyance and may not be prosecuted except by order of court so long as the medical director of the treatment facility certifies that the accused is cooperating in a prescribed treatment program and is benefiting from treatment. At the expiration of a certain period, the criminal charge is automatically dismissed. Pennsylvania statutes also provide limited ability for Expunging Criminal Records pursuant to § 780-119.

Under 35 P.S. § 807.1, Pennsylvania mandates school directors to prohibit steroids:

> The board of school directors in every school district in this Commonwealth shall prescribe, adopt and enforce rules and regulations to prohibit the use of anabolic steroids, except for a valid medical purpose, by any pupil involved in school-related athletics. **Bodybuilding, muscle enhancement, increasing muscle bulk or strength or the enhancement of athletic ability is not a valid medical purpose. Human Growth Hormone (HGH) shall not be included as an anabolic steroid under the provisions of this act.**

A drug court has recently been instituted in parts of Pennsylvania, though it is limited to individuals who have a drug or alcohol problem, who do not have a serious criminal conviction, and who have a minimum of three felonies, usually level 3 or 4 repeat offenders. First time possession cases may be eligible for a diversionary program known as Accelerated Rehabilitative Disposition. Another possibility is probation without verdict, though this is a remedy usually limited to marijuana cases.

Sale cases face a more limited set of options and they often go to trial. Depending on the level of cooperation and the individual's drug history, offenders may be able to receive a better deal.

In Pennsylvania there is mandatory license revocation for some drug convictions.

* * *

PUERTO RICO

Controlled substances are dealt with in the Laws of Puerto Rico Annotated, Title 24, Health and Sanitation, Part V, Controlled Substances Act of Puerto Rico. Under 24 L.P.R.A. § 2102(7), a controlled substance is a drug or substance included in the five schedules that have been created under § 2202. **Anabolic steroids are not a controlled substance under any of Puerto Rico's five schedules**. They are prescription drugs, pursuant to 24 L.P.R.A. § 712. Trafficking operations could be prosecuted under criminal enterprise or conspiracy theories, and, of course, anabolics remain controlled substances under federal law and both possession and distribution could be prosecuted in federal court.

RHODE ISLAND

In Rhode Island, steroids are classified as schedule III controlled substances under the Uniform Controlled Substances Act, General Laws of Rhode Island Title 21, Food and Drugs, Chapter 21-28. The classification of schedules is located in Article II. R.I. Gen. Laws § 21-28-2.08, Schedule III:

(d) Anabolic Steroids (AS) or Human Growth Hormone (HGH), excluding those compounds, mixtures, or preparations containing an anabolic steroid that because of its concentration, preparation, mixture or delivery system, has no significant potential for abuse, as published in the United States Code of Federal Regulations, 21 CFR Part 1308.34, including but not limited to the following: (1) Chorionic gonadotropin (2) Clostebol (3) Dehydrochlormethyltestosterone (4) Ethylestrenol (5) Fluoxymesterone (6) Mesterolone (7) Metenolone (8) Methandienone (9) Methandrostenolone (10) Methyltestosterone (11) Nandrolone decanoate (12) Nandrolone phenpropionate (13) Norethandrolone (14) Oxandrolone (15) Oxymesterone (16) Oxymetholone (17) Stanozolol (18) Testosterone propionate (19) Testosterone-like related compounds (20) Human Growth Hormone (HGH)

Rhode Island schedules not only steroids, but both HCG and hGH. While the law explicitly states that the brief list of compounds is all-inclusive, there are a few perplexing aspects. What are "testosterone-like related compounds"? If they mean testosterone esters, why include testosterone propionate, and why leave out the other popular esters? And why leave out stanolone? Obviously, Rhode Island constructed the language of its statute rather than parroting the federal list. How then did it repeat the federal error of redundantly including both methandienone and methandrostenolone?

Offenses and sentencing provisions for controlled substances in schedule III are set forth under the Rhode Island Uniform Controlled Substances Act, Title 21 Chapter 28. **Regarding simple unlawful possession, it's a felony with up to three years imprisonment** under R.I. Gen. Laws § 21-28-4.01(C) states:

(C) It shall be unlawful for any person knowingly or intentionally to possess a controlled substance unless the substance was obtained directly from or pursuant to, a valid prescription or order of a practitioner while acting in the course of his or her professional practice, or except as otherwise authorized by this chapter.

(1) Any person who violates this subsection with respect to:

(a) A controlled substance classified in [schedule III] is guilty of a crime and upon conviction may be imprisoned for not more than three (3) years or fined not less than five hundred dollars ($500) nor more than five thousand dollars ($5,000), or both;

... (2) Additionally every person convicted or who pleads nolo contendere under subsection (C)(1)(a) or convicted or who pleads nolo contendere a second or subsequent time under subsection (C)(1)(b) above, who is not sentenced to a term of imprisonment to serve for the offense, shall be required to:

(a) Perform no less than one hundred (100) hours of community service;

(b) Be referred to Treatment Alternatives to Street Crime (TASC) to determine the existence of problems of drug abuse. Should TASC determine the person needs treatment, it will arrange for said treatment to be provided and after completion of said treatment, the person shall perform his or her required community service and attend the drug education program.

(c) Attend and complete a drug counseling and education program as prescribed by the director of the department of health and pay the sum of four hundred dollars ($400) to help defray the costs of this program which shall be deposited as general revenues. Failure to attend may result after hearing by the court in jail sentence up to one year;

(d) The court shall not suspend any part or all of the imposition of the fee required by this subsection, unless the court finds an inability to pay.

(e) If the offense involves the use of any automobile to transport the substance or the substance is found within an automobile, then a person convicted or who pleads nolo contendere under those subsections shall be subject to a loss of license for a period of six (6) months for a first offense and one year for each offense thereafter.

A separate subsection (E) addresses physicians or other practitioners specifically with respect to anabolic steroids:

> (E) It shall be **unlawful for a practitioner to prescribe, order, distribute, supply, or sell an anabolic steroid or human growth hormone for (i) enhancing performance in an exercise, sport, or game, or (ii) hormonal manipulation intended to increase muscle mass, strength, or weight without a medical necessity**. Any person who violates this subsection is guilty of a misdemeanor and upon conviction may be imprisoned for not more than six (6) months or a fine of not more than one thousand dollars ($1,000), or both.

Distribution crimes involving schedule III drugs are proscribed under subsection (A) of R.I. Gen. Laws § 21-28-4.01, but steroids **are treated differently than other schedule III substances – the maximum first-offense penalty for anabolic steroids, HCG and hGH is five years** as compared to twenty years for other substances in the very same schedule:

> (A) Except as authorized by this chapter, it shall be unlawful for any person to manufacture, deliver, or possess with intent to manufacture or deliver a controlled substance.
>
> ... (2) Any person, except as provided for in subsection (A)(1) who violates this subsection with respect to:
>
> ...(b) A controlled substance classified in schedule III ... is guilty of a crime and upon conviction may be imprisoned for not more than twenty (20) years, or fined not more than forty thousand dollars ($40,000), or both; provided, however, with respect to a controlled substance classified in schedule III(d) [anabolic steroids and growth hormone] upon conviction may be imprisoned for not more than five (5) years, or fined not more than twenty thousand dollars ($20,000), or both.

Under § 21-28-4.11, second offenders face imprisonment for a term up to twice the term otherwise authorized, and under § 21-28-4.14, third or subsequent offenders may be imprisoned for a term up to three (3) times the term otherwise authorized.

R.I. Gen. Laws § 21-28-4.07 makes an adult who distributes a schedule III substance to a person under eighteen (18) years of age who is at least three (3) years his or her junior punishable by a prison term of between five and twenty years.

Mechanisms for leniency are found in Title 12, Criminal Procedure. Chapter 12-18, Probation provides, under § 12-18-3, for a plea of "nolo contendere" to be followed by probation. § 12-19-8 and 12-19-13 provide for suspension of sentence, in whole or in part, and a term of probation in lieu of imprisonment. Rhode Island makes a special statutory provision for snitches. § 21-28-4.19 permits reduction of an imposed sentence upon receipt motion by the department of the attorney general based upon the person's demonstrated cooperation with law enforcement authorities in the investigation and prosecution of drug violations.

SOUTH CAROLINA

The Code of Laws of South Carolina lists its Schedule III substances in 44-43-230, and anabolic steroids are not included. Although technically unscheduled, steroids are criminalized by a special article contained in the Code of Laws of South Carolina, Title 44, Health, Chapter 53 Poisons, Drugs, and other Controlled Substances. Article 14 of that Chapter is entitled Anabolic Steroids, and it covers definitions, offenses, and penalties. The definition (missing many common substances, and without a catch-all provision) is contained in S.C. Code Ann. § 44-53-1510:

(A) The term "anabolic steroid" includes any of the following or any isomer, ester, salt, or derivative of the following that acts in the same manner on the human body: (1) clostebol; (2) dehydrochlormethyltestosterone; (3) ethylestrenol; (4) fluoxymesterone;(5) mesterolone; (6) methandienone; (7) methandrostenolone; (8) methenolone; (9) methyltestosterone; (10) nandrolone; (11) norethandrolone; (12) oxandrolone; (13) oxymesterone; (14) oxymetholone; (15) stanozolol; and (16) testosterone.

(B) Anabolic steroids that are expressly intended for administration through implants to cattle or other nonhuman species, and that are approved by the federal Food and Drug Administration for this use, are not considered anabolic steroids as defined by this article and are not governed by its provisions.

Possessing anabolic steroids without a prescription is proscribed by S.C. Code Ann. § 44-53-1530(2). It is unlawful for any person who is not a practitioner, pharmacist, or veterinarian to knowingly or intentionally possess anabolic steroids unless obtained directly from, or pursuant to a valid prescription or order of, a practitioner while acting in the course of his professional practice. The seriousness of the offense is based on the quantity of dosage units possessed, and sets forth the potential prison terms:

(2) **possession of ten or fewer dosage units of anabolic steroids without a valid prescription is guilty of a misdemeanor** and, upon conviction, must be punished as follows:
   (a) for a **first offense, imprisoned for a term not to exceed six months** or fined in an amount not to exceed one thousand dollars;
   (b) for a second or subsequent offense, imprisoned for a term not to exceed one year or fined in an amount not to exceed two thousand dollars, or both;

(3) **possession of more than ten but fewer than one hundred dosage-units of anabolic steroids without a valid prescription is guilty of a misdemeanor** and, upon conviction, must be punished as follows:
   (a) for a **first offense, imprisoned for a term not to exceed one year** or fined in an amount not to exceed two thousand dollars, or both;
   (b) for a second or subsequent offense, imprisoned for a term not to exceed two years or fined in an amount not to exceed three thousand dollars, or both;

(4) **possession of more than one hundred dosage-units of anabolic steroids without a valid prescription is guilty of a felony** and, upon conviction, must be punished as follows:
   (a) for a **first offense, imprisoned for a term not to exceed five years** or fined in an amount not to exceed five thousand dollars, or both;
   (b) for a second or subsequent offense, imprisoned for a term not to exceed ten years or fined in an amount not to exceed ten thousand dollars, or both.

Dosage-units of anabolic steroids or even of controlled substances are not defined. Should they be measured by individual tablets or under the federal discount? Perhaps the following provision from Title 44, Health, Chapter 53, Poisons, Drugs and Other Controlled Substances, may weigh against the federal discount interpretation:

SECTION 44-53-360. Prescriptions.

(e) Prescriptions for controlled substances in Schedules II through V, inclusive, must not exceed one hundred twenty-four dosage units or a thirty-one day supply in accordance with dosage instructions, whichever quantity is the lesser....

Misdemeanor sentences may be suspended, in the discretion of the circuit judge, pursuant to Section 17-25-100, found in Title 17, Criminal Procedures; Chapter 25, Judgment and Execution.

Illegal distribution conduct is covered by S.C. Code Ann. § 44-53-1530(1), which makes it a felony for any person who is not a practitioner, pharmacist, or veterinarian to knowingly or intentionally prescribe, dispense, deliver, or administer anabolic steroids to a person. Any person who violates this article with respect to:

(1) prescription, dispensation, delivery, or administration of an anabolic steroid, or delivery of an anabolic steroid to a person for human use without any purpose other than a valid medical purpose, or the sale or delivery of an anabolic steroid to a person for human use without a valid prescription, or the prescription, dispensation, delivery, or administration of an anabolic steroid to a person by any person who is not a practitioner, pharmacist, or veterinarian, is guilty of a felony and, upon conviction, must be punished as follows:
(a) for a **first offense, imprisoned for a term not to exceed five years** or fined in an amount not to exceed five thousand dollars, or both;
(b) for a second or subsequent offense, imprisoned for a term not to exceed ten years or fined in an amount not to exceed ten thousand dollars, or both;

Chapter 1 of Title 16, Crimes and Offenses, Section 16-1-10(A) classifies felonies into six categories and misdemeanors into three categories. Under Section 16-1-90, first offenses under subsection § 44-53-1530(1)(a) are Class F felonies, while second or subsequent offenses are Class E felonies.

A separate section addresses the conduct of practitioners with respect to anabolic steroids:

§ 44-53-1520. Unprofessional conduct to dispense under certain circumstances.
It is unprofessional conduct, and is not a valid medical purpose, for a practitioner or veterinarian to prescribe, dispense, or administer an anabolic steroid, or a pharmacist to dispense an anabolic steroid, for the purpose of the hormonal manipulation that is intended to increase muscle mass, strength, or weight without a medical necessity to do so, or for the intended purpose of improving performance in any form of exercise, sport, or game.

South Carolina has a Pretrial Intervention Act. It's found in Title 17, Criminal Procedures, Chapter 22. Upon successful completion of the program, the offender receives a non-criminal disposition of case and may apply to the court for an order to destroy all official records relating to the arrest.

According to South Carolina criminal defense practitioners, it is unlikely that a first time steroid offender who possesses or possesses with intent to distribute will receive a jail sentence. What the defendant would most likely face is pre-trial intervention as stated above, or what is commonly known as a "PTI." PTI is a state and county diversionary program. There is no admission of guilt; however the agreement of the district attorney is required. PTI does not require approval or commitment by the judge. Nonetheless, the background of the individual must reflect that they have not previously been in the program. Essentially, the program is intense probation for 90-days which costs $400.00, requires the following: self-reporting and no probation agent, 100 hours of community service, a tour of a prison, random drug testing, drug counseling, a written paper by the defendant and that he remains out of trouble. If the program is completed successfully the record is subject to being expunged. If the defendant's record is sufficient to keep him from getting into PTI, he most likely will receive probation.

Nonetheless, despite the above punishment which appears less strict, the suspension of driving privileges can be quite harsh. *With regard to scheduled drugs, there is a mandatory driver's license suspension for a period of one year for each count.* If the defendant is a first time offender who is either a full-time student or full-time employee who lives or works more than one mile from school or work, and it would be impractical to use mass transit, they may apply for a provisional driver's license.

SOUTH DAKOTA

In the State of South Dakota, anabolic steroids are classified as a schedule III controlled substance. They are defined and listed under South Dakota Codified Laws, Title 34 Public Health and Safety; Chapter 34-20B, Drugs and Substances Control. Steroids are listed under S.D. Codified Laws § 34-20B-22:

> The following are included in Schedule III:
> ...(3) Anabolic steroids as listed in § 34-20B-4.1;

S.D. Codified Laws § 34-20B-4.1 defines the term:

> An anabolic steroid is any drug or hormonal substance, chemically and pharmacologically related to testosterone, other than estrogens, progestins and corticosteroids, that promotes muscle growth and includes: (1) Bolandiol (2) Bolasterone (3) Boldenone (4) Bolenol (5) Bolmantalate (6) Chlortestosterone (7) Clostebol (8) Dehydrochlormethyltestosterone (9) Dihydrotestosterone (10) Dimethazine (11) Drostanolone (12) Ethylestrenol (13) Fluoxymesterone (14) Formebolone (15) Mesterolone (16) Metanabol (17) Methandienone (18) Methandriol (19) Methandrostenolone (20) Methenolone (21) Methyltestosterone (22) Mibolerone (23) Nandrolone (24) Nisterime (25) Norethandrolone (26) Oxandrolone (27) Oxymesterone (28) Oxymetholone (29) Pizotyline (30) Silandrone (31) Stanolone (32) Stanozolol (33) Stenbolone (34) Testolactone (35) Testosterone (36) Tibolone (37) Trenbolone (38) Trestolone (39) Any salt, ester or isomer of a drug or substance described or listed in this section, if that salt, ester or isomer promotes muscle growth.
>
> The term anabolic steroid as defined in this section does not include an anabolic steroid which is expressly intended for administration through implants to cattle or other nonhuman species. However, if any person prescribes, dispenses or distributes such a steroid for human use, the person shall be considered to have prescribed, dispensed or distributed an anabolic steroid within the meaning of this section.

Possession of controlled substances including anabolic steroids without a prescription is a Class 4 felony, proscribed by S.D. Codified Laws, Title 22, Crimes; Chapter 42, Controlled Substances and Marijuana. Unlawful personal use possession is a felony under S.D. Codified Laws § 22-42-5:

> No person may knowingly possess a controlled drug or substance unless the substance was obtained directly or pursuant to a valid prescription or order from a practitioner, while acting in the course of the practitioner's professional practice or except as otherwise authorized by chapter 34-20B. A violation of this section is a Class 4 felony.

Surreptitiously seeing multiple doctors to get a greater quantity of steroids is a misdemeanor, even if you're not caught in possession of the tained concurrently from different medical practitioners – Misdemeanor. Any person who knowingly obtains a controlled substance from a medical practitioner and who knowingly withholds information from that medical practitioner that he has obtained a controlled substance of similar therapeutic use in a concurrent time period from another medical practitioner is guilty of a Class 1 misdemeanor.

Situations of manufacture, distribution or possession with intent to distribute are addressed in a separate section, and are Class 5 felonies, with a thirty day minimum sentence on a first offense:

> 22-42-3. Unauthorized manufacture, distribution, counterfeiting, or possession of substance with moderate potential for abuse as felony – Mandatory sentences. Except as authorized by this chap-

> ter or chapter 34-20B, no person may manufacture, distribute, or dispense a substance listed in Schedule III; possess with intent to manufacture, distribute, or dispense, a substance listed in Schedule III; create or distribute a counterfeit substance listed in Schedule III; or possess with intent to distribute a counterfeit substance listed in Schedule III. A violation of this section is a Class 5 felony. However, the distribution of a substance listed in Schedule III to a minor is a Class 3 felony. A first conviction under this section shall be punished by a mandatory sentence in the state penitentiary or county jail of at least thirty days, which sentence may not be suspended. A second or subsequent conviction under this section shall be punished by a mandatory penitentiary or county jail sentence of at least one year, which sentence may not be suspended. However, a first conviction for distribution to a minor under this section shall be punished by a mandatory sentence in the state penitentiary or county jail of at least ninety days, which sentence may not be suspended. A second or subsequent conviction for distribution to a minor under this section shall be punished by a mandatory sentence in the state penitentiary of at least two years, which sentence may not be suspended. A civil penalty may be imposed, in addition to any criminal penalty, upon a conviction of a violation of this section not to exceed ten thousand dollars.

It seems that under the strange laws of South Dakota, distributing steroids (a Class 5 felony) is viewed less seriously than simply possessing them for personal use (a Class 4 felony). Go figure.

Other sections exist by which aggravating circumstances can escalate the severity of a case:

> 22-42-19. Drug free zones created – Violation as felony – Sentence – Defense. Any person who commits a violation of [§ 22-42-3], if such activity has taken place:
> (1) In, on, or within one thousand feet of real property comprising a public or private elementary or secondary school or a playground; or
> (2) In, on, or within five hundred feet of real property comprising a public or private youth center, public swimming pool, or video arcade facility, is guilty of a Class 4 felony. The sentence imposed for a conviction under this section carries a minimum sentence of imprisonment in the state penitentiary of five years. Any sentence imposed under this section shall be consecutive to any other sentence imposed for the principal felony. The court may not place on probation, suspend the execution of the sentence, or suspend the imposition of the sentence of any person convicted of a violation of this section. However, the sentencing court may impose a sentence other than that specified in this section if the court finds that mitigating circumstances exist which require a departure from the mandatory sentence provided for in this section. The court's finding of mitigating circumstances allowed by this section and the factual basis relied upon by the court shall be in writing.It is not a defense to the provisions of this section that the defendant did not know the distance involved. It is not a defense to the provisions of this section that school was not in session.

It would seem that selling steroids in a school yard is the same level felony as personal use possession. Surely, there's an error here!

In South Dakota, felonies are as follows, in descending order of seriousness: classes A, B, 1, 2, 3, 4, 5, and 6. The sentencing section of South Dakota law is provided for in Title 22, Chapter 22-6, Authorized Punishments.

Felonies are addressed in S.D. Codified Laws § 22-6-1:

> (5) Class 3 felony: fifteen years imprisonment in the state penitentiary. In addition, a fine of fifteen thousand dollars may be imposed;
> (6) **Class 4 felony: ten years imprisonment** in the state penitentiary. In addition, a fine of ten thousand dollars may be imposed;
> (7) **Class 5 felony: five years imprisonment** in the state penitentiary. In addition, a fine of five thousand dollars may be imposed;

Misdemeanors are addressed in 22-6-2:

> 22-6-2. Misdemeanor classes and penalties – Restitution – Unclassified misdemeanors – Act prohibited without penalty. Except as otherwise provided by law, misdemeanors are divided into two classes which are distinguished from each other by the following maximum penalties which are authorized upon conviction:
> (1) Class 1 misdemeanor: one year imprisonment in a county jail or one thousand dollars fine, or both;
> (2) Class 2 misdemeanor: thirty days imprisonment in a county jail or two hundred dollars fine, or both.

Mechanisms for leniency exist, including these:

> 23A-27-13. Order suspending imposition of sentence and placing defendant on probation – Revocation of suspension. Upon receiving a verdict or plea of guilty for a misdemeanor or felony not punishable by death or life imprisonment by a person never before convicted of a crime which at the time of conviction thereof would constitute a felony in this state, a court having jurisdiction of the defendant, when satisfied that the ends of justice and the best interest of the public as well as the defendant will be served thereby may, without entering a judgment of guilt, and with the consent of the defendant, suspend the imposition of sentence and place the defendant on probation for such period and upon such terms and conditions as the court may deem best. A court may revoke such suspension at any time during the probationary period and impose and execute sentence without diminishment or credit for any of the probationary period.

> 23A-27-14. Discharge and dismissal of probationer on completion of conditions – No judgment entered – Limitation to one time. Upon completion of the observance of all conditions imposed pursuant to § 23A-27-13, the court services officer assigned to defendant's case shall bring the matter to the attention of the court, whereupon the defendant shall be discharged by the court. A formal entry of such discharge shall be entered by the clerk of courts. Discharge and dismissal under this section shall be without court adjudication of guilt and shall not be deemed a conviction for purposes of disqualifications or disabilities imposed by law upon conviction of a crime. Discharge and dismissal under this section may occur only once with respect to any person.

> 22-6-1.1. Sentence to jail in lieu of penitentiary in minor felonies. If a person is convicted of a Class 5 or Class 6 felony, the court may sentence the person so convicted to imprisonment in the county jail of the county where such person was convicted, for a term of not more than one year.

> 23A-27-18. Suspension of execution of sentence – Conditions imposed. Upon conviction, the court having jurisdiction to try the offense may suspend the execution of any sentence imposed during good behavior, subject to such conditions or restitutions as the court may impose. The suspension order or judgment can be made only by the court in which the conviction occurred.

In the simple first-time possession case involving an adult, it is likely that the defendant will be sent to a diversionary program. As part of the diversionary program, there will be a suspended imposition of sentence. There will be a conviction; however, the sentence will not be imposed. If the defendant follows the terms of the diversionary program they may then make an application to have the record sealed.

In the case of distribution, the state will most likely reduce the charge to a Class IV felony. As such, the defendant has a shot at a plea to straight possession.

If the defendant is arrested in their vehicle their driving privileges will be suspended for up to six months. A commercial driver's license will be suspended for up to one year.

TENNESSEE

The Tennessee Code, Title 39, Criminal Offenses; Chapter 17, Offenses Against Public Health, Safety, and Welfare addresses anabolic steroids. Part 4, Drugs, lists the schedules of controlled substances, and the State has categorized anabolic steroids as a schedule III substance under Tenn. Code Ann. § 39-17-410:

> (f) *Anabolic steroids.* Unless specifically excepted or unless listed in another schedule, any drug or hormonal substance, chemically and pharmacologically related to testosterone (other than estrogens, progestins, and corticosteroids) that promotes muscle growth, and includes: (1) Boldenone; (2) Chlorotestosterone; (3) Clostebol; (4) Dehydrochlormethyltestosterone; (5) Dihydratestosterone; (6) Drostanolone; (7) Ethylestrenol; (8) Fluoxymesterone; (9) Formebulone; (10) Mesterolone; (11) Methandienone; (12) Methandranone; (13) Methandriol; (14) Methandrostenolone; (15) Methenolone; (16) Methyltestosterone; (17) Mibolerone; (18) Nandrolone; (19) Norethandrolone; (20) Oxandrolone; (21) Oxymesterone; (22) Oxymetholone; (23) Stanolone; (24) Stanozolol; (25) Testolactone; (26) Testosterone; (27) Trenbolone; and (28) Any salt, ester, or isomer of a drug or substance described or listed in this subsection, if such salt, ester, or isomer promotes muscle growth.
>
> (g) (1) Except as provided in subdivision (g)(2), subsection (f) shall not be construed to include an anabolic steroid which is expressly intended for administration through implants to cattle or other nonhuman species and which has been approved by the United States secretary of health and human services for such administration. Also, except as provided in subdivision (g)(2), subsection (f) does not include an anabolic steroid which is a combination of estrogen with anabolic steroid and which is expressly intended for administration to hormone deficient women.
>
> (2) If any person prescribes, dispenses, or distributes a steroid described in subdivision (g)(1) for human use, such person shall be considered to have prescribed, dispensed, or distributed an anabolic steroid within the meaning of subsection (f). If any person prescribes, dispenses, or distributes an anabolic steroid which is a combination of estrogens with anabolic steroid and which is intended for administration to hormone deficient women, for use by persons who are not hormone deficient women, such person shall be considered to have prescribed, dispensed or distributed an anabolic steroid within the meaning of subsection (f).

First offense illegal possession of anabolic steroids without a prescription and their "casual exchange" (a small exchange with no intent to sell) are Class A misdemeanors under Tenn. Code Ann. § 39-17-418:

> (a) It is an offense for a person to knowingly possess or casually exchange a controlled substance unless the substance was obtained directly from, or pursuant to, a valid prescription or order of a practitioner while acting in the course of professional practice.
>
> ... (c) Except as provided in subsections (d) and (e), a violation of this section is a Class A misdemeanor.
>
> (d) A violation ... where there is casual exchange to a minor from an adult who is at least two (2) years such minor's senior, and knows that such person is a minor, is punished as a felony as provided in § 39-17-417.
>
> (e) A violation under this section is a Class E felony where the person has two (2) or more prior convictions under this section.
>
> (f) (1) In addition to the other penalties provided in this section, any person convicted of violating this section for possession of a controlled substance may be required to attend a drug offender school, if available, or may be required to perform community service work at a drug or alcohol rehabilitation or treatment center.
>
> (2) Any person required to attend a drug offender school pursuant to this subsection shall also be required to pay a fee for attending such school. If the court determines that such person by reason of indigency cannot afford to pay a fee to attend such school, the court shall waive the fee and the person shall attend the school without charge..

Distribution offenses are Class D felonies under Tenn. Code Ann. § 39-17-417:

(a) It is an offense for a defendant to knowingly:
(1) Manufacture a controlled substance;
(2) Deliver a controlled substance;
(3) Sell a controlled substance; or
(4) Possess a controlled substance with intent to manufacture, deliver or sell such controlled substance.
...(d) (1) A violation of subsection (a) with respect to a Schedule III controlled substance is a Class D felony and, in addition thereto, may be fined not more than fifty thousand dollars ($50,000).
(2) (A) Notwithstanding any other provision of law to the contrary, **a person charged for the first time with delivering an anabolic steroid or possessing an anabolic steroid with the intent to manufacture, deliver or sell such steroid shall be eligible for pretrial diversion** pursuant to title 40, chapter 15, and probation pursuant to § 40-35-313 and title 40, chapter 28.
(B) The inference permitted by the first sentence of § 39-17-419 does not apply to a person charged under subdivision (a)(4) with possession of an anabolic steroid with intent to sell or deliver such steroid. Unless the state can prove that an actual sale or delivery occurred, such person may only be convicted of simple possession and punished as provided in § 39-17-418.

Tennessee distinguishes anabolic steroids in its distribution section in two ways. First, it provides for pretrial diversion and probation in first time delivery situations (compare this leniency to the policy of the State of Virginia, which takes the opposite approach). Second, it makes the following inference in § 39-17-419 inapplicable unless there is an actual sale or delivery: "It may be inferred from the amount of a controlled substance or substances possessed by an offender, along with other relevant facts surrounding the arrest, that the controlled substance or substances were possessed with the purpose of selling or otherwise dispensing." So, **the state is restricted from using quantity to infer the intent to sell**.

Although Tennessee explicitly addresses steroids in its general distribution statute, it also covers them in a separate special section, Anabolic steroids – Prohibited activities, in Tenn. Code Ann. § 39-17-430:

(a) It is **unlawful for a practitioner to prescribe, order, distribute, supply or sell an anabolic steroid for**:
(1) **Enhancing performance** in an exercise, sport or game without medical necessity; or
(2) Hormonal manipulation intended **to increase muscle mass**, strength or weight without medical necessity.
(b) (1) It is unlawful for any person who is not a practitioner or lawful manufacturer of anabolic steroids to:
(A) Knowingly or intentionally manufacture or deliver an anabolic steroid, pure or adulterated; or
(B) Possess, with intent to manufacture or deliver, an anabolic steroid.
(2) As used in this subsection, "practitioner" means a physician, dentist or veterinarian.
(c) A person who knowingly violates this section shall be punished as provided in § 39-17-417(d) for a violation of a Schedule III controlled substance.

Subsection (a) restricts health practitioners from prescribing or dispensing steroids for muscle growth or sports performance, and subsection (b) deals with non-practitioners in a manner similar to the general distribution statute.

Distribution offenses under Tenn. Code Ann. § 39-17-417 are enhanced by one classification when they occur in a Drug-Free School Zone (within 1,000 feet of a school) under 39-17-432.

Authorized terms of imprisonment are set forth under Tenn. Code Ann. § 40-35-111:

(a) A sentence for a felony is a determinate sentence.
(b) The authorized terms of imprisonment and fines for felonies are:

...(4) **Class D felony, not less than two (2) years nor more than twelve (12) years**. In addition, the jury may assess a fine not to exceed five thousand dollars ($5,000), unless otherwise provided
(5) Class E felony, not less than one (1) year nor more than six (6) years. In addition, the jury may assess a fine not to exceed three thousand dollars ($3,000), unless otherwise provided by statute.

Sentencing for misdemeanor offenders under §39-17-418 is outlined under Tennessee Code Title 40 Criminal Procedure, Chapter 35 Criminal Sentencing Reform Act of 1989, Part 1 general Provisions.

Tenn. Code Ann. § 40-35-111:
(d) A sentence for a misdemeanor is a determinate sentence.
(e) The authorized terms of imprisonment and fines for misdemeanors are:
(1) **Class A misdemeanor, not greater than eleven (11) months twenty-nine (29) days** or a fine not to exceed two thousand five hundred dollars ($2,500), or both, unless otherwise provided by statute;
(2) Class B misdemeanor, not greater than six (6) months or a fine not to exceed five hundred dollars ($500), or both, unless otherwise provided by statute; and
(3) Class C misdemeanor, not greater than thirty (30) days or a fine not to exceed fifty dollars ($50.00), or both, unless otherwise provided by statute.

A mechanism for leniency is provided in for 40-15-105, Memorandum of understanding – Suspended prosecution, which allows prosecution to be suspended upon agreement for up to two years of supervisory monitoring. This is a form of pre-trial diversion.

First offenses may receive pre-trial diversion or probation with dismissal and in some cases, expungement. Second offenses can still receive probation, even on a felony charge. Sale cases can receive a one-time casual exchange treatment and be knocked down to possession.

There is no mandatory license suspension.

TEXAS

The Texas Code Title 6, Subtitle C, Chapter 481 outlines the Texas Controlled Substances Act and its penalty groups. Anabolic steroids have been listed under the Texas Controlled Substances Act under Penalty Group 3. Tex. Health & Safety Code § 481.104:

(a) Penalty Group 3 consists of:
...(9)an anabolic steroid or any substance that is chemically or pharmacologically related to testosterone, other than an estrogen, progestin, or corticosteroid, and promotes muscle growth, including: Boldenone; Chlorotestosterone (4-chlortestosterone); Clostebol; Dehydrochlormethyltestosterone; Dihydrotestosterone (4-dihydrotestosterone); Drostanolone; Ethylestrenol; Fluoxymesterone; Formebulone; Mesterolone; Methandienone; Methandranone; Methandriol; Methandrostenolone; Methenolone; Methyltestosterone; Mibolerone; Nandrolone; Norethandrolone; Oxandrolone; Oxymesterone; Oxymetholone; Stanolone; Stanozolol; Testolactone; Testosterone; and Trenbolone.

As in the federal regulations, Texas excludes from the schedules and application of the Act certain steroid products having no potential for abuse under Tex. Health & Safety Code § 481.033:

(g) An anabolic steroid product, which has no significant potential for abuse due to concentration, preparation, mixture, or delivery system, is exempted from Schedules I through V and the application of this chapter to the same extent that the substance has been exempted from the application of the Federal Controlled Substances Act, if the substance is listed as an exempt anabolic steroid product under 21 C.F.R. Section 1308.34 and its subsequent amendments.

Simple possession of anabolic steroids without a prescription is an offense under the Texas Controlled Substances Act, Chapter 481, Subchapter D Offenses and Penalties. Illegal possession carries a misdemeanor or felony penalty, depending on the weight under Tex. Health & Safety Code § 481.117:

(a) Except as authorized by this chapter, a person commits an offense if the person knowingly or intentionally possesses a controlled substance listed in Penalty Group 3, unless the person obtains the substance directly from or under a valid prescription or order of a practitioner acting in the course of professional practice.
(b) An offense under Subsection (a) is **a Class A misdemeanor if the amount of the controlled substance possessed is, by aggregate weight, including adulterants or dilutants, less than 28 grams.**
(c) An offense under Subsection (a) is **a felony of the third degree if the amount of the controlled substance possessed is, by aggregate weight, including adulterants or dilutants, 28 grams or more but less than 200 grams.**
(d) An offense under Subsection (a) is **a felony of the second degree, if the amount of the controlled substance possessed is, by aggregate weight, including adulterants or dilutants, 200 grams or more but less than 400 grams.**
(e) An offense under Subsection (a) is **punishable by imprisonment ... for life or for a term of not more than 99 years or less than five years, and a fine not to exceed $ 50,000, if the amount of the controlled substance possessed is, by aggregate weight, including adulterants or dilutants, 400 grams or more.**

The big question is, how does one measure anabolic steroids in *grams*? Is it based on potency (the AAS milligrams contained in a tablet or vial), or on the total weight including binders and fillers, or, in the case of injectables, the water or oil? For a disturbing example of how it was done in one Texas case, see *Wall v. Texas* in the Case Notes section of the Appendix.

Tex. Penal Code § 12.21 covers misdemeanors:

An individual adjudged guilty of a Class A misdemeanor shall be punished by:
(1) a fine not to exceed $ 4,000;
(2) confinement in jail for a term not to exceed one year; or
(3) both such fine and confinement.

Distribution offenses are also graded by weight, and are covered by § 481.114, Offense: Manufacture or Delivery of Substance in Penalty Group 3 or 4:

(a) Except as authorized by this chapter, a person commits an offense if the person knowingly or intentionally manufactures, delivers, or possesses with intent to manufacture or deliver a controlled substance listed in Penalty Group 3 or 4.
(b) An offense under Subsection (a) is a state jail felony [punishable by 180 days to two years] if the amount of the controlled substance to which the offense applies is, by aggregate weight, including adulterants or dilutants, less than 28 grams.
(c) An offense under Subsection (a) is a felony of the second degree if the amount of the controlled substance to which the offense applies is, by aggregate weight, including adulterants or dilutants, 28 grams or more but less than 200 grams.
(d) An offense under Subsection (a) is a felony of the first degree, if the amount of the controlled substance to which the offense applies is, by aggregate weight, including adulterants or dilutants, 200 grams or more but less than 400 grams.
(e) An offense under Subsection (a) is punishable by imprisonment in the institutional division of the Texas Department of Criminal Justice for life or for a term of not more than 99 years or less than 10 years, and a fine not to exceed $ 100,000, if the amount of the controlled substance to which the offense applies is, by aggregate weight, including any adulterants or dilutants, 400 grams or more.

It's a felony of the second degree to deliver any quantity to a minor under § 481.122.

Felonies of the third degree fall under Tex. Penal Code § 12.34:

(a) An individual adjudged guilty of **a felony of the third degree shall be punished by imprisonment in the institutional division for any term of not more than 10 years or less than 2 years.**

Felonies of the second degree fall under Tex. Penal Code § 12.33:

(a) An individual adjudged guilty of **a felony of the second degree shall be punished by imprisonment in the institutional division for any term of not more than 20 years or less than 2 years.**

Felonies of the first degree fall under Tex. Penal Code § 12.32:

(a) An individual adjudged guilty of **a felony of the first degree shall be punished by imprisonment in the institutional division for life or for any term of not more than 99 years or less than 5 years.**

In Texas, there are a number of diversionary programs available for simple possession cases, such as Dallas County's Divert Program. This program is available for felony possession of controlled substances and allows for alternatives such as a probationary period. These programs vary by jurisdiction, as does the availability of Drug Court, which is not an option is every county. In some counties, misdemeanor cases are eligible for pre-trial diversion.

There is mandatory driver's license revocation for conviction of drug offenses.

UTAH

The state of Utah defines anabolic steroids as a schedule III controlled substance under Utah Code Title 58, Occupations and Professions; Chapter 37 Controlled Substances Act.

Utah Code Ann. § 58-37-4(2):
(c) Schedule III:
...(vi)Unless specifically excepted or unless listed in another schedule, anabolic steroids including any of the following or any isomer, ester, salt, or derivative of the following that promotes muscle growth: (A) Boldenone; (B) Chlorotestosterone (4-chlortestosterone); (C) Clostebol; (D) Dehydrochlormethyltestosterone; (E) Dihydrotestosterone (4-dihydrotestosterone); (F) Drostanolone; (G) Ethylestrenol; (H) Fluoxymesterone; (I) Formebulone (formebolone); (J) Mesterolone; (K) Methandienone; (L) Methandranone;(M) Methandriol; (N) Methandrostenolone; (O) Methenolone; (P) Methyltestosterone; (Q) Mibolerone; (R) Nandrolone; (S) Norethandrolone; (T) Oxandrolone; (U) Oxymesterone; (V) Oxymetholone; (W) Stanolone; (X) Stanozolol; (Y) Testolactone; (Z) Testosterone; and (AA) Trenbolone.

Anabolic steroids expressly intended for administration through implants to cattle or other nonhuman species, and approved by the Secretary of Health and Human Services for use, may not be classified as a controlled substance.

Under Utah Code Ann. § 58-37-8, prohibited acts and penalties involving drugs are divided into categories. **First offenses for simple unlawful possession are a class B misdemeanor**:

(2) Prohibited acts B – Penalties:
(a) It is unlawful:
(i) for any person knowingly and intentionally to possess or use a controlled substance, unless

it was obtained under a valid prescription or order, directly from a practitioner while acting in the course of his professional practice, or as otherwise authorized by this chapter;...

(e) Any person who violates ... with respect to [steroids] is guilty of a class B misdemeanor. Upon a second conviction the person is guilty of a class A misdemeanor, and upon a third or subsequent conviction the person is guilty of a third degree felony.

Sentencing for misdemeanor offenses such as illegal possession of controlled substances is governed under Utah Code Title 76, Chapter 03, Punishments:

Utah Code Ann. § 76-3-204:

A person who has been convicted of a misdemeanor may be sentenced to imprisonment as follows:

(1) In the case of a class A misdemeanor, for a term not exceeding one year;
(2) In the case of a **class B misdemeanor, for a term not exceeding six months**;

Distribution offenses are covered in a separate subsection of Utah Code Ann. § 58-37-8:

(1) Prohibited acts A – Penalties:
(a) Except as authorized by this chapter, it is unlawful for any person to knowingly and intentionally:
(i) produce, manufacture, or dispense, or to possess with intent to produce, manufacture, or dispense, a controlled or counterfeit substance;
(ii) distribute a controlled or counterfeit substance, or to agree, consent, offer, or arrange to distribute a controlled or counterfeit substance;
(iii) possess a controlled or counterfeit substance with intent to distribute; or
(iv) engage in a continuing [drug conspiracy] criminal enterprise...

Under 76-3-103, felonies are classified into four categories:
(a) Capital felonies;
(b) Felonies of the first degree;
(c) Felonies of the second degree;
(d) Felonies of the third degree.

An offense designated as a felony without specification as to punishment or category is a felony of the third degree.

Violators for distribution offenses involving Schedule III substances like steroids face, under subsection (1)(b):

(ii) a substance classified in Schedule III ... is guilty of **a third degree felony**, and upon a second or subsequent conviction is guilty of a second degree felony;

Persons convicted of a violation of Subsection (1)(a)(ii) may be sentenced to imprisonment for an indeterminate term as provided by law, but if the trier of fact finds a firearm was used, carried, or possessed on his person or in his immediate possession during the commission or in furtherance of the offense, the court shall additionally sentence the person convicted for a term of one year to run consecutively and not concurrently; and the court may additionally sentence the person convicted for an indeterminate term not to exceed five years to run consecutively and not concurrently.

Under a separate subsection of prohibited acts (subd. 4), escalated felony levels and heavier punishments are meted out for drug crimes in or within 1,000 feet of certain schools, parks, stadiums, child-care facilities, houses of worship, shopping malls, movies houses, playhouses, public parking lots, churches, synagogues. Also, if in the immediate presence of a person younger than 18 years of age, regardless of where the act occurs.

Under 76-3-203, the following terms of imprisonment are authorized for felonies:

(2) A person who has been convicted of a felony may be sentenced to imprisonment for an indeterminate term as follows:
   (a) In the case of a felony of the first degree, for a term of not less than five years, unless otherwise specifically provided by law, and which may be for life, ...
   (b) In the case of a felony of the second degree, for a term of not less than one year nor more than 15 years, ...
   (c) In the case of **a felony of the third degree, for a term not to exceed five years,** ...

Heavier punishments apply if a dangerous weapon was used in the commission or furtherance of the felony.

Mechanisms exist for leniency, such as 76-3-402:

Conviction of lower degree of offense.

(1) If the court, having regard to the nature and circumstances of the offense of which the defendant was found guilty and to the history and character of the defendant, concludes it would be unduly harsh to record the conviction as being for that degree of offense established by statute and to sentence the defendant to an alternative normally applicable to that offense, the court may unless otherwise specifically provided by law enter a judgment of conviction for the next lower degree of offense and impose sentence accordingly.
(2) If a conviction is for a third degree felony the conviction is considered to be for a class A misdemeanor if:
   (a) the judge designates the sentence to be for a class A misdemeanor and the sentence imposed is within the limits provided by law for a class A misdemeanor; or
   (b) (i) the imposition of the sentence is stayed and the defendant is placed on probation, whether committed to jail as a condition of probation or not;
      (ii) the defendant is subsequently discharged without violating his probation; and
      (iii) the judge upon motion and notice to the prosecuting attorney, and a hearing if requested by either party or the court, finds it is in the interest of justice that the conviction be considered to be for a class A misdemeanor.
(3) An offense may be reduced only one degree under this section unless the prosecutor specifically agrees in writing or on the court record that the offense may be reduced two degrees. In no case may an offense be reduced under this section by more than two degrees.
(4) This section may not be construed to preclude any person from obtaining or being granted an expungement of his record as provided by law.

In some cases the option may be available for felony possession charges to plea to a class A misdemeanor after a six month probation. A misdemeanor can get reduced to probation.

Drug Court may be another option for offenders with at least one prior drug related offense and no history of violent crimes. That means that some sale or distribution cases are eligible for drug court, though "intent" cases are more likely candidates. Successful completion results in dismissal. Sale or distribution cases might be able to plead down to a third degree felony. They are not likely to spend time in prison, 6-8 months if at all.

There is mandatory license revocation by the DMV for any drug crime, usually for six months.

VERMONT

Vermont Statutes Title 18, Health; Part 5, Food and Drugs; Chapter 84, Possession and Control of Regulated Drugs deals with controlled substances, which in Vermont are called "regulated drugs." Take a look at the definition of "regulated drug" in 18 V.S.A. § 4201(29) and you'll see it means "(A) a narcotic drug;

(B) a depressant or stimulant drug; (C) a hallucinogenic drug; (D) Ecstasy; or (E) marijuana." Does that mean steroids are not controlled?

Well, in 18 V.S.A. § 4202, the Board of Health is authorized and empowered to pass regulations to supplement the provisions of the Vermont Statutes.

According to the Board of Health, ***no*** **regulations have been passed to address anabolic steroids. They remain *unregulated* under Vermont law.** Obviously they remain controlled under federal law. According to Vermont law enforcement authorities, serious offenses would be referred to the local U.S. Attorney for federal prosecution. One police spokesman remembered a few prosecutions of physicians for prescribing to bodybuilders, but could not recall any prosecutions of end users for simple possession.

VIRGINIA

In the state of Virginia, there are six classes of controlled substances (Schedule VI includes all prescription drugs). Anabolic steroids are defined as controlled substances in Schedule III of the Virginia Drug Control Act, Code of Virginia Title 51.4, Professions and Occupations, Chapter 34.

Va. Code Ann. § 54.1-3450:

The controlled substances listed in this section are included in Schedule III:

...5. Unless specifically excepted or unless listed in another schedule, any material, compound, mixture, or preparation containing any quantity of the following substances, including its salts, isomers, and salts of isomers whenever the existence of such salts of isomers is possible within the specific chemical designation: Anabolic steroids, including, but not limited to: Boldenone (Dehydrotestosterone); Clostebol (4-Chlorotestosterone) (Chlorotestosterone); Dromostanolone (Drostanolone); Ethylestrenol; Fluoxymesterone; Formyldienolone (Formebolone); Mesterolone; Methandriol (methylandrostenediol); Methandrostenolone (Methandienone) (Dehydromethyltestosterone); Methenolone; 17-Methyltestosterone (Methyltestosterone); Mibolerone; Nandrolone (19-Nortestosterone); Norethandrolone; Oxandrolone; Oxymesterone (Oxymestrone); Oxymetholone (Anasterone); Stanolone (4-Dihydrotestosterone) (Dihydrotestosterone); Stanozolol (Androstanazole); Testolactone (1-Dehydrotestololactone); Testosterone; Trenbolone (Trienbolone) (Trienolone); and

Any salt, ester, or isomer of a drug or substance described or listed in this paragraph, if that salt, ester, or isomer promotes muscle growth. However, such term does not include an anabolic steroid which is expressly intended for administration through implants to cattle or other nonhuman species and which has been approved by the United States Secretary of Health and Human Services for such administration. If any person prescribes, dispenses, or distributes any such steroid for human use, such person shall be considered to have prescribed, dispensed, or distributed an anabolic steroid within the meaning of this subdivision.

Penalties for possession of controlled substances in schedule III are outlined in the Code of Virginia, Title 18.2, Crimes and Offenses; Chapter 7, Crimes Involving Health and Safety; Article 1 Drugs. **Possession without a valid prescription is a Class 1 misdemeanor**.

Va. Code Ann. § 18.2-250:

A. It is unlawful for any person knowingly or intentionally to possess a controlled substance unless the substance was obtained directly from, or pursuant to, a valid prescription or order of a practitioner while acting in the course of his professional practice, or except as otherwise authorized .... Upon the prosecution of a person for a violation of this section, ownership or occupancy of premises or vehicle upon or in which a controlled substance was found shall not create a presumption that such person either knowingly or intentionally possessed such controlled substance.

...(b)Any person other than [a jail inmate or detainee] who violates this section with respect to a controlled substance classified in Schedule III shall be guilty of a Class 1 misdemeanor.

Virginia criminal sentencing is governed by Code of Virginia Title 18.2 Crimes and Offenses, Chapter 1, In General, Article 3. A Class 1 misdemeanor as described in § 18.2-250 can carry up to 1 year imprisonment and up to a $2,500 fine. Va. Code Ann. § 18.2-11:

> The authorized punishments for conviction of a misdemeanor are:
> (a) For Class 1 misdemeanors, confinement in jail for not more than twelve months and a fine of not more than $2,500, either or both.
> (b) For Class 2 misdemeanors, confinement in jail for not more than six months and a fine of not more than $1,000, either or both.

A provision exists for probation without adjudication for first offenders:

> § 18.2-251. Persons charged with first offense may be placed on probation; conditions; screening, assessment and education programs; drug tests; costs and fees; violations; discharge.
> Whenever any person who has not previously been convicted of any offense under this article or under any statute of the United States or of any state relating to narcotic drugs, marijuana, or stimulant, depressant, or hallucinogenic drugs, or has not previously had a proceeding against him for violation of such an offense dismissed as provided in this section, pleads guilty to or enters a plea of not guilty to possession of a controlled substance under § 18.2-250 ... the court, upon such plea if the facts found by the court would justify a finding of guilt, without entering a judgment of guilt and with the consent of the accused, may defer further proceedings and place him on probation upon terms and conditions.
> As a term or condition, the court shall require the accused to undergo a substance abuse assessment ... and enter a treatment and/or education program [if appropriate]. ...
> As a condition of probation, the court shall require the accused (i) to successfully complete the treatment or education program, (ii) to remain drug and alcohol free during the period of probation and submit to such tests during that period as may be necessary and appropriate to determine if the accused is drug and alcohol free, (iii) to make reasonable efforts to secure and maintain employment, and (iv) to comply with a plan of at least 100 hours of community service for a felony and up to twenty-four hours of community service for a misdemeanor. Such testing shall be conducted by personnel of the supervising probation agency or personnel of any program or agency approved by the supervising probation agency.
> The court shall, unless done at arrest, order the accused to report to the original arresting law-enforcement agency to submit to fingerprinting.
> Upon violation of a term or condition, the court may enter an adjudication of guilt and proceed as otherwise provided. Upon fulfillment of the terms and conditions, the court shall discharge the person and dismiss the proceedings against him. Discharge and dismissal under this section shall be without adjudication of guilt and is a conviction only for the purposes of applying this section in subsequent proceedings.
> Notwithstanding any other provision of this section, whenever a court places an individual on probation upon terms and conditions pursuant to this section, such action shall be treated as a conviction for purposes of [driver's license forfeiture]....

Under § 18.2-252, suspended sentences are conditioned upon substance abuse screening, assessment, testing, and treatment or education.

The forfeiture of an offender's driver's license results from most convictions and probation deferrals:

> § 18.2-259.1. Forfeiture of driver's license for violations of article.
> A. In addition to any other sanction or penalty imposed for a violation of this article, the (i) judgment of conviction under this article or (ii) placement on probation following deferral of further proceedings ...shall of itself operate to deprive the person ... of the privilege to drive or operate a motor vehicle, engine, or train in the Commonwealth for a period of six months from

the date of such judgment or placement on probation. Such license forfeiture shall be in addition to and shall run consecutively with any other license suspension, revocation or forfeiture in effect or imposed upon the person so convicted or placed on probation. However, a juvenile who has had his license suspended or denied pursuant to § 16.1-278.9 shall not have his license forfeited pursuant to this section for the same offense.

...C. In those cases where the court determines there are compelling circumstances warranting an exception, the court may provide that any individual be issued a restricted license to operate a motor vehicle for any of the purposes set forth in subsection E of § 18.2-271.1.

Now, when it comes to selling steroids, Virginia's laws get more interesting. Here's the law:

§ 18.2-248. Manufacturing, selling, giving, distributing or possessing with intent to manufacture, sell, give or distribute a controlled substance or an imitation controlled substance prohibited; penalties.

A. Except as authorized in the Drug Control Act (§ 54.1-3400 et seq.), it shall be unlawful for any person to manufacture, sell, give, distribute, or possess with intent to manufacture, sell, give or distribute a controlled substance or an imitation controlled substance...

..F. Any person who violates this section with respect to a controlled substance classified in Schedule III ... except for an anabolic steroid classified in Schedule III constituting a violation of § 18.2-248.5, shall be guilty of a Class 1 misdemeanor.

So, selling a Schedule III drug is only a misdemeanor, EXCEPT in the case of steroids:

§ 18.2-248.5. Illegal stimulants and steroids; penalty.

A. Except as authorized ... **it shall be unlawful for any person to knowingly manufacture, sell, give, distribute or possess with intent to manufacture, sell, give or distribute any anabolic steroid.**

A violation of subsection A shall be punishable by a term of imprisonment of not less than one year nor more than ten years or, in the discretion of the jury or the court trying the case without a jury, confinement in jail for not more than twelve months or a fine of not more than $20,000, either or both. **Any person violating the provisions of this subsection shall, upon conviction, be incarcerated for a minimum, mandatory term of six months which shall not be suspended** in whole or in part and shall be served consecutively with any other sentence.

Ouch! The Virginia legislature has decided that selling steroids should be punished more severely than selling any other drug in Schedule III. The approach goes in the opposite direction of a state like Tennessee, which goes out of its way to treat first time steroid sales *more* leniently than in the case of other schedule III drugs.

Distribution to minors significantly escalates the penalties:

§ 18.2-255. Distribution of certain drugs to persons under eighteen prohibited; penalty.

A. Except as authorized ... it shall be unlawful for any person who is at least eighteen years of age to knowingly or intentionally (i) distribute any [Schedule III drug] to any person under eighteen years of age who is at least three years his junior or (ii) cause any person under eighteen years of age to assist in such distribution.... Any person violating this provision shall upon conviction be imprisoned in a state correctional facility for a period not less than ten nor more than fifty years, and fined not more than $100,000....

§ 18.2-255.2 prohibits the sale of drugs on or near certain properties:

A. It shall be unlawful for any person to manufacture, sell or distribute or possess with intent to sell, give or distribute any controlled substance ... while (i) upon the property, including buildings and grounds, of any public or private elementary, secondary, or post secondary school, or any public or private two-year or four-year institution of higher education; (ii) upon public property or any property open to public use within 1,000 feet of such school property; (iii) on any school bus ...; (iv) upon a designated school bus stop, or upon either public property or any property open to public use which is within 1,000 feet of such school bus stop, during the time when school children are waiting to be picked up and transported to or are being dropped off from school or a school-sponsored activity; (v) upon the property, including buildings and grounds, of any publicly owned or publicly operated recreation or community center facility or any public library; or (vi) upon the property of any state hospital ... or upon public property or property open to public use within 1,000 feet of such an institution....

Under subsection (B), violation of this section is a separate and distinct felony, punishable by imprisonment of not less than one year or more than five years. A second or subsequent conviction for a Schedule III drug faces a minimum, mandatory term of imprisonment of one year which shall not be suspended in whole or in part and shall be served consecutively with any other sentence. However, if the accused proves that he sold the drug only as an accommodation to another individual and not with intent to profit thereby from any consideration received or expected nor to induce the recipient or intended recipient to use or become addicted to the drug, he's guilty of a Class 1 misdemeanor.

There is mandatory license suspension for six to twelve months with restricted licenses issued for exceptions such as work, doctor, etc.

WASHINGTON

In Washington State, anabolic steroids are defined as schedule III controlled substances under the Code of Washington Title 69, Food, Drugs, Cosmetics, and Poisons; Chapter 69.50, Uniform Controlled Substances Act; Article II, Standards and Schedules. Rev. Code Wash. (ARCW) § 69.50.208:

§ 69.50.208. Schedule III Unless specifically excepted by state or federal law or regulation or more specifically included in another schedule, the following controlled substances are listed in Schedule III:

...(d)Anabolic steroids. The term "anabolic steroid" means any drug or hormonal substance, chemically and pharmacologically related to testosterone (other than estrogens, progestins, and corticosteroids) that promotes muscle growth, and includes: (1) Boldenone; (2) Chlorotestosterone; (3) Clostebol; (4) Dehydrochlormethyltestosterone; (5) Dihydrotestosterone; (6) Drostanolone; (7) Ethylestrenol; (8) Fluoxymesterone; (9) Formebulone; (10) Mesterolone; (11) Methandienone; (12) Methandranone; (13) Methandriol; (14) Methandrostenolone; (15) Methenolone; (16) Methyltestosterone; (17) Mibolerone; (18) Nanrolone [nandrolone]; (19) Norethandrolone; (20) Oxandrolone; (21) Oxymesterone; (22) Oxymetholone; (23) Stanolone; (24) Stanozolol; (25) Testolactone; (26) Testosterone; (27) Trenbolone; and (28) Any salt, ester, or isomer of a drug or substance described or listed in this subsection, if that salt, ester, or isomer promotes muscle growth. Except such term does not include an anabolic steroid which is expressly intended for administration through implants to cattle or other nonhuman species and which has been approved by the secretary of health and human services for such administration. If any person prescribes, dispenses, or distributes such steroid for human use such person shall be considered to have prescribed, dispensed, or distributed an anabolic steroid within the meaning of this subsection.

Washington makes simple unlawful possession of controlled substances such as anabolic steroids a felony charge, with up to a 5 year prison sentence and up to a $10,000 fine. These penalties are listed under Chapter 69.50, Article IV Offenses and Penalties. Rev. Code Wash. (ARCW) § 69.50.401:

> d) It is unlawful for any person to possess a controlled substance unless the substance was obtained directly from, or pursuant to, a valid prescription or order of a practitioner while acting in the course of his or her professional practice, or except as otherwise authorized by this chapter. Any person who violates this subsection is guilty of a crime, and upon conviction may be imprisoned for not more than five years, fined not more than ten thousand dollars, or both, except as provided for in subsection (e) of this section.

The penalties for trafficking offenses are also a maximum of five years in prison, under subsection (a) of § 69.50.401:

> (a) Except as authorized by this chapter, it is unlawful for any person to manufacture, deliver, or possess with intent to manufacture or deliver, a controlled substance.
>
> (1) Any person who violates this subsection with respect to:
>
> ...(iii) any other controlled substance [in Schedule III], is guilty of a crime and upon conviction may be imprisoned for not more than five years, fined not more than ten thousand dollars, or both;

Unlike most states, Washington makes both delivering steroids and simply possessing them for personal use class E felonies punishable by the same maximum statutory penalty. **The actual penalties imposed, however, are determined not by the statute but by the State's sentencing guidelines**. Based on the federal guidelines and similar to the grid system used in Minnesota, the guidelines contain a table by which the presumptive sentences can be ascertained. Generally, first time offenders for simple possession may receive a felony conviction (with a possibility of future expungement) but no jail sentence, while first time traffickers may get a bit of jail time and a period of probation.

Washington has distinctly different sentencing systems for Superior Court felonies and District Court misdemeanors. Sometimes a felony possession charge can be negotiated down to a misdemeanor plea for solicitation. Unlike felonies, misdemeanor convictions allow for suspended sentences. Like most states, Washington has drug courts favoring treatment over incarceration. The specifics vary county by county depending on grant funding, but dismissal after 18 months of successful treatment is common.

Second or subsequent offenders for trafficking charges face doubled terms of imprisonment under RCW 69.50.408(a). Offenders eighteen years or older who distribute drugs to minors at least three years younger face doubled terms of imprisonment under RCW 69.50.406(b). Doubled terms of imprisonment also may apply, under RCW 69.50.435, for trafficking offenses in or near a school, on a school bus, within one thousand feet of a school bus stop, in a park, in a public housing project, on a public transit vehicle or stop shelter, or at a civic center.

Only simple possession cases are eligible for Drug Court. Drug Court is available to repeat offenders as well as first time offenders, as long as there is no history of violent crimes. Successful completion of the program results in dismissal, while failure to complete the program can get you a conviction. Outside of Drug Court, Washington strictly adheres to its guidelines-based sentencing system. Reportedly, a significant number of cases go to trial. One option for sale cases attempting to negotiate below the mandatory sentencing might be to try to plea down to a conspiracy charge.

Driver's license suspensions are only for minors under 21 years of age.

WEST VIRGINIA

West Virginia defines anabolic steroids as a controlled substance in schedule III of their Uniform Controlled Substances Act. The Act is located in West Virginia Code Chapter 60A. Article 2, Standards and Schedules, lists the controlled substances in schedule III, which states that anabolic steroids are part of the schedule, however the West Virginia Code does not list the specific substances considered to be anabolic steroids. Bizarrely, steroids (and growth hormones) are scheduled under depressants, then steroids are again listed on their own. W. Va. Code § 60A-2-208:

> (c) *Depressants* – Unless specifically excepted or unless listed in another schedule, any material, compound, mixture or preparation which contains any quantity of the following substances having a depressant effect on the central nervous system:
> ...(12) Human growth hormones or anabolic steroids.
> ...(f) *Anabolic steroids* – Unless specifically excepted or unless listed in another schedule, any material, compound, mixture, or preparation containing any quantity of the following substances, including its salts, isomers, and salts of isomers whenever the existence of such salts of isomers is possible within the specific chemical designation:
> (1) Anabolic steroids.

Possession of anabolic steroids or hGH without a valid prescription is a misdemeanor with an authorized sentence of 90 days to six months jail. W. Va. Code § 60A-4-401:

> (c) It is unlawful for any person knowingly or intentionally to possess a controlled substance unless the substance was obtained directly from, or pursuant to, a valid prescription or order of a practitioner while acting in the course of his professional practice, or except as otherwise authorized by this act. Any person who violates this subsection is guilty of a misdemeanor, and disposition may be made under section 407 [§ 60A-4-407], ... or upon conviction, such person may be confined in the county jail not less than ninety days nor more than six months, or fined not more than one thousand dollars, or both..

The Code provides for Conditional Discharge for first offenses of simple possession. W. Va. Code § 60A-4-407:

> Whenever any person who has not previously been convicted of any offense under this chapter or under any statute of the United States or of any state relating to narcotic drugs, marihuana, or stimulant, depressant, or hallucinogenic drugs, pleads guilty to or is found guilty of possession of a controlled substance under section 401 (c) [§ 60A-4-401 (c)], the court, without entering a judgment of guilt and with the consent of the accused, may defer further proceedings and place him on probation upon terms and conditions. Upon violation of a term or condition, the court may enter an adjudication of guilt and proceed as otherwise provided. Upon fulfillment of the terms and conditions, the court shall discharge the person and dismiss the proceedings against him. Discharge and dismissal under this section shall be without adjudication of guilt and is not a conviction for purposes of this section or for purposes of disqualifications or disabilities imposed by law upon conviction of a crime, including the additional penalties imposed for second or subsequent convictions under section 408 [§ 60A-4-408]. The effect of such dismissal and discharge shall be to restore such person in contemplation of law to the status he occupied prior to such arrest and trial. No person as to whom such dismissal and discharge have been effected shall be thereafter held to be guilty of perjury, false swearing, or otherwise giving a false statement by reason of his failure to disclose or acknowledge such arrest or trial in response to any inquiry made of him for any purpose. There may be only one discharge and dismissal under this section with respect to any person. After a period of not less than six months which shall begin to run immediately upon the expiration of a term of probation imposed upon any person under this chapter, such person may apply to the court for an order to expunge from all official records all recordations of his arrest, trial, and conviction, pursuant to this section. If the court determines after a hearing that such person during the period of such probation and during the period of time prior to his application to the court under this section has not been guilty of any serious or repeated violation of the conditions of such probation, it shall enter such order.

Manufacturing, delivering, or possessing with intent is a felony charge with an authorized sentence of

between one and five years in prison. W. Va. Code § 60A-4-401:

(a) Except as authorized by this chapter, it is unlawful for any person to manufacture, deliver, or possess with intent to manufacture or deliver, a controlled substance. Any person who violates this subsection with respect to:
...(ii)Any other controlled substance classified in Schedule I, II or III, is guilty of a felony, and, upon conviction, may be imprisoned in the penitentiary for not less than one year nor more than five years, or fined not more than fifteen thousand dollars, or both;

Possession with intent to deliver a controlled substance can be proven by establishing a number of circumstances including the quantity possessed and the presence of other paraphernalia customarily used in the packaging and delivery of controlled substances. [*See* State v. Drake, 170 W. Va. 169, 291 S.E.2d 484 (1982)]

Provisions exist for enhancement of penalties for aggravating factors. Second or subsequent offenders for trafficking charges face doubled terms of imprisonment under W. Va. Code §60A-4-408. W. Va. Code § 60A-4-406 increases the mandatory period of incarceration prior to parole eligibility for an offender twenty-one or older who distributes drugs to a person under eighteen, and for an offender eighteen or older who distributes on, or within one thousand feet of, a school or college.

There are currently no drug courts or diversionary programs in West Virginia, however, possession cases and some small quantity sale cases may receive probation with drug treatment.

There is only driver's license suspension for DUI or other driving related offenses.

WISCONSIN

Wisconsin deals with anabolic steroids in its Uniform Controlled Substances Act, Wisconsin Statutes Chapter 961. Wis. Stat. § 961.01, Definitions, provides under subsection (2m) that as used in this chapter:

(a) "Anabolic steroid" means any drug or hormonal substance, chemically or pharmacologically related to testosterone, except estrogens, progestin, and corticosteroids, that promotes muscle growth. The term includes all of the substances included in s. 961.18 (7), and any of their esters, isomers, esters of isomers, salts and salts of esters, isomers and esters of isomers, that are theoretically possible within the specific chemical designation, and if such esters, isomers, esters of isomers, salts and salts of esters, isomers and esters of isomers promote muscle growth.
(b) Except as provided in par. (c), the term does not include an anabolic steroid which is expressly intended for administration through implants to cattle or other nonhuman species and which has been approved by the United States Secretary of Health and Human Services for such administration.
(c) If a person prescribes, dispenses or distributes such steroid for human use, such person shall be considered to have prescribed, dispensed or distributed an anabolic steroid within the meaning of par. (a)

The definition references the provision that schedules anabolic steroids as a schedule III controlled substance. Wis. Stat. § 961.18:

(7) ANABOLIC STEROIDS. Any material, compound, mixture, or preparation containing any quantity of any of the following anabolic steroids, including any of their esters, isomers, esters of isomers, salts and salts of esters, isomers and esters of isomers that are theoretically possible within the specific chemical designation: (a) Boldenone; (b) 4-chlorotestosterone, which is also called clostebol; (c) Dehydrochloromethyltestosterone; (d) 4-dihydrotestosterone, which is also called stanolone; (e) Drostanolone; (f) Ethylestrenol; (g) Fluoxymesterone; (h) Formebulone, which is also called fromebolone; (i) Mesterolone; (j) Methandienone, which is also called methandrostenolone; (k) Methandriol; (L) Methenolone; (m) Methyltestosterone; (n) Mibolerone; (o) Nandrolone; (p) Nore-

thandrolone; (q) Oxandrolone; (r) Oxymesterone; (s) Oxymetholone; (t) Stanozolol; (u) Testolactone; (v) Testosterone; (w) Trenbolone.

Unlike most states, the Wisconsin legislature recognized that methandienone and methandrostenolone are one in the same, as are DHT and stanolone! But in the absence of a catch-all provision, the definition seems to exclude anabolic steroids that are not specifically mentioned on the list.

Possession of anabolic steroids without a valid prescription is a misdemeanor. Wis. Stat. § 961.41:

> (3g)POSSESSION. No person may possess or attempt to possess a controlled substance or a controlled substance analog unless the person obtains the substance or the analog directly from, or pursuant to a valid prescription or order of, a practitioner who is acting in the course of his or her professional practice, or unless the person is otherwise authorized by this chapter to possess the substance or the analog. Any person who violates this subsection is subject to the following penalties;
>
> ...(b)Except as provided ... if the person possesses or attempts to possess a [Schedule III controlled substance], the person is guilty of a misdemeanor, punishable under s. 939.61.

The misdemeanor possession charge carries the possibility of 30 days imprisonment under Wis. Stat. § 939.61(2):

> If a person is convicted of a misdemeanor under state law for which no penalty is expressed, the person may be fined not more than $500 or imprisoned not more than 30 days or both.

Wisconsin provides a conditional discharge for first offenders charged with possession or attempted possession under Wis. Stat. § 961.47:

> (1) Whenever any person who has not previously been convicted of any offense under this chapter, or of any offense under any statute of the United States or of any state or of any county ordinance relating to controlled substances or controlled substance analogs, narcotic drugs, marijuana or stimulant, depressant or hallucinogenic drugs, pleads guilty to or is found guilty of possession or attempted possession of a controlled substance or controlled substance analog under s. 961.41 (3g) (b), the court, without entering a judgment of guilt and with the consent of the accused, may defer further proceedings and place him or her on probation upon terms and conditions. Upon violation of a term or condition, the court may enter an adjudication of guilt and proceed as otherwise provided. Upon fulfillment of the terms and conditions, the court shall discharge the person and dismiss the proceedings against him or her. Discharge and dismissal under this section shall be without adjudication of guilt and is not a conviction for purposes of disqualifications or disabilities imposed by law upon conviction of a crime, including the additional penalties imposed for 2nd or subsequent convictions under s. 961.48. There may be only one discharge and dismissal under this section with respect to any person.

An alternative option in simple possession cases is provided under 961.475:

> Treatment option. Whenever any person pleads guilty to or is found guilty of possession or attempted possession of a controlled substance or controlled substance analog under s. 961.41 (3g), the court may, upon request of the person and with the consent of a treatment facility with special inpatient or outpatient programs for the treatment of drug dependent persons, allow the person to enter the treatment programs voluntarily for purposes of treatment and rehabilitation. Treatment shall be for the period the treatment facility feels is necessary and required, but shall not exceed the maximum sentence allowable unless the person consents to the continued treatment. At the end of the necessary and required treatment, with the consent of the court, the person may be released from sentence. If treatment efforts are ineffective or the person ceases to cooperate with treatment rehabilitation efforts, the person may be remanded to the court for completion of sentencing.

Trafficking offenses are punishable by up to a 7 and a half year sentence, under 961.41, Prohibited acts A penalties:

> (1) MANUFACTURE, DISTRIBUTION OR DELIVERY. Except as authorized by this chapter, it is unlawful for any person to manufacture, distribute or deliver a controlled substance or controlled substance analog. Any person who violates this subsection with respect to:
>
> ...(b)Except as provided ..., any other controlled substance included in [schedule III], may be fined not more than $15,000 or imprisoned for not more than 7 years and 6 months or both.

For whatever reason, Wisconsin enacted, under the same section and with the same penalties, one provision for the manufacture, distribution or delivery of controlled substances, and a different one for the offense of possessing with the intent to manufacture, distribute or deliver (which also supplies a guide as to what evidence demonstrates the requisite intent):

> ...(1m) POSSESSION WITH INTENT TO MANUFACTURE, DISTRIBUTE OR DELIVER. Except as authorized by this chapter, it is unlawful for any person to possess, with intent to manufacture, distribute or deliver, a controlled substance or a controlled substance analog. **Intent under this subsection may be demonstrated by, without limitation because of enumeration, evidence of the quantity and monetary value of the substances possessed, the possession of manufacturing implements or paraphernalia, and the activities or statements of the person in possession of the controlled substance or a controlled substance analog prior to and after the alleged violation**. Any person who violates this subsection with respect to:
>
> ...(b)Except as provided ..., any other controlled substance included in [schedule III], may be fined not more than $ 15,000 or imprisoned for not more than 7 years and 6 months or both.

An offender seventeen years or over convicted of distributing to a person seventeen or younger who is at least three years his or her junior is subject to a doubled term of imprisonment under Wis. Stat. § 961.46. Doubled terms of imprisonment also apply for distributing to prisoners under 961.465, and for second or subsequent distribution offenses under 961.48.

Several of the typical enhanced offenses under the controlled substances acts of other states do *not* apply to schedule III drugs in Wisconsin. These inapplicable sections include 961.495 (possession or attempted possession of a controlled substance on or near public housing, parks, jails, public pools, or youth centers), 961.492 (distribution or possession with intent to deliver on public transit vehicles), and 961.49 (distribution of or possession with intent to deliver on or near public housing, parks, jails, public pools, or youth centers).

First offenders for possession are eligible for expungement of the record, and Drug Courts are becoming increasingly popular. Typically, minor trafficking scenarios might incur a probation recommendation for a small stretch of jail time and a fine. A new Alternative to Prison Program for felony offenders with moderate prior criminal histories is very intensive, with a combination of some jail time with counseling and community service.

Wis. Stat. § 961.50 mandates the *suspension or revocation of driving privileges for between six months and five years, with limits on occupational license privileges.*

WYOMING

The Wyoming Statutes address anabolic steroid crimes in Title 35, Public Health and Safety; Chapter 7, Food and Drugs; Article 10, Controlled Substances. Wyo. Stat. § 35-7-1018 lists anabolic steroids as Schedule III controlled substances:

(g) Anabolic steroids – Unless specifically excepted or unless listed in another schedule, any of the following or any isomer, ester, salt or derivative of the following that acts in the same manner on the human body: (i) Bodenone; (ii) Chlorotestosterone; (iii) Clostebol; (iv) Dehydrochlormethyltestosterone; (v) Dihydrotestosterone; (vi) Drostanolone; (vii) Ethylestrenol; (viii) Fluoxymesterone; (ix) Mesterolone; (x) Methandienone; (xi) Methandranone; (xii) Methandriol; (xiii) Methandrostenolone; (xiv) Methyltestosterone;(xv) Mibolerone; (xvi) Nandrolone; (xvii) Norethandrolone; (xviii) Oxandrolone; (xix) Oxymesterone; (xx) Oxymetholone; (xxi) Stanolone; (xxii) Stanozolol; (xxiii) Testolactone; (xxiv) Testosterone; and (xxv) Trenbolone; (xxvi) Formebulone (formebolone); (xxvii) Methenolone; (xxviii) Any salt, ester or isomer of a drug or substance described or listed in this paragraph, if that salt, ester or isomer promotes muscle growth, except the term does not include an anabolic steroid which is expressly intended for administration through implants to cattle or other nonhuman species and which has been approved by the United States secretary of health and humans services for such administration. If any person prescribes, dispenses or distributes such steroid for human use, the person shall be considered to have prescribed, dispensed or distributed an anabolic steroid within the meaning of this paragraph.

Another example of poor draftsmanship: the lack of a catch-all provision would seem to exclude steroids that are not isomers, salts or derivatives of the listed substances. "Bodenone" is likely supposed to be boldenone.

Unlawful possession of anabolic steroids carries either a misdemeanor charge with up to 1 year imprisonment, or a felony charge with up to 5 years imprisonment, depending on the quantity of the controlled substance in possession. Wyo. Stat. § 35-7-1031:

(c) It is unlawful for any person knowingly or intentionally to possess a controlled substance unless the substance was obtained directly from, or pursuant to a valid prescription or order of a practitioner while acting in the course of his professional practice, or except as otherwise authorized by this act. Any person who violates this subsection:

(i) And has in his possession a controlled substance in the amount set forth in this paragraph is guilty of a misdemeanor punishable by imprisonment for not more than twelve (12) months, a fine of not more than one thousand dollars ($1,000.00), or both. Any person convicted for a third or subsequent offense under this paragraph shall be imprisoned for a term not more than five (5) years, fined not more than five thousand dollars ($5,000.00), or both. For purposes of this paragraph, the amounts of a controlled substance are as follows:

(A) For a controlled substance in plant form, no more than three (3) ounces;

(B) **For a controlled substance in liquid form, no more than three-tenths (3/10) of a gram;**

(C) For a controlled substance in powder or crystalline form, no more than three (3) grams;

(D) **For a controlled substance in pill or capsule form, no more than three (3) grams; ...**

...(iii)And has in his possession any other controlled substance classified in [Schedule III] in an amount greater than set forth in paragraph (c)(i) of this section, is **guilty of a felony** punishable by imprisonment for not more than five (5) years, a fine of not more than ten thousand dollars ($10,000.00), or both;

Wyo. Stat. § 35-7-1031(d) states:

"For purposes of determining the weights to be given the controlled substances under this section, the weights designated in this section shall include the weight of the controlled substance and the weight of any carrier element, cutting agent, diluting agent or any other substance excluding packaging material." Check out *Wall v. Texas* in the Case Notes section of the Appendix for how the State of Texas interpreted "adulterants and dilutents" as to anabolics steroids.

First offenders are eligible for probation and discharge pursuant to Wyo. Stat. § 35-7-1037:

Whenever any person who has not previously been convicted of any offense under this act or under any statute of the United States or of any state relating to narcotic drugs, marihuana, or stimulant, depressant, or hallucinogenic drugs, pleads guilty to or is found guilty of possession of a controlled substance under W.S. 35-7-1031(c), the court, without entering a judgment of guilt and with the consent of the accused, may defer further proceedings and place him on probation upon terms and conditions. Upon violation of a term or condition, the court may enter an adjudication of guilt and proceed as otherwise provided. Upon fulfillment of the terms and conditions, the court shall discharge the person and dismiss the proceedings against him. Discharge and dismissal under this section shall be without adjudication of guilt and is not a conviction for purposes of this section or for purposes of disqualifications or disabilities imposed by law upon conviction of a crime, including the additional penalties imposed for second or subsequent convictions under W.S. 35-7-1038. There may be only one (1) discharge and dismissal under this section with respect to any person. This section shall not be construed to provide an exclusive procedure. Any other procedure provided by law relating to suspension of trial or probation, may be followed, in the discretion of the trial court.

Trafficking offenses are punishable with up to ten years in prison under Wyo. Stat. § 35-7-1031:

(a) Except as authorized by this act, it is unlawful for any person to manufacture, deliver, or possess with intent to manufacture or deliver, a controlled substance. Any person who violates this subsection with respect to:
   (ii) Any other controlled substance classified in Schedule ... III, is guilty of a crime and upon conviction may be imprisoned for not more than ten (10) years, fined not more than ten thousand dollars ($10,000.00), or both;

Enhanced sentencing applies in certain distribution situations. Under Wyo. Stat. § 35-7-1038, second or subsequent offenders may face imprisonment of up to twice that otherwise authorized. Wyo. Stat. § 35-7-1036 sets forth the enhancements for distribution to minors under 18 and in drug free school zones.

On the other hand, Title 7, Criminal Procedure; Chapter 13, Sentence and Imprisonment; Article 3, Probation and Suspension of Sentence, provides mechanisms for leniency. Under Wyo. Stat. § 7-13-301:

(a) If a person who has not previously been convicted of any felony is charged with or is found guilty of or pleads guilty or no contest to any [drug charge, including a felony], the court may, with the consent of the defendant and the state and without entering a judgment of guilt or conviction, defer further proceedings and place the person on probation for a term not to exceed five (5) years upon terms and conditions set by the court. The terms of probation shall include that he:
   (i) Report to the court not less than twice in each year at times and places fixed in the order;
   (ii) Conduct himself in a law-abiding manner;
   (iii) Not leave the state without the consent of the court;
   (iv) Conform his conduct to any other terms of probation the court finds proper; ...
(b) If the court finds the person has fulfilled the terms of probation and that his rehabilitation has been attained to the satisfaction of the court, the court may at the end of five (5) years, or at any time after the expiration of one (1) year from the date of the original probation, discharge the person and dismiss the proceedings against him.
(c) If the defendant violates a term or condition of probation at any time before final discharge, the court may:
   (i) Enter an adjudication of guilt and conviction and proceed to impose sentence upon the defendant if he previously pled guilty to or was found guilty of the original charge for which probation was granted under this section; or
   (ii) Order that the trial of the original charge proceed if the defendant has not previously pled or been found guilty.
(d) Discharge and dismissal under this section shall be without adjudication of guilt and is not a conviction for any purpose.

(e) There shall be only one (1) discharge and dismissal under this section or under any similar section of the probationary statutes of any other jurisdiction.

Another provision, Wyo. Stat. § 7-13-302, permits placing a person convicted on probation or suspending imposition or execution of sentence:

(a) After conviction or plea of guilty for any offense, except crimes punishable by death or life imprisonment, and following entry of the judgment of conviction, the court may:
(i) Suspend the imposition or execution of sentence and place the defendant on probation; or
(ii) Impose a fine applicable to the offense and place the defendant on probation.

Drug Court is an option available primarily for second offense drug possession cases. It is generally an alternative to prison time, offering intensive drug treatment.

There is no mandatory driver's license suspension for conviction of drug crimes.

FIRST OFFENSE PERSONAL USE CHART

The following chart contains information regarding the scheduling status of anabolic steroids in all 50 states, the District of Columbia and Puerto Rico. Unless otherwise noted, when anabolic steroids are scheduled they are in Schedule III. The chart sets forth whether a first offense for a small personal use quantity of anabolic steroids is a misdemeanor or a felony, and also sets forth whether HCG and/or hGH are scheduled.

First Offense Personal Use Chart

STATE	STEROIDS (SCHEDULE III UNLESS OTHERWISE NOTED)	HCG AND hGH
ALABAMA	FELONY	NOT SCHEDULED
ALASKA	NOT SCHEDULED	NOT SCHEDULED
ARIZONA	FELONY	NOT SCHEDULED
ARKANSAS	MISD.	NOT SCHEDULED
CALIFORNIA	MISD.	HCG - INCORRECTLY LISTED AS "HGC"
COLORADO	"USE" IS MISD. BUT "POSS" IS *FELONY!*	HCG AND hGH
CONNECTICUT	MISD.	HCG
D.C.	MISD.	NOT SCHEDULED
DELAWARE	MISD.	NOT SCHEDULED
FLORIDA	FELONY	NOT SCHEDULED
GEORGIA	FELONY	NOT SCHEDULED
HAWAII	MISD. IF LESS THAN 25 TABS	NOT SCHEDULED
IDAHO	MISD.	hGH AND HCG
ILLINOIS	MISD.	NOT SCHEDULED; NON-MEDICAL DISTRIBUTION OF hGH IS CRIMINALIZED
INDIANA	FELONY, BUT COURT MAY ENTER JUDGMENT OF CONVICTION AS A MISDEMEANOR FOR 1ST OFFENSE	HCG UNDER LEGEND DRUG ACT
IOWA	MISD.	NOT SCHEDULED
KANSAS	MISD.	NOT SCHEDULED
KENTUCKY	MISD.	NOT SCHEDULED
LOUISIANA	FELONY, WITH UP TO 5 YEARS WITH OR WITHOUT HARD LABOR	HCG SCHEDULED TO PROHIBIT PRACTITIONERS FROM DISPENSING FOR BODYBUILDING
MAINE	CLASS E CRIME, ESSENTIALLY A MISD.	ALL PRESCRIPTION DRUGS
MARYLAND	"MISD.," BUT UP TO 4 YEARS IN JAIL!!!	NOT SCHEDULED
MASSACHUSETTS	MISD.	ALL PRESCRIPTION DRUGS
MICHIGAN	MISD.	NOT SCHEDULED
MINNESOTA	FELONY, UP TO 5 YEARS ON FIRST OFFENSE (SCHEDULE IV)	hGH

MISSISSIPPI	MISD. IF LESS THAN 50 GRAMS OR 100 DOSAGE UNITS AS DEFINED BY STATE LAW	NOT SCHEDULED
MISSOURI	FELONY, SUSP'D IMP. (UP TO 7 YEARS)	NOT SCHEDULED
MONTANA	MISD. 6 MONTHS, 1ST OFFENSE (EXCEPTION TO OTHER DRUGS - MORE LENIENT FOR AAS)	NOT SCHEDULED
NEBRASKA	FELONY	NOT SCHEDULED
NEVADA	FELONY, BUT SUSP'D SENTENCE AUTH'D	HCG – INCORRECTLY LISTED AS "HGC"
NEW HAMPSHIRE	FELONY	NOT SCHEDULED
NEW JERSEY	FELONY	NOT SCHEDULED
NEW MEXICO	MISD.	NOT SCHEDULED
NEW YORK	MISD. (SCHEDULE II)	HCG
NORTH CAROLINA	MISD., UNLESS OVER 100 TABS OR DOSAGE UNITS	HCG
NORTH DAKOTA	FELONY	NOT SCHEDULED
OHIO	MISD., IF UNDER 200 TABS, 16 GRAMS OR 16 ML	NOT SCHEDULED
OKLAHOMA	MISD.	NOT SCHEDULED
OREGON	MISD.	hGH
PENNSYLVANIA	MISD.	HCG
PUERTO RICO	NOT SCHEDULED	NOT SCHEDULED
RHODE ISLAND	FELONY	HCG AND hGH
SOUTH CAROLINA	MISD., UP TO 100 DOSAGE UNITS	NOT SCHEDULED
SOUTH DAKOTA	FELONY	NOT SCHEDULED
TENNESSEE	MISD.	NOT SCHEDULED
TEXAS	MISD. IF UNDER 28 GRAMS BY AGGREGATE WEIGHT	NOT SCHEDULED
UTAH	MISD.	NOT SCHEDULED
VERMONT	NOT SCHEDULED	NOT SCHEDULED
VIRGINIA	MISD.	NOT SCHEDULED
WASHINGTON	FELONY	NOT SCHEDULED
WEST VIRGINIA	MISD.	hGH
WISCONSIN	MISD.	NOT SCHEDULED
WYOMING	MISD. IF NOT OVER 3 GRAMS IN PILLS OR 3/10 GRAM OF LIQUID	NOT SCHEDULED

Appendix III

Case Notes

ATHLETE CASES

Univ. of Colo. ex rel. Regents of the Univ. of Colo. v. Derdeyn, 863 P.2d 929 (Colo. 1993).

Student athletes filed a class action suit regarding the constitutionality of the random, suspicionless drug-testing program of the University of Colorado. After several appeals, the Supreme Court balanced the privacy interests of the student athletes against the governmental interest of the university, and held the testing unconstitutional. The rationale was that the athletes did not have a lower expectation of privacy, and there was no compelling governmental interest to outweigh the significant intrusion on the reasonable privacy expectations of the student athletes.

Hill v. Nat'l Collegiate Athletic Ass'n, 865 P.2d 633 (Cal. 1994).

Defendant athletic association was granted a final judgment because defendant's drug-testing program did not violate plaintiff student athletes' state constitutional right to privacy. Plaintiffs had no right to participate in intercollegiate athletic competitions, and plaintiffs' reasonable expectation of privacy had been diminished by the notice and consent elements of defendant's testing program. The Court's rationale was that the testing furthers the legitimate interest of maintaining the integrity of intercollegiate athletic competitions as well as the protection of plaintiffs' health and safety.

Schulz v. U.S. Boxing Ass'n, 105 F.3d 127 (3d Cir. 1997).

After defeating plaintiff boxer in a championship fight, defendant boxer tested positive for steroid use. The District Court issued, and the Third Circuit upheld, a preliminary injunction mandating that defendant boxing federation disqualify defendant boxer. Since plaintiff's interests were sufficiently affected by the decision not to disqualify defendant boxer, and he was likely to prevail on the merits, the preliminary injunction was proper. In addition, the public policy of the state of New Jersey is to promote a public confidence and trust in boxing through strict control and regulation.

[On the general issue of suspicionless drug testing of students and Fourth Amendment protections, *see* the United States Supreme Court's recent opinion in *Board of Education of Independent School District No. 92 of Pottawatomie County v. Earls* (122 S. Ct. 2559; 153 L. Ed. 2d 735; 2002 U.S. LEXIS 4882), discussed in Chapter 11.]

POLICE OFFICER CASES

Grubb v. Borough of Hightstown, 802 A.2d 596 (N.J. Super. Ct. App. Div. 2002).

Plaintiff is a former municipal police officer who was convicted of possession of steroids and official misconduct, which led to his forfeiture of position. While his conviction was reversed on appeal, defendant initiated a disciplinary proceeding pursuant to a resolution which stated that "authorized action in no way constitute a waiver of the Borough's rights to institute departmental charges against Mr. Grubb, in the event of a successful appeal of the criminal conviction." Subsequently, plaintiff was permanently terminated from his job. Plaintiff appealed defendant's authority to bring disciplinary charges against him, which the Court rejected. The Borough's police department has the power to adopt additional rules, regulations, and procedures as shall be deemed necessary to promote the efficiency of the Department.

POSSESSION AND INTENT TO DELIVER CASES

Wall v. Texas, 878 S.W.2d 686 (Tex. Crim. App. 1994).

Donnie Keith Wall was found guilty of possessing, with intent to deliver, between 200 and 400 grams of anabolic steroids. The jury assessed punishment at *35 years in prison*. Wall had been stopped for a seat belt violation in Jackson County, at which time he had no identification. After falsely identifying himself, the officer learned his true identity as well as his criminal history that included a methamphetamine possession charge. After Wall refused a car search, the officer detained him until a search warrant could be issued. Upon obtaining the warrant, the officer found a variety of pills and liquids, which were later determined to be anabolic steroids. After unsuccessfully challenging the legality of the issued search warrant, the Court rejected Wall's argument that he was illegally detained until the warrant had been obtained because detention is legal when a driver does not have a valid driver's license.

The crucial issue in Wall's case was how to quantify the steroids under the Texas drug laws, which call for weighing controlled substances in grams *including adulterants and dilutants*. The Court held that when adulterants and dilutants constitute a part of the weight utilized to increase the punishment, the State must prove the following beyond a reasonable doubt: (1) the identity of the named illegal substance, (2) that the added remainder (adulterants and/or dilutants) has not affected the chemical activity of the named illegal substance, (3) that the remainder (adulterants and/or dilutants) was added to the named illegal substance with the intent to increase the bulk or quantity of the final product, (4) the weight of the illegal substance, including any adulterants and/or dilutants. Defense counsel argued that the evidence failed to show that adulterants and dilutants, if any, were identified or added to the steroids for the purpose of increasing the bulk or quantity of the final product, as required by *Cawthon v. State* [849 S.W.2d 346, 349 (Tex. Crim. App. 1992)]. At trial, the State and the defense each presented expert testimony, disagreeing on whether the non-steroid liquid (i.e., oils and/or water) and solid substances (tablet binders and fillers) in which the steroids were found constituted adulterants or dilutants under the definition set forth in *McGlothlin v. State* [749 S.W.2d 856, 860 (Tex.Crim. App. 1988)]. The defense expert stated that the non-steroid portions were carrying agents and were not added with the intent to increase the bulk. The State expert, however, disagreed, claiming that the non-steroid portions were added with the intent to increase the bulk. While reasonable for powdery substances like cocaine, where the black market quantity bought or sold inherently includes various fillers, such claims make virtually no sense for anabolic steroids.

The jury bought the prosecution's arguments. In fact, defense counsel told me that the defendant would have been sentenced to *life in prison* but for one holdout juror! On appellate review, the Court shrugged, claiming to be "jurists, not chemists." They affirmed the conviction. While Wall was clearly no choirboy, this case is an extreme example of an unduly harsh sentence based on bad information.

U.S. v. Roberts, 119 F.3d 1006 (1st Cir. 1997).

Daniel Roberts worked as a personal trainer at various gyms in the Lewiston-Aubrun area and was a member of a team of weightlifters. In addition, he purchased steroids from one Robert Tibbetts, who obtained his supply from a veterinary doctor in Maine by representing their intended use to be for draft horses. When this doctor cut off his supply because of concern of possible illicit purposes, Tibbetts sought a new source in New Hampshire. When large parts of orders were missing, Tibbetts and Roberts decided that Roberts should make the trips to New Hampshire. When a young boy's mother told local police that Tibbetts had sold her son steroids, an investigation ensued which led to the arrest of Roberts by Maine law enforcement authorities. Upon handing over a large box of steroids, Roberts told the officers that the steroids were for his own personal use. Nonetheless, Roberts was charged in a 2-count indictment with conspiracy to possess with intent to distribute anabolic steroids, and possession with intent to distribute anabolic steroids. Roberts was convicted and sentenced to concurrent sentences of 16 months in prison for each of the two counts, to be followed by 2 concurrent 3-year terms of supervised release. Robert's prosecutorial misconduct argument on appeal was denied.

U.S. v. Orduno-Aguilera, 183 F.3d 1138 (9th Cir. 1999).

Zeferino Orduno-Aguilera appealed his conviction of importing anabolic steroids and possessing anabolic steroids with intent to distribute. When attempting to enter the United States through the San Ysidro, California Port of Entry, customs searched his car and found small boxes containing over 400 vials of liquid in hidden compartments of the car. On appeal, Orduno-Aguilera successfully demonstrated that the Government failed to prove the substances in question were anabolic steroids under the statutory definition. In particular, the Government's DEA forensic chemist could not provide any evidence that the particular ester derivatives in question promoted muscle growth, so the conviction was reversed.

U.S. v. Steyskal, No. 00-1133, 2001 U.S. App. LEXIS 7256 (8th Cir. Apr. 19, 2001).

Steyskal was convicted and sentenced for a marijuana conspiracy and an anabolic steroid conspiracy. He received a 60-month sentence on the anabolic steroid conspiracy count, which went unchallenged, but his 210-month marijuana conspiracy sentence was reversed and remanded for resentencing consistent with the *Apprendi* rule.

POSSESSION CASES

U.S. v. Domitrovich, No. 95-35680, 1996 U.S. App. LEXIS 12641 (9th Cir. May 15, 1996).

A search warrant executed by the DEA at defendant's residence revealed a large marijuana grow operation. A superseding indictment was returned charging Domitrovich with manufacture of marijuana, forfeiture of the subject property, possession with intent to distribute marijuana, and possession of anabolic steroids. In exchange for dismissing the possession with intent to distribute count, and the possession of steroids count, defendant pled guilty to the manufacture charge and agreed to forfeit any interest in the property. He was sentenced to a 60-month term of imprisonment, to be followed by a 4-year term of supervised release.

Haddock v. Florida, 671 So. 2d 304 (Fla. Dist. Ct. App. 1996).

Haddock was originally charged with 5 counts of possession of anabolic steroids. The state nolle prossed counts II, III, and IV, but the jury convicted him of counts I and V. He was sentenced to 5 years probation on count I, and 4 years probation on count V.

McGarry v. Saint Anthony of Padua Roman Catholic Church, 704 A.2d 1353 (N.J. Super. Ct. App. Div. 1998).

Plaintiff, the Music Minister/Director of Music at Saint Anthony of Padua Roman Catholic Church, was indicted on two counts of possession of controlled dangerous substances after receiving shipments of anabolic steroids at the church. The package received on the date of McGarry's arrest contained 290 tablets of methandrostenolone, 240 tablets of oxandrolone, and 9 vials of nandrolone decanoate. Plaintiff admitted that he had been taking steroids to assist him with bodybuilding, even though he knew they were illegal. The remainder of the case focused on plaintiff's claims of breach of employment contract, wrongful discharge, and defamation and interference with prospective economic advantage, all of which were denied.

Ohio v. Hernon, No. 3081-M, 2001 Ohio App. LEXIS 1276 (Ct. App. Mar. 21, 2001).

Defendant bodybuilder and her bodybuilder husband were arrested after law enforcement officials executed a search warrant at their condominium and discovered anabolic steroids. Defendant was convicted of possession of anabolic steroids because her knowledge of their presence in her condominium, illegal or not, was enough to establish constructive possession.

DISTRIBUTION CASES

Nebraska v. Connely, 499 N.W.2d 65 (Neb. 1993).

Steven Connely was a college criminal justice major seeking to gain employment in one of the federal law enforcement agencies. In his desire to prepare to join the DEA, he researched using steroids and decided to try a short cycle of 8 weeks of use of the oral steroid methyltestosterone. Failing to achieve the results he sought out, he stopped taking this substance. A police informant was sent to the campus after learning of the possible sale of anabolic steroids on campus, and approached Connely to buy steroids. Connely contacted a source and then quoted prices to the informant. The informant made 2 purchases of the controlled substance steroid testosterone, after which Connely was arrested and sentenced. Connely's arguments of entrapment, vagueness, and insufficiency of evidence were all denied.

Ohio v. Singerman, No. 14497, 1995 Ohio App. LEXIS 3017 (Ct. App. Jul. 14, 1995).

Mark Singerman was convicted on two counts of aggravated trafficking for selling anabolic steroids to an agent of the police, and he was sentenced consecutively to one year of actual incarceration on the first count, and two to fifteen years on the second count, the first two years of which were to be actual incarceration. In addition, Singerman was fined $5,000.

Singerman was a member of Moore's Nautilus and was a friend of Doug Criffield, an employee of Moore's. While they had discussed steroids at the gym, neither ever revealed their own usage. In 1993 Criffield was arrested for aggravated trafficking after having been found with anabolic steroids in his possession. Criffield then made a deal with the district attorney that, in return for a lesser sentence, he would assist law enforcement officials in locating dealers of steroids. Several months later, Criffield informed Singerman that he had a friend who wanted to buy steroids in a taped conversation. Criffield's friend was Detective Loofboro of the Montgomery County Sheriff's Office. Singerman agreed to sell eleven vials of steroids for $225. Several weeks later, an agreement to sell 40 vials for $800 was made, and Singerman was arrested immediately after the exchange was made. On appeal, Singerman failed to prove the defense of entrapment because he could not show that he lacked the predisposition to sell steroids.

U.S. v. One Parcel Property Located at Lot 85, 894 F. Supp. 397 (D. Kan. 1995).

Pursuant to a valid court order intercepting phone communications on the line servicing the residence located at 8940 Hall, Lenexa, Kansas, law enforcement officers obtained evidence of a conspiracy to unlawfully sell and distribute cocaine, marijuana, diazepam, anabolic steroids, and 3,4-Methylene-dioxymethamphetamine, by the sole owner of said property, Steven Muchnick. In a 3-week period, 1,509 phone calls were intercepted. Of that total, 689 were calls placed or received in which an actual conversation ensued. Of those 689 calls, 154 conversations involved drugs and/or drug use. 94 conversations involved actual drug transactions. Despite claims that the drugs were intended for Muchnick's personal consumption, he could not defeat the finding of probable cause for forfeiture of his residence, and he could not prove that forfeiture of the property (worth $158,000) was an excessive fine in light of the fines, which could have been imposed upon him.

U.S. v. Smith, 105 F. Supp. 2d 446 (W.D. Pa. 2000).

Defendant Jason Smith was indicted on 8 separate charges of federal drug and firearms violations. He was convicted of conspiracy to distribute and possess with the intent to distribute marijuana, conspiracy to distribute anabolic steroids, distributing and possessing with the intent to distribute in excess of 100 kilograms of marijuana, possessing with the intent to distribute less than 50 kilograms of marijuana, and possessing with the intent to distribute anabolic steroids. Applying an adjusted offense level of 38 and a criminal history category of I, the Court sentenced Smith to an aggregate term of imprisonment of 240 months, to be followed by a 5-year term of supervised release.

PHYSICIAN CASES

Webb v. Jarvis, 575 N.E.2d 992 (Ind. 1991).

Dr. Webb was a family practitioner in Indiana who prescribed anabolic steroids to Michael Neal. Unknown to Dr. Webb, Neal battered his wife and once pointed a gun to her head. On a single day Neal twice threatened his wife with a knife and pulled the trigger of an unloaded gun pointed at her head. Mrs. Neal left her husband, and when she returned to obtain her clothes, she was escorted by Tom Jarvis, a state police officer. On that date, Michael Neal aimed a rifle at Jarvis but Jarvis was able to grab him, and Mrs. Neal was able to escape. When Michael Neal broke free of Jarvis' hold, Neal began shooting and hit Jarvis in the leg twice. Jarvis shot and killed a nurse at the county hospital before being apprehended by the police.

Jarvis sought recovery from Dr. Webb on the theory that his over-prescribing of anabolic steroids turned Neal into a toxic psychotic who was unable to control his rages. Dr. Webb was granted summary judgment because a physician owes no duty to a third-party who may have been injured by the physician's treatment of the patient. A professional only owes a duty to a third-party if the professional had actual knowledge that those persons would rely on his rendering of professional services. In addition, the Court stated that public policy and social requirements weigh most heavily against imposing a duty on physicians to consider unknown third persons in deciding whether to prescribe a course of drug therapy for a patient. Finally the Court stated that Jarvis was not a readily identifiable victim and the harm inflicted was not reasonably foreseeable.

U.S. v. Jekot, No. 93-50700 1995 U.S. App. LEXIS 3888 (9th Cir. 1995).

Walter Jekot, a pioneer in steroid therapies for AIDS patients, was found guilty of one count of conspiracy to obtain and distribute anabolic steroids and human growth hormone, pursuant to 21 USCS § 333(e) and (f). Jekot was found to have prescribed steroids without a genuine doctor-patient relationship, and the court found no error in his conviction.

Murray v. Cramblett, No. 95-3363, 1996 U.S. App. LEXIS 14459 (6th Cir. May 8, 1996).

After investigating allegations that then Dr. Murray, a physician, illegally prescribed anabolic steroids to his patients to increase their muscle mass and improve their athletic ability, the State Medical Board of Ohio revoked his license to practice medicine. After several appeals and rehearings, the revocation was upheld.

Ark. St. Bd. of Pharm. v. Fenwick, No. CA 95-904, 1996 Ark. App. LEXIS 603 (Ct. App. Oct. 2, 1996).

Plaintiff discovered that Fenwick, a pharmacist at National Family Pharmacy, had distributed anabolic steroids for the illicit purpose of body-building. The Board concluded that Fenwick's conduct constituted knowingly filling prescriptions not issued in the usual course of professional treatment; his conduct was in violation of Board regulations; that is was gross unprofessional conduct; and that it demonstrated he was unfit or incompetent to practice pharmacy by reason of the negligent performance of his duties. The

Board ordered that Fenwick pay a monetary penalty of $2000, his pharmacy license be suspended for 30 days, and he be placed on probation for one year. Pharmacists have a corresponding duty with physicians to insure that medications are properly proscribed and dispensed.

Chang v. Virginia, No. 2599-95-4, 1996 Va. App. LEXIS 691 (Ct. App. Nov. 5, 1996).

Samual Wise Chang, a general physician licensed to practice in Virginia, was convicted of unlawfully distributing anabolic steroids and unlawfully prescribing Schedule III controlled substances. From 1992-1994 he prescribed to various individuals anabolic steroids including Deca-durabolin, Halotestin, Testosterone Cypionate, Anadrol, and the drugs Vicodin and Hydrocodone. The Alexandria Police obtained a search warrant for Dr. Chang's office after gathering information in an undercover investigation that included drug purchases by undercover police officers and others who wore body wires. During the search, the police seized patient files as well as records of patients not specifically mentioned in the warrant. Dr. Chang was convicted of 17 counts of unlawfully and feloniously distributing anabolic steroids, and 7 counts of unlawfully prescribing a schedule III controlled substance.

Auge v. Ohio St. Med. Bd., No. 98AP-157, 1998 WL 808230 (Ohio Ct. App. Nov. 17, 1998).

Dr. Wayne Auge was indicted on two counts of illegal processing of drug documents by was convicted of only count two, which charged that Auge "did intentionally make, utter, or sell a false or forged prescription contrary to the statute". He was sentenced to one year at the Ohio Department of Rehabilitation and Corrections, but the sentence was suspended on condition of Auge's probation for a period of two years under specified terms and conditions. The Board issued a Notice of Immediate Suspension and Opportunity for Hearing because Dr. Auge wrote and signed a prescription for Winstrol, a schedule III steroid, for a fictitious patient, and he wrote and/or telephoned prescriptions for Profasi, an injectable form of human chorionic gonadotropin, on four different occasions without maintaining any patient records. The Board recommended that his certificate to practice medicine be suspended for two years and not be reinstated unless certain minimum requirements are met.

Ohio v. Spencer, 710 N.E.2d 352 (Ohio Ct. App. 1998).

Dr. Jeffrey Spencer was found in contempt of court in failing to produce the medical records containing prescriptions issued to a particular patient. A compliance agent for the Ohio Board of Pharmacy testified that a law enforcement coordinator for the state medical board presented to him several faxed prescriptions from the defendant to his patient for a large amount of anabolic steroids. An investigation revealed 20-30 similar prescriptions from three different pharmacies. When a sports medicine expert asked to view the patient's medical records, to determine what medical purpose the steroids were prescribed for, Dr. Spencer refused because of physician-patient confidentiality. The Court stated that when the unrebutted evidence supports the contention that prescribed pharmaceuticals far exceed the dosage levels generally accepted in the medical community, the circumstance takes the claimed communication outside the realm of privilege. Case was remanded for execution of sentence.

Appendix IV

THE *LEGAL MUSCLE* GLOSSARY

The public at large, including the academic, medical and legal communities, has little insight into the drug practices of hardcore bodybuilders. In one case I handled, the Customs agents attempted to identify the tablets they found by looking in the Physician's Desk Reference, an incomprehensible strategy since the fact that they were foreign drugs being imported made it almost certain that they wouldn't be in there. Most lawyers, judges and prosecutors would have little understanding of what the muscle folks that are being prosecuted are actually up to. I was recently contacted by a poor soul in Minnesota whose public defender kept referring to the steroid accusations against him as a "narcotics case." This basic glossary of terms is an attempt to shine just a little bit of light on what goes on in the underground of anabolic desperadoes.

ALPHA ALKYLATION, C-17: A structural modification that enables certain steroid compounds to be effective when taken by mouth. The placement of an alkyl substitute at the 17-carbon position of the molecule prevents these compounds from being inactivated upon the *first pass* through the liver that occurs with oral administration. Alpha alkylated chemical structures are toxic to the liver and can lead to conditions such as peliosis hepatitis (blood-filled cysts on the liver) and liver cancer. Alpha alkylated compounds include methyltestosterone, Anadrol-50® (oxymetholone), Dianabol (methandrostenolone) and Halotestin (fluoxymesterone).

ANABOL: See Dianabol.

ANABOLIC: The characteristic of building lean muscle mass through the increase of protein synthesis and other bodily processes (increased oxygen uptake, reduced need for sleep and reduced recovery time from workouts); often distinguished from the *androgenic* or masculinizing characteristic of steroids. Anabolic steroids may be simply called *anabolics.*

ANABOLIC STEROID: Any of a class of pharmaceutical drugs that contain a synthetically manufactured testosterone hormone, or a related compound that is similar in structure or in its action to testosterone. These drugs may be referred to as *anabolic-androgenic steroids (AAS)*, *anabolics*, *androgens* or *steroids*, or in the vernacular as *juice*, *gear*, *roids*, or *sauce*. Excluded from this definition are the other ancillary drugs used by muscle builders, which the uninitiated may refer to erroneously as steroids. This distinction is extremely important in terms of the potential legal consequences. Such excluded drugs include, but are not limited to: human growth hormone (hGH), human chorionic gonadotropin (HCG), clenbuterol, Clomid®, Nolvadex®, T-3, T-4, injectable Lasix®, insulin, Triacana, and insulin-like growth factor (IGF-1). Also excluded are popular over-the-counter products such as creatine monohydrate. *Anabolic steroids are federally classified as Schedule III controlled substances.*

ANADROL-50®: See oxymetholone.

ANAPHYLACTIC SHOCK: A potentially fatal allergic reaction by the body to a foreign protein or organism, characterized by difficulty breathing, bronchial spasm, dizziness, collapse, loss of consciousness, convulsions and ultimately death. This reaction may be precipitated in persons allergic to insect bites, chemicals, medications such as penicillin, and foods such as nuts and shellfish. It is extremely rare with hormone drugs such as steroids; however, it's a possibility if a contaminated or non-sterile substance is injected. This might be a concern because of the large number of counterfeit drugs, designer or basement drugs, impure veterinary and poorly manufactured drugs of third world origin that have flooded the market since the Anabolic Steroid Control Act.

ANAVAR: See oxandrolone.

ANCILLARY DRUG: Drugs that are not anabolics but may be used during and/or after a cycle to enhance the effects of the steroids or to prevent or minimize side effects. Such drugs may, for example, include diuretics, acne medications and estrogen blockers.

ANDRODERM® (Testosterone): A transdermal testosterone patch that delivers the drug into the bloodstream through the skin, fostering a time-released method of administration. The drug is in a gel on the center of the patch, with an adhesive around the perimeter to secure the patch to the patient's skin. The patches are available with different concentrations of testosterone and are distinguishable by their shape. The round patch contains 12.2 mg of testosterone that delivers approximately 2.5 mg of testosterone over a 24-hour period. The oval patch contains 24.3 mg of testosterone that delivers approximately 5 mg of testosterone over a 24-hour period. This item is prescribed for men who are testosterone deficient and can restore hormone levels to normal. This product is far too mild in its concentration to be useful for hardcore muscle enthusiasts. *Androderm® is available by prescription only and is a Schedule III controlled substance.*

ANDRODIOL: The trade name for a particular prohormone. The actual chemical name is 4-androstene-3beta,17beta-diol. *Androdiol is not a federal controlled substance.* [*See* prohormones]

ANDROGEL®: A clear, colorless testosterone gel (containing 1% testosterone) that is applied daily to the skin of the shoulders, upper arms and/or abdomen. AndroGel® is approved by the FDA for replacement therapy in men for conditions associated with low testosterone. Clinical studies have found that once-daily application raised circulating testosterone levels into the normal range and maintained these levels. This product is far too mild in its concentration to be useful for hardcore muscle enthusiasts. *AndroGel® is available by prescription only and contains a federal Schedule III controlled substance.*

ANDROGENIC: The masculinizing properties of testosterone which are associated with deepening of the voice, body and facial hair growth, development of the male sexual organs, libido and aggression. It is these androgenic properties that are responsible for some of the undesirable side effects of steroids, especially in women.

ANDROPAUSE: The unfortunate diminution of testosterone levels in older men, sometimes beginning as early as 35 or 40. The female converse to this condition is menopause. Decreased testosterone levels in men can result in loose skin, soft muscles, fatigue, listlessness and a lack of interest in and ability to perform sexually. Men who are suffering from the condition are candidates for hormone replacement therapy (HRT). Such therapy may include therapeutic doses of anabolic steroids and human growth hormone.

ANDROSTENEDIONE: A legal, orally administered, over-the-counter dietary supplement of the class commonly called *prohormones*. Popularized when baseball slugger Mark McGwire admitted its use, androstenedione is a molecule very similar to testosterone, the principal male sex hormone. Its sole difference is that where testosterone has a hydroxyl group in a certain position, androstenedione has a keto group. Most simply, you can think of it as "one step away" from testosterone – its "precursor." The body can convert androstenedione to testosterone (and vice versa) by use of a specific enzyme that is present in the body in fairly large amounts. Oral androstenedione supplementation very briefly increases blood levels of testosterone. It is this ability to act as a direct hormonal precursor (a "prohormone") of testosterone that makes it attractive to those seeking a sports aid. But while androstenedione is a precursor of testosterone, it is also, unfortunately, a precursor of estrone, an estrogenic hormone. As such, it can have adverse estrogenic effects similar to those of illegal anabolic steroids, such as gynecomastia (feminized swelling of the nipples). Also, testosterone itself not only converts to estrone, but also converts to a potent androgenic compound known as dihydrotestosterone (DHT), sometimes leading to hair and skin problems. In all mammals, androstenedione is produced in the gonads and adrenal glands. *Androstenedione is neither a federal controlled substance nor a prescription drug despite threats by government anti-drug czars and sports anti-doping officials to have it reclassified. A federal bill has recently been introduced to classify it as a controlled substance.*

ANEMIA: A condition in which the concentration of hemoglobin in the circulating blood is below normal. This condition may be caused by a deficient number of erythrocytes (commonly known as red blood cells), an abnormally low-level of hemoglobin in the individual cells, or both of these conditions simultaneously. All types of anemia are associated with similar signs and symptoms because of the blood's reduced capacity to carry oxygen. These symptoms include pallor of the skin and mucous membranes, weakness, dizziness, frequent fatigue, and drowsiness. Various anabolic steroids have been designated for use in treating certain anemias, such as anemia of renal insufficiency and those caused by insufficient red blood cell production.

ARIMIDEX® (Anastrozole): This drug is clinically used in the treatment of breast cancer. It is used as an ancillary drug in steroid cycles to control the side effects of excessive estrogens. It is an *anti-aromatase* – it blocks the enzyme aromatase, thereby suppressing the production of estrogen. *It is available by prescription only; however, it is not a federal controlled substance.*

AROMATIZATION: The conversion of androgenic hormones to the female hormone estrogen within the body, accomplished by the enzyme aromatase. Unusually high levels of estrogen in males can result in a number of highly undesirable and unpleasant side effects such as edema and gynecomastia. These effects are typically prevented or controlled with ancillary drugs such as Arimidex® and Nolvadex®.

BACNE: This is just what it sounds like, a slang term used to describe a severe case of back acne that some heavy AAS users may experience.

BLOOD DOPING: A banned sports practice, often referred to as induced erythrocythemia, which may be performed for athletes seeking greater endurance and oxygen uptake. In essence, it usually involves the drawing of one to four units of the athlete's blood (1 unit = 450 ml of blood) several weeks before a competition. That blood is then centrifuged and the plasma components are immediately re-infused, while the remaining red blood cells (RBCs) are placed in cold storage. The RBCs are later re-infused into the body, usually one to seven days before a high-endurance event. When done correctly, this process can increase the hemoglobin level and RBC count by up to twenty percent. The end result is that the athlete can have greater endurance through improved oxygen uptake.

BODYBUILDING: The practice of developing the skeletal muscles through the combined approach of progressive resistance exercise and nutrition. At the recreational level, size, shape, proportion and muscular definition are important qualities to bodybuilders. The emphasis is on *appearance*, with many non-competing bodybuilders shaving and tanning their bodies year-round. Power and strength are highly prized for ego gratification, but somewhat tangential to the main goal. To maximize gains, most bodybuilders consume a variety of nutritional supplements, and some take anabolic steroids to hasten progress or to overcome natural genetic limitations. As such, anabolics are a controversial but unequivocably *cosmetic* tool for the majority of bodybuilders.

BOLDENONE: *See* Equipoise.

BRO (Brother in iron): A slang term by which one musclehead refers to another, such as, "You're looking jacked, bro." Non-bodybuilders should refrain from using the term.

BUTANEDIOL (1,4-butanediol): One of various chemicals having similarities to GHB, 1,4-butanediol (1,4-BD) is a natural substance with widespread industrial uses in the manufacture of polyesters and plastics. It's found in corn, yeast and animal skin lipids. Although 1,4-BD is not a federal controlled substance, the government has recently taken the position that it's just as illegal as GHB *if sold for human consumption*, relying upon a federal law known as the Analogue Statute. A drug is legally an "analogue" if it has a *substantially similar chemical structure* to that of a controlled substance *and* either has a *substantially similar* *effect* on the user's central nervous system or is represented or intended by a particular person to have such an effect. An analogue intended for human consumption *is treated as a Schedule I controlled substance*. Contending that 1,4-BD is an analogue of GHB and that it's being sold for human consumption, the government is aggressively going after manufacturers and distributors. At the present time, courts are divided as to whether the Analogue Statute is properly applied to 1,4-butanediol. The issue is likely to be resolved soon, as numerous cases are being hotly contested on a variety of issues: for example, "substantial similarity" may be challenged as unconstitutionally vague (even expert chemists disagree about what "substantially similar" means). The structural difference in question, between GHB as an acid and 1,4-BD as an alcohol, is the same as between vinegar and beer.

CATABOLISM: The process by which complex body components are broken down into simpler ones, it is most often associated with the breakdown of muscle proteins for energy. This process is often accompanied by rising cortisol levels, and is a most undesirable state for physique enthusiasts who are seeking to promote muscle growth (anabolism).

CLENBUTEROL: Clenbuterol hydrochloride or "clen" is not a steroid hormone but a selective beta-2-sympathomimetic used to treat asthma in some foreign countries. It may be found under the following brand names: Broncodil, Broncoterol, Cesbron, Clenasma, Contrasmina, Contraspasmina, Oxibron, Spiropent, Spiropent mite, Spasmo-Mucosolvan, Monores, Ventolase, Novegam, Prontovent and Ventipulmin. While anabolic effects in humans are questionable, clenbuterol is sometimes used for anti-catabolic effect, which means it decreases the rate at which protein is reduced in the muscle cell, consequently causing an enlargement or maintenance of muscle cells. For this reason, numerous physique enthusiasts use clenbuterol after an AAS cycle to balance the resulting catabolic phase and thus obtain maximum strength and muscle mass. A further aspect of clenbuterol is its distinct fat-burning effect. Clenbuterol burns fat without dieting because it increases the body temperature slightly, forcing the body to burn fat. *Clenbuterol is not a controlled substance; however, it is not approved for use in the United States. An import alert to confiscate clenbuterol was issued by the FDA in 1989 and remains in effect. If Customs detects clenbuterol, it will be seized.*

CLOMID® (Clomiphene citrate): The most common brand name for this oral fertility drug. Other brand names: Arodomon, Clomifen, Clomiphen, Dufine, Dyneric, Gravosan, Indovar, Omifin, Pergotine, Pioner, Prolifen, Serofene, Serophene, Serpafar and Tokormon. Clomid® is not an anabolic steroid, but rather an ancillary drug used during or after a steroid cycle for two purposes. Firstly, it blocks the ability of estrogen to bind with its receptor, minimizing the effects of estrogen (such as edema and gynecomastia) when using androgenic drugs that are likely to aromatize. Secondly, it can "kick start" the body's endogenous production of testosterone upon the cessation of a steroid cycle by stimulating the production of luteinizing hormone (LH) and follicle stimulating hormone (FSH). *Clomid® is available by prescription; however, it is not a controlled substance.*

CORTISOL: Cortisol is the primary glucocorticoid steroid hormone produced by the adrenal cortex gland for the purpose of controlling blood glucose (blood sugar). Cortisol also stimulates the release of amino acids from muscle tissue and fatty acids from adipose tissue; these amino acids will be converted by the liver into glucose and used by the brain for energy. The fatty acids can then be used by skeletal muscles for energy instead of the glucose, thereby allowing the glucose to be available to the brain. Some of the cortisol is metabolized by the liver to produce 17 hydroxycorticosteroids, which is then excreted in the urine. Cortisol acts through specific intracellular receptors and affects numerous physiologic systems including immune function, glucose counter regulation, vascular tone, and bone metabolism. Certain events such as missed meals and strenuous weight training can increase cortisol levels in the blood.

COUNTERFEIT: An illegal reproduction of a legitimate pharmaceutical medication. This has partly been the result of the classification of steroids and their restricted availability, as well as simple greed. These items may or may not contain any active ingredient. Counterfeit tablets may be nothing more than filler;

injectables may be nothing more than sesame or peanut oil. At the worst, they may be contaminated and cause abscesses, hepatitis and flu-like symptoms. One of the persistent rumors circulating has surrounded a counterfeit of Winstrol suspension. The suspension, which appears as a milky-white liquid substance, has reportedly been counterfeited by filling vials with a well-known automotive detailing product. In terms of legal consequences, even a counterfeit item that contains nothing more than entirely inert ingredients could be the basis for a prosecution under various laws that punish the sale or possession of imitation controlled substances under certain circumstances.

CREATINE: Not a drug, creatine monohydrate is a natural compound that is synthesized in the liver and found in foods, especially red meats. In fact, the term creatine is derived from the Greek word *kreas,* meaning flesh. This crystallizable nitrogenous compound is converted into phosphocreatine in the body through a process known as phosphorylation. The end product, phosphocreatine, is then stored in the skeletal muscle where it acts in conjunction with adenosine triphosphate (ATP) as the energy source for muscular contractions. During muscular contractions, ATP is rapidly utilized and must be resynthesized in order for muscular contractions to continue. This is where creatine monohydrate exerts its effects. During bouts of maximal muscular contractions (such as lifting a weight or sprinting), creatine and glycogen act almost as the exclusive vehicle by which ATP is resynthesized. There is evidence to suggest that fatigue during intense muscular contractions is the result of the rapid utilization of muscular stores of phosphocreatine. Therefore, any mechanism that increases the stores of phosphocreatine in the muscle fibers can increase the intensity of muscular contractions and prolong their duration. There are research studies that have shown that oral creatine supplementation is effective in increasing muscular stores of phosphocreatine. What is most important to weight training athletes is that studies have demonstrated that creatine supplementation has resulted in increased muscular torque. Creatine is widely available as a legal, over-the-counter, dietary supplement and there are no restrictions on its sale in the United States. It is not banned for drug-tested athletic competition by the International Olympic Committee. While the media has sensationalized speculative concerns over health dangers, there is *no* evidence of deleterious effects in healthy individuals at this time.

CYCLE: A course of anabolics over a pre-determined time frame for the promotion of muscle size or strength. An AAS cycle is the illicit version of the legitimate use of prescribed medications over a course of time determined by a treating physician for the treatment of a condition or illness. In their most judicious use, steroids may be used in an "on" period of eight to sixteen weeks before taking an "off cycle." At its worst, steroid use may continue year-round. Such use can lead to undesirable side effects and health consequences long-term. A cycle may be further refined in terms of whether the desired effect is to gain weight and size or to get as lean as possible. These may be referred to as "bulking" or "cutting" cycles, respectively.

CYCLOFENIL: An oral, non-steroidal, ancillary drug that may be used by AAS users during and/or after their cycle. It may be identified by the brand names Fertodur, Neocym, Ondogyne, Rehibin or Sexovid. Males may use this drug at the cessation of an AAS cycle to stimulate endogenous testosterone production. Essentially, cyclofenil acts as an estrogen agonist/antagonist and affects the binding effectiveness of estrogen receptors in certain tissues to which it is targeted. *Cyclofenil is not a federally controlled substance.*

CYTADREN® (Aminoglutethimide): A non-steroidal, orally administered drug used clinically in the treatment of estrogen dependent breast cancer, as well as Cushing's Syndrome, a condition where the body produces excessive cortisol. Other brand names include: Mamomit, Orimeten, Orimetene Rodazol. It may be used in bodybuilding for the obvious reason of inhibiting cortisol, as well as for its antiestrogen action. *It is a prescription drug; however, it is not a federally controlled substance.*

CYTOMEL® (Liothyronine sodium): This is a thyroid hormone used to treat cases of hypothyroidism. Other brand names include: Cynomel, Linomel, T3, and Tiromel. It may be used by bodybuilders in a pre-contest phase in an effort to achieve a ripped condition. When used in a stack with clenbuterol, bodybuilders can burn a tremendous amount of body fat while sparing lean muscle tissue. The fat-burning effect can be achieved without severely limiting calories. Stacking it with anabolics appears to promote greater anabolism, possibly because of faster use of proteins within the body. However, excessive dosages can be highly catabolic to muscle, and dosages must be closely monitored. Cytomel® carries a number of serious side effects with its use, including but not limited to, heart palpitations, irregular heartbeat, shortness of breath, headaches and nausea. Taking high dosages of Cytomel® over extended periods of time risks the development of a chronic thyroid insufficiency requiring the administration of thyroid medication for the rest of your life. *Cytomel® is a prescription medication, but not a federally controlled substance.*

DAN DUCHAINE: (1952-2000) The original "Steroid Guru," Duchaine was a pioneer in anabolic science and a controversial and outspoken personality. He did two stints in federal prison for his involvements with bodybuilding drugs, and wrote the controversial high-fat diet tome *BodyOpus* while incarcerated. In 1997, he published a short-lived newsletter titled *Dirty Dieting.* As a liberal arts major with no formal scientific educational background, Duchaine nonetheless had an unprecedented talent for understanding what worked and what didn't in the juicer's quest for size and cuts. His wicked sense of humor, acerbic personality and mischievousness made for an enigmatic individual who very few people understood completely. He was bodybuilding's mad scientist. Plagued by health problems throughout this life, he ultimately succumbed to complications related to hereditary polycystic kidney disease, passing away at a mere 48 years of age.

DART: A slang term for a hypodermic instrument, also referred to as a "pin," used to administer injectable drugs either intramuscularly (into the muscle) or subcutaneously (under the epidermis). The instrument is comprised of a needle and a syringe. A one to one-and-half inch long needle is typically used for deep intramuscular injections of steroids. The diameter of the needle is called the "gauge," which can range from 21 to 28. The lower the gauge number, the larger the needle's diameter. The viscosity of the steroid dictates the optimal gauge, with 21 to 25 gauge needles most standard. When, out of necessity, an 18 gauge veterinary needle (resembling a carpentry finishing nail) is used, the injection can be quite painful. Conversely, using a very fine 25-gauge needle to inject oil-based steroids is a very slow, tedious process requiring a tremendous pressure on the syringe stopper. The syringe capacities most commonly used range from one cubic centimeter (cc) to three, with a 3 cc syringe most typical (one cc is equivalent to one ml). AAS users should be aware that the possession of syringes without a prescription for the purpose of unlawfully injecting steroids and associated drugs might be a criminal offense in many states.

DECA-DURABOLIN® (Nandrolone decanoate): The Organon brand name for an injectable, oil-based, steroid compound known as nandrolone decanoate, commonly called "Deca." Foreign versions include Extraboline, Norandren and Decanandrolen. This drug is immensely popular among muscle builders because it has low androgenic activity as well as a low propensity for conversion to estrogen. Although unsupported by clinical data, it is claimed to improve joint pain and connective tissue injuries. It is typically stacked with other steroids such as testosterone esters. Its affinity for the progesterone receptor may lead to progesterone-related gynecomastia, which may be difficult to prevent in predisposed individuals. Competitive athletes and others who may be drug tested should be aware that the nandrolone metabolites will be detectable for more than one year. *Nandrolone decanoate is a Schedule III federally controlled substance.*

DEFINITION: The sharp clarity of muscle achieved when body fat levels are reduced. Largely a product of diet and exercise, the use of bodybuilding chemicals, particularly diuretics, and certain supplements can also play a role. A bodybuilder who is highly defined may be called cut, ripped, shredded, or sliced.

DHEA: A legal, over-the-counter, oral dietary supplement, the unabbreviated chemical name of which is dehydroepiandrosterone. It is a naturally occurring steroidal hormone or "prohormone" produced in the adrenal gland that is a precursor to testosterone. In the biochemical pathway to testosterone, DHEA is two steps away. The exact physiological role of DHEA is not entirely known; however, research has shown that it decreases with age. Because aging is associated with a number of health ailments, including obesity, insulin resistance and arteriosclerosis, some researchers are exploring the interaction of DHEA supplementation with obesity and related physiological problems. This dietary supplement was one of the first prohormones to enter the market following the 1994 DSHEA. *DHEA is not a controlled substance.* [*See,* prohormones]

DHT (Dihydrotestosterone): Also known as 5-alpha-dihydrotestosterone and stanolone, dihydrotestosterone is a C-19 androgenic steroid hormone similar to testosterone and androstenedione. The bulk of the androgen production takes place mainly in the Leydig cells of the testes. Androgens circulate in the blood bound to proteins, especially sex hormone binding globulin (SHBG) and albumin. In males about 70% of DHT is derived from peripheral conversion of testosterone. However, in females most of the DHT is derived from androstenedione. This hormone is actually active in the prostate and stimulates the growth of the prostate gland. DHT is also the primary androgen hormone that triggers hair loss in androgenetic alopecia. When hair follicles that are genetically programmed to be receptive to androgens like DHT receive the DHT message over a long enough period of time, the follicle begins to produce less hair. *DHT is a Schedule III federally controlled substance.*

DIANABOL (Methandrostenolone): The original and long-discontinued Ciba brand name for the oral anabolic steroid methandrostenolone, also called methandienone. D-bol (D-ball) is the popular slang term. Dianabol is very popular because it gives great size and strength gains, but as an alpha alkylated compound it is stressful to the liver. It is most often used in conjunction with injectable anabolics. The most popular black market product is Anabol from Thailand, which is manufactured in pink, pentagonal 5 mg tablets typically purchased in tubs of 1,000 tablets but often shipped in smaller quantities to avoid mail seizure. Note that the tablet potency is only 10% of a tablet of Anadrol 50®, its chemical cousin. (For a fuller discussion of methandrostenolone in the context of "intent to sell" quantities, see Chapter 14.) *Methandrostenolone is a Schedule III federally controlled substance.*

DIURETIC: An oral or injectable medication that causes an increase in urine production. Diuretic medications may be used in the treatment of hypertension and conditions involving edema, such as congestive heart failure. Examples of diuretic medications include Lasix®, Dyazide®, hydrochlorothiazide, furosemide, chlorothiazide, Aldactone®, Aldactazide®, Bumex®, ethacrynic acid, and Maxzide®. Bodybuilders may use a diuretic prior to a physique show to rid the body of any excess water and achieve a truly "ripped" appearance. Athletes who compete in weight classes may use a diuretic prior to weigh-in to qualify for a lighter class. Diuretics are banned in drug-tested competition. *These prescription drugs are not anabolic steroids and are not controlled substances.*

DIMETHYL SULFOXIDE (DMSO): An industrial solvent that is a by-product of the paper manufactur-ing process. DMSO has the unique property of being able to pass through membranes, including the skin, and can carry other drugs with it. It is more successful at carrying some drugs, such as morphine sulfate, penicillin, steroids, and cortisone, than others, such as insulin. What it will carry depends on the molecular weight, shape, and electrochemistry of the molecules. This property would enable DMSO to act as a new drug delivery system that would lower the risk of infection occurring whenever skin is penetrated. Because of impurities, the vast majority of the DMSO sold contains a disclaimer to the effect that it is merely a mild solvent, may be unsafe, and is not approved for human use. In the United States, DMSO has FDA approval only for use as a preservative of organs for transplant and for interstitial cystitis, a bladder disease. DMSO is readily available OTC in liquid, gel and roll-on forms. *It is not a controlled substance.*

DNP (2,4-Dinitrophenol): 2,4-Dinitrophenol may be seen as a yellowish crystalline solid, powder or liquid and is the most important of the six possible dinitrophenol forms. It is used mostly as an intermediate to make dyes, photochemicals, pest control agents, wood preservatives, and explosives. Dinitrophenol is what is known as an uncoupler: it has the ability to separate the flow of electrons and the pumping of ions for ATP synthesis. In practice, this means that much of the food consumed would not be used for ATP synthesis, resulting in a loss of body fat. However, too little ATP can be deadly. The difference between weight loss and death is only a small change in DNP concentration, making the substance extremely dangerous. Fifty years ago, DNP was given as a drug to help patients lose weight, and some very daring cosmetic users have experimented with DNP for this purpose. Side effects may include cataracts, dermatitis and death. *DNP is not a controlled substance, but it is banned for human use.* An Indiana man was recently convicted of selling a misbranded drug after selling DNP to a Long Island man who died from using it.

DRIVE® (Boldenone undecylenate & methylandrostenediol dipropionate): The brand name for a veterinary, oil-based, injectable steroid compound that is a combination of boldenone undecyclenate (*see* Equipoise) and methylandrostenediol dipropionate. This compound is highly anabolic and has significant androgenic properties. As such, this compound can produce significant gains in lean muscle mass while also producing a number of unwanted side effects. This drug is manufactured in Australia and is not commonly found on the black market in the United States. *It is a Schedule III federally controlled substance.*

DSHEA (The Dietary Supplement Health and Education Act): The common name for Public Law 103-417 which was signed into law by President Clinton on October 25, 1994. For years, the Food and Drug Administration (FDA) regulated dietary supplements as foods, presumably to ensure that they were safe and wholesome, and that their labeling was truthful and not misleading. An important facet of ensuring safety was FDA's evaluation of the safety of all new ingredients, including those used in dietary supplements, under the 1958 Food Additive Amendments to the Federal Food, Drug, and Cosmetic Act (FD&C Act). However, with passage of the Dietary Supplements Health and Education Act of 1994, Congress amended the FD&C Act to include several provisions that apply only to dietary supplements and dietary ingredients of dietary supplements. As a result of these provisions, dietary ingredients used in dietary supplements are no longer subject to the pre-market safety evaluations required of other new food ingredients or for new uses of old food ingredients. However, they must meet the requirements of other safety provisions. The provisions of DSHEA define dietary supplements and dietary ingredients; establish a new framework for assuring safety; outline guidelines for literature displayed where supplements are sold; provide for use of claims and nutritional support statements; require ingredient and nutrition labeling; and grant FDA the authority to establish good manufacturing practice (GMP) regulations. The law also requires formation of an executive level Commission on Dietary Supplement Labels and an Office of Dietary Supplements within the National Institutes of Health. It is DSHEA that makes it possible for supplement manufacturers to sell prohormones. Recently, anti-supplement lobbyists and anti-doping crusaders are pushing to restrict DSHEA.

DURABOLIN® (Nandrolone phenylpropionate): This oil-based, injectable steroid compound is not unlike Deca-Durabolin® (see this glossary) in its properties; however, the primary difference is the duration during which the drug is released. Unlike Deca-Durabolin®, Durabolin® may be active for only a few days. *Durabolin® is a Schedule III federally controlled substance.*

DYAZIDE® (Triamterene and hydrochlorothiazide): An oral diuretic sometimes used by physique competitors seeking to get ripped or other athletes seeking to reduce bodyweight to qualify for a lighter weight class. *This item is available by prescription only; however, it is not a controlled substance.*

DYNABOL (Nandrolone cypionate): A veterinary, injectable nandrolone ester from Australia. This highly anabolic, mildly androgenic drug exerts effects similar to Deca-Durabolin®, but differs in release time. *It is a Schedule III federally controlled substance.*

DYNABOLON (Nandrolone undecanoate): A long-acting, oil-based, injectable nandrolone ester from Italy, also manufactured under the name Psychobolan. *It is a Schedule III federally controlled substance.*

ECA: The abbreviation for the commonly used stack of ephedrine, caffeine and aspirin, available as an OTC dietary supplement, for weight loss. It was discovered this stack has a profound effect upon lipolysis as well as having a central nervous system stimulatory effect.

ECSTASY: *see MDMA*

EDEMA: Water retention, commonly identified by a lack of muscular definition and a soft, puffy, bloated appearance, particularly of the face. It is an undesirable side effect of steroids with a high propensity to aromatize to estrogens. While genetic predisposition is a big factor, edema can be avoided or controlled by using less androgenic drugs, strict dieting, and limiting sodium intake.

ENDOGENOUS: Produced naturally by the body's own endocrine system, as the testes make testosterone. When androgens from outside the body (exogenous) are administered for a period of time, endogenous production can be suppressed.

EPHEDRA: Ephedra sinica, also known as ma huang, is the plant most commonly used as a source of ephedra products. Ma huang is a popular OTC dietary supplement in the United States and has been used for thousands of years in Chinese medicine. Ephedra includes "ephedrine alkaloids," which are naturally occurring compounds that are found in plants. Ephedra dietary supplements generally contain standardized extracts that have 6 to 8 percent ephedrine alkaloids. While controversy continues, scientific studies have confirmed that ephedra products are safe when used as part of an overall weight-loss program. However, it is very important to adhere to product directions and warnings. Ephedra and ephedrine are banned in many sports [*see* ephedrine].

EPHEDRINE: The synthetic drug ephedrine hydrochloride is based on ephedra, its herbal equivalent. It's a legal, OTC oral drug used in the treatment of paroxysms of bronchial asthma. It is most frequently packaged in 25mg, 100-tablet bottles. Common brand names include Primatene tablets and Dymetadrine-25. Ephedrine stimulates the central nervous system, burns fat, and suppresses the appetite, making it popular for bodybuilders as well as dieters. Athletes can benefit from the increased energy and more intense muscular contractions it offers, permitting them to train with heavier weights and for longer periods of time. For dieters and bodybuilders it is most often used in a stack with caffeine and aspirin (ECA). There are some commercially available over-the-counter products such as Xenadrine and Stacker 2, which are nothing more than a pre-prepared stack of these substances in capsule form. It is most often combined with guaifenesin (pronounced gwye-FEN-e-sin), an expectorant often used in over-the-counter cold medications to reduce coughs by thinning the mucus or phlegm in the lungs.

The FDA does not currently control ephedrine because it is considered a dietary supplement. This means the product is protected under DSHEA. According to the FDA, despite ephedrine's harmful side effects, the product has not been proven to be hazardous to one's health. Because the FDA does not regulate ephedrine, manufacturers do not need a background in medicine or pharmacology to produce it. Ephedrine's lack of regulation also means that companies do not have to test their product before releasing it. Some argue that manufacturers are able take advantage of ephedrine's current legal status by mixing the product with other stimulants. This attempt to produce a "legal amphetamine" represents negligence, according to many consumers and experts in the medical field. Opinions on ephedrine are mixed in professional sports; however, the product has been banned from most amateur sports. While ephedrine is still legal in professional baseball and basketball, it has long been banned from competition in the NCAA, CIS, and the Olympics. On September 27, 2001 the National Football League (NFL) banned ephedrine. Under this ban, no team or player may use, distribute, or promote ephedrine. If the product is even found on team property, players, management, or staff may be fined or suspended under the league's substance abuse policy. *Ephedrine is not a scheduled controlled substance; however, it is important to note that some states and local jurisdictions have imposed restrictions on its sale, particularly to minors.*

EPITESTOSTERONE: A biological form of testosterone that does not enhance performance. Drug tests for testosterone typically measure the ratio of testosterone to epitestosterone (T/E ratio). When the T/E ratio is above 6:1, the athlete fails. Testosterone and epitestosterone do not exist in the body in a 1:1 ratio. They are actually excreted in a 20:1 ratio, but by the time they are excreted in the urine they are in a 1:1 ratio. This is because testosterone is much more prone to metabolism than epitestosterone is.

EPO (Erythropoietin): This drug is a genetically engineered protein that is clinically used to treat certain anemias, such as those associated with chronic renal failure and those secondary to cancer chemotherapy, by stimulating the production of red blood cells. The brand name is Epogen®. In cases of renal failure, severe anemia is caused by the insufficient production of erythropoietin, a protein naturally produced in healthy kidneys, which circulates through the bloodstream to the bone marrow, stimulating the production of red blood cells. Without adequate amounts of erythropoietin, there are too few red blood cells to deliver oxygen sufficiently throughout the body. With fewer red blood cells, anemia develops, which can result in dialysis patients feeling fatigued to the point where they are unable to perform their usual daily activities. Healthy athletes, particularly those involved in endurance sports, may seek the red blood cell production that results from the use of EPO. The use of EPO by athletes is essentially an artificial method of blood doping (see this glossary for *blood doping*). Additionally, the use of EPO by athletes carries with it the same associated risk as blood doping, namely blood cell concentration. *EPO is not a controlled substance.*

EQUIPOISE® (Boldenone undecyclenate): A veterinary, oil-based, injectable steroid compound. Other brand names include Boldebal-H, Boldenon, Boldenone-50, Crecibol, Equi-gan, Ganabol, Mitgan 50, Maxigan, Pace, Sybolin, Ultragan, and Vebonol. This testosterone derivative is mildly androgenic while exhibiting high anabolic properties. It is typically used similarly to Deca as part of a testosterone-based stack. *Equipoise is a Schedule III federally controlled substance.*

ESICLENE (Formebolone): An uncommon anabolic steroid once used to cause localized swelling of a lagging muscle. It is the only available steroid that is water-soluble. Today, Synthol is the product of choice for this effect. *Formebolone is a Schedule III federally controlled substance.*

ESTER: An oil-based, injectable variation of a steroid, such as nandrolone decanoate or testosterone cypionate. Esterification is the process by which the molecule is made more soluble in oil than in water without any loss of efficacy or potential potency. The oil contained in a vial or ampoule is merely the delivery system for the drug. When the oil is injected intramuscularly, it creates a "depot" in the muscle. The oil, along with the drug it contains, will disperse into the bloodstream over time, usually seven to fourteen days. An esterified compound with a longer ester chain will dissipate more slowly and obviate the need for frequent injections. Accordingly, a fast-dispersing ester like testosterone propionate will require more frequent injections that a long-acting one like testosterone enanthate.

ESTRADIOL: Estradiol is a female steroid hormone that has a number of functions in females. Estradiol is mainly synthesized in and secreted from the placenta, ovarian follicle, and adrenal cortex. It is responsible for growth of the uterus, Fallopian tubes and vagina; promotion of breast development; maturation of the external genitalia; deposition of body fat in a female distribution; and termination of linear growth. Estradiol stimulates the proliferation of the endometrium in the first half of the menstrual cycle. This hormone can be found as a component in a number of the veterinary, subcutaneous, cattle growth implants, such as Synovex. The use of such products can have adverse results in males, such as a gynecomastia. *It is not a controlled substance.*

ESTROGEN: a collective term for the female steroid hormones estradiol, estrone and estriol.

EXOGENOUS: Originating outside the body and not produced by the body's own endocrine system.

Anabolic steroids are exogenous hormones. Administering exogenous androgens will suppress the body's own endogenous androgen production.

FINA KIT: An underground conversion kit that permits a home chemist to extract the anabolic steroids out of a bovine implant to make them available for human administration. The end result is a "home brew" of trenbolone or testosterone ready for intramuscular injection. The short-acting anabolics typically produced require frequent and often painful injections, and may be unsterile and contain impurities such as methanol. Would-be users may be taking substantial risks self-administering the results of this process. In and of itself, the kit merely contains some innocuous components. However, the facts and circumstances surrounding the possession of the kit may arguably be sufficient evidence of criminal intent to possess drug paraphernalia.

FINAPLIX®: A veterinary cattle implant containing trenbolone acetate, a potent androgen with little, if any, estrogenic activity. This item is commonly referred to as "Fina" among physique enthusiasts. The product is sold by feed stores and farm supply houses and is used to increase the weight of cattle prior to slaughter. It is dramatically effective at accomplishing that goal and significantly increases profits to cattle ranchers. It is manufactured in two forms, Finaplix-H (for heifers) and Finaplix-S (for steers), with differing total dosages. A competitor has manufactured two similar products: Component-TH and Component-TS. These trenbolone acetate implants must be distinguished from Revalor and Synovex plus implants, which contain a significant dose of estradiol in addition to trenbolone acetate. *Cattle implants are specifically excluded from the scheduling classifications of the Controlled Substances Act and are therefore regulated by the FDA instead of the DEA. They are legal to buy for administration to cattle. However, they may be treated as controlled substances where circumstances connect them to human use. See Chapter 4 for a full discussion.*

GANABOL: *See* boldenone.

GBL: Gamma-Butyrolactone is one of the two chemicals used to create GHB. Butyrolactone is converted into GHB in the body. Its effects are similar to GHB (see GHB). *GBL became a List 1 chemical on Feb 18, 2000.*

GEAR a.k.a. JUICE: The slang term used to identify anabolic steroids. Sometimes it encompasses all the related substances that will be used during one's cycle.

GHB: An abbreviation for the long chemical name, gamma hydroxybutyric acid, it's a carbohydrate that occurs naturally in the human body and in foods that we commonly eat. It was sold in health food stores during the late 1980s, purchased by bodybuilders for its ability to stimulate release of muscle-building human growth hormone. As a central nervous system depressant, it can promote relaxation and induce deep sleep. Police and regulatory agencies have referred to GHB as a deadly, addictive and brain-damaging "designer drug." Like rohypnol, it's been labeled a "date rape" drug by the media and has been presented as such to Congress. Regardless of the true dangers and merits of GHB, its current legal status is as a *controlled substance*. In February 2000, President Clinton signed the "Hillory J. Farias and Samantha Reid Date-Rape Drug Prohibition Act of 2000," ordering GHB to be added to the list of *Schedule I* controlled substances – those with the highest potential for abuse and no currently accepted medical use. The law took effect a month later, with GHB assuming the *most serious* drug status under federal law. (Anabolic steroids are only Schedule III substances.) It may be referred to by the slang terms Liquid X, G, Liquid Ecstasy, Grievous Bodily Harm, Georgia Home Boy, Scoop, Great Hormones at Bedtime, Salty Water, Water, Everclear, Aminos, GH Buddy, Blue Monster, Blue Nitro, Firewater, Remforce, Renewtrient, Firewater and Easy Lay. Its dose-dependent central nervous system effects include drowsiness, dizziness, nausea, amnesia, visual hallucinations, hypotension, bradycardia, and, in some cases, severe respiratory depression, and coma. The use of alcohol in combination with GHB greatly enhances its depressant effects. A victim of an overdose may not simply "sleep it off" and may require emergency room care. *Although GHB* *is a Schedule I controlled substance, the Orphan pharmaceutical company has been granted special approval to market a Schedule III version of the drug for sleep disorders.*

GLUCOPHAGE (Metformin HCL): A brand name for the oral, anti-hypoglycemic drug, metformin hydrochloride. Clinically, this drug is used in the control of mature onset, Type II diabetes, in those cases where diet and exercise are insufficient, yet injectable insulin is inappropriate. This ancillary drug is reportedly used for a mild anabolic effect. However, this drug has a number of risks associated with its use, the most serious of which is a potentially fatal metabolic condition known as lactic acidosis. *Glucophage is available by prescription only; however, it is not a controlled substance.*

GYNECOMASTIA: The feminization of the male chest, usually around the nipple, commonly caused by the use of drugs that convert into excessive estrogen, progesterone or prolactin. The slang term is "bitch tits." The condition may be visually subtle or quite obvious, and may be accompanied by sensitivity or even pain. If untreated, extreme cases may require a removal of the tissue and glands around the nipple. Fortunately, the condition can be prevented by the use of non-aromatizing steroids and through the administration of anti-estrogens such as Proviron®, Cytadren®, Nolvadex®, or Arimidex®.

HALOTESTIN® (Fluoxymesterone): Fluoxymesterone is a potent, highly androgenic oral steroid. It's alpha alkylated and liver stressful, particularly with long-term use. Not a good size builder, bodybuilders may use it pre-contest to achieve a harder, denser look. *This drug is a Schedule III controlled substance under federal law.*

HARDCORE: In bodybuilding parlance, this term may be used in reference to those who are fanatical about becoming as muscular as possible, often while reducing body fat levels to a severely low level. The term implies a devotion to massive training poundages, regulated eating habits, and, quite often, the use of anabolic steroids.

HEPATOTOXICITY: The potential to cause toxic damage to the liver. The liver, a solid organ located in the upper right quadrant of the abdomen, plays a major role in the metabolism, digestion, detoxification, and elimination of substances from the body. Hepatotoxicity from anabolic steroids is associated with the use of 17 alpha alkylated drugs. Oil-based injectable steroids have been shown to have little if any effect on the liver.

HMB: Beta-Hydroxy Beta-methylbutyrate, also shown as ß-hydroxy ß-methylbutyrate monohydrate. Not a drug, but a legal dietary supplement, now reportedly discredited as having no anabolic effects.

HORMONE REPLACEMENT THERAPY (HRT): The clinical use of therapeutic doses of anabolics and/or human growth hormone for medically evaluated individuals. It's important to understand that androgen therapy is a replacement for, not a supplement to, natural production. Once exogenous androgens have been administered in significant dosages for a sufficient period, believed to be about three weeks, the body shuts down its own production. The only androgens circulating in the body are those that are administered.

HUMAN CHORIONIC GONADOTROPIN (HCG): This hormone is not an anabolic steroid, and it is important not to confuse it with human growth hormone (hGH). Chorionic gonadotropin is a hormone that is found in females during pregnancy. This hormone, produced in the placenta, helps to maintain pregnancy once a fetus begins to develop. It appears in the urine in approximately the first week after the first missed menstrual period, and is the basis for two kinds of pregnancy tests. Its effect on physique enthusiasts is to stimulate the testes to produce testosterone. It is typically used at various points during an AAS cycle, particularly a long cycle, and/or at the end of the cycle. HCG is an effective tool against the endogenous suppression of testosterone that occurs from using steroids, and can prevent or alleviate testicular shrinkage. Popular brand names are Pregnyl® and Profasi®. *HCG is available by prescription only and is not a controlled substance under federal law. However, some states have classified it as a controlled substance under state law. (See State Laws appendix.)*

HUMAN GROWTH HORMONE (hGH): A natural hormone produced in the human body by the pituitary gland that has become available as an injectable, synthetically produced drug. It has become a popular but expensive hormone in anti-aging medicine, and is reported to have highly positive effects when used medically in this context. Physique athletes may use it to improve size and strength. Many bodybuilders report that hGH has limited effects on its own, but works synergistically with anabolics to produce dramatic gains. Excessive use can lead to significant side effects. Some of the brand names are Genotropin®, Humatrope®, Nutropin®, Protropin®, Saizen®, Serostim® and Somatotropin®. There is as yet no sports doping drug test to determine the exogenous use of this hormone. *HGH is available by prescription only; it is not a controlled substance under federal law. However, federal law prohibits the distribution or possession with the intent to distribute human growth hormone for use in humans other than for the treatment of a disease or other recognized medical condition under 21 U.S.C. § 333(e). Violations may be punishable by imprisonment of up to 5 years (10 years if to a person under 18 years old). Some states have classified hGH as a controlled substance [see State Laws appendix].*

HYPOGONADISM: In men, the decreased or absent secretion of androgens from the testes and a basis for testosterone replacement therapy. The average normal testosterone range for adult males is 278 to 1,000 ng/dl of blood.

INJECTABLE: Any of those drugs that are administered through the use of a needle and syringe. It is important to note that steroids are administered intramuscularly, not intravenously (into the vein) the way a heroin user would. Injectable steroids may be oil or water based.

INSULIN: Insulin is not an androgen or a steroid. It is what is known as a proteinaceous hormone and is responsible for regulating glucose levels in the body. Insulin or "slin" has both anabolic and anti-catabolic properties. It increases the uptake of compounds such as protein and carbohydrates into the cell. Using insulin in combination with anabolic steroids is a common practice of bodybuilders, as anabolic steroids increase protein synthesis and insulin increases the amount of protein that is shuttled to the muscle cells. Insulin has additional appeal in that it cannot be detected by urinalysis. Three types of non-prescription insulin are commonly used by bodybuilders and can be obtained at pharmacies. The first and most commonly used product is known as Humulin-R. It is fast acting, making it more desirable than other forms of insulin. Another, more intermediate form, is known as Humulin-N or Humulin-L, which can last almost three times as long as Humulin-R. Finally, there is Humulin-U, which has the characteristic of staying active more than 24 hours. This is more desirable for the diabetic than the bodybuilder, who prefers to have more control over his insulin spikes for safety and efficacy. Humalog is a prescription form of insulin, which is even more desirable than Humulin-R, as it is even faster acting. *Insulin is not a controlled substance.*

JACKED: Slang term used to describe a physique that is huge and muscular.

JUICER: A slang term to describe a bodybuilder who uses steroids. The term is most frequently associated with the heavy user.

LASIX® (Furosemide): Lasix® is the most powerful and effective diuretic available. Bodybuilders prefer the injectable version as it is fast acting and can remove intracellular and extracellular water almost immediately, which is ideal for pre-contest prep. However, it is also extremely dangerous. Along with the undesirable "water weight," key electrolytes such as sodium and potassium are lost as well. This can lead to severe muscle cramping among other undesirable side effects. Lasix® can be found in both a tablet and an injectable form. The tablets are 20 or 40mg and are taken orally, while the injectable version is more commonly administered intravenously, unlike most steroids, which are always injected intramuscularly. Lasix® is banned in drug-tested athletic competition. *It is available by prescription only; however, it is not a controlled substance.*

LAURABOLIN (Nandrolone laurate): This nandrolone ester is similar to Deca, but is an exclusively veterinary product made outside the United States. The characteristics that make it less popular than its counterpart are its lack of availability and that it is usually found in lesser concentrations, requiring more frequent injections. *It is a Schedule III controlled substance under federal law.*

LIQUIDEX: A liquid version of the prescription drug anastrozole (see Arimidex® in this glossary). This product is not produced by a legitimate pharmaceutical manufacturer, but by an underground lab and sold through the Internet as a "research chemical." *It is important to note that while this drug is not a controlled substance, it is nonetheless a prescription item.* Merely labeling it as intended "for research purposes only" does not purge the criminality of selling or possessing this item without a prescription.

MASTERON (Drostanolone propionate): Also known as drostanolone, Masteron has had limited availability in the last few years. Intended for oral administration, Masteron is a 2-methylated steroid often utilized by bodybuilders in the weeks prior to a contest, when shedding body fat while maintaining muscle mass is the main concern. It is a derivative of dihydrotestosterone (DHT) and a *schedule III controlled substance under federal law.*

MDMA (Ecstasy): This substance is a chemical variation of mescaline and amphetamine, which has been synthesized in underground laboratories. This is just one of a whole host of related chemicals which are illicitly manufactured. MDMA, which chemically is 3, 4-methylene-dioxymethamphetamine, is also referred to on the street as Ecstasy, E, Fantasy, XTC, Adam, Clarity, and Lover's Speed. They are all amphetamine variants for which there is no medical use. MDMA produces both amphetamine-like stimulation and mild mescaline-like hallucinations. MDMA may produce a sense of well-being and euphoria, increased energy, increased sensual arousal, and enhanced tactile sensations. Because these drugs are manufactured in underground labs, they are frequently impure. Furthermore, the dosage in a tablet, capsule or on a square of impregnated paper may be expected to vary considerably. MDMA users often experience muscle tension, involuntary teeth clenching (teens with infant pacifiers around their necks were either using it to avoid damage to their teeth or trying to pretend to be doing so), nausea, blurred vision, faintness, chills, and sweating. In addition, MDMA can produce significant increases in heart rate and blood pressure similar to those associated with amphetamine use. MDMA's effects may typically last anywhere from 3 to 6 hours, but users report that confusion, depression, insomnia, anxiety, and paranoia may occur even weeks after the drug is taken. Not only does MDMA do nothing to improve muscle-building efforts, in high doses it can cause extreme increases in body temperature that may lead to muscle breakdown and kidney and cardiovascular system failure. This condition, called "malignant hyperthermia," can be fatal. *MDMA is a Schedule I controlled substance.*

METABOLITE: Any substance produced by metabolism or by a metabolic process. In essence, this may describe the processes by which a particular substance is handled in the living body. In drug use, a metabolite usually refers to the end product (what remains after metabolism). With regard to anabolics, this term may often be heard when drug testing is discussed. Anabolics are transformed in structure in the body. This resulting end product is a metabolite. Metabolites may be disclosed through drug testing up to 18 months from the first administration of a steroid, depending upon the steroid used.

METHYLTESTOSTERONE: Methyltestosterone is an oral version of testosterone that utilizes a 17-alpha-methyl addition to the base hormone testosterone in order to make it orally active. Methyltestosterone is not a preferred steroid due to the fact that there are other injectable versions of testosterone that will produce similar or superior results while avoiding the more toxic alpha alkylated steroid. Additionally, this oral version is made less potent than testosterone due to the properties intrinsic to alpha alkylated compounds. *Methyltestosterone is a Schedule III controlled substance under federal law.*

MIOTOLAN (Furazabol): Furazabol is structurally similar to stanozolol (Winstrol) in that it is a DHT derivative that is C-17-alpha-methylated, making it orally bioavailable. It is manufactured only in Japan and found in 1mg tablets. Though slightly more potent than stanozolol, furazabol is more expensive and more difficult to procure than its counterpart, and therefore it is less likely to be chosen over the more available alternatives. *Furazabol is a Schedule III controlled substance under federal law.*

NATURAL: A term used to describe athletes or cosmetic physique enthusiasts who do not use steroids in their training. This term may be further refined to describe a "lifetime natural" as a person who has never used steroids, in contrast, with one who may be natural only for a given contest or event. For a full examination of the concept of "natural bodybuilding," see the articles section of www.steroidlaw.com.

NEOTEST 250 (Testosterone decanoate)**:** Exclusively produced by the Mexican pharmaceutical manufacturer Loeffler, Neotest 250 is unique in that it is the only product to include strictly testosterone decanoate, the slowest-acting ester of testosterone available. Neotest 250 is a viable alternative to Sustanon for those seeking the gradual increase in blood concentrations that the decanoate ester provides, but prefer to avoid the irritation associated with the propionate ester contained in Sustanon. Neotest 250 comes in a 10ml bottle and contains a concentration of 250mg/ml. *Testosterone decanoate is a Schedule III controlled substance under federal law.*

NILEVAR (Norethandrolone): Nilevar is an oral nortestosterone derivative, which has characteristics very much like Deca-durabolin®, however slightly weaker androgenically, a bit more potent estrogenically, and a lot more progestational (thus causing much more edema). As is characteristic of other nortestosterone derivatives, the nortestosterone metabolites can be detectable for a significant time after cessation of use. This is commonly the way that drug- tested athletes produce a positive urine analysis long after they have discontinued steroid use. The most ominous difference between nandrolone and norethandrolone is that it is C-17-alkylated in order to make it orally bioavailable. Consequently, norethandrolone is never used as a "base" compound in a steroid stack. Its alpha-alkylation increases its risk of hepatotoxicity and it is commonly limited to a much shorter duration of use than that of the injectable nandrolone. Common dosages are in the range of 30-40mg per day. *Norethandrolone is a Schedule III controlled substance under federal law.*

NOLVADEX® (Tamoxifen citrate): An estrogen antagonist with mixed agonist/antagonist properties. It reduces estrogenic activity by preventing estrogen from binding to the estrogen receptor. Reducing estrogenic activity is linked to reducing water retention, gynecomastia, and estrogen related (adipose tissue) fat gain. Nolvadex® can be utilized during a cycle of aromatizable steroids to reduce estrogen or at the end of a cycle to help recover natural testosterone production by stimulating leutinizing hormone while continuing to block estrogen. Additionally, being a mixed agonist/antagonist, Nolvadex® acts as an estrogen in the liver, improving HDL, the good cholesterol, and lowering LDL, the bad cholesterol. This is beneficial during a cycle of non-aromatizable androgens, where the lack of estrogen can lead to an unfavorable cholesterol profile. Nolvadex® can be found in 10mg and 20mg tablets. Nolvadex is banned from use in drug-tested athletic competition. *It is available by prescription only; however, it is not a controlled substance.*

NUBAIN® (Nalbuphine HCL): Nalbuphine is the chemical name for the extremely popular bodybuilding recreational drug known as Nubain or simply 'Bain.' In reality, this injectable drug is a synthetic opiate agonist/antagonist; this means that nalbuphine is a painkiller like morphine but, because nalbuphine is selectively agonistic, the drug lacks the euphoria (and theoretically the pleasurable experience) associated with morphine and other opiates. Unfortunately, nalbuphine is every bit as addictive as heroin or morphine. Nalbuphine is usually injected intravenously, intramuscularly or subcutaneously. Bodybuilders frequently begin at the 10mg dosage described above, yet as their experience increases and their bodies become more resistant, the dosages can edge up quickly. Not only do the dosages increase, but the frequency of injections may increase. An experienced user may use 2mls per injection several times a day. *Nalbuphine is specifically excluded from the list of Schedule II controlled substances; however it is still a prescription drug.*

OMNADREN (Testosterone blend): This is a blend of different forms of esterified testosterone, very similar to the combination used in Sustanon 250 (see Sustanon). The only difference is that 100mg/ml of testosterone hexanoate is substituted for the testosterone decanoate that is used in Sustanon. This results in a faster increase in blood levels and a shorter overall half-life for Omnadren. Omnadren injections are weekly although some effect will still be noticeable 2-3 weeks after the last injection. *Omnadren is a Schedule III controlled substance.*

ORABOLIN® (Ethylestrenol): Orabolin® is another of the nortestosterone derivatives. It was once available in the U.S. under the name Maxibolan. The C-17-alkylation presents greater potential for hepatotoxicity than injectables, therefore limiting the duration of use as well as the dosage, and hindering its desirability. *Ethylestrenol is a Schedule III controlled substance under federal law.*

ORALS: Anabolic steroids that are administered by mouth. These most commonly include Dianabol, Anadrol 50®, Anavar®, Andriol, Halotestin®, methyltestosterone and Winstrol® tabs. The most toxic steroids to the liver are those orals that are 17-alpha-alkylated.

OVER-THE-COUNTER (OTC): Legitimate pharmaceutical drugs which may be legally purchased without a medical doctor's prescription. Examples include: aspirin, acetaminophen, Ibuprofen, ephedrine hydrochloride and pseudoephedrine.

OXANDROLONE: Although it is alpha alkylated, this mild anabolic is commonly viewed as one of the safest steroids available. Brand names include Anavar, Oxandralone SPA, Oxandrin, Anatrophill, Lipidex, Lonavar and Vasorome. Typically used by bodybuilders during a "cutting" phase where the goal is the reduction of body fat, this steroid does not aromatize and as a result does not cause edema. Moreover, because it is low in androgenic activity it is popular with some female athletes who may use low doses with a limited risk of virilizing effects. *Oxandrolone is a federal Schedule III controlled substance.*

OXYCODONE: An analgesic-narcotic derived from the opiate alkaloid thebaine, it is the active ingredient in several painkillers, including OxyContin. This drug is available in time-release tablets that can last for as long as 12 hours. When used as prescribed, it helps cancer patients and chronic pain sufferers manage their pain. However, it is highly addictive and has been implicated in numerous overdose fatalities. *Oxycodone is a Schedule II controlled substance.*

OXYMETHOLONE: A highly anabolic and androgenic oral steroid. Brand names include: Anadrol 50®, Anapolon 50, Anasteron, Dynasten, Hemogenin, Oxitosona 50, Oxybolone, Oxylone, Plenastril, Roboral and Synasteron. Oxymetholone is a 17-alpha-alkylated compound (orally effective but potentially hepatotoxic) and can also be stressful to the kidneys through the associated edema and hypertension. However, recent studies with HIV+ patients seem to be supportive of safe use. Anadrol 50® is available in a 50mg tablet and packaged most often in bottles of 100. Because it contains so many milligrams per tablet, the typical dose is only one to four tablets daily. Dramatic gains in strength, size and body weight can be achieved in a short time, but the accompanying edema may cause a puffy, bloated appearance and post-cycle losses can be significant. *Oxymetholone is a federal Schedule III controlled substance.*

PAPER STEROIDS: A somewhat new method of avoiding detection involving the impregnation of blotter paper with anabolic steroids. This has been done in the past with LSD and MDMA. For example, a piece of blotter paper could be impregnated with oxymetholone, and the user would simply eat an appropriately sized piece of paper. Uniformity of potency is a key issue.

PARABOLAN (Trenbolone hexahydrobenzylcarbonate): Parabolan was a trenbolone product packaged in 1.5ml ampoules containing an ester that extends the steroid's activity for more than two weeks. Parabolan was a popular pre-contest drug but it is no longer in production. *Trenbolone esters are Schedule III federally controlled substances; however, black market products claiming to contain Parabolan most likely do not.*

PELIOSIS HEPATITIS: A condition in which the liver and, in some cases, splenic tissue is replaced with blood-filled cysts. This condition may be associated with the use of 17-alpha-alylated steroids, mostly in geriatric patients who are administered these drugs for prolonged periods. These cysts are sometimes present with minimal hepatic dysfunction, but at other times they have been associated with liver failure. They are often not recognized until life-threatening liver failure or intra-abdominal hemorrhage develops. The cessation of drug use most often results in a complete disappearance of lesions.

PRIMOBOLAN® (Methenolone acetate): This oral formulation of Primobolan or "primo" containing methenolone acetate is *not* C-17-alpha-alkylated, reducing the potential for liver toxicity. It is very similar in action to the Primobolan Depot. Considered to be one of the most "mild" steroids, Primobolan® is often utilized by those concerned with side effects. Primobolan® is an extremely mild androgen with mild anabolic properties as well. It is another of the non-aromatizable androgens, making it desirable for "cutting" purposes. A male bodybuilder will use doses in the range of 75mg to 150mg daily. Legitimate oral Primobolan® is found in 5mg and 25mg tablets. *Methenolone acetate is a Schedule III federally controlled substance.*

PRIMOBOLAN® DEPOT (Methenolone enanthate): This is the injectable form of methenolone with an added enanthate ester. This Depot version of Primobolan® has much of the same characteristics as the oral version. Bodybuilders will often choose Primobolan® Depot in place of a nandrolone injectable. Despite the fact that they are both relatively mild androgens, methenolone is reportedly not nearly as suppressive of endogenous testosterone levels as nandrolone. *Primobolan® Depot is Schedule III controlled substance under federal law.*

PROHORMONE: In December, 1996, chemist Patrick Arnold announced the public availability of androstenedione, a natural precursor to testosterone which could be legally sold for oral consumption. Prohormones remained largely unknown to the general public until August, 1998, when home-run slugger Mark McGwire publicly revealed that he used androstenedione as an athletic performance enhancer. Since then, various other prohormones have been produced and marketed for the purpose of enhancing testosterone and nortestosterone (nandrolone) levels, including, as examples, androstenediol, norandrostenedione, norandrostenediol, 1-androstenediol, and 5-alpha androstanediol. Government authorities have suggested restricting prohormones to prescription drug status or even scheduling them as controlled substances, but at the present time they remain available as over-the-counter dietary supplements.

PROSCAR® (Finasteride): This ancillary drug acts to inhibit the 5alpha-reductase enzyme from converting testosterone into dihydrotestosterone (DHT). DHT is thought to be implicated in male pattern baldness and benign prostate hyperplasia (BPH). Proscar® was the initial brand name used to market this product in treatment of BPH. Finasteride was later approved to treat hair loss and is marketed under the name Propecia®. This is of great utility to the bodybuilder, as many of the unwanted side effects such as oily skin, acne, body hair growth, and male pattern baldness are related to high levels of DHT built up in certain tissues. This product is most useful when using a synthetic testosterone, as testosterone has a high conversion to DHT. Finasteride can be found as 1mg tabs under the brand name Propecia® or as 5mg tabs under the brand name Proscar®. *Finasteride is a prescription medication; however, it is not a controlled substance.*

PROTEIN: The basic building blocks of muscle tissue, made of amino acids. Protein supplementation provides a positive environment for muscle growth. Protein supplementation can provide a positive nitrogen balance in the body, favorable to building muscle. However, protein in and of itself, without progressive resistance training, will not build muscle. A negative nitrogen balance puts the body in a catabolic state, wherein muscle protein is being used and broken down for energy. This catabolic state can result when a weight-trainer fails to consume adequate amounts of protein within a proper time frame. Protein may actually be used for fuel during intense exercise, particularly when carbohydrates are not available, and can provide as much as 10% of the energy during exercise when a person is carbohydrate depleted. The Recommended Dietary Allowance of 0.36 grams of protein per pound of body weight for sedentary adult individuals is an amount that is woefully inadequate for all active individuals, not only those engaged in weight training exercise. The total protein intake and total caloric intake will determine whether or not an anabolic state can exist. If the athlete consumes a lot of calories, carbohydrates and fats without eating sufficient protein, muscular growth will not occur. Studies by the world's top protein researchers, such as Dr. Peter Lemon, have determined that .8 grams per pound of body weight should be your *minimum* for protein if you exercise regularly. Optimal intake for hard-training athletes, such as bodybuilders, is still unknown and may be even higher. In one study of Polish weightlifters, 50% of the subjects were still in negative nitrogen balance, even while consuming 250% of the RDA. For bodybuilders, one gram per pound of body weight has been a rule of thumb for years, and it's close to the .8 grams per pound of body weight recommended in Lemon's research. Although no studies have been done, most bodybuilders believe that two grams per pound of body weight is needed to maximize gains on anabolic steroid cycles. Concerns about the safety of a typical high protein bodybuilder's diet appear completely unfounded [for a review of the studies, see *Sports Supplements*, edited by J. Antonio, Ph.D. and J. Stout, Ph.D. (Philadelphia, PA: Lipincott Williams, 2001)].

PROVIRON® (Mesterolone): Mesterolone is an orally active, 1-methylated DHT. Proviron® is made by Schering. It does not aromatize. Despite its strong androgenic properties, Proviron® is considered to exert a week anabolic effect, insufficient to promote muscle growth. Clinically, Proviron® has been prescribed to treat various forms of sexual dysfunction, but bodybuilders are more interested in its anti-aromatase properties which help to harden the physique's appearance at contest time. Proviron® is commonly used in doses ranging from one to four 25mg tablets per day. *Mesterolone is a Schedule III controlled substance federally.*

PYRAMID: A cycle theory whereby the steroid doses are incrementally increased to a maximum point over a predetermined weekly time frame, and then incrementally reduced (tapered) over a corresponding time frame. If we were to plot this cycle on a graph with the drug dosage on the "X" axis and the number of weeks on the "Y" axis, the resulting plotting of points would resemble a pyramid in appearance.

RIPPED: The term is the common parlance used by bodybuilders when referring to the physical appearance characterized by a high degree of muscle definition attributable to an extremely low body fat percentage and lack of water retention. A truly "ripped" bodybuilder will essentially be a walking anatomy chart of the body's skeletal-muscular system, coursing with veins that resemble a road atlas in appearance and with skin that is near-transparent.

ROID RAGE: Slang, derogatory term used in reference to the alleged out-of-control aggressive behavior associated with steroid use. The popular notion that most or all steroid users are prone to this behavior is completely a myth, perpetuated by certain publicity-seekers in the medical community and a hyperbolic press. Documented roid rage incidents are in fact extremely few and far between. Given the rarity of the condition, to what extent genetic predisposition and expectancy play a part is subject to speculation. The so-called "roid rage defense" has been attempted as an excuse for bad behavior in criminal cases. To the best of my knowledge, no jury has bought it.

SIDE EFFECT: Any undesirable effect that is attributable to a drug other than its desired therapeutic effect. Some are considered minor (acne), merely cosmetic (hair loss), and/or annoying (insomnia), but others can be life-threatening. Statistically, side effects that occur with an incidence of one percent or greater (1 out of 100 patients on the drug) are usually considered to be causally related to the use of that particular medication.

STACKING: This is a practice whereby athletes administer a combination of drugs to take advantage of a synergistic effect of these compounds and to minimize adverse consequences associated mostly with one or the other. It is important for the legal practitioner to note that the proper combination of the appropriate drugs can be far less toxic and produce far fewer side effects than the administration of high doses of a single drug. For example, milligram for milligram, a stack of drugs such as testosterone cypionate, nandrolone decanoate, and oxandrolone would be far less hepatotoxic and likely produce far fewer side effects than an equivalent dose of methandrostenolone alone. The significance of this fact is crucial when a prosecutor attempts to demonize a defendant specifically because of the variety of pharmaceuticals recovered in a search.

STEN (Testosterone propionate and testosterone cypionate): Sten is a blend of two testosterone esters intending to provide "sustained release" effect; however, there is a shorter active life than other blends such as Sustanon. This requires more frequent injections. *Sten contains Schedule III controlled substances.*

SUBCUTANEOUS: A term meaning beneath or under the skin. This term may be used in reference to injectable drug administrations that are typically made beneath the skin, such as insulin, insulin-like growth factor (IGF-1) and human growth hormone injections.

SUPPLEMENT: A legal, over-the-counter dietary product used by athletes to augment their diet and training program. These products are most commonly in powder, tablet or capsule form and are administered orally. They are not drugs but in essence food. One such well-known supplement among muscle enthusiasts and the public at large is the so-called "meal replacement powder." Some of the supplements physique athletes may currently be using include: creatine monohydrate (most frequently in powder form), protein powder, Vitamin C, flaxseed oil, saw palmetto and amino acids. The shelves of health food stores are chockfull of supplements which promise to do everything from promoting incredible gains in lean muscle mass and strength to making the user a sexual tyrannosaurus, but many of these products are of little or no value.

SUSTANON 250® (Testosterone blend): Sustanon (also manufactured as Durateston and Sostenon 250®) is a blend of typically four different types of testosterone esters, each with a different time released effect. One quite rare version, manufactured in India by Organon, is actually called *Sustaretard 250*. The combination provides a fast-acting dose of testosterone while concomitantly providing slower released testosterone esters that stay active for two and three weeks. It is likely the most popular testosterone product available, and comes in ampoules and preloaded redi-ject syringes. The side effects common to Sustanon, such as gynecomastia, oily skin, acne, increased body hair and accelerated hair loss, are similar to that of other aromatizable androgens. Many of these side effects can be avoided or reduced by using anti-estrogens, anti-aromatase, and finasteride. *Sustanon contains federal Schedule III controlled substances.*

SYNOVEX® (Testosterone propionate & estradiol): Synovex® is another cattle implant preparation, but it should not be confused with Synovex plus (which contains trenbolone). Synovex® has no trenbolone, but comes in the form of small pellets containing 25mg of testosterone propionate and 2.5mg of estradiol benzoate. Synovex-H implants are intended for feedlot heifers and contain 80 pellets per package. Bodybuilders do not find Synovex to be the most desirable hormone for human administration due to the estradiol content, which is responsible for many undesirable estrogen-related side effects. Currently there are "conversion kits" available on the black market that presumably remove the estradiol from the preparation leaving only the testosterone propionate. There is another "kit" that allows conversion of the residual testosterone propionate into a form for injectable administration. *Cattle implants are specifically excluded from the scheduling classifications of the Controlled Substances Act and are therefore regulated by the FDA instead of the DEA. They are legal to buy for administration to cattle. However, they may be treated as controlled substances where circumstances connect them to human use. See Chapter 4 for a full discussion.*

SYNTHOL: An alluring drug-like name for nothing more than an exorbitantly overpriced bottle of what appears to be MCT (medium chain triglyceride) oil. It may be identified by the names Pump N' Pose, Liquid Muscle or Esik-Clean. This item is sold as "posing oil" and, according to most product labels and the web sites selling it, is for external use only. However, this is not how the oil is used. Bodybuilders may inject the oil locally into muscle groups to gain a swift, dramatic increase in lagging body parts. The increases are not the result of muscle hypertrophy; however, they are merely the result of the oil becoming encapsulated in the muscle with the effect of stretching the muscle fascia, sometimes permanently. Most commonly the injections are made into the biceps, triceps, calves, and rear deltoids. Some bodybuilders have injected so much oil into the muscle so as to create absolutely ridiculous proportions and lose the natural muscle shape. The end result for some users can be hideously disproportionate muscle groups. *This item is not a prescription drug or controlled substance.*

SYNTHROID® (Levothyroxine sodium): This is a synthetic thyroid hormone having the effect of the endogenous thyroid hormone T-4. Bodybuilders use thyroid hormones such as Synthroid® to stimulate metabolic rate. Synthroid is similar to another thyroid hormone known as Cytomel®, the synthetic preparation of the thyroid hormone T-3. Synthroid (T-4), however, has a much weaker effect than Cytomel (T-3), which derives much of its effect from conversion of T-4 to T-3. Consequently, T-4 users need to take the thyroid hormone for a longer duration in order to achieve the same results had they taken T-3. *Synthroid® is a prescription medication; however, it is not a controlled substance under federal law.*

TESLAC: Testolactone is considered neither an anabolic nor an androgenic steroid. Rather its attributes are that of an anti-aromatase, much like Proviron® or Arimidex®. It also has gonadotropin stimulating properties. Testolactone is not a very popular drug as there are cheaper alternatives available that are proven to be effective. *Testolactone is a federally controlled substance.*

TEST 400: A testosterone blend produced by the Mexican pharmaceutical manufacturer Denkall, Test 400 contains 400mg of testosterone per each ml of oil and comes in a 10ml vial. It includes 25mg of testosterone propionate, 187mg of testosterone cypionate, and 188mg of testosterone enanthate. This combination allows for a mix of fast and slow acting esters, although testosterone cypionate and testosterone enanthate are nearly identical in the structure of their esters. *Test 400 contains federal Schedule III controlled substances.*

TESTICULAR ATROPHY: A highly undesirable side effect, shrunken testicles can result when exogenous androgens are introduced into the body, causing the body's feedback mechanism to shut down natural production of testosterone. With little to do, the testes shrink. This side-effect has been highly exaggerated by the media. It generally occurs only after prolonged use, and can usually be easily avoided or treated by the administration of HCG.

TESTOSTERONE CYPIONATE: Probably the most popular form of testosterone, cypionate is a single-ester, long acting, oil based injectable form of testosterone that will keep levels elevated for nearly two weeks. Despite its long duration of action, users often prefer to administer injections up to twice weekly. It is commonly used as a base upon which to stack other steroids. Currently, a number of pharmaceutical companies have produced their own versions of this popular testosterone product, which commonly comes in 10ml vials but may also be packaged in ampoules, smaller vials, and larger vials. *Testosterone cypionate is a Schedule III federally controlled substance.*

TESTOSTERONE ENANTHATE: Very similar to testosterone cypionate, testosterone enanthate is another long lasting, oil-based injectable steroid. This is the most popular form of synthetic testosterone utilized by the medical community in treating disorders such as hypogonadism (usually as Delatestryl). One of the most appealing attributes to physicians and patients, who are treated with Hormone Replacement Therapy, is that it does not necessitate frequent injections in order to keep blood concentrations consistently elevated. The most popular products available today include Mexican generics from the veterinary firms of Brovel and Tornel. These products come in 200mg/ml concentrations, packaged in 10ml vials. Loeffler offers a 250mg/ml enanthate in a 10ml vial. Other popular brands are Primotesten from Mexico and Testoviron (1ml ampoules) from Schering in Spain. *Testosterone enanthate is a Schedule III controlled substance under federal law.*

TESTOSTERONE PROPIONATE: Another of the oil-based injectable versions of synthetic testosterone, testosterone propionate utilizes a much faster-acting ester when compared to the cypionate and enanthate esters. This requires more frequent injections ranging from every day to every third day, in order to maintain steady blood concentrations. Additionally, the propionate ester is notoriously irritating to the injection site and it is not uncommon for soreness and a fever to result. The propionate ester is included in most testosterone blends as it provides the user with a fast-acting form of testosterone so results may be seen more quickly. Some common brand name propionate products are Testex, Testoviron, Ara-Test, Testogan and Testopro L/A. *Testosterone propionate is a Schedule III federally controlled substance.*

TESTOSTERONE SUSPENSION: This is an injectable, water-based version of testosterone that does not contain an ester; meaning that 100mg of testosterone suspension equates to 100mg of pure testosterone whereas with most injectables, the total number of milligrams includes the weight of the ester. Considered to be the most powerful injectable steroid available, testosterone suspension is extremely fast acting. Aptly labeled, testosterone "suspension" actually separates from the water within the vial, with the steroid settling to the bottom. Administration daily or every other day is the most common course of action as suspension only keeps blood levels elevated for 2-3 days. Some of the most popular brands of testosterone suspension are Testotus100 an Australian product manufacture by Jurox, Anabolic-TS by Grupo Comercial Tarasco, and Uni-Test Suspension by the Canadian manufacturer Univet. Product concentrations range from 25mg/ml to 100mg/ml. *Testosterone suspension is a Schedule III controlled substance under federal law.*

TESTOSTERONE UNDECANOATE: An oral steroid preparation based in oil and sealed in a gelcap. Brand names include Andriol, Androxon, Panteston, Restandol, Undestor and Virigen. Importantly, it is one of the few orally effective compounds that is not 17-alpha-alkylated. Additionally, there is only mild aromatization with its use. However, its weak anabolic properties make it unpopular for muscle builders. *Testosterone undecanoate is a federal Schedule III controlled substance.*

TESTOVIRON® (Testosterone blend): Not to be confused with the pure testosterone enanthate preparation also produced by Schering and also called Testoviron, Schering has produced another product which is a blend of the injectables testosterone propionate and enanthate under the brand name Testoviron®. The product is packaged in 1ml ampoules, and intended to produce a fast acting response from the propionate while blood concentrations from the enanthate are building. The approach is similar to that of other products such as Sten and Sustanon. *Testoviron is a Schedule III federally controlled substance.*

TRANSDERMAL: This term describes a method of delivering a drug into the bloodstream by its application on the skin, fostering a time-release effect. Simply, "trans" means "across" and "derma" means "skin." The drug is delivered across the skin barrier into the bloodstream. This may be effectuated by compounding the drug with a carrier agent such as isopropyl myris-tate, dimethlsulfoxide (DMSO), or pleuronic lecithinic organogel (PLO). One of the most common transdermal drug applications is the nicotine patch. However, less commonly known is a transdermal testosterone compound known as Androderm® which may be prescribed for males with low testosterone levels and a fear of needles. There is ongoing research into developing transdermals for insulin-dependent diabetics who must endure the unpleasantness of daily injections.

TRENBOLONE ACETATE: A powerful non-aromatizable androgen, trenbolone or simply "tren" is a very popular steroid used during a dieting phase or contest preparation, as it is not likely to produce water retention. Finaject was one of the most infamous trenbolone products on the market, though it is no longer in production. Trenbolone may still be found in some cattle implants such as Finaplix, Synovex plus and Revalor, which require conversion into an injectable; however the Mexican manufacturer Ttokkyo recently produced a pure trenbolone product known as Trenbol 75. Trenbolone is a unique steroid, as it is a 19-nor derivative, however it is a much more potent androgen than other nandrolone-like steroids yet it maintains anabolic properties as well. Trenbolone requires administration daily or every other day. *Trenbolone is a Schedule III controlled substance under federal law.*

TRIACANA (Tiratricol): Unlike the synthetic thyroid preparations Cytomel® (T-3) and Synthroid® (T-4), tiratricol is a naturally occurring metabolite of the endogenous hormone T-3. As a result, tiratricol is much weaker than either of the synthetic preparations and is generally considered to be a safer alternative. Several years ago, Triacana, which is the product's trade name, was available legally as a dietary supplement and sold over the counter for about 8 months before the FDA designated it an unapproved new drug and demanded it be removed from the market. The French pharmaceutical manufacturing company Medgenix is likely the only name brand tiratricol product available today. *Triacana is not a controlled substance.*

TRISORALEN®® (Trioxsalen): Trisoralen is a synthetic version of the melanizing agent trioxsalen. Bodybuilders may use Trisoralen to facilitate a deeper, darker tan, which plays an important role in stage presentation. The mechanism of action is a bit unclear; however the effect is an increased rate of skin pigmentation. *Trisoralen is a prescription drug; however, it is not a federally controlled substance.*

WATER RETENTION: *See* Edema.

WINSTROL® (STANOZOLOL): Also known as "Winny," Winstrol® is the brand name for the popular anabolic steroid stanozolol. It is a relatively mild steroid, predominantly anabolic in nature, with mild androgenic properties despite being a derivative of dihydrotestosterone. Winstrol is manufactured in both an oral and injectable form; however both preparations contain the C-17-alkylation that allows steroids to survive first pass metabolism and become orally active. This is unique in that most injectable steroids are considered to be safer as they lack the methylation characteristic, hence putting less stress on the liver. Winstrol is a drug of choice for "cutting cycles" as well as for endurance athletes, as it is incapable of aromatization. The most notorious case of Winstrol being used by an athlete is that of Olympic sprinter Ben Johnson, who tested positive for stanozolol during the 1988 Olympics and was stripped of his gold medals. The most popular injectable brands available today are Stanol-V by Ttokkyo, Anabolic-ST (formerly Stanosus) from Grupo Comercial Tarasco, Stanazolic from Ilium, and Winstrol Depot by Zambon. The most popular oral brands are Stanol-V by Ttokkyo and Winstrol by Zambon. *Stanozolol is a Schedule III federally controlled substance.*

Index

A

B

C

D

E

F

G

H

I

J

K

L

M